VOLUME EIGHTY-SIX

VITAMINS AND HORMONES

Vitamins and the Immune System

VOLUME EIGHTY-SIX

VITAMINS AND HORMONES

Vitamins and the Immune System

Editor-in-Chief

GERALD LITWACK

Founding Chair, Department of Basic Sciences
The Commonwealth Medical College
Scranton, Pennsylvania

ELSEVIER

AMSTERDAM • BOSTON • HEIDELBERG • LONDON
NEW YORK • OXFORD • PARIS • SAN DIEGO
SAN FRANCISCO • SINGAPORE • SYDNEY • TOKYO
Academic Press is an imprint of Elsevier

Cover photo credit:
Hewison, M.
Vitamin D and innate and adaptive immunity.
Vitamins and Hormones (2011) **86**, pp. 23-62.

Academic Press is an imprint of Elsevier
32 Jamestown Road, London, NW1 7BY, UK
Radarweg 29, PO Box 211, 1000 AE Amsterdam, The Netherlands
Linacre House, Jordan Hill, Oxford OX2 8DP, UK
30 Corporate Drive, Suite 400, Burlington, MA 01803, USA
525 B Street, Suite 1900, San Diego, CA 92101-4495, USA

First edition 2011

ISBN: 978-0-12-386960-9
ISSN: 0083-6729

For information on all Academic Press publications
visit our website at elsevierdirect.com

Printed and bound by CPI Group (UK) Ltd, Croydon, CR0 4YY

Transferred to Digital Print 2011

Contents

Contributors

Luciano Adorini
Intercept Pharmaceuticals, Corciano (Perugia), Italy

Lokman Alpsoy
Fatih University, Science and Art Faculty, Department of Biology, Buyukcekmece, Istanbul, Turkey

Sandro Ardizzone
Department of Gastroenterology, "L. Sacco" University Hospital, Milan, Italy

Zsolt Barta
Division of Clinical Immunology, 3rd Department of Medicine, Medical and Health Science Center, University of Debrecen, Debrecen, Hungary

Maurizio Bevilacqua
Endocrinology Unit, Department of Clinical Science, "L. Sacco" University Hospital, Milan, Italy

Daniel D. Bikle
Department of Medicine and Dermatology, Veterans Affairs Medical Center, University of California, San Francisco, California, USA

Edit Bodolay
Division of Clinical Immunology, 3rd Department of Medicine, Medical and Health Science Center, University of Debrecen, Debrecen, Hungary

Steven Boonen
Division for Geriatric Medicine and Center of Metabolic Bone Diseases, University of Leuven, Belgium

Kyra Borchhardt
Division of Nephrology and Dialysis, Department of Internal Medicine III, Medical University of Vienna, Währinger Gürtel, Vienna, Austria

Nwaru I. Bright
Tampere School of Public Health, University of Tampere, Finland

Andrea Cassinotti
Department of Gastroenterology, "L. Sacco" University Hospital, Milan, Italy

Qiuyan Chen
Department of Nutritional Sciences, Pennsylvania State University, University Park, Pennsylvania, USA

Mogens Helweg Claesson
Institute of International Health, Immunology and Microbiology, Faculty of Health Sciences, University of Copenhagen, Copenhagen, Denmark

Mario Clerici
Chair of Immunology, DISP LITA Vialba, and DISTeB LITA Segrate, University of Milan, Milan, Italy

Maurizio Cutolo
Rheumatology, Research Laboratories and Academic Unit of Clinical Rheumatology, Postgraduate Academic School of Rheumatology, University of Genova, Genova, Italy

Jan Damoiseaux
Laboratory of Clinical Immunology, Maastricht University Medical Center, Maastricht, The Netherlands

Marc Decramer
Respiratory Division, University of Leuven, Herestraat 49, Leuven, Belgium

Nikolai Engedal
Centre for Molecular Medicine Norway, Nordic EMBL Partnership, University of Oslo, Oslo, Norway

Geneviève Fortin
Department of Experimental Medicine, McGill University, Montreal, Quebec, Canada

Sif Hansdottir
Department of Medicine, University of Iowa Carver College of Medicine and Veterans Administration Medical Center, Iowa City, Iowa, USA

Viljakainen T. Heli
Hospital for Children and Adolescents, HUS, Finland

Martin Hewison
Department of Orthopaedic Surgery and Molecular Biology Institute, David Geffen School of Medicine at UCLA, Los Angeles, California, USA

Makoto Iwata
Laboratory of Immunology, Faculty of Pharmaceutical Sciences at Kagawa Campus, Tokushima Bunri University, Sanuki-shi, Kagawa, Japan, and Japan Science and Technology Agency, CREST, Chiyoda-ku, Tokyo, Japan

Wim Janssens
Respiratory Division, University of Leuven, Herestraat 49, Leuven, Belgium

Chang H. Kim
Laboratory of Immunology and Hematopoiesis, Department of Comparative Pathobiology, School of Veterinary Medicine and Center for Cancer Research, Purdue University, West Lafayette, Indiana, USA

Yifan Ma
Department of Nutritional Sciences, Pennsylvania State University, University Park, Pennsylvania, USA

Erkkola Maijaliisa
Division of Nutrition, Department of Food and Environmental Sciences, University of Helsinki, Finland

Chantal Mathieu
Division of Endocrinology, University of Leuven, Belgium

Martha M. Monick
Department of Medicine, University of Iowa Carver College of Medicine and Veterans Administration Medical Center, Iowa City, Iowa, USA

Ayako Wakatsuki Pedersen
DanDrit Biotech A/S, Symbion Science Park, Copenhagen, Denmark

Didem Pekmezci
Department of Internal Medicine, Faculty of Veterinary Medicine, University of Ondokuz Mayıs, Kurupelit, Samsun, Turkey

M. Plebani
Department of Laboratory Medicine, University Hospital of Padova, Padova, Italy

Gabriele Bianchi Porro
Department of Gastroenterology, "L. Sacco" University Hospital, Milan, Italy

A. Catharine Ross
Department of Nutritional Sciences, and Huck Institute for Life Sciences, Pennsylvania State University, University Park, Pennsylvania, USA

P. Selvaraj
Department of Immunology, Tuberculosis Research Centre, Indian Council of Medical Research, Chennai, India

Yehuda Shoenfeld
Department of Medicine 'B', Zabludowicz Center for Autoimmune Diseases, Sheba Medical Center (Affiliated to Tel-Aviv University), Tel-Hashomer, Israel, and Incumbent of the Laura Schwarz-Kipp Chair for Research of Autoimmune Diseases, Tel-Aviv University, Tel-Aviv, Israel

Joost Smolders
School for Mental Health and Neuroscience, and Department of Internal Medicine, Division of Clinical and Experimental Immunology, Maastricht University Medical Center, Maastricht, The Netherlands

Ursula Thiem
Division of Nephrology and Dialysis, Department of Internal Medicine III, Medical University of Vienna, Währinger Gürtel, Vienna, Austria

Angela Tincani
Rheumatology and Clinical Immunology, Spedali Civili and University of Brescia, Brescia, Italy

Mehmet Emir Yalvac
Yeditepe University, Faculty of Engineering and Architecture, Department of Genetics and Bioengineering, Istanbul, Turkey

Aya Yokota
Laboratory of Immunology, Faculty of Pharmaceutical Sciences at Kagawa Campus, Tokushima Bunri University, Sanuki-shi, Kagawa, Japan, and Japan Science and Technology Agency, CREST, Chiyoda-ku, Tokyo, Japan

Mai-Britt Zocca
DanDrit Biotech A/S, Symbion Science Park, Copenhagen, Denmark

Eva Zold
Division of Clinical Immunology, 3rd Department of Medicine, Medical and Health Science Center, University of Debrecen, Debrecen, Hungary

Preface

The relationship of vitamin intake to the functioning of the immune system has been emphasized in recent times. A prime example is the linkage between vitamin D deficiency and the genesis of colon cancer. It is now known that there are many such linkages between vitamin deficiencies and various disease conditions. Much of these phenomena can be related to the effects of vitamins on the functionality of the immune system, the system by which beginning cancers are removed. In this volume is reviewed the recent knowledge of these relationships involving vitamin D, vitamin A, vitamin E, vitamin C, and even L-carnitine which, itself, is not classified as a vitamin but has interesting effects on immunity and inflammation.

I have tried to arrange the contributions so that more general discussions appear at first and more specific discussions about individual disease conditions are presented afterward. Accordingly, the first chapter is entitled "Vitamin D Regulation of Immune Function" by D. D. Bikle. This is followed by "Vitamin D and Innate and Adaptive Immunity" by M. Hewison. This is followed by "Dendritic Cells Modified by Vitamin D: Future Immunotherapy for Autoimmune Diseases" by A. W. Pedersen, M. H. Claesson, and M.-B. Zocca. C. H. Kim reviews "Retinoic Acid, Immunity, and Inflammation." A. C. Ross, Q. Chen, and Y. Ma follow with "Vitamin A and Retinoic Acid in the Regulation of B Cell Development and Antibody Production." Retinoic acid is also the topic of M. Iwata and A. Yokota who introduce "Retinoic Acid Production by Intestinal Dendritic Cells." N. Engedal reviews "Immune Regulator Vitamin A and T Cell Death." Vitamin E comes into the picture with "Vitamin E and Immunity" by D. Pekmezci, and this completes the general topics.

Relating to more specific diseases, S. Hansdottir and M. M. Monick offer "Vitamin D Effects on Lung Immunity and Respiratory Diseases." "Maternal Vitamin D During Pregnancy and Its Relation to Immune-Mediated Diseases in the Offspring" is the subject of E. Maijaliisa, N. Bright I, and H. T. Viljakainen. "Vitamin D Deficiency and Connective Tissue Disease" is by E. Zold, Z. Barta, and E. Bodolay. L. Alpsoy and M. E. Yalvac introduce "Key Roles of Vitamin A, C, and E in Aflatoxin B_1-Induced Oxidative Stress." "Vitamin D, Vitamin D Receptor, and Cathelicidin in the Treatment of Tuberculosis" is the contribution of P. Selvaraj. M. Cutolo, M. Plebani, Y. Shoenfeld, L. Adorini, and A. Tincani write about "Vitamin D Endocrine System and the Immune Response in Rheumatic Diseases." G. Fortin introduces "L-Carnitine and Intestinal

Inflammation." Bowel disease is discussed by S. Ardizzone, A. Cassinotti, M. Bevilacqua, M. Clerici, and G. B. Porro. W. Janssens, C. Mathieu, S. Boonen, and M. Decramer describe "Vitamin D Deficiency and Chronic Obstructive Pulmonary Disease: A Vicious Circle." J. Smolders and J. Damoiseaux introduce "Vitamin D as a T Cell Modulator in Multiple Sclerosis." Finally, U. Thiem and K. Borchhardt detail "Vitamin D in Solid Organ Transplantation with Special Emphasis on Kidney Transplantation."

Key roles in the final processing of this volume have been played by Delsy Retchagar with oversight by Lisa Tickner and lately by Mary Ann Zimmerman and others at Elsevier.

The cover figure is reproduced from Figure 2.2 from the contribution entitled "Vitamin D and innate and adaptive immunity" by Martin Hewison.

Gerald Litwack
Scranton, PA

CHAPTER ONE

Vitamin D Regulation of Immune Function

Daniel D. Bikle

Contents

Abstract

Although the best known actions of vitamin D involve its regulation of bone mineral homeostasis, vitamin D exerts its influence on many physiologic processes. One of these processes is the immune system. Both the adaptive and innate immune systems are impacted by the active metabolite of vitamin D, 1,25 $(OH)_2D$. These observations have important implications for understanding the predisposition of individuals with vitamin D deficiency to infectious diseases such as tuberculosis as well as to autoimmune diseases such as type 1 diabetes mellitus and multiple sclerosis. However, depending on the disease process not all actions of vitamin D may be beneficial. In this review, I examine the

Department of Medicine and Dermatology, Veterans Affairs Medical Center, University of California, San Francisco, California, USA

Vitamins and Hormones, Volume 86

ISSN 0083-6729, DOI: 10.1016/B978-0-12-386960-9.00001-0

regulation by $1,25(OH)_2D$ of immune function, then assess the evidence implicating vitamin D deficiency in human disease resulting from immune dysfunction.

I. Introduction

The potential role for vitamin D and its active metabolite $1,25(OH)_2D$ in modulating the immune response has long been recognized since the discovery of vitamin D receptors (VDRs) in macrophages, dendritic cells (DCs), and activated T and B lymphocytes, the ability of macrophages and DCs as well as activated T and B cells to express CYP27B1, the enzyme that produces $1,25(OH)_2D$, and the ability of $1,25(OH)_2D$ to regulate the proliferation and function of these cells. While these are the key cells mediating the adaptive immune response, $1,25(OH)_2D$, VDR, and CYP27B1 are also expressed in a large number of epithelial cells which along with the aforementioned members of the "professional" immune system contribute to host defense by their innate immune response. The totality of the immune response involves both types of responses in complex interactions involving numerous cytokines. The regulation by $1,25(OH)_2D$ of these different responses and their interactions is nuanced. In general, $1,25(OH)_2D$ enhances the innate immune response primarily via its ability to stimulate cathelicidin, an antimicrobial peptide (AMP) important in defense against invading organisms, whereas it inhibits the adaptive immune response primarily by inhibiting the maturation of DCs important for antigen presentation, reducing T cell proliferation, and shifting the balance of T cell differentiation from the Th1 and Th17 pathways to Th2 and regulatory T cells (Treg) pathways. Impairment of the innate immune system in vitamin D deficiency predisposes to tuberculosis, whereas an overactive adaptive immune system in vitamin D deficiency may account for the higher incidence of type 1 diabetes mellitus in children born to vitamin D deficient mothers or the increased incidence of multiple sclerosis in young adults.

II. $1,25(OH)_2D$ Production in Cells of the Immune System: Comparisons to Renal Production

Before reviewing the regulation by $1,25(OH)_2D$ of immune function, the importance of the ability of cells involved with the immune response to produce their own $1,25(OH)_2D$ needs to be emphasized. $1,25(OH)_2D$ is produced from 25OHD by the enzyme 25OHD-1α-hydroxylase (CYP27B1). Mutations in this gene are responsible for the rare autosomal

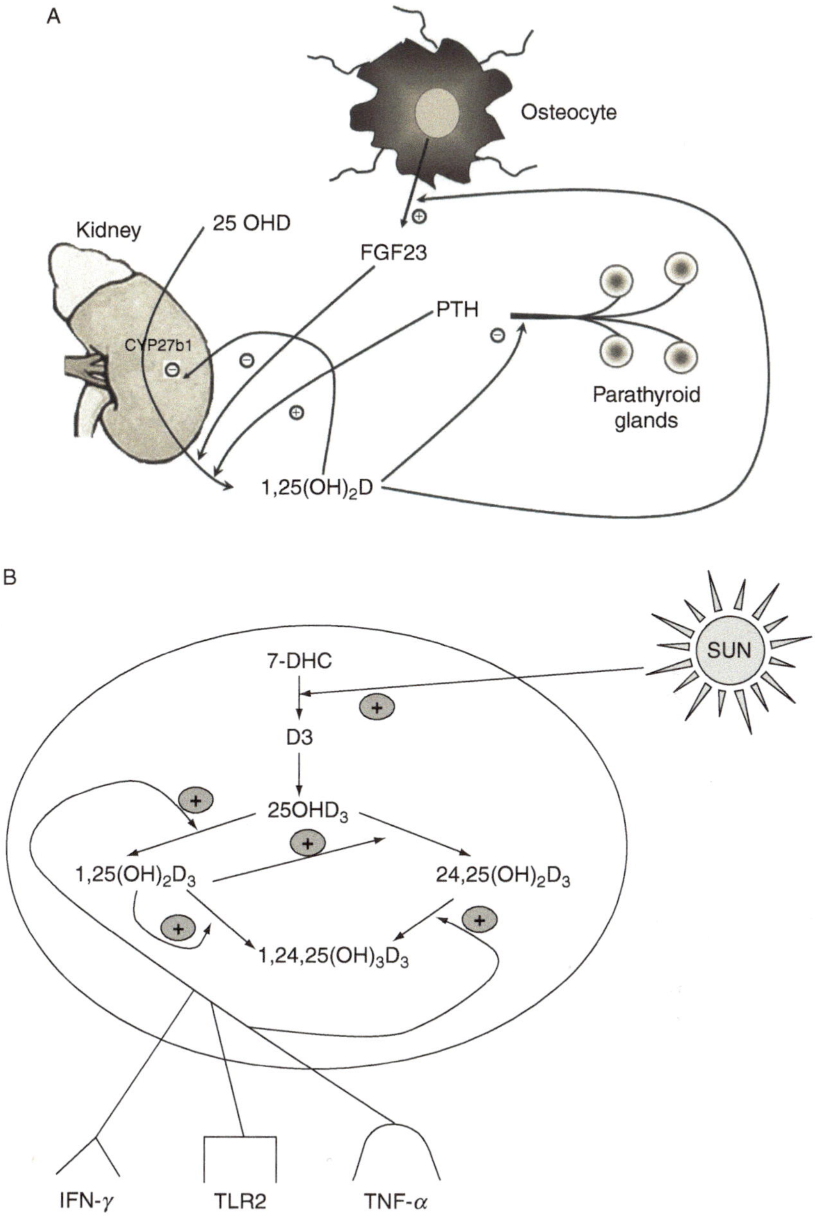

Figure 1.1 *Comparison of the regulation of CYP27B1 in the kidney with that in the keratinocyte.* (A) CYP27B1 in the kidney is regulated principally by three hormones: PTH, FGF23, and its product $1,25(OH)_2D$. PTH stimulates, while FGF23 and $1,25(OH)_2D$ inhibit CYP27B1. $1,25(OH)_2D$ in turn inhibits PTH production while stimulating that of FGF23. Calcium and phosphate likewise regulate PTH and FGF23 production, providing feedback loops that tightly control CYP27B1 activity and maintain normal calcium and phosphate homeostasis. Adapted from Figure 2 in Bikle (2009). (B) In the keratinocyte and other extrarenal sites of CYP27B1 expression, $1,25(OH)_2D_3$ production is controlled primarily by cytokines such as IFN-γ and TNF-α and activation of toll-like receptors (TLRs). Unlike the kidney, $1,25(OH)_2D_3$ regulates its own levels within the cell primarily by induction of CYP24, which catabolizes both the substrate ($25OHD_3$) and product ($1,25(OH)_2D_3$) of CYP27B1. In the macrophage, this latter mechanism is lax, and conditions of increased macrophage activation can lead to excess $1,25(OH)_2D_3$ production and hypercalcemia.

disease of pseudovitamin D deficiency (Fu *et al.*, 1997; Kitanaka *et al.*, 1998; St-Arnaud *et al.*, 1997; Wang *et al.*, 1998). An animal model in which the gene is knocked out by homologous recombination reproduces the clinical features of this disease including retarded growth, rickets, hypocalcemia, hyperparathyroidism, and undetectable 1,25$(OH)_2$D (Dardenne *et al.*, 2001), although the immune system has received little study in this model so far. CYP27B1 is a mitochondrial mixed function oxidase with significant homology to other mitochondrial steroid hydroxylases. These mitochondrial P450 enzymes are located in the inner membrane of the mitochondrion, and serve as the terminal acceptor for electrons transferred from NADPH through ferrodoxin reductase and ferrodoxin. Expression of CYP27B1 is highest in epidermal keratinocytes (Fu *et al.*, 1997; Liu *et al.*, 2007a), but it is well expressed in the epithelium of other organs including the prostate, lungs, intestine, and breast (Bikle, 2010) as well as macrophages, DCs, T, and B lymphocytes (Chen *et al.*, 2007; Sigmundsdottir *et al.*, 2007), but only when these cells are activated. However, the kidney is the major source of circulating 1,25$(OH)_2$D.

The principal regulators of CYP27B1 activity in the kidney are parathyroid hormone (PTH), FGF23, calcium, phosphate, and 1,25$(OH)_2$D itself. Extrarenal production tends to be stimulated by cytokines such as interferon-γ (IFN-γ) and tumor necrosis factor-α (TNF-α) more effectively than PTH (Bikle and Pillai, 1993), as these cells are not known to express the PTH receptor, and may be less inhibited by calcium, phosphate, and 1,25$(OH)_2$D depending on the tissue. Only cells expressing both the FGF receptor and Klotho respond to FGF23; the presence of these coreceptors has not been evaluated in cells of the immune system. Administration of PTH *in vivo* (Horiuchi *et al.*, 1977) or *in vitro* (Rasmussen *et al.*, 1972; Rost *et al.*, 1981) stimulates renal production of 1,25$(OH)_2$D. This action of PTH can be mimicked by cAMP (Horiuchi *et al.*, 1977; Rost *et al.*, 1981) and forskolin (Armbrecht *et al.*, 1984; Henry, 1985) indicating that at least part of the effect of PTH is mediated via its activation of adenylate cyclase. However, PTH activation of protein kinase C (PKC) also appears to be involved (Janulis *et al.*, 1992, 1993). Calcium suppresses CYP27B1 directly and indirectly by inhibiting PTH secretion. FGF23 inhibits CYP27B1 activity in vivo and in vitro and impairs phosphate reabsorption in the kidney (Saito *et al.*, 2003). FGF23 has been implicated as at least one of the factors responsible for impaired phosphate reabsorption and 1,25 $(OH)_2$D production in conditions such as X-linked and autosomal dominant hypophosphatemic rickets and oncogenic osteomalacia (Shimada *et al.*, 2001; White *et al.*, 2000). The immune function in these individuals has received little attention. 1,25$(OH)_2$D administration leads to an apparent reduction in CYP27B1 activity. It was initially thought that this feedback inhibition was mediated at the level of gene expression. However, no vitamin D response element (VDRE) has been identified in the promoter of the 1α-hydroxylase gene (Brenza *et al.*, 1998). In keratinocytes, 1,25 $(OH)_2D$ has little or no effect on CYP27B1 mRNA and protein levels when given *in vitro*. When 24-hydroxylase activity (the major catabolic pathway for 1,25$(OH)_2D$) is blocked, 1,25$(OH)_2D$ administration fails to reduce the levels of 1,25$(OH)_2D$ produced (Schuster *et al.*, 2001; Xie *et al.*, 2001). Thus the apparent feedback regulation of CYP27B1 activity by 1,25 $(OH)_2D$ appears to be due to its stimulation of CYP24A1 (24-hydroxylase) and subsequent catabolism, not to a direct effect on CYP27B1 expression or activity at least in keratinocytes. However, in one renal cell line, a chromatin remodeling complex (WINAC) has been described that mediates the ability of the VDR to regulate CYP27B1 gene expression in a nonclassic manner enabling 1,25$(OH)_2D$ suppression of this gene (Kato *et al.*, 2007); whether this mechanism is operative in other cells including normal kidney or immune cells remains to be demonstrated.

For most cells, the substrate for CYP27B1, 25OHD, is produced from vitamin D by the liver. 25OHD is the major circulating form of vitamin D and provides a clinically useful marker for vitamin D status. 25-Hydroxylase activity has been found in both the liver mitochondria and endoplasmic reticulum, and the enzymatic activities differ, indicating different proteins. Indeed, the mitochondrial 25-hydroxylase is CYP27A1 and the major microsomal 25-hydroxylase is CYP2R1. However, in mouse knockout studies and in humans with mutations in these enzymes, only CYP2R1 loss is clearly associated with changes in vitamin D metabolite production. These are mixed function oxidases, but differ in apparent K_ms and substrate specificities. The mitochondrial CYP27A1 was first identified as catalyzing a critical step in the bile acid synthesis pathway. This is a high capacity, low affinity enzyme consistent with the observation that 25-hydroxylation is not generally rate limiting in vitamin D metabolism (Andersson *et al.*, 1989; Cali and Russell, 1991; Usui *et al.*, 1990). CYP27A1 is widely distributed throughout different tissues with highest levels not only in liver and muscle but also in kidney, intestine, lung, skin, bone, and some immune cells (Andersson *et al.*, 1989; Cali and Russell, 1991; Cali *et al.*, 1991; Ichikawa *et al.*, 1995; Leitersdorf *et al.*, 1993; Usui *et al.*, 1990). Mutations in CYP27A1 lead to cerebrotendinous xanthomatosis (Cali *et al.*, 1991; Leitersdorf *et al.*, 1993), and is associated with abnormal vitamin D and/or calcium metabolism in some but not all of these patients (Berginer *et al.*, 1993; Leitersdorf *et al.*, 1993, 1994). CYP2R1, like that of CYP27A1, is widely distributed, although it is most abundantly expressed in liver, skin, and testes (Cheng *et al.*, 2003). The skin expresses less and the testes lack CYP27A1 expression (Cheng *et al.*, 2003). Unlike CYP27A1, CYP2R1 25-hydroxylates D_2 and D_3 equally (Cheng *et al.*, 2003). A patient with an inactivating mutation in CYP2R1 has been described with rickets and reduced 25OHD levels, reduced serum calcium and phosphate, but normal 1,25$(OH)_2D$ levels (Cheng *et al.*, 2004). No comment was made regarding immune deficiencies in this patient. The subject responded to D_2 therapy (Cheng *et al.*, 2004). Thus CYP27A1 and CYP2R1 by themselves do not account for all 25-hydroxyase activity in the body, but each most likely contributes and together may account for most if not all of the 25-hydroxylase activity in humans.

Keratinocytes, DCs but not T cells also express CYP27A1, and both DCs and T cells express CYP2R1 (Lehmann *et al.*, 2004; Sigmundsdottir *et al.*, 2007). However, only DCs produce $1,25(OH)_2D$ from vitamin D_3, suggesting that the CYP2R1 is not functional in the T cells (Sigmundsdottir *et al.*, 2007). Furthermore, CYP24A1 expression and activity, the 1,25 $(OH)_2D$-inducible enzyme that catabolizes 25OHD and $1,25(OH)_2D$, in activated macrophages and DCs is either absent (Sigmundsdottir *et al.*, 2007) or blocked (Ren *et al.*, 2005; Vidal *et al.*, 2002), removing this feedback control of the $1,25(OH)_2D$ produced. Diseases associated with immune activation can and do lead to hypercalcemia and hypercalciuria as a result of increased circulating levels of $1,25(OH)_2D$ (reviewed in Bikle, 2010). The mechanisms for this lack of feedback control are several. First, the major drivers for CYP27B1 expression and activity in these cells are cytokines, not PTH, and cytokines are not regulated by calcium and phosphate. Second, CYP24A1 induction and/or function in macrophages in response to 1,25 $(OH)_2D$ is blunted. One mechanism appears to involve the expression of a truncated form of CYP24A1, which includes the substrate binding domain but not the mitochondrial targeting sequence. This truncated form is postulated to act as a dominant negative form of CYP24A1, binding 1,25 $(OH)_2D$ within the cytoplasm and preventing its catabolism (Ren *et al.*, 2005). A second mechanism involves the ability of STAT-1 (induced by IFN-γ) to complex with VDR blocking its ability to bind to and activate the VDRE in the CYP24A1 promoter (Vidal *et al.*, 2002).

As noted above, epithelia are key players in the initiation of the innate immune response, the first line of defense to invading microorganisms, and CYP27B1 expression and activity have been found in most epithelia where they have been sought (Bikle, 2010). Epidermal keratinocytes also express CYP27A1 enabling them to produce $1,25(OH)_2D$ from endogenous sources of vitamin D_3 (Lehmann *et al.*, 2004). Ultraviolet B (UVB) radiation, which increases vitamin D and subsequently $1,25(OH)_2D$ production in epidermal keratinocytes, suppresses the adaptive immune response mediating contact hypersensitivity (Loser *et al.*, 2006), while increasing the innate immune response (Zasloff, 2005). Suppression of the adaptive immune response is at least partially attributable to $1,25(OH)_2D$-induced expression of RANKL in keratinocytes leading to activation of Langerhans cells, and the subsequent induction of Treg (Loser *et al.*, 2006). Activation of the innate immune response is due to $1,25(OH)_2D$ induced cathelicidin production (Zasloff, 2005). Unlike macrophages, these epithelia also express CYP24A1, which limits the levels of $1,25(OH)_2D$ within these tissues such that the $1,25(OH)_2D$ produced is likely to play primarily a paracrine or an autocrine role in these tissues and not lead to systemic effects on calcium metabolism.

Regulation of CYP27B1 in these cells differs from that of the kidney (Fig. 1.1). Pulmonary alveolar macrophage production of $1,25(OH)_2D$ requires activation by IFN-γ and TNF-α, and is inhibited by dexamethasone (Pryke *et al.*, 1990). The production of $1,25(OH)_2D$ by circulating monocytes can be stimulated by IFN-γ and other cytokines including TNF-α, interleukin (IL)-1 and IL-2 (Gyetko *et al.*, 1993). Lipopolysaccharide (LPS) has also been shown to induce CYP27B1 (Stoffels *et al.*, 2006). LPS stimulates through specific toll-like receptors (TLRs) in association with the coreceptor CD14, an important trigger of the innate immune response. Such stimulation involves signaling through the JAK/STAT, p38 MAPK, and nuclear factor (NF)-κB pathways, and implicates CEBPβ as a key transcription factor (Stoffels *et al.*, 2006). Like the macrophage, TNF (Bikle *et al.*, 1991) and IFN (Bikle *et al.*, 1989) are potent inducers of CYP27B1 activity in the keratinocyte. In pulmonary epithelial cells, double-stranded RNA (poly I:C) and the RSV virus, also ligands for specific TLRs, induce CYP27B1 (Hansdottir *et al.*, 2008), again illustrating the importance of the innate immune response in activating $1,25(OH)_2D$ production.

III. Role of Vitamin D in the Adaptive Immune Response (Fig. 1.2)

The adaptive immune response is initiated by cells specialized in antigen presentation, DCs and macrophages in particular, activating the cells responsible for subsequent antigen recognition, T and B lymphocytes. These cells are capable of a wide repertoire of responses that ultimately determine the nature and duration of the immune response. Activation of T and B cells occurs after a priming period in tissues of the body, for example, lymph nodes, distant from the site of the initial exposure to the antigenic substance, and is marked by proliferation of the activated T and B cells accompanied by posttranslational modifications of immunoglobulin production that enable the cellular response to adapt specifically to the antigen presented. Importantly, the type of T cell activated, CD4 or CD8, or within the helper T cell class Th1, Th2, Th17, Treg, and subtle variations of those, is dependent on the context of the antigen presented by which cell and in what environment. Systemic factors such as vitamin D influence this process. Vitamin D in general exerts an inhibitory action on the adaptive immune system. $1,25(OH)_2D$ decreases the maturation of DCs as marked by inhibited expression of the costimulatory molecules HLA-DR, CD40,

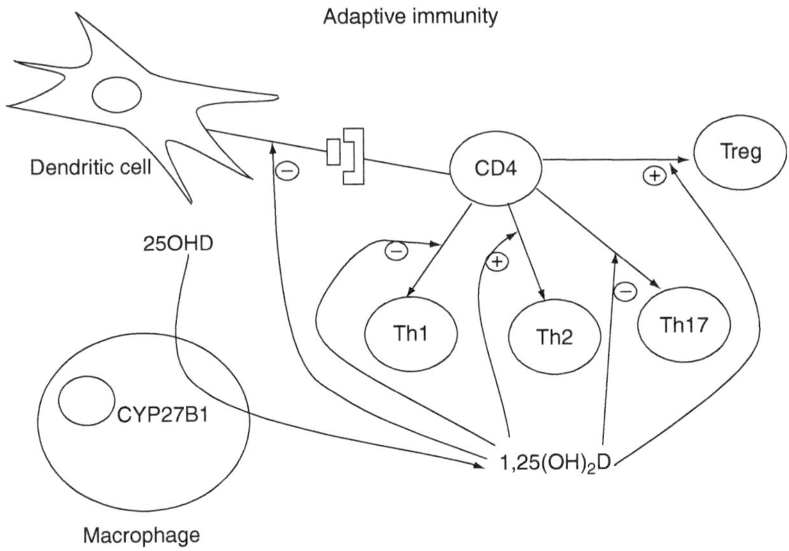

Figure 1.2 *1,25(OH)$_2$D regulates adaptive immunity.* CYP27B1 activity in either the macrophage or the keratinocyte is increased by cytokines. The 1,25(OH)$_2$D produced then serves to inhibit the adaptive response by suppressing Th1 and Th17 proliferation and function while promoting Th2 and Treg functions. Adapted from Figure 3 in Bikle (2009).

CD80, and CD86, decreasing their ability to present antigen and so activate T cells (van Etten and Mathieu, 2005). Furthermore, by suppressing IL-12 production, important for Th1 development, and IL-23 and IL-6 production, important for Th17 development and function, 1,25(OH)$_2$D inhibits the development of Th1 cells capable of producing IFN-γ and IL-2 and of Th17 cells producing IL-17 (Daniel *et al.*, 2008). These actions prevent further antigen presentation to and recruitment of T lymphocytes (role of IFN-γ), and T lymphocyte proliferation (role of IL-2). Furthermore, suppression of IL-12 increases the development of Th2 cells leading to increased IL-4, IL-5, and IL-13 production, which further suppresses Th1 development shifting the balance to a Th2 cell phenotype. Treatment of DCs with 1,25(OH)$_2$D can also induce CD4+/CD25+ regulatory T cells (Treg) (Gregori *et al.*, 2001) as shown by increased FoxP3 expression, critical for Treg development (Daniel *et al.*, 2008). These cells produce IL-10, which suppresses the development of the other Th subclasses. Treg are critical for the induction of immune tolerance (Sakaguchi *et al.*, 2008). In addition, 1,25(OH)$_2$D alters the homing properties of T cells, for example, by inducing expression of CCR10, the receptor for CCL27, a keratinocyte specific cytokine, while suppressing that of CCR9, a gut homing receptor (Sigmundsdottir *et al.*, 2007). The actions of 1,25

$(OH)_2D$ on B cells have received less attention, but recent studies have demonstrated a reduction in proliferation, maturation to plasma cells and immunoglobulin production (Chen *et al.*, 2007).

1,25$(OH)_2D$ has both direct and indirect effects on regulation of a number of cytokines involved with the immune response (reviewed in Bouillon *et al.*, 2008). TNF has a VDRE in its promoter to which the VDR/retinoid X receptor (RXR) complex binds. 1,25$(OH)_2D$ both blocks the activation of NF-κB via an increase in IκBα expression and impedes its binding to its response elements in the genes such as IL-8 and IL-12 that it regulates. 1,25$(OH)_2D$ has also been shown to bring an inhibitor complex containing histone deacetylase 3 (HDAC3) to the promoter of rel B, one of the members of the NF-κB family, thus suppressing gene expression. Thus, TNF/NF-κB activity is markedly impaired by 1,25 $(OH)_2D$ at multiple levels. In VDR null fibroblasts, NF-κB activity is enhanced. Furthermore, 1,25$(OH)_2D$ suppresses IFN-γ and a negative VDRE has been found in the IFN-γ promoter. Granulocyte/macrophage colony-stimulating factor (GM-CSF) is regulated by VDR monomers binding to a repressive complex in the promoter of this gene, competing with nuclear factor of T cells 1 (NFAT1) for binding to the promoter.

IV. Clinical Implications of the Inhibition of the Adaptive Immune Response

A. Inhibition by vitamin D of autoimmunity

The ability of 1,25$(OH)_2D$ to suppress the adaptive immune system appears to be beneficial for a number of conditions in which the immune system is directed at self, that is, autoimmunity (reviewed in Adorini and Penna, 2008). In a number of experimental models including inflammatory arthritis, psoriasis, autoimmune diabetes (e.g., NOD mice), systemic lupus erythematosus (SLE), experimental allergic encephalitis (EAE) (a model for multiple sclerosis), inflammatory bowel disease (IBD), prostatitis, and thyroiditis, VDR agonist administration has prevented and/or treated the disease process. These actions of 1,25$(OH)_2D$ were originally ascribed to inhibition of Th1 function, but Th17 cells have recently been shown to play important roles in a number of these conditions including psoriasis (Adamopoulos and Bowman, 2008), experimental colitis (Daniel *et al.*, 2008), and rheumatoid arthritis (Adamopoulos and Bowman, 2008), conditions that respond to 1,25$(OH)_2D$ and its analogs. Although few prospective, randomized, placebo controlled trials in humans have been performed, epidemiologic and case-control studies indicate that a number of these diseases in humans are favorably impacted by adequate vitamin D levels.

For example, the incidence of multiple sclerosis correlates inversely with 25OHD levels and vitamin D intake (Ascherio *et al.*, 2010), and early studies suggested benefit in the treatment of patients with rheumatoid arthritis and multiple sclerosis with VDR agonists (Adorini and Penna, 2008; Bouillon *et al.*, 2008). Children who are vitamin D deficient have a higher risk of developing type 1 diabetes mellitus, and supplementation with vitamin D during early childhood and/or of mothers during pregnancy may reduce the risk of developing type 1 diabetes (Knip *et al.*, 2010; van Etten and Mathieu, 2005). In VDR null mice, myelopoiesis and the composition of lymphoid organs are normal, although a number of abnormalities in the immune response have been found. Some of the abnormalities in macrophage function and T cell proliferation in response to anti-CD3 stimulation in these animals could be reversed by placing the animals on a high calcium diet to normalize serum calcium (Mathieu *et al.*, 2001). These results indicate the important role of calcium in vitamin D-regulated immune function as in skeletal development and maintenance, an area that has received limited investigation. Other studies have noted an increased number of mature DCs in the lymph nodes of VDR null mice, which would be expected to promote the adaptive immune response (O'Kelly *et al.*, 2002). Somewhat surprisingly, RANKL also increases the number and retention of DCs in lymph nodes (Josien *et al.*, 2000), suggesting that at least this mechanism is not mediated via the RANKL/RANK system in VDR null mice, which would be expected to reduce RANKL signaling. In contrast to these inhibitory actions of $1,25(OH)_2D$, Th2 function, as indicated by increased IgE stimulated histamine from mast cells, is increased in VDR null mice (Baroni *et al.*, 2007). The IL-10 null mouse model of IBD shows an accelerated disease profile when bred with the VDR null mouse with increased expression of Th1 cytokines (Froicu *et al.*, 2003). Surprisingly, despite a reduction in natural killer T cells and Treg and a decreased number of mature DCs, VDR null mice bred with NOD mice do not show accelerated development of diabetes (Gysemans *et al.*, 2008). Part of the difference in tissue response in VDR null mice may relate to differences in the ability of $1,25(OH)_2D$ to alter the homing of T cells to the different tissues (Sigmundsdottir *et al.*, 2007).

B. Vitamin D protection of tissue transplants

Inhibition of the adaptive immune response may also have benefit in transplantation procedures (Adorini, 2005). In experimental allograft models of the aorta, bone, bone marrow, heart, kidney, liver, pancreatic islets, skin, and small bowel, VDR agonists have shown benefit generally in combination with other immunosuppressive agents such as cyclosporine, tacrolimus, sirolimus, and glucocorticoids (Adorini, 2005). Much of the effect could be attributed to a reduction in infiltration of Th1 cells, macrophages, and DCs into the grafted tissue associated with a reduction in chemokines such as CXCL10, CXCL9, CCL2, and CCL5. CXCL10, the ligand for CXCR3, may be of particular importance for acute rejection in a number of tissues, whereas CXCL9 as well as CXCL10 (both CXCR3 ligands) may be more important for chronic rejection at least in the heart and kidney, respectively. A recent report noted that vitamin D supplementation to individuals following liver transplantation to prevent osteoporosis was associated with fewer episodes of acute rejection (Bitetto *et al.*, 2010). However, the results of large-scale prospective randomized control trials have not been reported.

C. Vitamin D inhibition of adaptive immunity may have adverse effects

Suppression of the adaptive immune system may not be without a price. Several publications have demonstrated that for some infections including *Leishmania major* (Ehrchen *et al.*, 2007) and toxoplasmosis (Rajapakse *et al.*, 2005), $1,25(OH)_2D$ promotes the infection (Rajapakse *et al.*, 2005), while the mouse null for VDR is protected (Ehrchen *et al.*, 2007). This may be due at least in part to the loss of IFN-γ stimulation of reactive oxygen species (ROS) and nitric oxide (NO) production required for macrophage antimicrobial activity (Ehrchen *et al.*, 2007). In allergic airway disease (asthma), Th2 cells, not Th1 cells, dominate the inflammatory response. $1,25(OH)_2D$ administration to normal mice protected these mice from experimentally induced asthma in one study, blocking eosinophil infiltration, IL-4 production, and limiting histologic evidence of inflammation (Topilski *et al.*, 2004). Furthermore, in humans, vitamin D deficiency is associated with increased risk of severe asthmatic exacerbations (Brehm *et al.*, 2010). However, a study with VDR null mice using a comparable method of inducing asthma showed that lack of VDR also protected the mice from an inflammatory response in their lungs (Wittke *et al.*, 2004). Furthermore, atopic dermatitis, a disease associated with increased Th2 activity (Soumelis *et al.*, 2002), and allergic airway disease, likewise associated with increased Th2 activity, (Topilski *et al.*, 2004; Wittke *et al.*, 2004, 2007), may be aggravated by $1,25(OH)_2D$ and less severe in animals null for VDR. These concerns are supported by one small clinical study in which higher vitamin D intake during infancy was associated with increased incidence of atopic allergies (Back *et al.*, 2009). These results will need confirmation in larger randomized placebo controlled prospective trials. However, at this point, the role of vitamin D in allergic diseases in humans remains unclear, with evidence for both benefit and harm.

V. Role of Vitamin D in the Innate Immune Response (Fig. 1.3)

The innate immune response involves the activation of TLRs in polymorphonuclear cells (PMNs), monocytes, and macrophages as well as in a number of epithelial cells including those of the epidermis, gingiva, intestine, vagina, bladder, and lungs (reviewed in Liu *et al.*, 2007a). There are 10 functional TLRs in human cells (of 11 known mammalian TLRs). TLRs are an extended family of host noncatalytic transmembrane pathogen-recognition receptors that interact with specific membrane patterns (PAMP) shed by infectious agents that trigger the innate immune response in the host. A number of these TLRs signal through adapter molecules such as myeloid differentiation factor-88 (MyD88) and the TIR-domain containing adapter inducing IFN-β (TRIF). MyD88 signaling includes translocation of NF-κB to the nucleus, leading to the production and secretion of a number of inflammatory cytokines. TRIF signaling leads to the activation of interferon regulatory factor-3 (IRF-3) and the induction of type 1 interferons such as IFN-β. MyD88 mediates signaling from TLR 2, 4, 5, 7,

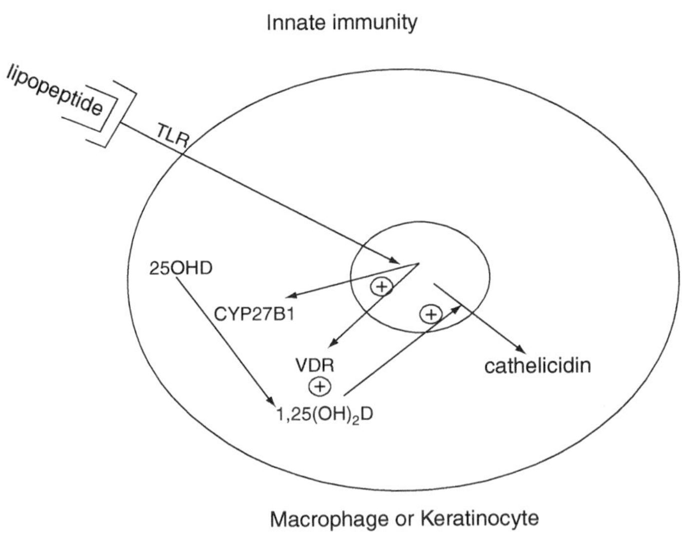

Figure 1.3 *$1,25(OH)_2D$ regulates innate immunity*. CYP27B1 and the VDR in either the macrophage or the keratinocyte are induced by activation of TLR by foreign proteins such as the lipopeptide of *M. tuberculosis*. The $1,25(OH)_2D$ produced from either endogenous or exogenous 25OHD promotes innate immunity by increasing cathelicidin expression, which kills the invading microorganism. Adapted from Figure 3 in Bikle (2009).

and 9, whereas TRIF mediates signaling from TLR 3 and 4. TLR1/2, TLR4, TLR5, and TLR2/6 respond to bacterial ligands, whereas TLR3, TLR7, and TLR 8 respond to viral ligands. The TLR response to fungi is less well defined. CD14 serves as a coreceptor for a number of these TLRs. Activation of TLRs leads to the induction of AMPs and ROS, which kill the organism. Among those AMPs is cathelicidin. Cathelicidin plays a number of roles in the innate immune response. The precursor protein, hCAP18, must be cleaved to its major peptide LL-37 to be active. In addition to its antimicrobial properties, LL-37 can stimulate the release of cytokines such as IL-6 and IL-10 through G protein-coupled receptors, and IL-18 through ERK/P38 pathways, stimulate the EGF receptor leading to activation of STAT1 and 3, induce the chemotaxis of neutrophils, monocytes, macrophages, and T cells into the skin, and promote keratinocyte proliferation and migration (Schauber and Gallo, 2008). The expression of this AMP is induced by 1,25$(OH)_2$D in both myeloid and epithelial cells (Gombart *et al.*, 2005; Wang *et al.*, 2004). In addition, 1,25$(OH)_2$D induces the coreceptor CD14 in keratinocytes (Schauber *et al.*, 2007). Stimulation of TLR2 by an AMP in macrophages (Liu *et al.*, 2006) or stimulation of TLR2 in keratinocytes by wounding the epidermis (Schauber *et al.*, 2007) results in increased expression of CYP27B1, which in the presence of adequate substrate (25OHD) stimulates the expression of cathelicidin. Lack of substrate (25OHD) or lack of CYP27B1 blunts the ability of these cells to respond to a challenge with respect to cathelicidin and/or CD14 production (Liu *et al.*, 2006; Schauber *et al.*, 2007; Wang *et al.*, 2004). In diseases such as atopic dermatitis, the production of cathelicidin and other AMPs is reduced, predisposing these patients to microbial superinfections (Ong *et al.*, 2002). Th2 cytokines such as IL-4 and 13 suppress the induction of AMPs (Howell *et al.*, 2006). Since 1,25$(OH)_2$D stimulates the differentiation of Th2 cells, in this disease 1,25$(OH)_2$D administration may be harmful. An important role of these AMPs besides their antimicrobial properties is to help link the innate and adaptive immune response.

Although many cells are capable of the innate immune response, most studies have focused on the macrophage and the keratinocyte. Vitamin D regulation of the innate immune response in these two cell types is comparable, but differences exist.

A. Macrophages

The importance of adequate vitamin D nutrition for resistance to certain infections has long been appreciated but poorly understood. This has been especially true for tuberculosis. Indeed, prior to the development of specific drugs for the treatment of tuberculosis, getting out of the city into fresh air and sunlight was the treatment of choice. In a recent survey of patients with tuberculosis in London (Ustianowski *et al.*, 2005), 56% had undetectable

25OHD levels and an additional 20% had detectable levels but below 9 ng/ml (22 nM). In 1986, Rook *et al.* demonstrated that 1,25$(OH)_2$D could inhibit the growth of *Mycobacterium tuberculosis*. The mechanism for this remained unclear until the publication by Liu *et al.* (2006) of their results in macrophages. They observed that activation of the toll-like receptor TLR2/1 by a lipoprotein extracted from *M. tuberculosis* reduced the viability of intracellular *M. tuberculosis* in human monocytes and macrophages concomitant with increased expression of the VDR and of CYP27B1 in these cells. Killing of *M. tuberculosis* occurred only when the serum in which the cells were cultured contained adequate levels of 25OHD, the substrate for CYP27B1. This provided clear evidence for the importance of vitamin D nutrition (as manifested by adequate serum levels of 25OHD) in preventing and treating this disease, and demonstrated the critical role for endogenous production of 1,25$(OH)_2$D by the macrophage to enable its antimycobacterial capacity. Activation of TLR2/1 or directly treating these cells with 1,25$(OH)_2$D induced the AMP cathelicidin, which is toxic for *M. tuberculosis*. If induction of cathelicidin is blocked as with siRNA, the ability of 1,25$(OH)_2$D to enhance the killing of *M. tuberculosis* is prevented (Liu *et al.*, 2007b). Furthermore, 1,25$(OH)_2$D also induces the production of ROS which if blocked likewise prevents the antimycobacterial activity of 1,25$(OH)_2$D-treated macrophages (Sly *et al.*, 2001). The murine cathelicidin gene lacks a known VDRE in its promoter, and so might not be expected to be induced by 1,25$(OH)_2$D in mouse cells, yet 1,25$(OH)_2$D stimulates antimycobacterial activity in murine macrophages. Murine macrophages, unlike human macrophages, utilize inducible nitric oxide synthase (iNOS) for their TLR- and 1,25$(OH)_2$D-mediated killing of *M. tuberculosis* (Brightbill *et al.*, 1999; Sly *et al.*, 2001).

B. Keratinocytes

Cathelicidin and CD14 expression in epidermal keratinocytes is also induced by 1,25$(OH)_2$D (Schauber and Gallo, 2008; Schauber *et al.*, 2007, 2008). In these cells, butyrate, which by itself has little effect, potentiates the ability of 1,25$(OH)_2$D to induce cathelicidin (Schauber *et al.*, 2008). Keratinocytes treated with 1,25$(OH)_2$D are substantially more effective in killing *Staphylococcus aureus* than are untreated keratinocytes. Wounding the epidermis induces the expression of TLR2 and that of its coreceptor CD14 and cathelicidin (Schauber *et al.*, 2007). This does not occur in mice lacking CYP27B1 (Schauber *et al.*, 2007). Unlike macrophages, 1,25$(OH)_2$D stimulates TLR2 expression in keratinocytes as well as in the epidermis when applied topically (Schauber *et al.*, 2007) providing a feed forward loop to amplify the innate immune response. Wounding also increases the expression of CYP27B1, the enzyme that produces 1,25$(OH)_2$D. This may occur as a result of increased levels of cytokines such as TNF-α and IFN-γ, both of which we have shown stimulate 1,25$(OH)_2$D production as well as TGF-β and the TLR2 ligand Malp-2 (Schauber *et al.*, 2007). When the levels of VDR or one of its principal coactivators, SRC3, are reduced using siRNA technology, the ability of 1,25$(OH)_2$D to induce cathelicidin and CD14 expression in human keratinocytes is markedly blunted (Schauber *et al.*, 2008).

C. Vitamin D stimulation of the innate immune response may have adverse effects

The innate immune system is the first line of defense against invading pathogens. This mechanism initiates the inflammatory response and activates the adaptive arm of the immune defense mechanism (Oppenheim *et al.*, 2007). However, chronic activation of the innate immune response can be deleterious. Cathelicidin has been shown to bind self-DNA forming a complex that is detected by plasmacytoid DCs, perhaps contributing to the psoriatic process (Lande *et al.*, 2007). IL-8/CXCL8, a chemoattractant for polymorphonuclear leukocytes (PMNs), is found in normal gingival tissue. In early stages of periodontitis, IL-8/CXCL8 levels are increased and PMNs are the first cells to respond (Garlet *et al.*, 2005). However, with increasing severity of the infection, IL-8 levels and PMN numbers increase leading to periodontal tissue destruction (Waddington *et al.*, 2000). That said, vitamin D analogs and 1,25$(OH)_2$D itself have proven useful in the treatment of psoriasis, although their role in periodontal disease and other chronic infections has not been established.

VI. Conclusion

The immune system defends the body against microbial invasion by activation of both adaptive and innate mechanisms. The innate immune system is the more primitive system prebuilt into cells that are on the front line for defense against bacterial and viral invasion, including epithelial cells in the skin, gut, and lung as well as macrophages and neutrophils. The adaptive immune system provides a more specific response, but takes longer to develop, although once developed provides a powerful response against invading organisms. Vitamin D, via its active metabolite 1,25$(OH)_2$D, regulates both types of immunity, suppressing adaptive immunity but potentiating the innate immune response. Suppression of the adaptive immune response is likely to be useful in combating a variety of autoimmune diseases, and protecting transplanted organs from rejection. Stimulation of the innate immune response at those surfaces exposed to the environment provides a first line of defense against pathogens in the environment, and so would be expected to enhance the resistance to acute infections in the skin, lungs, gastrointestinal tract, bladder, and other epithelial surfaces. However, vitamin D signaling may have its down side. As 1,25(OH)$_2$D shifts the repertoire of T cells from Th1/Th17 to Th2, the potential for aggravating atopic diseases such as asthma and atopic dermatitis needs to be considered. Resistance to infections by organisms such as leishmaniasis in which an intact adaptive immune response is crucial for their prevention/treatment may be compromised by vitamin D. In chronic inflammatory states, persistent activation of the innate immune system may perpetuate the inflammatory condition as in psoriasis and periodontal disease. However, the bulk of the evidence supports the concept that vitamin D regulation of the immune system is beneficial, and provides an important rationale to maintain vitamin D sufficiency on a year round basis.

ACKNOWLEDGMENTS

This work was supported by Grants RO1 AR050023 and AR051930 from the National Institutes of Health, a Merit Review from the Department of Veterans Affairs, and Grant 07A140 from the American Institute of Cancer Research.

REFERENCES

Adamopoulos, I. E., and Bowman, E. P. (2008). Immune regulation of bone loss by Th17 cells. *Arthritis Res. Ther.* **10,** 225.

Adorini, L. (2005). Intervention in autoimmunity: The potential of vitamin D receptor agonists. *Cell. Immunol.* **233,** 115–124.

Adorini, L., and Penna, G. (2008). Control of autoimmune diseases by the vitamin D endocrine system. *Nat. Clin. Pract. Rheumatol.* **4,** 404–412.

Andersson, S., Davis, D. L., Dahlbäck, H., Jörnvall, H., and Russell, D. W. (1989). Cloning, structure, and expression of the mitochondrial cytochrome P-450 sterol 26-hydroxylase, a bile acid biosynthetic enzyme. *J. Biol. Chem.* **264,** 8222–8229.

Armbrecht, H. J., Forte, L. R., Wongsurawat, N., Zenser, T. V., and Davis, B. B. (1984). Forskolin increases 1,25-dihydroxyvitamin D3 production by rat renal slices in vitro. *Endocrinology* **114,** 644–649.

Ascherio, A., Munger, K. L., and Simon, K. C. (2010). Vitamin D and multiple sclerosis. *Lancet Neurol.* **9,** 599–612.

Back, O., Blomquist, H. K., Hernell, O., and Stenberg, B. (2009). Does vitamin D intake during infancy promote the development of atopic allergy? *Acta Derm. Venereol.* **89,** 28–32.

Baroni, E., Biffi, M., Benigni, F., Monno, A., Carlucci, D., Carmeliet, G., Bouillon, R., and D'Ambrosio, D. (2007). VDR-dependent regulation of mast cell maturation mediated by 1,25-dihydroxyvitamin D3. *J. Leukoc. Biol.* **81,** 250–262.

Berginer, V. M., Shany, S., Alkalay, D., Berginer, J., Dekel, S., Salen, G., Tint, G. S., and Gazit, D. (1993). Osteoporosis and increased bone fractures in cerebrotendinous xanthomatosis. *Metabolism* **42,** 69–74.

Bikle, D. D. (2009). Nonclassical actions of vitamin D. *J. Endocrinol. Metab.* **94,** 26–34.

Bikle, D. (2010). Extra renal synthesis of 1,25-dihydroxyvitamin D and its health implications. *In* "Vitamin D: Physiology, Molecular Biology, and Clinical Applications," (M. Holick, Ed.), pp. 277–295. Humana Press, New York.

Bikle, D. D., and Pillai, S. (1993). Vitamin D, calcium, and epidermal differentiation. *Endocr. Rev.* **14,** 3–19.

Bikle, D. D., Pillai, S., Gee, E., and Hincenbergs, M. (1989). Regulation of 1,25-dihydroxyvitamin D production in human keratinocytes by interferon-gamma. *Endocrinology* **124,** 655–660.

Bikle, D. D., Pillai, S., Gee, E., and Hincenbergs, M. (1991). Tumor necrosis factor-alpha regulation of 1,25-dihydroxyvitamin D production by human keratinocytes. *Endocrinology* **129,** 33–38.

Bitetto, D., Fabris, C., Falleti, E., Fornasiere, E., Fumolo, E., Fontanini, E., Cussigh, A., Occhino, G., Baccarani, U., Pirisi, M., and Toniutto, P. (2010). Vitamin D and the risk of acute allograft rejection following human liver transplantation. *Liver Int.* **30,** 417–444.

Bouillon, R., Carmeliet, G., Verlinden, L., van Etten, E., Verstuyf, A., Luderer, H. F., Lieben, L., Mathieu, C., and Demay, M. (2008). Vitamin D and human health: Lessons from vitamin D receptor null mice. *Endocr. Rev.* **29,** 726–776.

Brehm, J. M., Schuemann, B., Fuhlbrigge, A. L., Hollis, B. W., Strunk, R. C., Zeiger, R. S., Weiss, S. T., and Litonjua, A. A. (2010). Serum vitamin D levels and severe asthma exacerbations in the Childhood Asthma Management Program study. *J. Allergy Clin. Immunol.* **126,** 52–58.

Brenza, H. L., Kimmel-Jehan, C., Jehan, F., Shinki, T., Wakino, S., Anazawa, H., Suda, T., and DeLuca, H. F. (1998). Parathyroid hormone activation of the 25-hydroxyvitamin D3-1alpha-hydroxylase gene promoter. *Proc. Natl. Acad. Sci. USA* **95,** 1387–1391.

Brightbill, H. D., Libraty, D. H., Krutzik, S. R., Yang, R. B., Belisle, J. T., Bleharski, J. R., Maitland, M., Norgard, M. V., Plevy, S. E., Smale, S. T., Brennan, P. J., Bloom, B. R., *et al.* (1999). Host defense mechanisms triggered by microbial lipoproteins through toll-like receptors. *Science* **285,** 732–736.

Cali, J. J., and Russell, D. W. (1991). Characterization of human sterol 27-hydroxylase. A mitochondrial cytochrome P-450 that catalyzes multiple oxidation reaction in bile acid biosynthesis. *J. Biol. Chem.* **266,** 7774–7778.

Cali, J. J., Hsieh, C. L., Francke, U., and Russell, D. W. (1991). Mutations in the bile acid biosynthetic enzyme sterol 27-hydroxylase underlie cerebrotendinous xanthomatosis. *J. Biol. Chem.* **266,** 7779–7783.

Chen, S., Sims, G. P., Chen, X. X., Gu, Y. Y., Chen, S., and Lipsky, P. E. (2007). Modulatory effects of 1,25-dihydroxyvitamin D3 on human B cell differentiation. *J. Immunol.* **179,** 1634–1647.

Cheng, J. B., Motola, D. L., Mangelsdorf, D. J., and Russell, D. W. (2003). De-orphanization of cytochrome P450 2R1: A microsomal vitamin D 25-hydroxilase. *J. Biol. Chem.* **278,** 38084–38093.

Cheng, J. B., Levine, M. A., Bell, N. H., Mangelsdorf, D. J., and Russell, D. W. (2004). Genetic evidence that the human CYP2R1 enzyme is a key vitamin D 25-hydroxylase. *Proc. Natl. Acad. Sci. USA* **101,** 7711–7715.

Daniel, C., Sartory, N. A., Zahn, N., Radeke, H. H., and Stein, J. M. (2008). Immune modulatory treatment of trinitrobenzene sulfonic acid colitis with calcitriol is associated with a change of a T helper (Th) 1/Th17 to a Th2 and regulatory T cell profile. *J. Pharmacol. Exp. Ther.* **324,** 23–33.

Dardenne, O., Prud'homme, J., Arabian, A., Glorieux, F. H., and St-Arnaud, R. (2001). Targeted inactivation of the 25-hydroxyvitamin D(3)-1(alpha)-hydroxylase gene (CYP27B1) creates an animal model of pseudovitamin D-deficiency rickets. *Endocrinology* **142,** 3135–3141.

Ehrchen, J., Helming, L., Varga, G., Pasche, B., Loser, K., Gunzer, M., Sunderkotter, C., Sorg, C., Roth, J., and Lengeling, A. (2007). Vitamin D receptor signaling contributes to susceptibility to infection with *Leishmania major*. *FASEB J.* **21,** 3208–3218.

Froicu, M., Weaver, V., Wynn, T. A., McDowell, M. A., Welsh, J. E., and Cantorna, M. T. (2003). A crucial role for the vitamin D receptor in experimental inflammatory bowel diseases. *Mol. Endocrinol.* **17,** 2386–2392.

Fu, G. K., Lin, D., Zhang, M. Y., Bikle, D. D., Shackleton, C. H., Miller, W. L., and Portale, A. A. (1997). Cloning of human 25-hydroxyvitamin D-1 alpha-hydroxylase and mutations causing vitamin D-dependent rickets type 1. *Mol. Endocrinol.* **11,** 1961–1970.

Garlet, G. P., Avila-Campos, M. J., Milanezi, C. M., Ferreira, B. R., and Silva, J. S. (2005). Actinobacillus actinomycetemcomitans-induced periodontal disease in mice: Patterns of cytokine, chemokine, and chemokine receptor expression and leukocyte migration. *Microbes Infect.* **7,** 738–747.

Gombart, A. F., Borregaard, N., and Koeffler, H. P. (2005). Human cathelicidin antimicrobial peptide (CAMP) gene is a direct target of the vitamin D receptor and is strongly up-regulated in myeloid cells by 1,25-dihydroxyvitamin D3. *FASEB J.* **19,** 1067–1077.

Gregori, S., Casorati, M., Amuchastegui, S., Smiroldo, S., Davalli, A. M., and Adorini, L. (2001). Regulatory T cells induced by 1 alpha,25-dihydroxyvitamin D3 and mycophenolate mofetil treatment mediate transplantation tolerance. *J. Immunol.* **167,** 1945–1953.

Gyetko, M. R., Hsu, C. H., Wilkinson, C. C., Patel, S., and Young, E. (1993). Monocyte 1 alpha-hydroxylase regulation: Induction by inflammatory cytokines and suppression by dexamethasone and uremia toxin. *J. Leukoc. Biol.* **54,** 17–22.

Gysemans, C., van Etten, E., Overbergh, L., Giulietti, A., Eelen, G., Waer, M., Verstuyf, A., Bouillon, R., and Mathieu, C. (2008). Unaltered diabetes presentation in NOD mice lacking the vitamin D receptor. *Diabetes* **57,** 269–275.

Hansdottir, S., Monick, M. M., Hinde, S. L., Lovan, N., Look, D. C., and Hunninghake, G. W. (2008). Respiratory epithelial cells convert inactive vitamin D to its active form: Potential effects on host defense. *J. Immunol.* **181,** 7090–7099.

Henry, H. L. (1985). Parathyroid hormone modulation of 25-hydroxyvitamin D3 metabolism by cultured chick kidney cells is mimicked and enhanced by forskolin. *Endocrinology* **116,** 503–510.

Horiuchi, N., Suda, T., Takahashi, H., Shimazawa, E., and Ogata, E. (1977). In vivo evidence for the intermediary role of 3′,5′-cyclic AMP in parathyroid hormone-induced stimulation of 1alpha,25-dihydroxyvitamin D3 synthesis in rats. *Endocrinology* **101,** 969–974.

Howell, M. D., Gallo, R. L., Boguniewicz, M., Jones, J. F., Wong, C., Streib, J. E., and Leung, D. Y. (2006). Cytokine milieu of atopic dermatitis skin subverts the innate immune response to vaccinia virus. *Immunity* **24,** 341–348.

Ichikawa, F., Sato, K., Nanjo, M., Nishii, Y., Shinki, T., Takahashi, N., and Suda, T. (1995). Mouse primary osteoblasts express vitamin D3 25-hydroxylase mRNA and convert 1 alpha-hydroxyvitamin D3 into 1 alpha,25-dihydroxyvitamin D3. *Bone* **16,** 129–135.

Janulis, M., Tembe, V., and Favus, M. J. (1992). Role of protein kinase C in parathyroid hormone stimulation of renal 1,25-dihydroxyvitamin D3 secretion. *J. Clin. Invest.* **90,** 2278–2283.

Janulis, M., Wong, M. S., and Favus, M. J. (1993). Structure-function requirements of parathyroid hormone for stimulation of 1,25-dihydroxyvitamin D3 production by rat renal proximal tubules. *Endocrinology* **133,** 713–719.

Josien, R., Li, H. L., Ingulli, E., Sarma, S., Wong, B. R., Vologodskaia, M., Steinman, R. M., and Choi, Y. (2000). TRANCE, a tumor necrosis factor family member, enhances the longevity and adjuvant properties of dendritic cells in vivo. *J. Exp. Med.* **191,** 495–502.

Kato, S., Fujiki, R., Kim, M. S., and Kitagawa, H. (2007). Ligand-induced transrepressive function of VDR requires a chromatin remodeling complex, WINAC. *J. Steroid Biochem. Mol. Biol.* **103,** 372–380.

Kitanaka, S., Takeyama, K., Murayama, A., Sato, T., Okumura, K., Nogami, M., Hasegawa, Y., Niimi, H., Yanagisawa, J., Tanaka, T., and Kato, S. (1998). Inactivating mutations in the 25-hydroxyvitamin D3 1alpha-hydroxylase gene in patients with pseudovitamin D-deficiency rickets. *N. Engl. J. Med.* **338,** 653–661.

Knip, M., Virtanen, S. M., and Akerblom, H. K. (2010). Infant feeding and the risk of type 1 diabetes. *Am. J. Clin. Nutr.* **91,** 1506S–1513S.

Lande, R., Gregorio, J., Facchinetti, V., Chatterjee, B., Wang, Y. H., Homey, B., Cao, W., Wang, Y. H., Su, B., Nestle, F. O., Zal, T., Mellman, I., *et al.* (2007). Plasmacytoid dendritic cells sense self-DNA coupled with antimicrobial peptide. *Nature* **449,** 564–569.

Lehmann, B., Querings, K., and Reichrath, J. (2004). Vitamin D and skin: New aspects for dermatology. *Exp. Dermatol.* **13**(Suppl. 4), 11–15.

Leitersdorf, E., Reshef, A., Meiner, V., Levitzki, R., Schwartz, S. P., Dann, E. J., Berkman, N., Cali, J. J., Klapholz, L., and Berginer, V. M. (1993). Frameshift and splice-junction mutations in the sterol 27-hydroxylase gene cause cerebrotendinous xanthomatosis in Jews or Moroccan origin. *J. Clin. Invest.* **91,** 2488–2496.

Leitersdorf, E., Safadi, R., Meiner, V., Reshef, A., Björkhem, I., Friedlander, Y., Morkos, S., and Berginer, V. M. (1994). Cerebrotendinous xanthomatosis in the Israeli Druze: Molecular genetics and phenotypic characteristics. *Am. J. Hum. Genet.* **55,** 907–915.

Liu, P. T., Stenger, S., Li, H., Wenzel, L., Tan, B. H., Krutzik, S. R., Ochoa, M. T., Schauber, J., Wu, K., Meinken, C., Kamen, D. L., Wagner, M., *et al.* (2006). Toll-like receptor triggering of a vitamin D-mediated human antimicrobial response. *Science* **311,** 1770–1773.

Liu, P. T., Krutzik, S. R., and Modlin, R. L. (2007a). Therapeutic implications of the TLR and VDR partnership. *Trends Mol. Med.* **13,** 117–124.

Liu, P. T., Stenger, S., Tang, D. H., and Modlin, R. L. (2007b). Cutting edge: Vitamin D-mediated human antimicrobial activity against *Mycobacterium tuberculosis* is dependent on the induction of cathelicidin. *J. Immunol.* **179,** 2060–2063.

Loser, K., Mehling, A., Loeser, S., Apelt, J., Kuhn, A., Grabbe, S., Schwarz, T., Penninger, J. M., and Beissert, S. (2006). Epidermal RANKL controls regulatory T-cell numbers via activation of dendritic cells. *Nat. Med.* **12,** 1372–1379.

Mathieu, C., Van Etten, E., Gysemans, C., Decallonne, B., Kato, S., Laureys, J., Depovere, J., Valckx, D., Verstuyf, A., and Bouillon, R. (2001). In vitro and in vivo analysis of the immune system of vitamin D receptor knockout mice. *J. Bone Miner. Res.* **16,** 2057–2065.

O'Kelly, J., Hisatake, J., Hisatake, Y., Bishop, J., Norman, A., and Koeffler, H. P. (2002). Normal myelopoiesis but abnormal T lymphocyte responses in vitamin D receptor knockout mice. *J. Clin. Invest.* **109,** 1091–1099.

Ong, P. Y., Ohtake, T., Brandt, C., Strickland, I., Boguniewicz, M., Ganz, T., Gallo, R. L., and Leung, D. Y. (2002). Endogenous antimicrobial peptides and skin infections in atopic dermatitis. *N. Engl. J. Med.* **347,** 1151–1160.

Oppenheim, J. J., Tewary, P., de la Rosa, G., and Yang, D. (2007). Alarmins initiate host defense. *Adv. Exp. Med. Biol.* **601,** 185–194.

Pryke, A. M., Duggan, C., White, C. P., Posen, S., and Mason, R. S. (1990). Tumor necrosis factor-alpha induces vitamin D-1-hydroxylase activity in normal human alveolar macrophages. *J. Cell. Physiol.* **142,** 652–656.

Rajapakse, R., Mousli, M., Pfaff, A. W., Uring-Lambert, B., Marcellin, L., Bronner, C., Jeanblanc, M., Villard, O., Letscher-Bru, V., Klein, J. P., and Candolfi, E. (2005).

1, 25-Dihydroxyvitamin D3 induces splenocyte apoptosis and enhances BALB/c mice sensitivity to toxoplasmosis. *J. Steroid Biochem. Mol. Biol.* **96,** 179–185.

Rasmussen, H., Wong, M., Bikle, D., and Goodman, D. B. (1972). Hormonal control of the renal conversion of 25-hydroxycholecalciferol to 1,25-dihydroxycholecalciferol. *J. Clin. Invest.* **51,** 2502–2504.

Ren, S., Nguyen, L., Wu, S., Encinas, C., Adams, J. S., and Hewison, M. (2005). Alternative splicing of vitamin D-24-hydroxylase: A novel mechanism for the regulation of extrarenal 1,25-dihydroxyvitamin D synthesis. *J. Biol. Chem.* **280,** 20604–20611.

Rook, G. A., Steele, J., Fraher, L., Barker, S., Karmali, R., O'Riordan, J., and Stanford, J. (1986). Vitamin D3, gamma interferon, and control of proliferation of *Mycobacterium tuberculosis* by human monocytes. *Immunology* **57,** 159–163.

Rost, C. R., Bikle, D. D., and Kaplan, R. A. (1981). In vitro stimulation of 25-hydroxycholecalciferol 1alpha-hydroxylation by parathyroid hormone in chick kidney slices: Evidence for a role for adenosine 3′,5′-monophosphate. *Endocrinology* **108,** 1002–1006.

Saito, H., Kusano, K., Kinosaki, M., Ito, H., Hirata, M., Segawa, H., Miyamoto, K., and Fukushima, N. (2003). Human fibroblast growth factor-23 mutants suppress Na^+-dependent phosphate co-transport activity and 1alpha,25-dihydroxyvitamin D3 production. *J. Biol. Chem.* **278,** 2206–2211.

Sakaguchi, S., Yamaguchi, T., Nomura, T., and Ono, M. (2008). Regulatory T cells and immune tolerance. *Cell* **133,** 775–787.

Schauber, J., and Gallo, R. L. (2008). The vitamin D pathway: A new target for control of the skin's immune response? *Exp. Dermatol.* **17,** 633–639.

Schauber, J., Dorschner, R. A., Coda, A. B., Buchau, A. S., Liu, P. T., Kiken, D., Helfrich, Y. R., Kang, S., Elalieh, H. Z., Steinmeyer, A., Zugel, U., Bikle, D. D., *et al.* (2007). Injury enhances TLR2 function and antimicrobial peptide expression through a vitamin D-dependent mechanism. *J. Clin. Invest.* **117,** 803–811.

Schauber, J., Oda, Y., Buchau, A. S., Yun, Q. C., Steinmeyer, A., Zugel, U., Bikle, D. D., and Gallo, R. L. (2008). Histone acetylation in keratinocytes enables control of the expression of cathelicidin and CD14 by 1,25-dihydroxyvitamin D(3). *J. Invest. Dermatol.* **128,** 816–824.

Schuster, I., Egger, H., Astecker, N., Herzig, G., Schussler, M., and Vorisek, G. (2001). Selective inhibitors of CYP24: Mechanistic tools to explore vitamin D metabolism in human keratinocytes. *Steroids* **66,** 451–462.

Shimada, T., Mizutani, S., Muto, T., Yoneya, T., Hino, R., Takeda, S., Takeuchi, Y., Fujita, T., Fukumoto, S., and Yamashita, T. (2001). Cloning and characterization of FGF23 as a causative factor of tumor-induced osteomalacia. *Proc. Natl. Acad. Sci. USA* **98,** 6500–6505.

Sigmundsdottir, H., Pan, J., Debes, G. F., Alt, C., Habtezion, A., Soler, D., and Butcher, E. C. (2007). DCs metabolize sunlight-induced vitamin D3 to 'program' T cell attraction to the epidermal chemokine CCL27. *Nat. Immunol.* **8,** 285–293.

Sly, L. M., Lopez, M., Nauseef, W. M., and Reiner, N. E. (2001). 1alpha,25-Dihydroxyvitamin D3-induced monocyte antimycobacterial activity is regulated by phosphatidylinositol 3-kinase and mediated by the NADPH-dependent phagocyte oxidase. *J. Biol. Chem.* **276,** 35482–35493.

Soumelis, V., Reche, P. A., Kanzler, H., Yuan, W., Edward, G., Homey, B., Gilliet, M., Ho, S., Antonenko, S., Lauerma, A., Smith, K., Gorman, D., *et al.* (2002). Human epithelial cells trigger dendritic cell mediated allergic inflammation by producing TSLP. *Nat. Immunol.* **3,** 673–680.

St-Arnaud, R., Messerlian, S., Moir, J. M., Omdahl, J. L., and Glorieux, F. H. (1997). The 25-hydroxyvitamin D 1-alpha-hydroxylase gene maps to the pseudovitamin D-deficiency rickets (PDDR) disease locus. *J. Bone Miner. Res.* **12,** 1552–1559.

Stoffels, K., Overbergh, L., Giulietti, A., Verlinden, L., Bouillon, R., and Mathieu, C. (2006). Immune regulation of 25-hydroxyvitamin-D3-1alpha-hydroxylase in human monocytes. *J. Bone Miner. Res.* **21,** 37–47.

Topilski, I., Flaishon, L., Naveh, Y., Harmelin, A., Levo, Y., and Shachar, I. (2004). The anti-inflammatory effects of 1,25-dihydroxyvitamin D3 on Th2 cells in vivo are due in part to the control of integrin-mediated T lymphocyte homing. *Eur. J. Immunol.* **34,** 1068–1076.

Ustianowski, A., Shaffer, R., Collin, S., Wilkinson, R. J., and Davidson, R. N. (2005). Prevalence and associations of vitamin D deficiency in foreign-born persons with tuberculosis in London. *J. Infect.* **50,** 432–437.

Usui, E., Noshiro, M., and Okuda, K. (1990). Molecular cloning of cDNA for vitamin D3 25-hydroxylase from rat liver mitochondria. *FEBS Lett.* **262,** 135–138.

van Etten, E., and Mathieu, C. (2005). Immunoregulation by 1,25-dihydroxyvitamin D3: Basic concepts. *J. Steroid Biochem. Mol. Biol.* **97,** 93–101.

Vidal, M., Ramana, C. V., and Dusso, A. S. (2002). Stat1-vitamin D receptor interactions antagonize 1,25-dihydroxyvitamin D transcriptional activity and enhance stat1-mediated transcription. *Mol. Cell. Biol.* **22,** 2777–2787.

Waddington, R. J., Moseley, R., and Embery, G. (2000). Reactive oxygen species: A potential role in the pathogenesis of periodontal diseases. *Oral Dis.* **6,** 138–151.

Wang, J. T., Lin, C. J., Burridge, S. M., Fu, G. K., Labuda, M., Portale, A. A., and Miller, W. L. (1998). Genetics of vitamin D 1alpha-hydroxylase deficiency in 17 families. *Am. J. Hum. Genet.* **63,** 1694–1702.

Wang, T. T., Nestel, F. P., Bourdeau, V., Nagai, Y., Wang, Q., Liao, J., Tavera-Mendoza, L., Lin, R., Hanrahan, J. W., Mader, S., and White, J. H. (2004). Cutting edge: 1,25-dihydroxyvitamin D3 is a direct inducer of antimicrobial peptide gene expression. *J. Immunol.* **173,** 2909–2912.

White, K. E., Evans, W. E., O'Riordan, J. L. H., Speer, M. C., Econs, M. J., Lorenz-Depiereux, B., Grabowski, M., Meitinger, T., and Strom, T. M. (2000). Autosomal dominant hypophosphataemic rickets is associated with mutations in FGF23. *Nat. Genet.* **26,** 345.

Wittke, A., Weaver, V., Mahon, B. D., August, A., and Cantorna, M. T. (2004). Vitamin D receptor-deficient mice fail to develop experimental allergic asthma. *J. Immunol.* **173,** 3432–3436.

Wittke, A., Chang, A., Froicu, M., Harandi, O. F., Weaver, V., August, A., Paulson, R. F., and Cantorna, M. T. (2007). Vitamin D receptor expression by the lung micro-environment is required for maximal induction of lung inflammation. *Arch. Biochem. Biophys.* **460,** 306–313.

Xie, Z., Munson, S., Huang, N., Schuster, I., Portale, A. A., Miller, W. L., and Bikle, D. D. (2001). The mechanism of 1,25-dihydroxyvitamin D3 auto-regulation in keratinocytes. *J. Bone Miner. Res.* **16**(Suppl. 1), S556.

Zasloff, M. (2005). Sunlight, vitamin D, and the innate immune defenses of the human skin. *J. Invest. Dermatol.* **125,** xvi–xvii.

CHAPTER TWO

Vitamin D and Innate and Adaptive Immunity

Martin Hewison

Contents

Abstract

In the last 5 years there has been renewed interest in the health benefits of vitamin D. A central feature of this revival has been new information concerning the nonclassical effects of vitamin D. In particular, studies of the interaction

Department of Orthopaedic Surgery and Molecular Biology Institute, David Geffen School of Medicine at UCLA, Los Angeles, California, USA

Vitamins and Hormones, Volume 86
ISSN 0083-6729, DOI: 10.1016/B978-0-12-386960-9.00002-2

between vitamin D and the immune system have highlighted the importance of localized conversion of precursor 25-hydroxyvitamin D (25OHD) to active 1,25-dihydroxyvitamin D (1,25$(OH)_2$D) as a mechanism for maintaining antibacterial activity in humans. The clinical relevance of this has been endorsed by increasing evidence of suboptimal 25OHD status in populations across the globe. Collectively these observations support the hypothesis that vitamin D insufficiency may lead to dysregulation of human immune responses and may therefore be an underlying cause of infectious disease and immune disorders. The current review describes the key mechanisms associated with vitamin D metabolism and signaling for both innate immune (antimicrobial activity and antigen presentation) and adaptive immune (T and B lymphocyte function) responses. These include coordinated actions of the vitamin D-activating enzyme, 1α-hydroxylase (CYP27B1), and the vitamin D receptor (VDR) in mediating intracrine and paracrine actions of vitamin D. Finally, the review will consider the role of immunomodulatory vitamin D in human health, with specific emphasis on infectious and autoimmune disease.

I. Introduction

In the last 5 years vitamin D has undergone a renaissance. A simple search of Pubmed from 2000 to 2005 identifies approximately 8000 entries for the term "vitamin D." This is almost identical to the number of entries for "thyroid hormone" over the same period. A similar search for "vitamin D" over the years 2005–2010 shows 11,200 entries, a 40% increase on the previous 5 years. This contrasts with 9000 entries for "thyroid hormone," a 12% increase over the previous 5 years. Two key factors have contributed to this. The first concerns our current view of what constitutes adequate vitamin D status. Until recently, the vitamin D status of an individual was defined simply by presence or absence of the bone disease rickets (osteomalacia in adults). Rachitic bone disease associated with vitamin D deficiency is relatively rare but it is now clear that suboptimal vitamin D status can occur in the absence of rachitic bone disease. This new perspective on vitamin D status arose from the observation that serum levels of the main circulating form of vitamin D (25OHD) as high as 75 nM correlate inversely with serum parathyroid hormone (PTH) concentrations (Chapuy *et al.*, 1997). As a result, new terminology for suboptimal vitamin D status has been introduced. Vitamin D "insufficiency" now refers to serum levels of 25OHD that are suboptimal (<75 nM) but not necessarily rachitic (<20 nM; Holick, 2007). Circulating levels of 25OHD are a direct reflection of vitamin D status, which for any given individual will depend on access to vitamin D either through exposure to ultraviolet (UV) light and epidermal synthesis of vitamin D or as a result of dietary intake. Consequently vitamin D status can vary significantly in populations depending on geographical, social, or economic factors. Moreover, recent studies of populations in the USA suggest that in the last 10 years alone, serum vitamin D levels have on average fallen by approximately 20% (Ginde *et al.*, 2009).

The key question now being considered is what is the physiological and clinical impact of global vitamin D insufficiency beyond classical bone diseases such as rickets? Part of the answer to this has been provided by the second recent development in vitamin D research. A potential role for vitamin D as a modulator of the immune system has been postulated for many years. Until recently, this was considered to simply be a manifestation of granulomatous diseases such as sarcoidosis, where synthesis of the active form of vitamin D, 1,25-dihydroxyvitamin D ($1{,}25(OH)_2D$) from precursor 25OHD is known to be dysregulated. However, in the last 5 years a wealth of *in vitro*, *in vivo* and clinical association studies have provided new evidence to support a role for 25OHD and $1{,}25(OH)_2D$ in mediating normal function of both the innate and adaptive immune systems. These new developments and the studies that preceded them are discussed in more detail in the following review with specific emphasis on different facets of the immune system.

II. Antibacterial Actions of Vitamin D

One of the earliest observations linking vitamin D with the innate immune system arose from a 1985 paper by Rook *et al.* who showed that treatment with the active form of vitamin D, $1{,}25(OH)_2D$, inhibited growth of the microbial pathogen *Mycobacterium tuberculosis* in human monocytes (Rook *et al.*, 1986). At the time, the authors were unable to define a mechanism for this effect and it was another 20 years before an explanation was finally published. The paper in question by Liu *et al.* (2006) has become a cornerstone in our understanding of how vitamin D is able to influence immune function. In this study the authors investigated the mechanisms by which monocytes and macrophages manage pathogens such as *M. tuberculosis*. Consistent with their phagocytic phenotype, monocytes are able to internalize pathogens but if left unchecked the pathogen can then replicate, leading to the possible death of the host cell. However, monocytes and macrophages can sense and respond to organisms such as *M. tuberculosis* by utilizing pathogen-recognition receptors (PRR; Janeway and Medzhitov, 2002; Kumar *et al.*, 2009). These include the large family of toll-like receptors (TLR; Anderson, 2000; Medzhitov and Janeway, 2000), that are able to initiate innate immune defense mechanisms in response to infection (Brightbill and Modlin, 2000; Brightbill *et al.*, 1999; Modlin *et al.*, 1999; Thoma-Uszynski *et al.*, 2001). The pathogen *M. tuberculosis* is known to interact with a dimer of TLR2 and TLR1 (TLR2/1) expressed by innate immune cells such as monocytes and dendritic cells (DCs). Liu *et al.* (2006) treated cultures of monocytes or DCs with a mimic to *M. tuberculosis* (19 kDa lipoprotein) which also binds and activates TLR2/1. They then used DNA array profiles to identify TLR2/1-activated genes specifically regulated in monocytes relative to DCs. The phagocytic nature of the monocytes meant that resulting cluster of regulated genes was more representative of an antibacterial response, rather than antigen presentation.

Amongst the genes identified as being induced in this study were the vitamin D receptor (VDR) and the vitamin D-activating enzyme 1α-hydroxylase (CYP27B1; Liu *et al.*, 2006). It was therefore proposed that TLR2/1-mediated responses to *M. tuberculosis* by monocytes included increased capacity for localized metabolism of substrate 25OHD and subsequent stimulation of VDR signaling following binding to the receptor of product $1,25(OH)_2D$. The viability of this intracrine pathway was initially validated by experiments showing that cotreatment of monocytes with TLR2/1 ligand and 25OHD induced expression of the VDR-target gene 24-hydroxylase (CYP24A1). Intracrine activation of monocytic VDR in the presence of 25OHD also stimulated expression of the cationic antibacterial agent, LL37, a C-terminal product of the propeptide cathelicidin (hCAP; Sorensen *et al.*, 2001). Previous studies using a variety of cell types indicated that expression of hCAP is directly induced by $1,25(OH)_2D$ acting via vitamin D response elements (VDREs) in the proximal promoter of the gene for hCAP (Gombart *et al.*, 2005; Wang *et al.*, 2004). The importance of intracrine induction of LL37 was underlined by two further experiments by Liu *et al.* (2006). In the first of these, siRNA knockdown of LL37 was shown to diminish monocyte capacity for killing of *M. tuberculosis*, indicating that induction of this antimicrobial protein is a pivotal step in the host response to this pathogen. In the second experiment, monocytes were cultured in growth medium supplemented with serum from either vitamin D-sufficient white subjects or vitamin D-insufficient black subjects. Following TLR2/1 challenge, cells cultured with vitamin D-sufficient serum showed levels of LL37 expression that were three times higher than cells cultured with vitamin D-insufficient serum. The singular importance of serum 25OHD as a determinant of this difference was illustrated by add-back of exogenous 25OHD which "rescued" the low levels of LL37 in cells cultured with serum from black donors. The studies outlined above provide a core pathway by which vitamin D is able to promote antibacterial activity (see Fig. 2.1). Subsequent reports have expanded the scope of this mechanism and its potential biological impact and these new observations are outlined in the following sections.

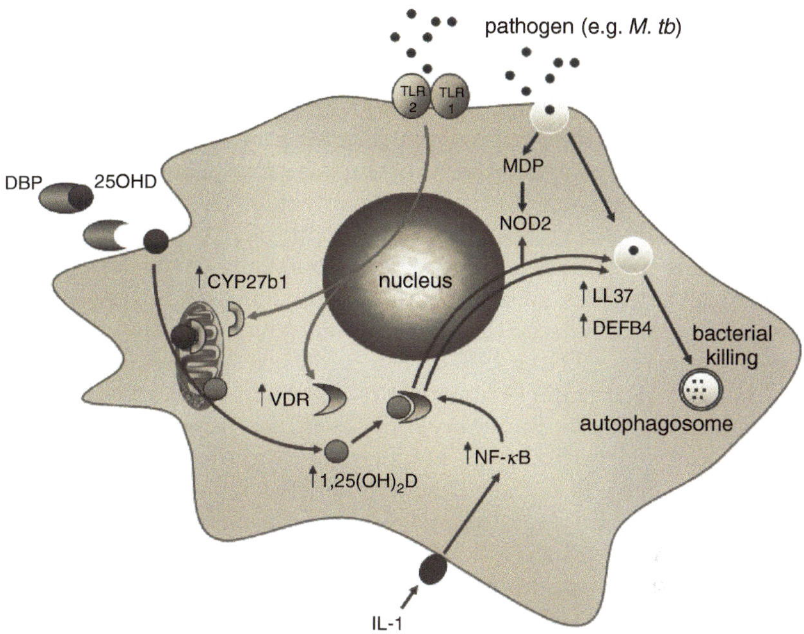

Figure 2.1 *Vitamin D and monocyte antibacterial responses.* Schematic representation showing mechanisms associated with the intracrine regulation of bacterial killing mechanisms by vitamin D in response to a pathogen such as *Mycobacterium tuberculosis*. Monocyte sensing of *M. tuberculosis* via toll-like receptor (TLR) 2 and 1 enhances expression of the vitamin D-activating enzyme 1α-hydroxylase (CYP27B1) and the vitamin D receptor (VDR). CYP27B1 catalyzes synthesis of active 1,25-dihydroxyvitamin D (1,25(OH)$_2$D) from substrate 25-hydroxyvitamin D (25OHD), the main circulating form of vitamin D. Bioavailability of 25OHD is dependent on vitamin D status and the action of serum vitamin D-binding protein (DBP). 1,25(OH)$_2$D synthesized by monocyte CYP27B1 binds to VDR and regulates transcription of target genes such as the antimicrobial protein cathelicidin (LL37). Other antibacterial proteins such as β-defensin 2 (DEFB4) are also induced by 1,25(OH)$_2$D but require adjunct signaling via nuclear factor-kappa B (NF-κB), involving signaling via interleukin-1 (IL-1) or nucleotide-binding oligomerization domain containing 2 (NOD2) and muramyl dipeptide (MDP). Intracrine synthesis of 1,25(OH)$_2$D is also associated with the induction of autophagy, a cytoplasmic process known to enhance bacterial killing. (See Color Insert.)

A. Vitamin D bioavailability and antibacterial activity

A key finding from the original studies of TLR-triggered action of vitamin D in monocytes was that antibacterial function is dependent on levels of prohormone 25OHD. This was initially based on differential induction of LL37 in monocytes exposed to serum from two populations whose vitamin D status was at opposite ends of the spectrum. However, more recent reports have shown that similar responses can also be demonstrated using serum from individuals supplemented with vitamin D *in vivo* (Adams *et al.*, 2009). In this instance, subjects identified as being vitamin D-insufficient (<75 nM serum 25OHD) were supplemented with vitamin D_2 (100,000 IU per week for 5 weeks). This restored vitamin D sufficiency in the patients, and serum collected following this restoration supported higher TLR2/1 induction of LL37 under autologous conditions when compared to collected prior to supplementation (Adams *et al.*, 2009).

It is therefore clear that induction of VDR and CYP27B1 following TLR signaling is sufficient to sensitize monocytes to relatively modest physiological differences in serum 25OHD concentrations. Given that this may vary considerably from one person to another depending on access to dietary vitamin D_2 or D_3, or UV-driven epidermal synthesis of vitamin D_3, it seems likely that vitamin D status *per se* will be a major determinant of this particular facet of innate immunity. However, it is important to recognize that circulating levels of vitamin D metabolites may not necessarily reflect their bioavailability. In common with other steroids and sterol-like compounds, 25OHD and 1,25$(OH)_2$D circulate bound to serum proteins. Vitamin D metabolites show low affinity binding to albumin but serum also contains a more specific vitamin D-binding protein (DBP), originally referred to as group-specific component (Gc; White and Cooke, 2000). DBP is known to play a key role in the renal homeostasis of vitamin D as a result of facilitated renal reabsorption of DBP-bound vitamin D metabolites via the DBP receptors megalin (Nykjaer *et al.*, 1999) and cubilin (Nykjaer *et al.*, 2001). This mechanism is particular important for 25OHD which shows higher affinity binding to DBP than active 1,25$(OH)_2$D. In the kidney, retention of 25OHD by DBP is likely to be a key factor in optimizing endocrine synthesis of 1,25$(OH)_2$D given that this organ is the major contributor to circulating levels of active vitamin D.

Outside the kidney, the impact of DBP on vitamin D responses is less clear. Studies of vitamin D responses in CYP27B1-expressing breast epithelial cells suggest that they also utilize megalin–cubilin-mediated uptake of 25OHD, although in this instance the subsequent synthesis of 1,25 $(OH)_2$D is intracrine rather than paracrine (Rowling *et al.*, 2006). Monocytes are also able to internalize DBP but this does not appear to involve megalin–cubilin (Chun *et al.*, 2010). Moreover, in contrast to its effects on kidney and breast cells, monocyte uptake of DBP is not associated with concomitant internalization of vitamin D metabolites. Instead in this setting DBP appear to attenuate the bioavailability of 25OHD and 1,25$(OH)_2$D (Chun *et al.*, 2010). Monocytes cultured in medium containing serum from DBP knockout (−/−) mice were more able to induce LL37 in response to vitamin D metabolites than equivalent cultures using serum from $DBP^{+/-}$ mice. This effect was more pronounced for 25OHD compared to 1,25 $(OH)_2$D, consistent with the higher affinity binding of 25OHD to DBP (Chun *et al.*, 2010). Further studies showed that well-established genotypic variations in human DBP known to be associated with diminished affinity for vitamin D metabolites also supported enhanced monocyte induction of LL37 in response to 25OHD. With these observations in mind it seems likely that vitamin D-mediated antibacterial activity will not only be dependent on serum 25OHD status, but will also reflect the bioavailability of "free" 25OHD to target cells such as monocytes.

The effects of DBP on monocyte responses to vitamin D have important implications for supplementation strategies because, in addition to their effects on vitamin D-binding affinity, the main allelic forms of the *DBP* gene also show distinct patterns of racial distribution (Kamboh and Ferrell, 1986; Westwood *et al.*, 1987). With this in mind, it is possible to speculate that a specific serum level of 25OHD for one individual will be less effective in supporting innate immune function than the same level in another person. It is also interesting to note that the lower affinity forms of DBP (Gc2 and Gc1S) arose from the parental higher affinity forms of DBP (Gc1F). Such a change has the potential to compromise renal homeostasis of vitamin D where binding to DBP is central to urinary megalin–cubilin reclamation of 25OHD. However, in early humans this may have had a negligible impact provided serum vitamin D status was optimal. Instead a biological advantage of lower affinity forms of DBP may have stemmed from the migration of humans to more northerly geographical locations where UV-induced generation of vitamin D was less effective. Under these conditions we can speculate that decreased DBP binding and increased bioavailability of 25OHD to cells such as monocytes may have conferred a significant advantage with respect to infectious diseases. The alternative actions of DBP and its role in human immune disease are discussed in more detail in later sections.

B. Innate immune responses and the regulation of vitamin D metabolism

As outlined above, the ability of vitamin D to promote antibacterial responses to a pathogenic challenge appears to be highly dependent on tissue-specific synthesis of $1,25(OH)_2D$. Although, this is clearly linked to the bioavailability of substrate 25OHD, it is also likely to be strongly influenced by activity of the vitamin D-activating enzyme CYP27B1. Induction of this enzyme following TLR2/1 activation was one of the pivotal observations linking vitamin D with antibacterial activity (Liu *et al.*, 2006). However, many previous reports have documented alternative immune regulators of vitamin D metabolism, and these are discussed in the following section.

One of the initial observations linking vitamin D with immune function was the abundant synthesis of $1,25(OH)_2D$ by macrophages isolated from patients with sarcoidosis (Adams and Gacad, 1985; Adams *et al.*, 1983).

Similar observations have also been reported for macrophages associated with other granulomatous disorders (reviewed in Kallas *et al.*, 2010), inflammatory arthritis (Mawer *et al.*, 1991), and tumor (Townsend *et al.*, 2005), indicating that dysregulation of vitamin D metabolism is a common feature of several human diseases. Nevertheless, it is important to recognize that extrarenal expression of CYP27B1 is not restricted exclusively to pathogenic scenaria (Zehnder *et al.*, 2001). Notably, in the context of monocytes and macrophages, studies carried out using peripheral blood-derived monocytes from normal donors have shown that these cells are also able to convert 25OHD to $1,25(OH)_2D$. In this instance, the monocytes were treated *in vitro* with either the cytokine interferon gamma (IFNγ; Koeffler *et al.*, 1985), or the TLR4 ligand lipopolysaccharide (LPS; Reichel *et al.*, 1987). Since then other monocyte models and treatment regimes have also been reported to stimulate CYP27B1 activity (Hayes *et al.*, 1992; Hewison *et al.*, 1989; Yuan *et al.*, 1992), further underlining the importance of this enzyme as a target for the modulation of immunoactive $1,25(OH)_2D$. A key consideration for extrarenal activation of 25OHD under normal physiological conditions is that, unlike renal CYP27B1 activity, tissue-specific synthesis of $1,25(OH)_2D$ is unlikely to be manifested by alterations in circulating levels of the hormone. Instead it is predicted that extrarenal CYP27B1 acts in an intracrine or paracrine fashion (Hewison, 2010).

The vitamin D-activating enzyme CYP27B1 is a mitochondrial cytochrome P450 that catalyzes conversion of prohormone 25OHD to hormonal $1,25(OH)_2D$. In a classical renal setting, expression and activity of CYP27B1 is regulated in a sensitive fashion by endocrine factors associated with calcium and phosphate homeostasis such as PTH and fibroblast growth factor 23 (FGF23; Quarles, 2008). Similar mechanisms do not appear to be relevant to extrarenal sources of CYP27B1. Monocytes do not express a viable PTH signaling pathway for induction of CYP27B1 and, to date, there have been no reports of FGF23-mediated suppression of monocyte $1,25(OH)_2D$ production despite its potent actions in suppressing CYP27B1 activity in proximal tubule kidney cells (Shimada *et al.*, 2004). This occurs despite the fact that synthesis of $1,25(OH)_2D$ in renal and extrarenal tissues involves the same *CYP27B1* gene product (Fu *et al.*, 1997). The presence of a single enzyme for activation of vitamin D throughout the body has therefore shifted attention to tissue- and cell-specific regulatory mechanisms. Analysis of CYP27B1 transcription using promoter–reporter models has shown that the JAK–STAT, p38 MAP kinase, and nuclear factor-kappa B (NF-κB) pathways are all involved in mediating the effects of IFNγ and LPS in stimulating monocyte synthesis of $1,25(OH)_2D$, with CCAAT/enhancer-binding protein β (C/EBPβ) being the most important single transcription factor for induction of CYP27B1 (Stoffels *et al.*, 2006). Similar studies have yet to be performed for TLR2/1 induction of monocyte CYP27B1 but this may involve a still more complex mechanism.

Monocytes treated with the 19 kDa lipoprotein ligand for TLR2/1 appear to require stimulation of IL-15 expression in order to induce CYP27B1 and VDR expression; antibodies to IL-15 suppressed TLR2/1-mediated upregulation of both the enzyme and receptor (Krutzik *et al.*, 2008). The precise mechanism by which IL-15 promotes CYP27B1 transcription in monocytes has yet to be defined but data from other cell models indicated that the JAK–STAT pathway is the most likely candidate (Waldmann, 2006).

The ability of IL-15 and IFNγ to induce CYP27B1 expression independent of TLRs suggests that monocyte synthesis of $1,25(OH)_2D$ is not exclusively regulated by innate pathogen recognition. IFNγ is produced by natural killer (NK) and NK T-cells, as well as CD4 and CD8-positive T-cells (Schoenborn and Wilson, 2007). Conversely, T-cells expressing factors such as IFNγ are known to stimulate IL-15 synthesis by DCs (Josien *et al.*, 1999). The induction of monocyte CYP27B1 activity by either of these cytokines may therefore act as a novel mechanism by which the adaptive immune system is able to enhance innate immune response to infection. Indeed, in the case of IL-15, it may be possible to stimulate vitamin D-mediated antibacterial activity independent of any actual innate pathogen recognition, simply by T-cell-stimulated DCs providing the cytokine stimulus required for adequate expression of monocyte CYP27B1. This is endorsed by the fact that innate immune responses alone are not sufficient to combat infectious diseases, as evidenced by the high rates of TB infection in people who are positive for the human immunodeficiency virus (HIV).

Although tissue-specific regulation of CYP27B1 transcription appears to be a central feature of monocyte innate immune response to infection, other mechanisms may also impact on the final capacity for $1,25(OH)_2D$ production by these cells. For example, while mRNA for CYP27b1 is expressed by many tissues (Hewison *et al.*, 2007), these transcripts include an array of noncoding splice variants that act to attenuate expression of wild-type CYP27B1 protein, thereby limiting the accumulation of $1,25(OH)_2D$ at these sites (Wu *et al.*, 2007). A second mechanism for attenuating local concentrations of $1,25(OH)_2D$ involves the catabolic enzyme for vitamin D, CYP24A1, which catalyzes synthesis of less active forms of vitamin D such as 1,24,25-trihydroxyvitamin D ($1,24,25(OH)_2D$). Monocytes and macrophages express low levels of CYP24A1 but this is readily induced following treatment with 25OHD or $1,25(OH)_2D$, consistent with its role as a feedback regulator of $1,25(OH)_2D$ production (Sakaki *et al.*, 2005). However, even under stimulatory conditions, monocytes and macrophages exhibit very low levels of actual 24-hydroxylase activity relative to other CYP24A-positive cells. This appears to be due to expression of a truncated splice variant form of CYP24A1 (CYP24-SV) encoding a translated protein that lacks a mitochondrial targeting sequence and is therefore functionally inactive (Ren *et al.*, 2005). Despite its metabolic inactivity, CYP24-SV retains its substrate-binding pocket and is therefore able to bind either 25OHD or 1,25(OH)$_2$D. Consequently, expression of CYP24-SV by monocytes may act to attenuate local synthesis of 1,25(OH)$_2$D by acting as a decoy for the CYP27B1 substrate 25OHD. Conversely, expression of CYP24-SV may help to sustain local concentrations of 1,25(OH)$_2$D by acting as decoy for the wild-type catabolic enzyme CYP24A1. In this way, the splice variant form of CYP24A1 may provide a versatile and metabolically economic mechanism for controlling monocyte handling of vitamin D metabolites.

C. VDR expression and innate immune responses

The VDR is a phylogenetically ancient member of the nuclear receptor superfamily which is highly conserved in vertebrates, and which shows homology with receptors that bind bile acids such as the farnesoid X receptor (FXR) and the liver X receptor (LXR; Jurutka *et al.*, 2007). Following binding of its natural ligand, 1,25(OH)$_2$D, the occupied VDR forms a heterodimer with the retinoid X receptor (RXR) and undergoes conformational changes that allow it to interact with a diverse array of accessory proteins and enzymes required for chromatin remodeling and transcriptional activity (Jurutka *et al.*, 2007). Initial studies of innate immune responses to vitamin D showed that the ability of vitamin D metabolites to promote antituberculosis activity correlated closely with their VDR binding affinity (Rook *et al.*, 1986). However, because expression of VDR is ubiquitous, the factors that influence its expression have been less well documented than those associated with the induction of CYP27B1.

In a seminal study, Reichel *et al.* assessed the nuclear binding of 1,25 (OH)$_2$D and VDR mRNA expression in monocytes at various stages of differentiation to a mature macrophage phenotype (Kreutz *et al.*, 1993). The VDR was abundantly expressed in immature monocytes but these levels declined during macrophage differentiation. Conversely, expression of CYP27B1 and 1α-hydroxylation increased as monocytes differentiate (Kreutz *et al.*, 1993). The underlying mechanism for this remains unclear but it is notable that a similar pattern of divergent expression for VDR and CYP27B1 has also been reported for immature DCs as they differentiate toward a mature antigen-presenting cell (Hewison *et al.*, 2003). The significance of this is discussed in greater detail in later sections of the review (see Section III.A). Although levels of VDR in monocytes appear to decline as they mature, this is not necessarily directly linked to altered cell proliferation. Indeed, studies using myelomonocytic cell lines have reported increased nuclear binding of 1,25(OH)$_2$D following differentiation with antiproliferative phorbol esters (Hewison *et al.*, 1989, 1992). Thus, even in the absence of pathogen, the regulation of VDR expression is complex and is likely to reflect input by a variety of stimuli including cytokines and colony stimulating factors. What is more clear is that pathogen recognition in the form of TLR-activation acts to enhance VDR expression (Adams *et al.*, 2009; Liu *et al.*, 2006). As with TLR induction of CYP27B1, the mechanism by which this occurs is as yet unclear but is likely to involve a similar combination of JAK–STAT, p38 MAP kinase, and NF-κB pathways.

In common with other nuclear receptors, much interest has focused on the biological impact of disruption to VDR signaling. In humans, mutations in the *VDR* gene associated with hereditary vitamin D resistant rickets (HVDRR) are characteristically associated with rachitic bone disease and, in some cases, alopecia (Malloy *et al.*, 1999). However, because relatively few affected kindreds have been described worldwide, the potential impact of VDR dysfunction on human immune responses has yet to be documented. Studies using cells from different HVDRR patients have highlighted differential effects of VDR mutations on target gene transactivation (Nguyen *et al.*, 2006), and it seems likely that VDR mutations will have a similar variable impact on patient immune response to vitamin D. This is further complicated by the fact that most HVDRR patients are treated with high doses of 1,25$(OH)_2D$ as therapy for their underlying bone disease. Additional perspectives on how variations in VDR signaling can affect immune responses have been provided by analysis of *VDR* gene ablation in mice, and *VDR* gene single nucleotide polymorphisms (SNPs) in humans. These issues are discussed in later sections of the review.

D. Antibacterial targets for vitamin D

Perhaps the most significant advance in our understanding of how vitamin D promotes innate immune responses to infection has been the identification of molecular mechanisms for VDR-mediated transactivation of antibacterial proteins. Initial screening of human DNA sequences identified candidate VDREs in the gene promoters for LL37 and another antibacterial protein β-defensin 2 (DEFB4; Wang *et al.*, 2004). Subsequent functional studies demonstrated direct interaction between the gene promoter for LL37 and liganded VDR, leading to dose-dependent induction of transcription by 1,25 $(OH)_2D$ (Gombart *et al.*, 2005; Wang *et al.*, 2004). Intriguingly, the VDRE initially identified within the proximal gene promoter for LL37 appears to specific for primates, as there is no similar motif within the equivalent gene sequences for other mammals (Gombart *et al.*, 2005). Acquisition of this VDRE appears to have occurred following the introduction of an Alu short interspersed nuclear element (SINE) that placed the *LL37* gene under the control of the liganded VDR (Gombart *et al.*, 2009b). This primate-specific modification has been conserved in humans and apes as well as old world and new world primates, suggesting that a mechanism for vitamin D-mediated induction of LL37 confers biological advantages. Initially, such a mechanism would be readily supported by the relatively high circulating levels of 25OHD that are characteristic of nonhuman primates. However, in less vitamin D-replete modern man this pathway for induction of an antibacterial agent may be less effective, thus providing a key argument for the improvement of human vitamin D status.

In common with LL37, the gene promoter for DEFB4 also includes a functional VDRE although in contrast to LL37 this is not part of a primate SINE. However, whereas treatment with 1,25$(OH)_2D$ potently induces LL37 in a variety of cell types its effects on DEFB4 expression are much less pronounced (Gombart *et al.*, 2005; Liu *et al.*, 2006; Wang *et al.*, 2004). One possible explanation for this is that transcriptional activity of the DEFB4 VDRE requires additional stimuli for functional efficacy. In contrast to LL37, DEFB is sensitively induced by the cytokine interleukin-1 in gastrointestinal epithelial cells (IL-1β; O'Neil *et al.*, 1999), and similar results have also been described for monocytes (Liu *et al.*, 2009b) and keratinocytes (Wang *et al.*, 2004), with 1,25 $(OH)_2D$ cotreatment further enhancing the actions of IL-1β (Wang *et al.*, 2004). Based on these observations it has been proposed that IL-1β signaling interacts with the vitamin D pathway to facilitate transactivation via the DEFB4 VDRE (Liu *et al.*, 2009b) (see Fig. 2.1). The convergence of these two pathways probably involves NF-κB-binding sites that flank the DEFB4 VDRE; monocytes transfected with the p65 subunit of NF-κB showed sensitization to 1,25$(OH)_2D$-induced expression of DEFB4 (Liu *et al.*, 2009b).

A fresh perspective on the induction of DEFB4 by 1,25$(OH)_2D$ has been provided by studies of another innate immunity protein, nucleotide-binding oligomerization domain containing 2 (NOD2). In contrast to extracellular PRR such as TLR2 and TLR4, NOD2 acts as an intracellular PRR by binding muramyl dipeptide (MDP), a cell membrane product from $Gram^{+ve}$ and $Gram^{-ve}$ bacteria (Strober *et al.*, 2006). Following binding of MDP, NOD2 signals by activating the NF-κB pathway in a similar fashion to that observed with IL-1β. Recent studies by Wang *et al.* (2009) have shown that expression of NOD2 is potently induced by 1,25$(OH)_2D$ in a variety of cell types. Furthermore, combined treatment with 1,25$(OH)_2D$ and the NOD2 ligand MDP synergistically induced NF-κB activity, as well as expression of DEFB4 and LL37 (Wang *et al.*, 2009). Thus, NOD2 activation may provide an additional signaling mechanism by which NF-κ B is able to converge with the vitamin D pathway to induce DEFB4 (see Fig. 2.1). This may be particularly important in the gastrointestinal tract because inactivating mutations in the gene for NOD2 are associated with an inherited form of Crohn's disease (Hugot *et al.*, 2001; Ogura *et al.*, 2001). Polymorphic variations in the *NOD2* gene have also been described (Hugot *et al.*, 2001), and in these patients it is possible to speculate that low 25OHD levels may further complicate SNP-associated variations in NOD2 by compromising the efficacy of its transcription. In this way, vitamin D status may act as a key environmental trigger for those individuals who are genetically predisposed to Crohn's disease. The induction of NOD2, an inflammatory bowel disease susceptibility gene, also suggests that the antibacterial activity of vitamin D is not restricted to infectious diseases such as TB. The broader importance of tissue-specific vitamin D-induced innate immunity is discussed in further detail in Section II.E.

Initial studies of the effects of 25OHD and 1,25$(OH)_2$D on monocytes concluded that vitamin D-mediated innate immune response to *M. tuberculosis* infection was highly dependent on induction of LL37 (Liu *et al.*, 2006, 2007). However, the parallel stimulation of DEFB4 in concert with other stimulatory mechanisms suggests that this may also be pivotal to vitamin D-induced innate immunity. Knockdown of either LL37 or DEFB4 completely abrogated the ability of 1,25$(OH)_2$D to promote killing of intracellular *M. tuberculosis* in monocytes, indicating that both proteins play a role in mediating the antibacterial effects of vitamin D (Liu *et al.*, 2009b). As outlined earlier, the induction of LL37 and DEFB4 by 1,25 $(OH)_2$D appears to be restricted to higher primates that express consensus VDREs within their proximal gene promoters (Gombart *et al.*, 2005; Wang *et al.*, 2004). Although these VDREs are absent in the equivalent mouse genes, it is possible that vitamin D-inducibility will still be present if alternative VDREs are present in more distal areas of the LL37 or DEFB4 promoter. Another likely scenario is that vitamin D-induced responses to infection in mice will involve a different array of antibacterial targets. Recent DNA array analysis of colon tissue from vitamin D-sufficient and vitamin D-deficient mice has shown that expression of the mouse antimicrobial protein angiogenin-4 (Ang4) is potently suppressed under conditions of low serum 25OHD levels (Lagishetty *et al.*, 2010). Although the function of Ang4 appears to be restricted to specific areas of the gastrointestinal tract such as Paneth cells, this observation underlines the versatility of vitamin D as a promoter of antibacterial activity in different types of animals.

Another mechanism by which vitamin D may be able to exert more generalized antimicrobial activity is via nonspecific bacterial killing. This is best illustrated by studies of the relationship between vitamin D and reactive oxygen species (ROS), which can act as bacteriocides. Initial analysis of *M. tuberculosis* killing in response to 1,25$(OH)_2$D suggested that this probably did not involve ROS (Rook *et al.*, 1986). However, subsequent studies have reported that macrophages infected with *M. tuberculosis* in the presence of 1,25$(OH)_2$D produce high levels of superoxide anions via the NADPH-oxidase system (Sly *et al.*, 2001). More recently, attention has focused on nitric oxide (NO), which is produced by macrophages as part of innate immune response to infection. In addition to its established vascular activity, NO can function as an ROS and thus exert bacteriocidal effects (Kohchi *et al.*, 2009). The NO pathway appears to play a pivotal role in mouse responses to *M. tuberculosis* infection (Chan *et al.*, 1992), but its importance to humans is less clear. The relationship between vitamin D and NO is also uncertain. In neuronal cells, $1,25(OH)_2D$ has been reported to suppress the NO-generating enzyme, inducible nitric oxide synthase (iNOS; Garcion *et al.*, 1997). However, studies using monocytic cell lines have shown the opposite, in that induction of NO via either iNOS (Rockett *et al.*, 1998) or NADPH-oxidase 2 (Yang *et al.*, 2009) has been linked to suppression of *M. tuberculosis* growth. This effect would appear to be pathogen specific as macrophages infected with the intracellular protozoan *Leishmania major* showed decreased NO production and bacterial killing when treated with $1,25(OH)_2D$ (Ehrchen *et al.*, 2007). In this instance, it was suggested that vitamin D may enhance, rather than suppress, *L. major* infection.

In recent years, it has become clear that factors beyond the actual bacteriocidal agent are crucial for effective innate immune responses to infection. In particular, attention has focused on the environment in which bacterial killing takes place. Classic immunology indicates that following phagocytosis by macrophages, pathogens such as *M. tuberculosis* are confined to phagosomes. In the absence of any further response, the pathogen would still be able to function within this environment, and its proliferation would lead to host cell death. However, fusing of phagosomes with lysosomes produces a phagolysosomal environment that is more conducive to bacterial killing. This is due in part to the strongly acidic nature of the fused lysosome/phagosome, but may also involve incorporation of specific antibacterial factors such as LL37 and DEFB4 (Sorensen *et al.*, 2001). The efficacy of such a mechanism is far from clear and recent attention has focused on an additional facet of cellular function—autophagy—that may enhance the processing of phagocytosed pathogens. Autophagy is a cellular mechanism common to all eukaryotic organisms that involves membrane encapsulation of organelles or cell proteins in an autophagosome prior to fusion with lysosomes and degradation of the autolysosomal contents. It is well recognized that autophagy is a pivotal factor in the maintenance of cytosolic homeostasis, particularly under conditions of nutrient starvation (Klionsky and Emr, 2000). However, more recently, a role for autophagy in cellular response to infection has also been proposed, with pathogens contained in autophagosomes being either eliminated or degraded prior to presentation to PRRs such as TLRs (Deretic and Levine, 2009; Gutierrez *et al.*, 2004). Like the vitamin D system, autophagy is regulated by TLR signaling (Delgado *et al.*, 2009), and it was therefore interesting to note recent elegant studies by Yuk *et al.* (2009) who have shown that induction of autophagy is an essential feature of $1,25(OH)_2D$-induced antibacterial response to *M. tuberculosis* infection. In this particular study, the authors proposed an indirect model for vitamin D-induced autophagy involving elevated expression of LL37. However, direct effects on autophagy by vitamin D may also be possible. Synthetic analogs of 1,25 $(OH)_2D$ have been shown to inhibit the mammalian target of rapamycin (mTOR) pathway (O'Kelly *et al.*, 2006), a response known to promote autophagy (Sanjuan *et al.*, 2009). More recent studies have shown that induction of CYP27B1 is associated with TLR-induced autophagy, indicating that this mechanism is also likely to be strongly influenced by bioavailability of 25OHD (Shin *et al.*, 2010).

E. Antibacterial effects of vitamin D in neutrophils and other cell types

To date, the induction of antibacterial proteins such as LL37 by vitamin D metabolites has focused primarily on monocytes and macrophages and infection by *M. tuberculosis*. However, it is important to recognize that a wide range of cell types express PRRs and have the necessary machinery to exert innate immune responses to infection. Prominent amongst these are granulocytic cells such as neutrophils which are the most abundant of all the leukocytes and provide a rapid response to infection and inflammation. Although neutrophils and other granulocytes express VDR (Takahashi *et al.*, 2002), studies *in vitro* using precursor blast cells have tended to suggest that treatment with 1,25(OH)$_2$D promotes monocytopoiesis and suppresses granulocytopoiesis (Bunce *et al.*, 1997). Nevertheless, early reports of 1,25 (OH)$_2$D-induced expression of LL37 *in vitro* indicated that this response occurred in neutrophils as well as monocytes (Wang *et al.*, 2004). The physiological significance of this is not yet clear. Unlike monocytes and macrophages, there is no clear evidence that neutrophils express a functional CYP27B1 enzyme and so it is possible that these cells act as systemic responders to hormonal 1,25(OH)$_2$D. Despite this, the abundance of neutrophils indicates that they are likely to be the major source of serum hCAP (Sorensen *et al.*, 1997). Recent studies have described a link between low serum hCAP and disease mortality in patients with chronic kidney disease (Gombart *et al.*, 2009a). In this case, circulating levels of hCAP correlated with serum 1,25(OH)$_2$D rather than 25OHD, and it is interesting to speculate that this may represent an endocrine-regulated innate immune response, possibly involving VDR-positive, CYP27B1-negative neutrophils. By contrast, in patients with sepsis, a systemic inflammatory responses associated with infection and the sustained presence of neutrophils, circulating levels of hCAP (LL37) are lower in more critically ill patients and this is associated with low serum levels of 25OHD (Jeng *et al.*, 2009).

Antibacterial responses to vitamin D have also been described for a wide range of cell types outside the conventional immune system, although this is not always identical to the TLR-mediated mechanism originally described by Liu *et al.* (2006). In the skin, 1,25(OH)$_2$D induces keratinocyte expression of LL37 in a similar fashion to that observed in monocytes (Gombart *et al.*, 2005; Wang *et al.*, 2004) However, the intracrine mechanism underpinning this is relatively complex and involves initial signaling via transforming growth factor beta 1 (TGFβ1). Schauber *et al.* (2007) showed that treatment of keratinocytes with TGFβ1 increases expression of CYP27B1 and that this in turn facilitates enhanced local levels of 1,25$(OH)_2$D. By binding to endogenous VDR the 1,25$(OH)_2$D then stimulates transcriptional upregulation of TLR2 in keratinocytes, thereby enabling further enhancement of CYP27B1 and VDR, and concomitant production of LL37 via the conventional TLR-mediated pathway characteristic of monocytes. In this way, cells in the skin will only initiate vitamin D-mediated immunity provided there is sufficient TGFβ1 to support enhanced TLR expression. Expression of TGFβ1 is increased following epidermal wounding, underlining the potential importance of vitamin D-induced antibacterial activity as a mechanism for maintaining tissue "barrier integrity." The requirement for a "secondary" mechanism to mediate vitamin D induction of LL37 in the skin is endorsed by the fact that increased epidermal expression of LL37 is associated with inflammatory disorders such as psoriasis and atopic dermatitis (Ong *et al.*, 2002). Given that cathelicidins can promote inflammation by stimulating the release of cytokines and chemokines (Schauber and Gallo, 2007), it may be beneficial to have additional mechanism sensitive to tissue injury that will moderate the localized synthesis of LL37.

Other tissues that have been shown to induce LL37 in response to 1,25 $(OH)_2$D include respiratory epithelial cells (Hansdottir *et al.*, 2008; Yim *et al.*, 2007), and cells from both the decidual (maternal; Evans *et al.*, 2006) and trophoblastic (fetal) sides of the human placenta (Liu *et al.*, 2009a), with the latter being linked to increased bacterial killing. In the decidual and trophoblastic cells induction of LL37 was also observed with added 25OHD highlighting a similar intracrine mechanism to that observed in monocytes and keratinocytes. Interestingly, 25OHD induction of antibacterial activity by placental cells does not appear to require the same TLR-mediated upregulation of CYP27B1 and/or VDR that is characteristic of other tissues. This may be due to the fact that expression of these genes is elevated very early in gestation providing the placenta with a relatively high baseline level of constitutively synthesized 1,25$(OH)_2$D (Evans *et al.*, 2004; Zehnder *et al.*, 2002). Such a mechanism would be advantageous in maintaining optimal antibacterial responses within the fetal-maternal environment provided the maternal 25OHD availability was adequate. However, the absence of a TLR-mediated mechanism for enhancing placental VDR and CYP27B1 expression would clearly be disadvantageous under conditions of vitamin D deficiency as tissue levels of 1,25$(OH)_2$D, and therefore LL37, would decrease proportionally.

III. Vitamin D and Antigen Presentation

The cellular responses described for the interaction between vitamin D and innate immunity provide the first-line of defense following a pathogenic challenge, but the ultimate success of this response is also dependent on efficient incorporation of responses by other immune cell types, notably cells from the adaptive immune system. In this regard, a key interface between innate and adaptive immunity is that provided by antigen-presenting cells (APCs). Most cells in the body can present antigen to cytotoxic T-cells via the class I major histocompatibility complex (MHC class I). However, professional APCs such as DCs and macrophages are also able to present antigen via MHC class II and are therefore able to interact with both cytotoxic T-cells and helper T-cells. All of these actions may be influenced by vitamin D but following section will focus specifically on the proposed functions of vitamin D with respect to DCs.

A. Vitamin D and DC maturation

Early studies using DCs purified from human lymphatic tissue indicated that these cells express VDR (Brennan *et al.*, 1987). However, the functional significance of this was only addressed much later with the advent of improved selection methods and peripheral blood-derived culture models. Initial studies using DCs isolated from human epidermis (Langerhans cells; Dam *et al.*, 1996), or murine bone marrow (Griffin *et al.*, 2000) showed that treatment with 1,25$(OH)_2$D or a synthetic vitamin D analog suppressed antigen presentation. This effect was lost in VDR knockout mice (Griffin *et al.*, 2000), confirming the role of VDR in mediating DC responses to vitamin D metabolites. Subsequent reports revealed that suppression of antigen presentation by 1,25$(OH)_2$D or its analogs involves inhibition of DC maturation (Griffin *et al.*, 2001; Penna and Adorini, 2000; Piemonti *et al.*, 2000). Mice lacking the VDR were unable to demonstrate this response and presented with increased numbers of mature DCs in hypertrophic lymph nodes (Griffin *et al.*, 2001). A key molecular target for the inhibitory effects of 1,25$(OH)_2$D on DC maturation is relB, a NF-κB family member known to be intimately involved in DC differentiation (Dong *et al.*, 2003, 2005). NF-κB signaling is also known to play a pivotal role in the differential sensitivity of different DC subgroups to 1,25$(OH)_2$D. Myeloid DCs (mDC) demonstrate tolerogenic responses to treatment with 1,25$(OH)_2$D, whereas plasmacytoid DCs (pDC) do not (Penna *et al.*, 2007). This appears to be due to the fact that, in contrast to pDCs, mDCs treated with 1,25$(OH)_2$D show inhibition of NF-κB p65 subunit phosphorylation and nuclear translocation (Penna *et al.*, 2007).

A key facet of antigen presentation is the ability of DCs to migrate from the circulation to peripheral tissues where they encounter antigen, and from there to the lymph nodes where they interface with other leukocytes. This "trafficking" of DCs is dependent on the coordinated expression of chemokine ligands (CCL) and corresponding chemokine receptors (CCR; Cyster, 1999). Prominent amongst these is CCL22 which is constitutively produced by DCs and chemotactic for activated T-cells expressing CCR4 (Tang and Cyster,

1999). Treatment of mDCs with 1,25$(OH)_2$D increased CCL22 production, but had no effect on another cytokine CCL17 which is also known to bind to CCR4 (Penna *et al.*, 2007). In contrast to mDCs, vitamin D insensitive pDCs showed no changes in CCL22 expression following treatment with 1,25 $(OH)_2$D. These observations underline the versatile effects of 1,25$(OH)_2$D as a regulator of DC function, and the cell selectivity of its effects further emphasize a role in mediating tolerogenic immunity. Unlike mDCs, pDCs exhibit intrinsic tolerance under baseline conditions, promoting the development of suupressor regulatory T-cells (Tregs; Bilsborough *et al.*, 2003; Liu, 2005). Under these conditions no further input from 1,25$(OH)_2$D is required to enhance pDC function. By contrast, mDCs are not inherently tolerogenic but can be induced to promote suppressor T-cell function in the presence of 1,25$(OH)_2$D (Penna *et al.*, 2007).

B. Vitamin D metabolism and DC function

A key development in our understanding of how vitamin D status may be able to modulate DC function arose from studies of vitamin D metabolism. Studies using monocyte-derived DCs demonstrated expression of CYP27B1 and a capacity for synthesis of 1,25$(OH)_2$D similar to that observed for macrophages (Fritsche *et al.*, 2003; Hewison *et al.*, 2003). Moreover, the concomitant expression of VDR by these DCs suggested another intracrine vitamin D pathway similar to that described for macrophages. Treatment of DCs with either active 1,25$(OH)_2$D or inactive precursor 25OHD suppressed expression of markers of mature DC function such as CD80, CD83, CD86, and HLA-DR and, in doing so, inhibited antigen presentation and T-cell proliferation (Hewison *et al.*, 2003). These studies preceded description of a TLR-mediated intracrine system in monocytes by almost 3 years and provided the first real evidence of an intracrine system by which vitamin D can influence T-cell activity. The efficacy of this mechanism is illustrated by the fact that changes in DC maturation markers and associated effects on T-cell proliferation were observed with physiological doses of 25OHD compared to supraphysiological levels of 1,25$(OH)_2$D (Hewison *et al.*, 2003). Indeed, subsequent analysis of cellular vitamin D metabolism showed DC intracrine levels of 1,25$(OH)_2$D that were less than 5 nM following treatment with 150 nM 25OHD (Hewison *et al.*, 2007). Nevertheless, this treatment produced the same degree of CD80, CD83, and HLA-DR suppression as 100 nM exogenous 1,25$(OH)_2$D, indicating that that the intracrine pathway was more effective in modulating DC function.

Another important feature of vitamin D metabolism in DCs is that while expression of CYP27B1 and synthesis of 1,25$(OH)_2$D increases with DC maturation, there is a corresponding decline in expression of VDR and capacity for 1,25$(OH)_2$D binding (Fritsche *et al.*, 2003; Hewison *et al.*, 2003). This is similar to the reciprocal relationship reported for CYP27B1 and VDR in differentiating macrophages (Kreutz *et al.*, 1993), and provides a potential mechanism for the fine tuning of antigen presentation by vitamin D. Specifically, to initiate adaptive immune responses mature DCs present antigen to T-cells. These cells also have a high capacity for synthesis of 1,25 $(OH)_2D$ but if they also express high levels of VDR this would favor intracrine inhibition of DC maturation and thus suppression of antigen presentation. The chance of such a scenario is decreased if the mature DCs have lower levels of VDR. Instead the 1,25$(OH)_2D$ produced by mature DCs is more likely to act on less mature DCs which express higher levels of VDR. In this way, local synthesis of 1,25$(OH)_2D$ by DCs can act in a paracrine fashion to allow some antigen presentation to take place, while preventing an overelaboration of adaptive immune responses by suppressing further differentiation of immature DCs (Hewison *et al.*, 2004) (see Fig. 2.2). This may be particularly important as a mechanism

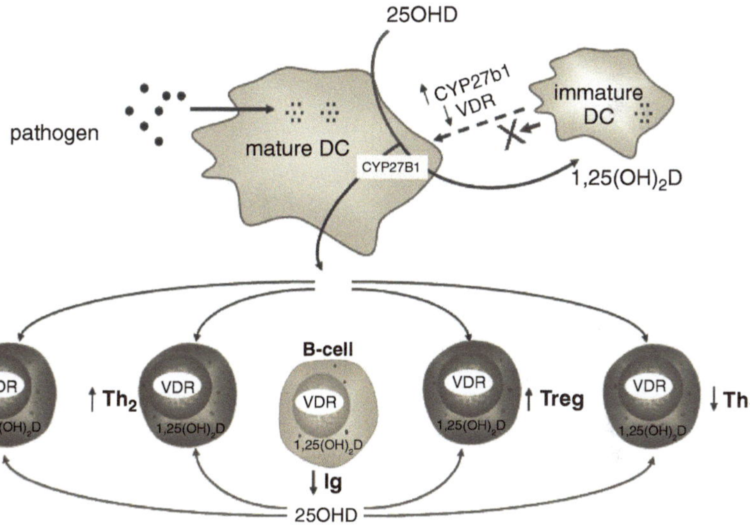

Figure 2.2 *Vitamin D, dendritic cell function and adaptive immunity.* Schematic representation showing the paracrine synthesis of 1,25-dihydroxyvitamin D (1,25$(OH)_2D$) by antigen-presenting dendritic cells (DCs) and the impact of this on the function of DCs as well and T- and B-cells. Mature DCs present antigen from pathogens to T- and B-cells. Mature DCs also express high levels of the vitamin D-activating enzyme 1α-hydroxylase (CYP27B1). 1,25$(OH)_2D$ synthesized from 25-hydroxyvitamin D (25OHD) by mature DCs acts on immature DCs which express higher levels of the vitamin D receptor (VDR). Using this mechanism, paracrine synthesis of 1,25$(OH)_2D$ acts to suppress maturation of DCs, thereby attenuating antigen presentation and enhancing a tolerogenic immune response. Paracrine synthesis of 1,25(OH)2D by DCs can also act on VDR-expressing T- and B-cells to promote a variety of adaptive immune responses. T- and B-cells have also been reported to express CYP27B1 and may therefore be regulated by vitamin D via intracrine conversion of 25OHD to 1,25 $(OH)_2D$. (See Color Insert.)

by which vitamin D is able to support tolerogenic adaptive immunity give that immature DCs have been reported to support the generation of immunosuppressive Tregs (Dhodapkar *et al.*, 2001; Jonuleit *et al.*, 2000).

IV. Vitamin D and Adaptive Immunity

As outlined above, the regulation of antigen presentation by DCs or other APCs such as macrophages is a pivotal facet of the interaction between vitamin D and the immune system. Although this represents another innate immune response to vitamin D, its downstream actions will clearly affect cells that interact with APCs, namely the adaptive immune system. This therefore raises two further questions about the immunomdulatory effects of vitamin D: (1) what are the adaptive immunity effects of vitamin D? (2) are these effects mediated via antigen presentation or as a consequence of direct interaction with T- and B-cells?

A. Vitamin D, T-cell activation and proliferation

One of the initial observations linking vitamin D with the immune system was the detection of VDR in lymphocytes. The development of T-cells and B-cells takes place in the thymus with VDR being expressed in medullary thymocytes but not in the less mature cortical thymocytes (Ravid *et al.*, 1984). This is in contrast to other nuclear receptors such as the glucocorticoid receptor which is expressed only in cortical thymocytes. Further studies showed that 1,25$(OH)_2$D inhibited proliferation of cytokine-activated medullary thymocytes, which are resistant to glucocorticoids (Koizumi *et al.*, 1985; Ravid *et al.*, 1984). VDR expression is lost once cells leave the thymus and enter the circulation as T- or B-cells but is then reinstated in T-cell cultures which have been activated to proliferate by treatment with mitogens (Bhalla *et al.*, 1983; Provvedini *et al.*, 1983). *In vitro*, immunoactivators such as phytohaemmaglutinin induce VDR expression within 24 h of treatment, coinciding with the transition of T-cells from a resting (Go) phase of the cell cycle into early G1 phase (Yu *et al.*, 1991).

Subsequent studies showed that 1,25$(OH)_2$D is a potent inhibitor of T-cell proliferation (Bhalla *et al.*, 1984; Nunn *et al.*, 1986). Fluorescence activated cell sorting (FACS) showed that 1,25$(OH)_2$D blocks the transition of cells from early G1 phase to late G1 phase. However, 1,25$(OH)_2$D had no effect on movement from Go (resting) to early G1 or from late G1 to S phase (Rigby *et al.*, 1985), and consequently had no effect on expression of the receptor for IL-2 (an early G1 event), but inhibited expression of the transferrin receptor (a late G1 event). Much of this work was initially carried using T-cells isolated from peripheral blood, a heterogeneous population of cells with varying degrees of inherent activation. Subsequent analysis of specific subsets of T-cells with more uniform patterns of proliferation was initially addressed using cells from lymphoid tissue, such as tonsils, where T-cells can be separated by centrifugation into different density populations: low density cells represent activated, proliferating T-cells, and high density T-cells correspond to resting T-cells. Studies using the latter showed that expression of VDR and responsiveness to 1,25$(OH)_2$D is proportional to the rate of cell proliferation (Karmali *et al.*, 1991).

T-cell activation is associated with the early induction of a large number of genes such as *c-myc* which like the VDR shows low levels of expression in resting T-cells. This increases rapidly following T-cell activation and parallels levels of proliferation and VDR expression (Karmali *et al.*, 1991), with *c-myc* expression in activated T-cells being inhibited by 1,25$(OH)_2$D. During early G1 phase induction of IL-2 receptor (IL-2R) expression enables the cell to respond to IL-2 and thus promote long-term growth of the T-cell population. Transcription of IL-2 mRNA is induced immediately after IL-2R and, initially, this appeared to be a target for the T-cell effects of 1,25 $(OH)_2$D. However, although 1,25$(OH)_2$D rapidly downregulates IL-2 expression in T-cells, there appears to be no abrogation of this response following treatment with exogenous cytokine (Rigby *et al.*, 1987a, 1990). Since these early studies, it has become clear that vitamin D modulates a much more complex network of cytokine than previously thought. The implications of this for effects of vitamin D on T-cell phenotype are discussed in the next section of the review.

B. Vitamin D, T-helper cells and cytotoxic T-cells

The population of lymphocytes commonly referred to as T-cells consists of several subgroups of cells including cytotoxic $CD8^+$ T-cells, NK cells, $\gamma\delta$ T-cells, memory cells, $CD4^+$ helper T-cells (Th cells), and regulatory T-cells (Treg). Initial studies of T-cell proliferation did not delineate between these different subgroups but it is now clear that 1,25$(OH)_2$D can act on each of these cell types. The most prominent responses have been described for Th cells, with 1,25$(OH)_2$D exerting effects on T-cell proliferation and cytokine production (Lemire *et al.*, 1985). Activation of naïve Th cells by antigen leads to the generation of pluripotent Th_0 cells which can then differentiate into further Th subgroups based on distinct cytokine profiles. The first two subgroups to be characterized were Th_1 (IL-2, IFNγ, tumor necrosis factor alpha) and Th_2 (IL-3, IL-4, IL-5, IL-10) cells. These two Th cell populations respectively support cell mediated and humoral immunity (Abbas *et al.*, 1996; Romagnani, 2006), with 1,25$(OH)_2$D acting to inhibit expression of Th_1 cytokines (Lemire *et al.*, 1995), while promoting Th_2 cytokines (Boonstra *et al.*, 2001). The shift from a Th_1 to Th_2 profile was originally proposed as a key mechanism by which vitamin D could exert beneficial effects on autoimmune disease (Overbergh *et al.*, 2000), with 1,25(OH)$_2$D acting either directly on T-cells (Boonstra *et al.*, 2001) or indirectly via APCs (Piemonti *et al.*, 2000). However, more recent studies have identified other Th cell subgroups such as interleukin-17 (IL-17)-secreting T-cells (Th_{17} cells) and these may also be targets for vitamin D (see Fig. 2.2). For example, it is notable that autoimmune disease-susceptible nonobese diabetic (NOD) mice treated with a synthetic analog of 1,25 (OH)$_2$D exhibit lower levels of IL-17 expression (Penna *et al.*, 2006). In a similar fashion, 1,25(OH)$_2$D suppression of murine retinal autoimmunity appears to involve inhibition of Th_{17} activity (Tang *et al.*, 2009).

Early studies of vitamin D and T-cell function suggested that 1,25(OH)$_2$D could act on both $CD4^+$ Th cells and $CD8^+$ cytotoxic T-cells (Provvedini and Manolagas, 1989; Rigby *et al.*, 1987b). The precise relevance of this with respect to cytotoxic T-cells has still to be determined, despite the fact that at least one report has shown higher levels of VDR expression in these cells (Veldman *et al.*, 2000). Cytotoxic T-cells are known to be involved in some forms of autoimmune disease such as multiple sclerosis (MS; Babbe *et al.*, 2000). It was therefore interesting to note that $CD8^+$ cells were not required for 1,25(OH)$_2$D to suppress the murine form of MS, experimental autoimmune encephalomyelitis (EAE; Meehan and DeLuca, 2002). A more recent link between vitamin D and CD8 has been provided by studies of CD8$\alpha\alpha$ cells, intraepithelial lymphocytes that express a homodimeric form of CD8. Unlike cytotoxic T-cells, CD8$\alpha\alpha$ cells are not self-destructive and may play a role in suppressing gastrointestinal inflammation (Cheroutre and Lambolez, 2008). It was therefore interesting to note that *VDR* gene knockout mice had decreased numbers of CD8$\alpha\alpha$ cells (Yu *et al.*, 2008). This was due to decreased T-cell expression of the chemokine receptor CCR9 which prevented T-cell homing to the gastrointestinal tract. Such a defect in T-cell homing provides a potential explanation for the exacerbation of gastrointestinal inflammation observed in VDR knockout mice (Froicu *et al.*, 2003). Vitamin D may also affect T-cell homing to other tissues. Recent data have shown that 1,25(OH)$_2$D stimulates expression of the chemokine receptor 10 (CCR10) which recognizes the chemokine CCL27 secreted by keratinocytes (Sigmundsdottir *et al.*, 2007). In this way, 1,25(OH)$_2$D$_3$ may act to promote T-cell translocation to the skin.

C. Vitamin D and regulatory T-cells

As well as acting as a modulator of Th cell proliferation and phenotype, vitamin D can also influence adaptive immunity by regulating the expression and activity of suppressor T-cells also known as Treg. Seminal studies by O'Garra and colleagues showed that $1,25(OH)_2D$ in combination with glucocorticoids was able to generate IL-10-producing $CD4^+$ $CD25^+$ Treg from naïve Th cells, in the absence of any antiproliferative actions (Barrat *et al.*, 2002). The ability of $1,25(OH)_2D$ to support differentiation of Treg was initially thought to be mediated via its effects on DCs. By suppressing maturation of DCs and by enhancing expression of DC cytokines such as CCL22 (particularly in mDC as opposed to pDCs), $1,25(OH)_2D$ has the potential to enhance tolerogenic responses by suppressing Th_1 cells and promoting $CD4^+$ $CD25^+$ Treg (Penna *et al.*, 2007). However, more recent studies have reported direct effects of $1,25(OH)_2D$ on T-cells to generate CTLA4-positive Treg (Jeffery *et al.*, 2009). This responses was synergistically enhanced in the presence of IL-2, which also promoted FoxP3 expression of the resulting Tregs (Jeffery *et al.*, 2009). Collectively these observations suggest that vitamin D can exert both direct and indirect effects on Treg generation, and it is tempting to speculate that these may involve both 25OHD (intracrine activity on DCs) and 1,25(OH)2D (endocrine/paracrine effects of $1,25(OH)_2D$).

Other studies have highlighted the importance of Treg induction in mediating the immunoregulatory actions of vitamin D. Systemic administration of $1,25(OH)_2D$ to patients with renal disease has been shown to increase numbers of circulating Tregs (Ardalan *et al.*, 2007). Similarly, topical application of $1,25(OH)_2D$ (Gorman *et al.*, 2007) or its synthetic analog calcipotriol (Ghoreishi *et al.*, 2009) increased the numbers of Treg in mice. In patients with MS, serum concentrations of 25OHD have been shown to correlate with Treg activity (Royal *et al.*, 2009; Smolders *et al.*, 2009b), emphasizing the importance of patient vitamin D status and effective local conversion of 25OHD to $1,25(OH)_2D$ as a facet of Treg adaptive immunity. As outlined above, Treg generation appears to be enhanced by either 25OHD or $1,25(OH)_2D$, with former acting in an intracrine fashion to modulate maturation of CYP27B1-expressing APCs. It is assumed that the direct induction of Tregs by $1,25(OH)_2D$ also involves APC synthesis of $1,25(OH)_2D$ but in this case acting in a paracrine fashion on T-cells. However, it is interesting to note studies describing CYP27B1 expression by T-cells, suggesting a potential intracrine mechanism by which 25OHD can influence these cells (Sigmundsdottir *et al.*, 2007).

D. Vitamin D and B-cell function

Analysis of B-cell responses *in vitro* initially showed that $1,25(OH)_2D$ suppresses the development of Ig-secreting B-cells following pokeweed mitogen stimulation (Iho *et al.*, 1986; Shiozawa *et al.*, 1985). Subsequent studies then suggested that this was likely to be mediated via inhibition of T-helper cells (Lemire *et al.*, 1985). However, more recent reports have reinstated a model for direct effects of $1,25(OH)_2D$ on B-cell homeostasis

(Chen *et al.*, 2007). This study also highlighted the ability of 1,25$(OH)_2D$ to suppress the differentiation of plasma cells and class-switched memory cells, suggesting a potential role for vitamin D in B-cell-related autoimmune disorders such as systemic lupus erythamtosus (SLE), and this is discussed in the next section of the review. More recent reports have shown that 1,25 $(OH)_2D$ also regulates B-cell IL-10 (Heine *et al.*, 2008) and CCR10 (Shirakawa *et al.*, 2008), indicating that the breadth of B-cell responses to vitamin D is likely to be much greater than previously thought.

V. Vitamin D, the Immune System and Human Health

The wide array of immune responses to vitamin D outlined in previous sections of this review suggests that vitamin D may exert similarly diverse effects on human health. Initial links between vitamin D and human immune function were centered on the aberrant extrarenal synthesis of 1,25$(OH)_2D$ that is characteristic of many patients with the granulomatous disease sarcoidosis (Fuss *et al.*, 1992). Similar dysregulation of extrarenal CYP27B1 has been described for other granulomatous diseases and some tumors (Hewison *et al.*, 2007), and may be a key consideration in the clinical management of these disorders. However, more recent data highlighting a role for CYP27B1 as an intracrine activator of vitamin D as part of normal innate and adaptive immunity suggests that vitamin D may be a contributory factor for some immune disorders. In particular, it has been hypothesized that impaired vitamin D status *in vivo* may act to compromise the innate and adaptive immune mechanism known to be regulated by vitamin D *in vitro*. Prominent examples of these are detailed in the following section of the review.

A. Vitamin D and tuberculosis

Vitamin D has a long-standing association with tuberculosis infection. Studies carried out many decades ago described the beneficial effects of UV light exposure on TB, with the 1903 Nobel Prize being awarded to Niels Finsen for demonstrating the treatment of Lupus Vulgaris, the epidermal forms of TB, with concentrated light (Moller *et al.*, 2005). However, the most recent impetus to study innate immune responses to vitamin D stemmed from studies 25 years ago to assess the effects of 1,25$(OH)_2D$ on monocyte infection by *M. tuberculosis* (Rook *et al.*, 1986). A potential role for vitamin D in the disease TB was then revived by the more recent observation that vitamin D acts to promote innate immune responses to TLR-activation by *M. tuberculosis* (Liu *et al.*, 2006).

Although, the vitamin D–TB link has become the most well studied facet of vitamin D and innate immunity (Martineau *et al.*, 2007a), clinical evidence of a role for vitamin D in TB progression and the possible benefits of vitamin D as treatment for the disease is still somewhat limited. Recent association studies have reaffirmed the proposed link between impaired vitamin D status and TB infection (Talat *et al.*, 2010; Wejse *et al.*, 2007), with low levels of vitamin D being also associated with increased risk of progression to active TB (Talat *et al.*, 2010). In supplementation studies, a single oral dose of vitamin D (2.5 mg) has been shown to enhance *ex vivo* macrophage immune response to infection with the weakened *M. tuberculosis* strain Bacille Calmette-Guérin (Martineau *et al.*, 2007b) while another study showed that adjunct vitamin D supplementation (0.25 mg vitamin D/day) of TB patients receiving conventional disease therapy reduced the time for sputum smear conversion from acid fast bacteria (AFB)-positive to AFB-negative status (Nursyam *et al.*, 2006). By contrast, a more recent placebo-controlled trial concluded that vitamin D supplementation had no effect on clinical outcomes or mortality amongst TB patients (Wejse *et al.*, 2009). However, it is important to recognize that none of the supplemented patients in this study showed a significant rise in serum vitamin D levels (Wejse *et al.*, 2009).

B. Vitamin D and type 1 diabetes

The effects of vitamin D on adaptive immune responses suggest a potential link between vitamin D and autoimmune diseases (Adorini and Penna, 2008). Although these disorders are characterized by an underlying genetic predisposition, it is likely that environmental factors such as vitamin D may contribute significantly to the manifestation of these diseases. Prominent amongst these is the link between vitamin D deficiency type 1 diabetes (reviewed in Mathieu *et al.*, 2005). Low serum concentrations of 25OHD have been reported in adolescents at the time of diagnosis of type 1 diabetes (Littorin *et al.*, 2006), and other studies have postulated beneficial effects of vitamin D supplementation in protecting against type 1 diabetes (Harris, 2005). Vitamin D may also be a factor in the genetics of type 1 diabetes in that some *VDR* gene haplotypes confer protection against diabetes (Ramos-Lopez *et al.*, 2006). More recent reports suggest that *CYP27b1* gene variation may also affect susceptibility to type 1 diabetes (Bailey *et al.*, 2007). Finally, studies *in vivo* using the NOD mouse model of type 1 diabetes have shown increased disease severity of the disease under conditions of dietary vitamin D restriction (Giulietti *et al.*, 2004).

C. Vitamin D and MS

Several epidemiology studies have described an association between vitamin D insufficiency and the autoimmune neurodegenerative disorder MS (reviewed in Ascherio *et al.*, 2010; Pierrot-Deseilligny and Souberbielle, 2010;

Raghuwanshi *et al.*, 2008; Solomon and Whitham, 2010). This has stemmed in part from geographical data showing a significant increase in areas of the world with low exposure to UV light which is required for epidermal synthesis vitamin D (Beretich and Beretich, 2009). However, it is important to recognize that in some cases the protective effects of UV light on EAE mice were independent of significant elevation in serum 25OHD levels (Becklund *et al.*, 2010) suggesting a vitamin D-independent mechanism. Other publications have reported association between MS and established polymorphic variations in the genes for VDR (Mamutse *et al.*, 2008; Tajouri *et al.*, 2005) or CYP27B1 (Sundqvist *et al.*, 2010). However, this is not a universally consistent observation (Simon *et al.*, 2010; Smolders *et al.*, 2009a), and it is important to recognize that some SNPs can act as potential markers of serum vitamin D status (Orton *et al.*, 2008) or dietary vitamin D intake (Simon *et al.*, 2010).

Epidemiological and genetic data from humans observations are supported by studies of animal models such as the EAE mouse, which exhibit increased disease severity under conditions of dietary vitamin D restriction (Spach and Hayes, 2005). Conversely EAE mice treated with active 1,25 $(OH)_2D$ are protected against the disease (Pedersen *et al.*, 2007; Spach *et al.*, 2004). This response appears to be mediated via effects on the synthesis of cytokines such as IL-10 as well as the apoptosis of inflammatory cells (Spach *et al.*, 2006), and has also been shown to be specific for female mice (Spach and Hayes, 2005). The latter appears to be due, at least in part, to estrogen-mediated enhancement of VDR expression within the mouse CNS system (Nashold *et al.*, 2009). In humans, MS shows a strong female gender bias and it is therefore tempting to speculate that low exposure to UV light and concomitant impairment of vitamin D status may be a particularly important factor in determining immune function in women.

D. Vitamin D and inflammatory bowel disease

The enzyme CYP27B1 is detectable in the human colon (Zehnder *et al.*, 2001), and its expression is elevated in affected tissue from patients with Crohn's disease, a form of inflammatory bowel disease (Abreu *et al.*, 2004). This has been linked to the increased serum $1,25(OH)_2D$ that is occasionally observed in these patients. Thus it appears that localized gastrointestinal synthesis of $1,25(OH)_2D$ in Crohn's disease patients can spill-over into the general circulation in a similar fashion to that observed in patients with sarcoidosis (Abreu *et al.*, 2004). However, it is also important to recognize that patients with Crohn's disease frequently present with decreased circulating levels of 25OHD (Pappa *et al.*, 2006a,b; Vagianos *et al.*, 2007). For many years this was considered to be due primarily to dietary malabsorption as a consequence of gastrointestinal inflammation (Davies *et al.*, 1980; Leichtmann *et al.*, 1991; Lo *et al.*, 1985), but recent research supports a more causative role for vitamin D.

Studies *in vivo* have shown that VDR and CYP27B1 knockout mice are more susceptible to experimentally induced forms of IBD (Froicu and Cantorna, 2007; Froicu *et al.*, 2003; Kong *et al.*, 2008; Liu *et al.*, 2008). This appears to involve dysregulation of several gastrointestinal mechanisms including the maintenance of mucosal barrier function (Kong *et al.*, 2008) and normal submucosal adaptive immunity (Froicu and Cantorna, 2007; Froicu *et al.*, 2003; Yu *et al.*, 2008). Mice raised on a vitamin D-deficient diet are also more susceptible to experimental IBD (Lagishetty *et al.*, 2010). In this instance, low serum 25OHD appears to predispose mice to the onset of disease as a result of decreased expression of the colonic antimicrobial-protein angionenin-4, a key regulator of tissue invasion by enteric bacteria (Hooper *et al.*, 2003). Vitamin D may therefore play a pivotal role in maintaining innate immune surveillance of enteric bacteria within the gastrointestinal tract—the microbiota—and this may be compromised under conditions of vitamin D insufficiency. It is therefore interesting to note recent studies that have implicated aberrant innate immune handling of enteric microbiota as an initiator of the adaptive immune damage associated with Crohn's disease (Packey and Sartor, 2009). Based on these observations it is possible to speculate that the association between vitamin D and Crohn's disease may involve both the activation of innate immune responses, together with the suppression of adaptive immunity and associated inflammation. A role for vitamin D as a regulator of innate immune function in Crohn's disease is further supported by the recent studies showing that $1,25(OH)_2D$ is a potent inducer of NOD2 (Wang *et al.*, 2009), the first susceptibility gene to be documented for Crohn's disease (Cuthbert *et al.*, 2002; see Section II.D).

VI. Conclusions and Future Directions

Recent studies have shown clearly that vitamin D is a pluripotent regulator of both innate and adaptive immune responses. Although elements of this story were first described almost 25 years ago, our current perspective on vitamin D and the immune system is characterized by two crucial new developments. The first is that the immune function of vitamin D is no longer considered to simply be a pathological feature of inflammatory disorders, notably granulomatous disease. As outlined in Section IV, there is now strong evidence to suggest that vitamin D contributes to normal immune responses and in doing so may be a key factor in protecting against both infectious and autoimmune disease. The current review documents the four most prominent immune diseases to be linked to vitamin D but it is important to recognize that this list continues to grow. For example, recent studies have linked vitamin D to infections associated with pregnancy

(Bodnar *et al.*, 2009). This may be particularly important as infections are a major cause of adverse preterm birth and pregnant women are known to be at high risk of vitamin D insufficiency (Bodnar *et al.*, 2007).

There is also increasing interest in the immunomodulatory function of vitamin D with respect to respiratory disorders, notably chronic obstructive pulmonary disease (Chishimba *et al.*, 2010). Further analysis of complex diseases such as this will shed more light on the ability of vitamin D to orchestrate adequate innate and adaptive immune activity, as well as clarifying the antiinflammatory functions of vitamin D. Other studies of respiratory disorders suggest that the innate immune actions of vitamin D may not be restricted to bacterial infection. Epidemiology has linked seasonal variations in vitamin D status with the infections such as influenza (Cannell *et al.*, 2006), and randomized clinical studies have reported effects of vitamin D supplementation in protecting against colds and influenza (Aloia and Li-Ng, 2007). As yet there is no clear mechanism by which vitamin D can protect against colds or flu, but the fact that LL37 exhibits antiviral as well as antibacterial properties (Bergman *et al.*, 2007), suggests that vitamin D supplementation may have a broader range of therapeutic applications than initially thought.

The second major change to our perspective on vitamin D and the immune system is the increasing awareness that tissue-specific synthesis of $1,25(OH)_2D$, rather classical endocrine production of the hormone, is the most likely mode of action. The advantage of intracrine or paracrine activity of CYP27B1 is this it provides a flexible and sensitive system for localized accumulation of $1,25(OH)_2D$, without the potential problems associated with endocrine homeostasis. Significantly, such a mechanism will also be more sensitive to alterations in vitamin D (25OHD) status. This has been identified as a potential explanation for the link between vitamin D insufficiency and immune diseases although, as outlined in this review, there may be other factors such as genetic variations in the VDR, CYP27B1, and DBP that will also influence the efficacy of vitamin D function at a tissue-specific level. The next major challenge in defining a role for vitamin D in normal human immunity will depend on the outcome of effective randomized clinical trials for vitamin D supplementation. As yet, there is little reported data regarding the disease protective or therapeutic effects of improved vitamin D status. However, given the quantum leap in vitamin D studies over the last 5 years, it seems likely that this will change in the near future.

REFERENCES

Abbas, A. K., Murphy, K. M., and Sher, A. (1996). Functional diversity of helper T lymphocytes. *Nature* **383,** 787–793.

Abreu, M. T., Kantorovich, V., Vasiliauskas, E. A., Gruntmanis, U., Matuk, R., Daigle, K., Chen, S., Zehnder, D., Lin, Y. C., Yang, H., Hewison, M., and Adams, J. S. (2004).

Measurement of vitamin D levels in inflammatory bowel disease patients reveals a subset of Crohn's disease patients with elevated 1,25-dihydroxyvitamin D and low bone mineral density. *Gut* **53,** 1129–1136.

Adams, J. S., and Gacad, M. A. (1985). Characterization of 1 alpha-hydroxylation of vitamin D3 sterols by cultured alveolar macrophages from patients with sarcoidosis. *J. Exp. Med.* **161,** 755–765.

Adams, J. S., Sharma, O. P., Gacad, M. A., and Singer, F. R. (1983). Metabolism of 25-hydroxyvitamin D3 by cultured pulmonary alveolar macrophages in sarcoidosis. *J. Clin. Invest.* **72,** 1856–1860.

Adams, J. S., Ren, S., Liu, P. T., Chun, R. F., Lagishetty, V., Gombart, A. F., Borregaard, N., Modlin, R. L., and Hewison, M. (2009). Vitamin d-directed rheostatic regulation of monocyte antibacterial responses. *J. Immunol.* **182,** 4289–4295.

Adorini, L., and Penna, G. (2008). Control of autoimmune diseases by the vitamin D endocrine system. *Nat. Clin. Pract. Rheumatol.* **4,** 404–412.

Aloia, J. F., and Li-Ng, M. (2007). Correspondence. *Epidemiol. Infect.* **135,** 1095–1096.

Anderson, K. V. (2000). Toll signaling pathways in the innate immune response. *Curr. Opin. Immunol.* **12,** 13–19.

Ardalan, M. R., Maljaei, H., Shoja, M. M., Piri, A. R., Khosroshahi, H. T., Noshad, H., and Argani, H. (2007). Calcitriol started in the donor, expands the population of $CD4^{+}CD25^{+}$ T cells in renal transplant recipients. *Transplant. Proc.* **39,** 951–953.

Ascherio, A., Munger, K. L., and Simon, K. C. (2010). Vitamin D and multiple sclerosis. *Lancet Neurol.* **9,** 599–612.

Babbe, H., Roers, A., Waisman, A., Lassmann, H., Goebels, N., Hohlfeld, R., Friese, M., Schroder, R., Deckert, M., Schmidt, S., Ravid, R., and Rajewsky, K. (2000). Clonal expansions of CD8(+) T cells dominate the T cell infiltrate in active multiple sclerosis lesions as shown by micromanipulation and single cell polymerase chain reaction. *J. Exp. Med.* **192,** 393–404.

Bailey, R., Cooper, J. D., Zeitels, L., Smyth, D. J., Yang, J. H., Walker, N. M., Hypponen, E., Dunger, D. B., Ramos-Lopez, E., Badenhoop, K., Nejentsev, S., and Todd, J. A. (2007). Association of the vitamin D metabolism gene CYP27B1 with type 1 diabetes. *Diabetes* **56,** 2616–2621.

Barrat, F. J., Cua, D. J., Boonstra, A., Richards, D. F., Crain, C., Savelkoul, H. F., de Waal-Malefyt, R., Coffman, R. L., Hawrylowicz, C. M., and O'Garra, A. (2002). In vitro generation of interleukin 10-producing regulatory CD4(+) T cells is induced by immunosuppressive drugs and inhibited by T helper type 1 (Th1)- and Th2-inducing cytokines. *J. Exp. Med.* **195,** 603–616.

Becklund, B. R., Severson, K. S., Vang, S. V., and DeLuca, H. F. (2010). UV radiation suppresses experimental autoimmune encephalomyelitis independent of vitamin D production. *Proc. Natl. Acad. Sci. USA* **107,** 6418–6423.

Beretich, B., and Beretich, T. (2009). Explaining multiple sclerosis prevalence by ultraviolet exposure: A geospatial analysis. *Mult. Scler.* **15,** 891–898.

Bergman, P., Walter-Jallow, L., Broliden, K., Agerberth, B., and Soderlund, J. (2007). The antimicrobial peptide LL-37 inhibits HIV-1 replication. *Curr. HIV Res.* **5,** 410–415.

Bhalla, A. K., Amento, E. P., Clemens, T. L., Holick, M. F., and Krane, S. M. (1983). Specific high-affinity receptors for 1,25-dihydroxyvitamin D3 in human peripheral blood mononuclear cells: Presence in monocytes and induction in T lymphocytes following activation. *J. Clin. Endocrinol. Metab.* **57,** 1308–1310.

Bhalla, A. K., Amento, E. P., Serog, B., and Glimcher, L. H. (1984). 1,25-Dihydroxyvitamin D3 inhibits antigen-induced T cell activation. *J. Immunol.* **133,** 1748–1754.

Bilsborough, J., George, T. C., Norment, A., and Viney, J. L. (2003). Mucosal $CD8alpha^{+}$ DC, with a plasmacytoid phenotype, induce differentiation and support function of T cells with regulatory properties. *Immunology* **108,** 481–492.

Bodnar, L. M., Simhan, H. N., Powers, R. W., Frank, M. P., Cooperstein, E., and Roberts, J. M. (2007). High prevalence of vitamin D insufficiency in black and white pregnant women residing in the northern United States and their neonates. *J. Nutr.* **137,** 447–452.

Bodnar, L. M., Krohn, M. A., and Simhan, H. N. (2009). Maternal vitamin D deficiency is associated with bacterial vaginosis in the first trimester of pregnancy. *J. Nutr.* **139,** 1157–1161.

Boonstra, A., Barrat, F. J., Crain, C., Heath, V. L., Savelkoul, H. F., and O'Garra, A. (2001). 1alpha, 25-Dihydroxyvitamin d3 has a direct effect on naive CD4(+) T cells to enhance the development of Th2 cells. *J. Immunol.* **167,** 4974–4980.

Brennan, A., Katz, D. R., Nunn, J. D., Barker, S., Hewison, M., Fraher, L. J., and O'Riordan, J. L. (1987). Dendritic cells from human tissues express receptors for the immunoregulatory vitamin D3 metabolite, dihydroxycholecalciferol. *Immunology* **61,** 457–461.

Brightbill, H. D., and Modlin, R. L. (2000). Toll-like receptors: Molecular mechanisms of the mammalian immune response. *Immunology* **101,** 1–10.

Brightbill, H. D., Libraty, D. H., Krutzik, S. R., Yang, R. B., Belisle, J. T., Bleharski, J. R., Maitland, M., Norgard, M. V., Plevy, S. E., Smale, S. T., Brennan, P. J., Bloom, B. R., *et al.* (1999). Host defense mechanisms triggered by microbial lipoproteins through toll-like receptors. *Science* **285,** 732–736.

Bunce, C. M., Brown, G., and Hewison, M. (1997). Vitamin D and haematopoiesis. *Trends Endocrinol. Metab.* **8,** 245–251.

Cannell, J. J., Vieth, R., Umhau, J. C., Holick, M. F., Grant, W. B., Madronich, S., Garland, C. F., and Giovannucci, E. (2006). Epidemic influenza and vitamin D. *Epidemiol. Infect.* **134,** 1129–1140.

Chan, J., Xing, Y., Magliozzo, R. S., and Bloom, B. R. (1992). Killing of virulent Mycobacterium tuberculosis by reactive nitrogen intermediates produced by activated murine macrophages. *J. Exp. Med.* **175,** 1111–1122.

Chapuy, M. C., Preziosi, P., Maamer, M., Arnaud, S., Galan, P., Hercberg, S., and Meunier, P. J. (1997). Prevalence of vitamin D insufficiency in an adult normal population. *Osteoporos. Int.* **7,** 439–443.

Chen, S., Sims, G. P., Chen, X. X., Gu, Y. Y., Chen, S., and Lipsky, P. E. (2007). Modulatory effects of 1,25-dihydroxyvitamin d3 on human B cell differentiation. *J. Immunol.* **179,** 1634–1647.

Cheroutre, H., and Lambolez, F. (2008). Doubting the TCR coreceptor function of CD8alphaalpha. *Immunity* **28,** 149–159.

Chishimba, L., Thickett, D. R., Stockley, R. A., and Wood, A. M. (2010). The vitamin D axis in the lung: A key role for vitamin D-binding protein. *Thorax* **65,** 456–462.

Chun, R. F., Lauridsen, A., Suon, L., Zella, L. A., Pike, J. W., Modlin, R. L., Martineau, A. R., Wilkinson, R. J., Adams, J. S., and Hewison, M. (2010). Vitamin D binding protein directs monocyte responses to 25-hydroxy- and 1,25-dihydroxyvitamin D. *J. Clin. Endocrinol. Metab.* **95,** 3368–3376.

Cuthbert, A. P., Fisher, S. A., Mirza, M. M., King, K., Hampe, J., Croucher, P. J., Mascheretti, S., Sanderson, J., Forbes, A., Mansfield, J., Schreiber, S., Lewis, C. M., *et al.* (2002). The contribution of NOD2 gene mutations to the risk and site of disease in inflammatory bowel disease. *Gastroenterology* **122,** 867–874.

Cyster, J. G. (1999). Chemokines and the homing of dendritic cells to the T cell areas of lymphoid organs. *J. Exp. Med.* **189,** 447–450.

Dam, T. N., Moller, B., Hindkjaer, J., and Kragballe, K. (1996). The vitamin D3 analog calcipotriol suppresses the number and antigen-presenting function of Langerhans cells in normal human skin. *J. Investig. Dermatol. Symp. Proc.* **1,** 72–77.

Davies, M., Mawer, E. B., and Krawitt, E. L. (1980). Comparative absorption of vitamin D3 and 25-hydroxyvitamin D3 in intestinal disease. *Gut* **21,** 287–292.

Delgado, M., Singh, S., De Haro, S., Master, S., Ponpuak, M., Dinkins, C., Ornatowski, W., Vergne, I., and Deretic, V. (2009). Autophagy and pattern recognition receptors in innate immunity. *Immunol. Rev.* **227,** 189–202.

Deretic, V., and Levine, B. (2009). Autophagy, immunity, and microbial adaptations. *Cell Host Microbe* **5,** 527–549.

Dhodapkar, M. V., Steinman, R. M., Krasovsky, J., Munz, C., and Bhardwaj, N. (2001). Antigen-specific inhibition of effector T cell function in humans after injection of immature dendritic cells. *J. Exp. Med.* **193,** 233–238.

Dong, X., Craig, T., Xing, N., Bachman, L. A., Paya, C. V., Weih, F., McKean, D. J., Kumar, R., and Griffin, M. D. (2003). Direct transcriptional regulation of RelB by 1alpha, 25-dihydroxyvitamin D3 and its analogs: Physiologic and therapeutic implications for dendritic cell function. *J. Biol. Chem.* **278,** 49378–49385.

Dong, X., Lutz, W., Schroeder, T. M., Bachman, L. A., Westendorf, J. J., Kumar, R., and Griffin, M. D. (2005). Regulation of relB in dendritic cells by means of modulated association of vitamin D receptor and histone deacetylase 3 with the promoter. *Proc. Natl. Acad. Sci. USA* **102,** 16007–16012.

Ehrchen, J., Helming, L., Varga, G., Pasche, B., Loser, K., Gunzer, M., Sunderkotter, C., Sorg, C., Roth, J., and Lengeling, A. (2007). Vitamin D receptor signaling contributes to susceptibility to infection with *Leishmania major*. *FASEB J.* **21,** 3208–3218.

Evans, K. N., Bulmer, J. N., Kilby, M. D., and Hewison, M. (2004). Vitamin D and placental-decidual function. *J. Soc. Gynecol. Investig.* **11,** 263–271.

Evans, K. N., Nguyen, L., Chan, J., Innes, B. A., Bulmer, J. N., Kilby, M. D., and Hewison, M. (2006). Effects of 25-hydroxyvitamin D3 and 1,25-dihydroxyvitamin D3 on cytokine production by human decidual cells. *Biol. Reprod.* **75,** 816–822.

Fritsche, J., Mondal, K., Ehrnsperger, A., Andreesen, R., and Kreutz, M. (2003). Regulation of 25-hydroxyvitamin D3–1 alpha-hydroxylase and production of 1 alpha, 25-dihydroxyvitamin D3 by human dendritic cells. *Blood* **102,** 3314–3316.

Froicu, M., and Cantorna, M. T. (2007). Vitamin D and the vitamin D receptor are critical for control of the innate immune response to colonic injury. *BMC Immunol.* **8,** 5.

Froicu, M., Weaver, V., Wynn, T. A., McDowell, M. A., Welsh, J. E., and Cantorna, M. T. (2003). A crucial role for the vitamin D receptor in experimental inflammatory bowel diseases. *Mol. Endocrinol.* **17,** 2386–2392.

Fu, G. K., Lin, D., Zhang, M. Y., Bikle, D. D., Shackleton, C. H., Miller, W. L., and Portale, A. A. (1997). Cloning of human 25-hydroxyvitamin D-1 alpha-hydroxylase and mutations causing vitamin D-dependent rickets type 1. *Mol. Endocrinol.* **11,** 1961–1970.

Fuss, M., Pepersack, T., Gillet, C., Karmali, R., and Corvilain, J. (1992). Calcium and vitamin D metabolism in granulomatous diseases. *Clin. Rheumatol.* **11,** 28–36.

Garcion, E., Nataf, S., Berod, A., Darcy, F., and Brachet, P. (1997). 1,25-Dihydroxyvitamin D3 inhibits the expression of inducible nitric oxide synthase in rat central nervous system during experimental allergic encephalomyelitis. *Brain Res. Mol. Brain Res.* **45,** 255–267.

Ghoreishi, M., Bach, P., Obst, J., Komba, M., Fleet, J. C., and Dutz, J. P. (2009). Expansion of antigen-specific regulatory T cells with the topical vitamin d analog calcipotriol. *J. Immunol.* **182,** 6071–6078.

Ginde, A. A., Liu, M. C., and Camargo, C. A., Jr. (2009). Demographic differences and trends of vitamin D insufficiency in the US population, 1988–2004. *Arch. Intern. Med.* **169,** 626–632.

Giulietti, A., Gysemans, C., Stoffels, K., van Etten, E., Decallonne, B., Overbergh, L., Bouillon, R., and Mathieu, C. (2004). Vitamin D deficiency in early life accelerates Type 1 diabetes in non-obese diabetic mice. *Diabetologia* **47,** 451–462.

Gombart, A. F., Borregaard, N., and Koeffler, H. P. (2005). Human cathelicidin antimicrobial peptide (CAMP) gene is a direct target of the vitamin D receptor and is strongly upregulated in myeloid cells by 1,25-dihydroxyvitamin D3. *FASEB J.* **19,** 1067–1077.

Gombart, A. F., Bhan, I., Borregaard, N., Tamez, H., Camargo, C. A., Jr., Koeffler, H. P., and Thadhani, R. (2009a). Low plasma level of cathelicidin antimicrobial peptide (hCAP18) predicts increased infectious disease mortality in patients undergoing hemodialysis. *Clin. Infect. Dis.* **48,** 418–424.

Gombart, A. F., Saito, T., and Koeffler, H. P. (2009b). Exaptation of an ancient Alu short interspersed element provides a highly conserved vitamin D-mediated innate immune response in humans and primates. *BMC Genomics* **10,** 321.

Gorman, S., Kuritzky, L. A., Judge, M. A., Dixon, K. M., McGlade, J. P., Mason, R. S., Finlay-Jones, J. J., and Hart, P. H. (2007). Topically applied 1,25-dihydroxyvitamin D3 enhances the suppressive activity of $CD4^+CD25^+$ cells in the draining lymph nodes. *J. Immunol.* **179,** 6273–6283.

Griffin, M. D., Lutz, W. H., Phan, V. A., Bachman, L. A., McKean, D. J., and Kumar, R. (2000). Potent inhibition of dendritic cell differentiation and maturation by vitamin D analogs. *Biochem. Biophys. Res. Commun.* **270,** 701–708.

Griffin, M. D., Lutz, W., Phan, V. A., Bachman, L. A., McKean, D. J., and Kumar, R. (2001). Dendritic cell modulation by 1alpha, 25 dihydroxyvitamin D3 and its analogs: A vitamin D receptor-dependent pathway that promotes a persistent state of immaturity in vitro and in vivo. *Proc. Natl. Acad. Sci. USA* **98,** 6800–6805.

Gutierrez, M. G., Master, S. S., Singh, S. B., Taylor, G. A., Colombo, M. I., and Deretic, V. (2004). Autophagy is a defense mechanism inhibiting BCG and Mycobacterium tuberculosis survival in infected macrophages. *Cell* **119,** 753–766.

Hansdottir, S., Monick, M. M., Hinde, S. L., Lovan, N., Look, D. C., and Hunninghake, G. W. (2008). Respiratory epithelial cells convert inactive vitamin D to its active form: Potential effects on host defense. *J. Immunol.* **181,** 7090–7099.

Harris, S. S. (2005). Vitamin D in type 1 diabetes prevention. *J. Nutr.* **135,** 323–325.

Hayes, M. E., Rai, A., Cooper, R. G., Bayley, D., Freemont, A. J., and Mawer, E. B. (1992). Inhibition by prostaglandin E1 and E2 of 1,25-dihydroxyvitamin D3 synthesis by synovial fluid macrophages from arthritic joints. *Ann. Rheum. Dis.* **51,** 632–637.

Heine, G., Niesner, U., Chang, H. D., Steinmeyer, A., Zugel, U., Zuberbier, T., Radbruch, A., and Worm, M. (2008). 1,25-dihydroxyvitamin D(3) promotes IL-10 production in human B cells. *Eur. J. Immunol.* **38,** 2210–2218.

Hewison, M. (2010). Vitamin D and the intracrinology of innate immunity. *Mol. Cell. Endocrinol.* **321,** 103–111.

Hewison, M., Barker, S., Brennan, A., Nathan, J., Katz, D. R., and O'Riordan, J. L. (1989). Autocrine regulation of 1,25-dihydroxycholecalciferol metabolism in myelomonocytic cells. *Immunology* **68,** 247–252.

Hewison, M., Brennan, A., Singh-Ranger, R., Walters, J. C., Katz, D. R., and O'Riordan, J. L. (1992). The comparative role of 1,25-dihydroxycholecalciferol and phorbol esters in the differentiation of the U937 cell line. *Immunology* **77,** 304–311.

Hewison, M., Freeman, L., Hughes, S. V., Evans, K. N., Bland, R., Eliopoulos, A. G., Kilby, M. D., Moss, P. A., and Chakraverty, R. (2003). Differential regulation of vitamin D receptor and its ligand in human monocyte-derived dendritic cells. *J. Immunol.* **170,** 5382–5390.

Hewison, M., Zehnder, D., Chakraverty, R., and Adams, J. S. (2004). Vitamin D and barrier function: A novel role for extra-renal 1 alpha-hydroxylase. *Mol. Cell. Endocrinol.* **215,** 31–38.

Hewison, M., Burke, F., Evans, K. N., Lammas, D. A., Sansom, D. M., Liu, P., Modlin, R. L., and Adams, J. S. (2007). Extra-renal 25-hydroxyvitamin D3-1alpha-hydroxylase in human health and disease. *J. Steroid Biochem. Mol. Biol.* **103,** 316–321.

Holick, M. F. (2007). Vitamin D deficiency. *N. Engl. J. Med.* **357,** 266–281.

Hooper, L. V., Stappenbeck, T. S., Hong, C. V., and Gordon, J. I. (2003). Angiogenins: A new class of microbicidal proteins involved in innate immunity. *Nat. Immunol.* **4,** 269–273.

Hugot, J. P., Chamaillard, M., Zouali, H., Lesage, S., Cezard, J. P., Belaiche, J., Almer, S., Tysk, C., O'Morain, C. A., Gassull, M., Binder, V., Finkel, Y., *et al.* (2001). Association of NOD2 leucine-rich repeat variants with susceptibility to Crohn's disease. *Nature* **411,** 599–603.

Iho, S., Takahashi, T., Kura, F., Sugiyama, H., and Hoshino, T. (1986). The effect of 1,25-dihydroxyvitamin D3 on in vitro immunoglobulin production in human B cells. *J. Immunol.* **136,** 4427–4431.

Janeway, C. A., Jr., and Medzhitov, R. (2002). Innate immune recognition. *Annu. Rev. Immunol.* **20,** 197–216.

Jeffery, L. E., Burke, F., Mura, M., Zheng, Y., Qureshi, O. S., Hewison, M., Walker, L. S., Lammas, D. A., Raza, K., and Sansom, D. M. (2009). 1,25-Dihydroxyvitamin D(3) and IL-2 combine to inhibit T cell production of inflammatory cytokines and promote development of regulatory T cells expressing CTLA-4 and FoxP3. *J. Immunol.* **183,** 5458–5467.

Jeng, L., Yamshchikov, A. V., Judd, S. E., Blumberg, H. M., Martin, G. S., Ziegler, T. R., and Tangpricha, V. (2009). Alterations in vitamin D status and anti-microbial peptide levels in patients in the intensive care unit with sepsis. *J. Transl. Med.* **7,** 28.

Jonuleit, H., Schmitt, E., Schuler, G., Knop, J., and Enk, A. H. (2000). Induction of interleukin 10-producing, nonproliferating CD4(+) T cells with regulatory properties by repetitive stimulation with allogeneic immature human dendritic cells. *J. Exp. Med.* **192,** 1213–1222.

Josien, R., Wong, B. R., Li, H. L., Steinman, R. M., and Choi, Y. (1999). TRANCE, a TNF family member, is differentially expressed on T cell subsets and induces cytokine production in dendritic cells. *J. Immunol.* **162,** 2562–2568.

Jurutka, P. W., Bartik, L., Whitfield, G. K., Mathern, D. R., Barthel, T. K., Gurevich, M., Hsieh, J. C., Kaczmarska, M., Haussler, C. A., and Haussler, M. R. (2007). Vitamin D receptor: Key roles in bone mineral pathophysiology, molecular mechanism of action, and novel nutritional ligands. *J. Bone Miner. Res.* **22**(Suppl. 2), V2–V10.

Kallas, M., Green, F., Hewison, M., White, C., and Kline, G. (2010). Rare causes of calcitriol-mediated hypercalcemia: A case report and literature review. *J. Clin. Endocrinol. Metab.* **95,** 3111–3117.

Kamboh, M. I., and Ferrell, R. E. (1986). Ethnic variation in vitamin D-binding protein (GC): A review of isoelectric focusing studies in human populations. *Hum. Genet.* **72,** 281–293.

Karmali, R., Hewison, M., Rayment, N., Farrow, S. M., Brennan, A., Katz, D. R., and O'Riordan, J. L. (1991). 1,25(OH)2D3 regulates c-myc mRNA levels in tonsillar T lymphocytes. *Immunology* **74,** 589–593.

Klionsky, D. J., and Emr, S. D. (2000). Autophagy as a regulated pathway of cellular degradation. *Science* **290,** 1717–1721.

Koeffler, H. P., Reichel, H., Bishop, J. E., and Norman, A. W. (1985). gamma-Interferon stimulates production of 1,25-dihydroxyvitamin D3 by normal human macrophages. *Biochem. Biophys. Res. Commun.* **127,** 596–603.

Kohchi, C., Inagawa, H., Nishizawa, T., and Soma, G. (2009). ROS and innate immunity. *Anticancer Res.* **29,** 817–821.

Koizumi, T., Nakao, Y., Matsui, T., Nakagawa, T., Katakami, Y., and Fujita, T. (1985). Effect of 1,25-dihydroxyvitamin D3 on cytokine-induced thymocyte proliferation. *Cell. Immunol.* **96,** 455–461.

Kong, J., Zhang, Z., Musch, M. W., Ning, G., Sun, J., Hart, J., Bissonnette, M., and Li, Y. C. (2008). Novel role of the vitamin D receptor in maintaining the integrity of the intestinal mucosal barrier. *Am. J. Physiol. Gastrointest. Liver Physiol.* **294,** G208–G216.

Kreutz, M., Andreesen, R., Krause, S. W., Szabo, A., Ritz, E., and Reichel, H. (1993). 1,25-dihydroxyvitamin D3 production and vitamin D3 receptor expression are developmentally regulated during differentiation of human monocytes into macrophages. *Blood* **82,** 1300–1307.

Krutzik, S. R., Hewison, M., Liu, P. T., Robles, J. A., Stenger, S., Adams, J. S., and Modlin, R. L. (2008). IL-15 links TLR2/1-induced macrophage differentiation to the vitamin D-dependent antimicrobial pathway. *J. Immunol.* **181,** 7115–7120.

Kumar, H., Kawai, T., and Akira, S. (2009). Pathogen recognition in the innate immune response. *Biochem. J.* **420,** 1–16.

Lagishetty, V., Misharin, A. V., Liu, N. Q., Lisse, T. S., Chun, R. F., Ouyang, Y., McLachlan, S. M., Adams, J. S., and Hewison, M. (2010). Vitamin D deficiency in mice impairs colonic antibacterial activity and predisposes to colitis. *Endocrinology* **151,** 2423–2432.

Leichtmann, G. A., Bengoa, J. M., Bolt, M. J., and Sitrin, M. D. (1991). Intestinal absorption of cholecalciferol and 25-hydroxycholecalciferol in patients with both Crohn's disease and intestinal resection. *Am. J. Clin. Nutr.* **54,** 548–552.

Lemire, J. M., Adams, J. S., Kermani-Arab, V., Bakke, A. C., Sakai, R., and Jordan, S. C. (1985). 1,25-Dihydroxyvitamin D3 suppresses human T helper/inducer lymphocyte activity in vitro. *J. Immunol.* **134,** 3032–3035.

Lemire, J. M., Archer, D. C., Beck, L., and Spiegelberg, H. L. (1995). Immunosuppressive actions of 1,25-dihydroxyvitamin D3: Preferential inhibition of Th1 functions. *J. Nutr.* **125,** 1704S–1708S.

Littorin, B., Blom, P., Scholin, A., Arnqvist, H. J., Blohme, G., Bolinder, J., Ekbom-Schnell, A., Eriksson, J. W., Gudbjornsdottir, S., Nystrom, L., Ostman, J., and Sundkvist, G. (2006). Lower levels of plasma 25-hydroxyvitamin D among young adults at diagnosis of autoimmune type 1 diabetes compared with control subjects: Results from the nationwide Diabetes Incidence Study in Sweden (DISS). *Diabetologia* **49,** 2847–2852.

Liu, Y. J. (2005). IPC: Professional type 1 interferon-producing cells and plasmacytoid dendritic cell precursors. *Annu. Rev. Immunol.* **23,** 275–306.

Liu, P. T., Stenger, S., Li, H., Wenzel, L., Tan, B. H., Krutzik, S. R., Ochoa, M. T., Schauber, J., Wu, K., Meinken, C., Kamen, D. L., Wagner, M., *et al.* (2006). Toll-like receptor triggering of a vitamin D-mediated human antimicrobial response. *Science* **311,** 1770–1773.

Liu, P. T., Stenger, S., Tang, D. H., and Modlin, R. L. (2007). Cutting edge: Vitamin D-mediated human antimicrobial activity against mycobacterium tuberculosis is dependent on the induction of cathelicidin. *J. Immunol.* **179,** 2060–2063.

Liu, N., Nguyen, L., Chun, R. F., Lagishetty, V., Ren, S., Wu, S., Hollis, B., Deluca, H. F., Adams, J. S., and Hewison, M. (2008). Altered endocrine and autocrine metabolism of vitamin d in a mouse model of gastrointestinal inflammation. *Endocrinology* **149,** 4799–4808.

Liu, N., Kaplan, A. T., Low, J., Nguyen, L., Liu, G. Y., Equils, O., and Hewison, M. (2009a). Vitamin D induces innate antibacterial responses in human trophoblasts via an intracrine pathway. *Biol. Reprod.* **80,** 398–406.

Liu, P. T., Schenk, M., Walker, V. P., Dempsey, P. W., Kanchanapoomi, M., Wheelwright, M., Vazirnia, A., Zhang, X., Steinmeyer, A., Zugel, U., Hollis, B. W., Cheng, G., *et al.* (2009b). Convergence of IL-1beta and VDR activation pathways in human TLR2/1-induced antimicrobial responses. *PLoS ONE* **4,** e5810.

Lo, C. W., Paris, P. W., Clemens, T. L., Nolan, J., and Holick, M. F. (1985). Vitamin D absorption in healthy subjects and in patients with intestinal malabsorption syndromes. *Am. J. Clin. Nutr.* **42,** 644–649.

Malloy, P. J., Pike, J. W., and Feldman, D. (1999). The vitamin D receptor and the syndrome of hereditary 1,25-dihydroxyvitamin D-resistant rickets. *Endocr. Rev.* **20,** 156–188.

Mamutse, G., Woolmore, J., Pye, E., Partridge, J., Boggild, M., Young, C., Fryer, A., Hoban, P. R., Rukin, N., Alldersea, J., Strange, R. C., and Hawkins, C. P. (2008). Vitamin D receptor gene polymorphism is associated with reduced disability in multiple sclerosis. *Mult. Scler.* **14,** 1280–1283.

Martineau, A. R., Honecker, F. U., Wilkinson, R. J., and Griffiths, C. J. (2007a). Vitamin D in the treatment of pulmonary tuberculosis. *J. Steroid Biochem. Mol. Biol.* **103,** 793–798.

Martineau, A. R., Wilkinson, R. J., Wilkinson, K. A., Newton, S. M., Kampmann, B., Hall, B. M., Packe, G. E., Davidson, R. N., Eldridge, S. M., Maunsell, Z. J., Rainbow, S. J., Berry, J. L., *et al.* (2007b). A single dose of vitamin d enhances immunity to mycobacteria. *Am. J. Respir. Crit. Care Med.* **176,** 208–213.

Mathieu, C., Gysemans, C., Giulietti, A., and Bouillon, R. (2005). Vitamin D and diabetes. *Diabetologia* **48,** 1247–1257.

Mawer, E. B., Hayes, M. E., Still, P. E., Davies, M., Lumb, G. A., Palit, J., and Holt, P. J. (1991). Evidence for nonrenal synthesis of 1,25-dihydroxyvitamin D in patients with inflammatory arthritis. *J. Bone Miner. Res.* **6,** 733–739.

Medzhitov, R., and Janeway, C., Jr. (2000). The toll receptor family and microbial recognition. *Trends Microbiol.* **8,** 452–456.

Meehan, T. F., and DeLuca, H. F. (2002). CD8(+) T cells are not necessary for 1 alpha,25-dihydroxyvitamin D(3) to suppress experimental autoimmune encephalomyelitis in mice. *Proc. Natl. Acad. Sci. USA* **99,** 5557–5560.

Modlin, R. L., Brightbill, H. D., and Godowski, P. J. (1999). The toll of innate immunity on microbial pathogens. *N. Engl. J. Med.* **340,** 1834–1835.

Moller, K. I., Kongshoj, B., Philipsen, P. A., Thomsen, V. O., and Wulf, H. C. (2005). How Finsen's light cured lupus vulgaris. *Photodermatol. Photoimmunol. Photomed.* **21,** 118–124.

Nashold, F. E., Spach, K. M., Spanier, J. A., and Hayes, C. E. (2009). Estrogen controls vitamin D3-mediated resistance to experimental autoimmune encephalomyelitis by controlling vitamin D3 metabolism and receptor expression. *J. Immunol.* **183,** 3672–3681.

Nguyen, M., d'Alesio, A., Pascussi, J. M., Kumar, R., Griffin, M. D., Dong, X., Guillozo, H., Rizk-Rabin, M., Sinding, C., Bougneres, P., Jehan, F., and Garabedian, M. (2006). Vitamin D-resistant rickets and type 1 diabetes in a child with compound heterozygous mutations of the vitamin D receptor (L263R and R391S): Dissociated responses of the CYP-24 and rel-B promoters to 1,25-dihydroxyvitamin D3. *J. Bone Miner. Res.* **21,** 886–894.

Nunn, J. D., Katz, D. R., Barker, S., Fraher, L. J., Hewison, M., Hendy, G. N., and O'Riordan, J. L. (1986). Regulation of human tonsillar T-cell proliferation by the active metabolite of vitamin D3. *Immunology* **59,** 479–484.

Nursyam, E. W., Amin, Z., and Rumende, C. M. (2006). The effect of vitamin D as supplementary treatment in patients with moderately advanced pulmonary tuberculous lesion. *Acta Med. Indones.* **38,** 3–5.

Nykjaer, A., Dragun, D., Walther, D., Vorum, H., Jacobsen, C., Herz, J., Melsen, F., Christensen, E. I., and Willnow, T. E. (1999). An endocytic pathway essential for renal uptake and activation of the steroid 25-(OH) vitamin D3. *Cell* **96,** 507–515.

Nykjaer, A., Fyfe, J. C., Kozyraki, R., Leheste, J. R., Jacobsen, C., Nielsen, M. S., Verroust, P. J., Aminoff, M., de la Chapelle, A., Moestrup, S. K., Ray, R., Gliemann, J., *et al.* (2001). Cubilin dysfunction causes abnormal metabolism of the steroid hormone 25(OH) vitamin D(3). *Proc. Natl. Acad. Sci. USA* **98,** 13895–13900.

Ogura, Y., Bonen, D. K., Inohara, N., Nicolae, D. L., Chen, F. F., Ramos, R., Britton, H., Moran, T., Karaliuskas, R., Duerr, R. H., Achkar, J. P., Brant, S. R., *et al.* (2001). A frameshift mutation in NOD2 associated with susceptibility to Crohn's disease. *Nature* **411,** 603–606.

O'Kelly, J., Uskokovic, M., Lemp, N., Vadgama, J., and Koeffler, H. P. (2006). Novel Gemini-vitamin D3 analog inhibits tumor cell growth and modulates the Akt/mTOR signaling pathway. *J. Steroid Biochem. Mol. Biol.* **100,** 107–116.

O'Neil, D. A., Porter, E. M., Elewaut, D., Anderson, G. M., Eckmann, L., Ganz, T., and Kagnoff, M. F. (1999). Expression and regulation of the human beta-defensins hBD-1 and hBD-2 in intestinal epithelium. *J. Immunol.* **163,** 6718–6724.

Ong, P. Y., Ohtake, T., Brandt, C., Strickland, I., Boguniewicz, M., Ganz, T., Gallo, R. L., and Leung, D. Y. (2002). Endogenous antimicrobial peptides and skin infections in atopic dermatitis. *N. Engl. J. Med.* **347,** 1151–1160.

Orton, S. M., Morris, A. P., Herrera, B. M., Ramagopalan, S. V., Lincoln, M. R., Chao, M. J., Vieth, R., Sadovnick, A. D., and Ebers, G. C. (2008). Evidence for genetic regulation of vitamin D status in twins with multiple sclerosis. *Am. J. Clin. Nutr.* **88,** 441–447.

Overbergh, L., Decallonne, B., Waer, M., Rutgeerts, O., Valckx, D., Casteels, K. M., Laureys, J., Bouillon, R., and Mathieu, C. (2000). 1alpha, 25-dihydroxyvitamin D3 induces an autoantigen-specific T-helper 1/T-helper 2 immune shift in NOD mice immunized with GAD65 (p524–543). *Diabetes* **49,** 1301–1307.

Packey, C. D., and Sartor, R. B. (2009). Commensal bacteria, traditional and opportunistic pathogens, dysbiosis and bacterial killing in inflammatory bowel diseases. *Curr. Opin. Infect. Dis.* **22,** 292–301.

Pappa, H. M., Gordon, C. M., Saslowsky, T. M., Zholudev, A., Horr, B., Shih, M. C., and Grand, R. J. (2006a). Vitamin D status in children and young adults with inflammatory bowel disease. *Pediatrics* **118,** 1950–1961.

Pappa, H. M., Grand, R. J., and Gordon, C. M. (2006b). Report on the vitamin D status of adult and pediatric patients with inflammatory bowel disease and its significance for bone health and disease. *Inflamm. Bowel Dis.* **12,** 1162–1174.

Pedersen, L. B., Nashold, F. E., Spach, K. M., and Hayes, C. E. (2007). 1,25-dihydroxyvitamin D3 reverses experimental autoimmune encephalomyelitis by inhibiting chemokine synthesis and monocyte trafficking. *J. Neurosci. Res.* **85,** 2480–2490.

Penna, G., and Adorini, L. (2000). 1 Alpha, 25-dihydroxyvitamin D3 inhibits differentiation, maturation, activation, and survival of dendritic cells leading to impaired alloreactive T cell activation. *J. Immunol.* **164,** 2405–2411.

Penna, G., Amuchastegui, S., Cossetti, C., Aquilano, F., Mariani, R., Sanvito, F., Doglioni, C., and Adorini, L. (2006). Treatment of experimental autoimmune prostatitis in nonobese diabetic mice by the vitamin D receptor agonist elocalcitol. *J. Immunol.* **177,** 8504–8511.

Penna, G., Amuchastegui, S., Giarratana, N., Daniel, K. C., Vulcano, M., Sozzani, S., and Adorini, L. (2007). 1,25-dihydroxyvitamin d3 selectively modulates tolerogenic properties in myeloid but not plasmacytoid dendritic cells. *J. Immunol.* **178,** 145–153.

Piemonti, L., Monti, P., Sironi, M., Fraticelli, P., Leone, B. E., Dal Cin, E., Allavena, P., and Di Carlo, V. (2000). Vitamin D3 affects differentiation, maturation, and function of human monocyte-derived dendritic cells. *J. Immunol.* **164,** 4443–4451.

Pierrot-Deseilligny, C., and Souberbielle, J. C. (2010). Is hypovitaminosis D one of the environmental risk factors for multiple sclerosis? *Brain* **133,** 1869–1888.

Provvedini, D. M., and Manolagas, S. C. (1989). 1 Alpha,25-dihydroxyvitamin D3 receptor distribution and effects in subpopulations of normal human T lymphocytes. *J. Clin. Endocrinol. Metab.* **68,** 774–779.

Provvedini, D. M., Tsoukas, C. D., Deftos, L. J., and Manolagas, S. C. (1983). 1,25-dihydroxyvitamin D3 receptors in human leukocytes. *Science* **221,** 1181–1183.

Quarles, L. D. (2008). Endocrine functions of bone in mineral metabolism regulation. *J. Clin. Invest.* **118,** 3820–3828.

Raghuwanshi, A., Joshi, S. S., and Christakos, S. (2008). Vitamin D and multiple sclerosis. *J. Cell. Biochem.* **105,** 338–343.

Ramos-Lopez, E., Jansen, T., Ivaskevicius, V., Kahles, H., Klepzig, C., Oldenburg, J., and Badenhoop, K. (2006). Protection from type 1 diabetes by vitamin D receptor haplotypes. *Ann. NY Acad. Sci.* **1079,** 327–334.

Ravid, A., Koren, R., Novogrodsky, A., and Liberman, U. A. (1984). 1,25-Dihydroxyvitamin D3 inhibits selectively the mitogenic stimulation of mouse medullary thymocytes. *Biochem. Biophys. Res. Commun.* **123,** 163–169.

Reichel, H., Koeffler, H. P., Bishop, J. E., and Norman, A. W. (1987). 25-Hydroxyvitamin D3 metabolism by lipopolysaccharide-stimulated normal human macrophages. *J. Clin. Endocrinol. Metab.* **64,** 1–9.

Ren, S., Nguyen, L., Wu, S., Encinas, C., Adams, J. S., and Hewison, M. (2005). Alternative splicing of vitamin D-24-hydroxylase: A novel mechanism for the regulation of extrarenal 1,25-dihydroxyvitamin D synthesis. *J. Biol. Chem.* **280,** 20604–20611.

Rigby, W. F., Noelle, R. J., Krause, K., and Fanger, M. W. (1985). The effects of 1,25-dihydroxyvitamin D3 on human T lymphocyte activation and proliferation: A cell cycle analysis. *J. Immunol.* **135,** 2279–2286.

Rigby, W. F., Denome, S., and Fanger, M. W. (1987a). Regulation of lymphokine production and human T lymphocyte activation by 1,25-dihydroxyvitamin D3. Specific inhibition at the level of messenger RNA. *J. Clin. Invest.* **79,** 1659–1664.

Rigby, W. F., Yirinec, B., Oldershaw, R. L., and Fanger, M. W. (1987b). Comparison of the effects of 1,25-dihydroxyvitamin D3 on T lymphocyte subpopulations. *Eur. J. Immunol.* **17,** 563–566.

Rigby, W. F., Hamilton, B. J., and Waugh, M. G. (1990). 1,25-Dihydroxyvitamin D3 modulates the effects of interleukin 2 independent of IL-2 receptor binding. *Cell. Immunol.* **125,** 396–414.

Rockett, K. A., Brookes, R., Udalova, I., Vidal, V., Hill, A. V., and Kwiatkowski, D. (1998). 1,25-Dihydroxyvitamin D3 induces nitric oxide synthase and suppresses growth of Mycobacterium tuberculosis in a human macrophage-like cell line. *Infect. Immun.* **66,** 5314–5321.

Romagnani, S. (2006). Regulation of the T cell response. *Clin. Exp. Allergy* **36,** 1357–1366.

Rook, G. A., Steele, J., Fraher, L., Barker, S., Karmali, R., O'Riordan, J., and Stanford, J. (1986). Vitamin D3, gamma interferon, and control of proliferation of Mycobacterium tuberculosis by human monocytes. *Immunology* **57,** 159–163.

Rowling, M. J., Kemmis, C. M., Taffany, D. A., and Welsh, J. (2006). Megalin-mediated endocytosis of vitamin D binding protein correlates with 25-hydroxycholecalciferol actions in human mammary cells. *J. Nutr.* **136,** 2754–2759.

Royal, W., 3rd, Mia, Y., Li, H., and Naunton, K. (2009). Peripheral blood regulatory T cell measurements correlate with serum vitamin D levels in patients with multiple sclerosis. *J. Neuroimmunol.* **213,** 135–141.

Sakaki, T., Kagawa, N., Yamamoto, K., and Inouye, K. (2005). Metabolism of vitamin D3 by cytochromes P450. *Front. Biosci.* **10,** 119–134.

Sanjuan, M. A., Milasta, S., and Green, D. R. (2009). Toll-like receptor signaling in the lysosomal pathways. *Immunol. Rev.* **227,** 203–220.

Schauber, J., and Gallo, R. L. (2007). Expanding the roles of antimicrobial peptides in skin: Alarming and arming keratinocytes. *J. Invest. Dermatol.* **127,** 510–512.

Schauber, J., Dorschner, R. A., Coda, A. B., Buchau, A. S., Liu, P. T., Kiken, D., Helfrich, Y. R., Kang, S., Elalieh, H. Z., Steinmeyer, A., Zugel, U., Bikle, D. D., *et al.* (2007). Injury enhances TLR2 function and antimicrobial peptide expression through a vitamin D-dependent mechanism. *J. Clin. Invest.* **117,** 803–811.

Schoenborn, J. R., and Wilson, C. B. (2007). Regulation of interferon-gamma during innate and adaptive immune responses. *Adv. Immunol.* **96,** 41–101.
Shimada, T., Kakitani, M., Yamazaki, Y., Hasegawa, H., Takeuchi, Y., Fujita, T., Fukumoto, S., Tomizuka, K., and Yamashita, T. (2004). Targeted ablation of Fgf23 demonstrates an essential physiological role of FGF23 in phosphate and vitamin D metabolism. *J. Clin. Invest.* **113,** 561–568.
Shin, D. M., Yuk, J. M., Lee, H. M., Lee, S. H., Son, J. W., Harding, C. V., Kim, J. M., Modlin, R. L., and Jo, E. K. (2010). Mycobacterial lipoprotein activates autophagy via TLR2/1/CD14 and a functional vitamin D receptor signaling. *Cell. Microbiol.* **12,** 1648–1665.
Shiozawa, K., Shiozawa, S., Shimizu, S., and Fujita, T. (1985). 1 alpha, 25-dihydroxyvitamin D3 inhibits pokeweed mitogen-stimulated human B-cell activation: An analysis using serum-free culture conditions. *Immunology* **56,** 161–167.
Shirakawa, A. K., Nagakubo, D., Hieshima, K., Nakayama, T., Jin, Z., and Yoshie, O. (2008). 1,25-dihydroxyvitamin D3 induces CCR10 expression in terminally differentiating human B cells. *J. Immunol.* **180,** 2786–2795.
Sigmundsdottir, H., Pan, J., Debes, G. F., Alt, C., Habtezion, A., Soler, D., and Butcher, E. C. (2007). DCs metabolize sunlight-induced vitamin D3 to 'program' T cell attraction to the epidermal chemokine CCL27. *Nat. Immunol.* **8,** 285–293.
Simon, K. C., Munger, K. L., Xing, Y., and Ascherio, A. (2010). Polymorphisms in vitamin D metabolism related genes and risk of multiple sclerosis. *Mult. Scler.* **16,** 133–138.
Sly, L. M., Lopez, M., Nauseef, W. M., and Reiner, N. E. (2001). 1alpha, 25-Dihydroxyvitamin D3-induced monocyte antimycobacterial activity is regulated by phosphatidylinositol 3-kinase and mediated by the NADPH-dependent phagocyte oxidase. *J. Biol. Chem.* **276,** 35482–35493.
Smolders, J., Damoiseaux, J., Menheere, P., Tervaert, J. W., and Hupperts, R. (2009a). Association study on two vitamin D receptor gene polymorphisms and vitamin D metabolites in multiple sclerosis. *Ann. NY Acad. Sci.* **1173,** 515–520.
Smolders, J., Thewissen, M., Peelen, E., Menheere, P., Cohen Tervaert, J. W., Damoiseaux, J., and Hupperts, R. (2009b). Vitamin D status is positively correlated with regulatory T cell function in patients with multiple sclerosis. *PLoS ONE* **4,** e6635.
Solomon, A. J., and Whitham, R. H. (2010). Multiple sclerosis and vitamin D: A review and recommendations. *Curr. Neurol. Neurosci. Rep.* **10,** 389–396.
Sorensen, O., Cowland, J. B., Askaa, J., and Borregaard, N. (1997). An ELISA for hCAP-18, the cathelicidin present in human neutrophils and plasma. *J. Immunol. Methods* **206,** 53–59.
Sorensen, O. E., Follin, P., Johnsen, A. H., Calafat, J., Tjabringa, G. S., Hiemstra, P. S., and Borregaard, N. (2001). Human cathelicidin, hCAP-18, is processed to the antimicrobial peptide LL-37 by extracellular cleavage with proteinase 3. *Blood* **97,** 3951–3959.
Spach, K. M., and Hayes, C. E. (2005). Vitamin D3 confers protection from autoimmune encephalomyelitis only in female mice. *J. Immunol.* **175,** 4119–4126.
Spach, K. M., Pedersen, L. B., Nashold, F. E., Kayo, T., Yandell, B. S., Prolla, T. A., and Hayes, C. E. (2004). Gene expression analysis suggests that 1,25-dihydroxyvitamin D3 reverses experimental autoimmune encephalomyelitis by stimulating inflammatory cell apoptosis. *Physiol. Genomics* **18,** 141–151.
Spach, K. M., Nashold, F. E., Dittel, B. N., and Hayes, C. E. (2006). IL-10 signaling is essential for 1,25-dihydroxyvitamin D3-mediated inhibition of experimental autoimmune encephalomyelitis. *J. Immunol.* **177,** 6030–6037.
Stoffels, K., Overbergh, L., Giulietti, A., Verlinden, L., Bouillon, R., and Mathieu, C. (2006). Immune regulation of 25-hydroxyvitamin-D3-1alpha-hydroxylase in human monocytes. *J. Bone Miner. Res.* **21,** 37–47.
Strober, W., Murray, P. J., Kitani, A., and Watanabe, T. (2006). Signalling pathways and molecular interactions of NOD1 and NOD2. *Nat. Rev. Immunol.* **6,** 9–20.

Sundqvist, E., Baarnhielm, M., Alfredsson, L., Hillert, J., Olsson, T., and Kockum, I. (2010). Confirmation of association between multiple sclerosis and CYP27B1. *Eur. J. Hum. Genet.* **18,** 1349–1352.

Tajouri, L., Ovcaric, M., Curtain, R., Johnson, M. P., Griffiths, L. R., Csurhes, P., Pender, M. P., and Lea, R. A. (2005). Variation in the vitamin D receptor gene is associated with multiple sclerosis in an Australian population. *J. Neurogenet.* **19,** 25–38.

Takahashi, K., Nakayama, Y., Horiuchi, H., Ohta, T., Komoriya, K., Ohmori, H., and Kamimura, T. (2002). Human neutrophils express messenger RNA of vitamin D receptor and respond to 1alpha, 25-dihydroxyvitamin D3. *Immunopharmacol. Immunotoxicol.* **24,** 335–347.

Talat, N., Perry, S., Parsonnet, J., Dawood, G., and Hussain, R. (2010). Vitamin D deficiency and tuberculosis progression. *Emerg. Infect. Dis.* **16,** 853–855.

Tang, H. L., and Cyster, J. G. (1999). Chemokine up-regulation and activated T cell attraction by maturing dendritic cells. *Science* **284,** 819–822.

Tang, J., Zhou, R., Luger, D., Zhu, W., Silver, P. B., Grajewski, R. S., Su, S. B., Chan, C. C., Adorini, L., and Caspi, R. R. (2009). Calcitriol suppresses antiretinal autoimmunity through inhibitory effects on the Th17 effector response. *J. Immunol.* **182,** 4624–4632.

Thoma-Uszynski, S., Stenger, S., Takeuchi, O., Ochoa, M. T., Engele, M., Sieling, P. A., Barnes, P. F., Rollinghoff, M., Bolcskei, P. L., Wagner, M., Akira, S., Norgard, M. V., *et al.* (2001). Induction of direct antimicrobial activity through mammalian toll-like receptors. *Science* **291,** 1544–1547.

Townsend, K., Evans, K. N., Campbell, M. J., Colston, K. W., Adams, J. S., and Hewison, M. (2005). Biological actions of extra-renal 25-hydroxyvitamin D-1alpha-hydroxylase and implications for chemoprevention and treatment. *J. Steroid Biochem. Mol. Biol.* **97,** 103–109.

Vagianos, K., Bector, S., McConnell, J., and Bernstein, C. N. (2007). Nutrition assessment of patients with inflammatory bowel disease. *JPEN J. Parenter. Enteral Nutr.* **31,** 311–319.

Veldman, C. M., Cantorna, M. T., and DeLuca, H. F. (2000). Expression of 1,25-dihydroxyvitamin D(3) receptor in the immune system. *Arch. Biochem. Biophys.* **374,** 334–338.

Waldmann, T. A. (2006). The biology of interleukin-2 and interleukin-15: Implications for cancer therapy and vaccine design. *Nat. Rev. Immunol.* **6,** 595–601.

Wang, T. T., Nestel, F. P., Bourdeau, V., Nagai, Y., Wang, Q., Liao, J., Tavera-Mendoza, L., Lin, R., Hanrahan, J. W., Mader, S., and White, J. H. (2004). Cutting edge: 1,25-dihydroxyvitamin D3 is a direct inducer of antimicrobial peptide gene expression. *J. Immunol.* **173,** 2909–2912.

Wang, T. T., Dabbas, B., Laperriere, D., Bitton, A. J., Soualhine, H., Tavera-Mendoza, L. E., Dionne, S., Servant, M. J., Bitton, A., Seidman, E. G., Mader, S., Behr, M. A., *et al.* (2009). Direct and indirect induction by 1,25-dihydroxyvitamin D3 of the NOD2/CARD15-beta defensin 2 innate immune pathway defective in Crohn's disease. *J. Biol. Chem.* **285,** 2227–2231.

Wejse, C., Olesen, R., Rabna, P., Kaestel, P., Gustafson, P., Aaby, P., Andersen, P. L., Glerup, H., and Sodemann, M. (2007). Serum 25-hydroxyvitamin D in a West African population of tuberculosis patients and unmatched healthy controls. *Am. J. Clin. Nutr.* **86,** 1376–1383.

Wejse, C., Gomes, V. F., Rabna, P., Gustafson, P., Aaby, P., Lisse, I. M., Andersen, P. L., Glerup, H., and Sodemann, M. (2009). Vitamin D as supplementary treatment for tuberculosis: A double-blind, randomized, placebo-controlled trial. *Am. J. Respir. Crit. Care Med.* **179,** 843–850.

Westwood, S. A., Seaman, P. J., O'Brien, C., and Thorogood, L. J. (1987). The phenotypic frequencies of group specific component and alpha-2-HS-glycoprotein in three ethnic groups. The use of these proteins as racial markers in forensic biology. *Forensic Sci. Int.* **35,** 197–207.

White, P., and Cooke, N. (2000). The multifunctional properties and characteristics of vitamin D-binding protein. *Trends Endocrinol. Metab.* **11,** 320–327.

Wu, S., Ren, S., Nguyen, L., Adams, J. S., and Hewison, M. (2007). Splice variants of the CYP27b1 gene and the regulation of 1,25-dihydroxyvitamin D3 production. *Endocrinology* **148,** 3410–3418.

Yang, C. S., Shin, D. M., Kim, K. H., Lee, Z. W., Lee, C. H., Park, S. G., Bae, Y. S., and Jo, E. K. (2009). NADPH oxidase 2 interaction with TLR2 is required for efficient innate immune responses to mycobacteria via cathelicidin expression. *J. Immunol.* **182,** 3696–3705.

Yim, S., Dhawan, P., Ragunath, C., Christakos, S., and Diamond, G. (2007). Induction of cathelicidin in normal and CF bronchial epithelial cells by 1,25-dihydroxyvitamin D(3). *J. Cyst. Fibros.* **6,** 403–410.

Yu, X. P., Mocharla, H., Hustmyer, F. G., and Manolagas, S. C. (1991). Vitamin D receptor expression in human lymphocytes. Signal requirements and characterization by western blots and DNA sequencing. *J. Biol. Chem.* **266,** 7588–7595.

Yu, S., Bruce, D., Froicu, M., Weaver, V., and Cantorna, M. T. (2008). Failure of T cell homing, reduced CD4/CD8alphaalpha intraepithelial lymphocytes, and inflammation in the gut of vitamin D receptor KO mice. *Proc. Natl. Acad. Sci. USA* **105,** 20834–20839.

Yuan, J. Y., Freemont, A. J., Mawer, E. B., and Hayes, M. E. (1992). Regulation of 1 alpha, 25-dihydroxyvitamin D3 synthesis in macrophages from arthritic joints by phorbol ester, dibutyryl-cAMP and calcium ionophore (A23187). *FEBS Lett.* **311,** 71–74.

Yuk, J. M., Shin, D. M., Lee, H. M., Yang, C. S., Jin, H. S., Kim, K. K., Lee, Z. W., Lee, S. H., Kim, J. M., and Jo, E. K. (2009). Vitamin D3 induces autophagy in human monocytes/macrophages via cathelicidin. *Cell Host Microbe* **6,** 231–243.

Zehnder, D., Bland, R., Williams, M. C., McNinch, R. W., Howie, A. J., Stewart, P. M., and Hewison, M. (2001). Extrarenal expression of 25-hydroxyvitamin d(3)-1 alpha-hydroxylase. *J. Clin. Endocrinol. Metab.* **86,** 888–894.

Zehnder, D., Evans, K. N., Kilby, M. D., Bulmer, J. N., Innes, B. A., Stewart, P. M., and Hewison, M. (2002). The ontogeny of 25-hydroxyvitamin D(3) 1alpha-hydroxylase expression in human placenta and decidua. *Am. J. Pathol.* **161,** 105–114.

CHAPTER THREE

Dendritic Cells Modified by Vitamin D: Future Immunotherapy for Autoimmune Diseases

Ayako Wakatsuki Pedersen,* Mogens Helweg Claesson,† *and* Mai-Britt Zocca*

Contents

Abstract

Dendritic cells (DCs), the most potent antigen-presenting cells of the immune system, express nuclear receptors for 1,25-dihydroxyvitamin D_3 (VD3) and they are one of its main targets. In the presence of VD3, DCs differentiate into a phenotype that resembles semimature DCs, with reduced T cell costimulatory molecules and hampered IL-12 production. These VD3-modulated DCs induce T cell tolerance *in vitro* using multiple mechanisms such as rendering T cells anergic, dampening of Th1 responses, and recruiting and differentiating regulatory T cells. Due to their ability to specifically target pathological T cells, VD3-modulated DCs are safe and potentially more effective alternatives to currently available immunoregulatory therapies. While a number of considerations remain, including the establishment of a reliable quality control measure to ensure the safety and efficacy of VD3-DCs *in vivo* and the optimal frequency, dose, and route of DC administration to achieve therapeutic effects in humans,

* DanDrit Biotech A/S, Symbion Science Park, Copenhagen, Denmark
† Institute of International Health, Immunology and Microbiology, Faculty of Health Sciences, University of Copenhagen, Copenhagen, Denmark

Vitamins and Hormones, Volume 86
ISSN 0083-6729, DOI: 10.1016/B978-0-12-386960-9.00003-4

adoptive VD3-DC transfer represents one of the most promising approaches to future treatment of autoimmune diseases.

I. Introduction

To date, the majority of immunotherapies that have been clinically approved for autoimmune diseases focus on the systemic inhibition of immune responses. Although such drugs are partially effective in the inhibition of pathology-causing cells, the nonspecific suppression of the immune response is associated with numerous side effects and therefore continuous long-term therapy is not plausible. In contrast, antigen-specific tolerance strategy specifically prevents the generation of autoantigen-specific effector cells and/or blocks their harmful effects without interfering with the normal function of the immune system to clear infection. One of the most promising strategies under development so far is the induction of antigen-specific tolerance by the use of immunoregulatory dendritic cells (DCs) (Morelli and Thomson, 2007; Xiao *et al.*, 2003). In this chapter, we discuss the biology of 1,25-dihydroxyvitamin D_3 (VD3)-modified DCs and their potential clinical application in the control of autoimmune diseases.

II. DCs and Their Role in the Immune System

DCs, often termed "nature's adjuvant," are $CD34^+$ hematopoietic stem cell-derived specialized antigen-presenting cells (APCs) and considered to be the most powerful regulators of the immune system (Banchereau and Steinman, 1998). DCs consist of heterogeneous populations and are found in circulation as well as in lymphoid and nonlymphoid organs.

In humans, two subsets of DCs can be found in blood: conventional myeloid DCs (often denoted as mDC or DC1) and lymphoid or plasmacytoid DCs (pDC or DC2). Myeloid DCs are characterized by a monocytic morphology with myeloid markers such as CD13, CD33, CD11c, and low levels of the IL-3 receptor α-chain CD123. Conversely, plasmacytoid DCs have a plasma cell-like morphology, and express high levels of CD4, CD62L, and CD123, but lack the expression of myeloid markers. Upon functional maturation, mDCs produce IL-12 (Rissoan *et al.*, 1999) and induce Th1 and Th17 cell differentiation, while pDCs secrete high levels of type I interferon (IFN) particularly in response to viruses or TLR9 ligands (Colonna *et al.*, 2004; Kadowaki and Liu, 2002) and can selectively induce Th2 cells (Colonna *et al.*, 2004; Rissoan *et al.*, 1999).

DCs found in peripheral tissues are efficient at taking up antigens, while expressing low levels of antigen presenting and costimulatory molecules on the cell surface, and are poor stimulator of T cells. Upon antigen uptake DCs migrate through the afferent lymph to T-dependent areas of secondary lymphoid organs where they can initiate adaptive immune responses. During migration to lymphoid organs, DCs mature into potent APCs by increasing their immunostimulatory properties while decreasing antigen-capturing capacity. This functional maturation is essential for the initiation of acquired immune response and is dependent on exposure to exogenous microbial products (collectively known as PAMP, pathogen-associated molecular pattern) such as bacterial lipopolysaccharides (LPS) and viral double-stranded RNA, as well as endogenous inflammatory factors (e.g., proinflammatory cytokines, heat shock proteins).

For a long time, it has been considered that the chief function of DCs in the immune system is to induce immunity. However, more recent studies have revealed another equally important role of DCs in the immune system, namely, to induce immunological tolerance. Antigen uptake in the absence of this functional maturation can result in DCs that have semimature phenotype (Lutz and Schuler, 2002), which migrate to the second lymphoid organs and induce tolerance instead of immunity. The ability of DC to induce tolerance was initially demonstrated by experiments on immature mDC residing in peripheral lymphoid tissues (Steinman and Nussenzweig, 2002; Steinman *et al.*, 2003). Under steady-state conditions, immature DCs capture apoptotic bodies derived from natural cell turnover and, after migration to the draining LNs, DCs present self antigens to induce tolerance (Steinman *et al.*, 2000). This process involves partial maturation of DCs into a semimature phenotype (Lutz and Schuler, 2002), where DCs can migrate, process, and present antigens without being able to produce IL-12 or induce T cell activation.

These semimature, conventional mDCs have been shown to suppress various autoimmune diseases (Li *et al.*, 2005; Steptoe *et al.*, 2005) as well as to prolong organ graft survival after their adoptive transfer across MHC barriers in the absence of immunosuppressive therapy (Lu *et al.*, 1995; Lutz *et al.*, 2000). In addition, human immature mDCs can drive the generation of T regulatory cells (Levings *et al.*, 2005) and induce antigen-specific T cells tolerance to model antigens *in vivo* (Dhodapkar *et al.*, 2001).

In contrast to mDCs, human pDCs activated by CD40 ligand (Gilliet and Liu, 2002) or CPG (Moseman *et al.*, 2004) induce regulatory T cells (Tregs). Interestingly, the Treg subsets induced by immature mDCs or pDCs appear to differ functionally, whereas regulatory mDCs induce differentiation of IL-10 producing Treg cells (Jonuleit *et al.*, 2000), activated pDCs preferentially induce the development of cell contact-dependent Treg cells (Gilliet and Liu, 2002).

Thus, DCs play key roles not only as an initiator of the immune response but also as a regulator of adaptive responses, ensuring to regulate the balance between immunity and maintenance of peripheral tolerance. This dual functionality of DCs is achieved by both the differential maturation of DCs and the subset-specific differentiation of DCs.

III. Vitamin D Metabolism in DCs

The biologically active form of vitamin D, VD3, is a secosteroid hormone that binds to the vitamin D receptor (VDR), a member of the superfamily of nuclear receptors for steroid hormones, thyroid hormone, and retinoic acid. The VDR is expressed in most nucleated cells of the body and the VDR ligation regulates multiple physiological functions, including the regulation of calcium/phosphate metabolism, control of cell proliferation and differentiation and immunoregulatory activities (Adorini *et al.*, 2003; van Etten and Mathieu, 2005; VanAmerongen *et al.*, 2004; Zella and DeLuca, 2003). Indeed, direct administration of VD3 or its analogs results in protection from or reduces severity of animal model of autoimmune diseases such as experimental autoimmune encephalomyelitis (EAE) (Cantorna *et al.*, 1996; Nashold *et al.*, 2000) and diabetes (Decallonne *et al.*, 2005; Gregori *et al.*, 2002; Mathieu *et al.*, 1994), and prolongs allograft survival (Gregori *et al.*, 2001).

In addition to their direct effects on T cell activation (Boonstra *et al.*, 2001; Takeuchi *et al.*, 1998), VDR ligands modulate phenotype and function of APCs, and in particular DCs. Whereas the expression of VDR is inducibly regulated in lymphocytes upon activation, VDR is expressed constitutively by APCs (Veldman *et al.*, 2000). The ligand–VDR complex first heterodimerizes with the retinoid X receptor, before acting as a transcription factor on vitamin D_3-responsive elements in target gene promoters (Schrader *et al.*, 1993). These genes include IL-12p35 and p40 (D'Ambrosio *et al.*, 1998) that are expressed upon functional maturation of DCs. Thus, the repressive effect of VD3 upon IL-12 secretion is lost in DCs derived from VDR knockout mice (Griffin *et al.*, 2001).

In the above study that examined the physiological significance of VD3/VDR interaction by deletion of the VDR gene (Griffin *et al.*, 2001), it was demonstrated that the immune system was overall intact with little effect on the number of $CD11c^+$ DCs in VDR-deficient mice compared to wild-type animals. However, these deficient mice showed enlarged lymph nodes containing a larger proportion of mature DCs, suggesting that VD3 may exert negative regulatory role in the physiologic control of immune responses.

The influence of VD3 on DC function is not restricted to their cellular expression of VDR but also includes local synthesis and/or breakdown of VD3. In macrophages, $25(OH)D_3$ 1-α-hydroxylase, the enzyme responsible for the final hydroxylation step in the synthesis of biologically active

VD3 ($1{,}25(OH)_2D_3$), is induced upon cell activation (Reichel *et al.*, 1987). It was shown more recently that DCs can regulate the expression of this enzyme in a similar fashion (Hewison *et al.*, 2003; Sigmundsdottir *et al.*, 2007). Thus, both macrophages and DCs are capable of regulating the synthesis and secretion of VD3. The upregulation of 1-α-hydroxylase expression is associated with the p38 mitogen-activated protein kinase- and the nuclear factor (NF)-κB-dependent maturation of DCs. This suggests that the DC differentiation process may be regulated by VDR/1-α-hydroxylase negative feedback mechanisms where activation of DC is carefully controlled (Hewison *et al.*, 2003). Furthermore, DCs in the skin hydroxylate sunlight-induced vitamin D3 into active hormone, which in turn induces the expression of the CC-chemokine CCR10 on activated T cells (including Treg). This enables homing of these T cells to chemokine CCL27 secreted by keratinocytes of the epidermis (Sigmundsdottir *et al.*, 2007), and may illustrate one of the mechanisms by which the immune system counteracts with the proinflammatory effects induced in the skin by sun exposure.

IV. Modulation of DC Function by VDR

The regulatory influence of exogenous VDR ligands upon DCs in culture has been clearly demonstrated in many studies, both in DCs derived from human peripheral blood monocytes (Berer *et al.*, 2000; Canning *et al.*, 2001; Gauzzi *et al.*, 2005; Penna and Adorini, 2000; Piemonti *et al.*, 2000; van Halteren *et al.*, 2004) and in mouse bone marrow-derived DCs (Griffin *et al.*, 2000, 2001). These studies have consistently shown that *in vitro* treatment of DCs with VDR agonists leads to differentiation of DC function toward an immature phenotype, consisting of downregulated expression of the costimulatory molecules CD40, CD80, and CD86; the upregulation of inhibitory molecules ILT3; impaired production of Th1-polarizing cytokine IL-12; and enhanced IL-10 production, resulting in decreased T cell activation. In addition, chemotaxis in response to CCL4 and CCL19 is abrogated by VD3 treatment in DCs differentiated in the presence of type I IFN and granulocyte/macrophage colony stimulating factor (GM-CSF) (Gauzzi *et al.*, 2005). The phenotype of VD3-modulated DCs, particularly of those that are derived from human peripheral blood monocytes, is described in numerous studies and is summarized in Table 3.1.

Addition of VD3 or its analogs (either alone or in combination with other immunosuppressive/modulatory substance, e.g., glucocorticoids) to DC cultures early during their differentiation results in DCs with reduced

Table 3.1 Effects of VDR ligands on human myeloid dendritic cells

Phenotype and function affected by VDR ligands	Effects	References
Antigen uptake		
Mannose receptor-mediated endocytosis	↑	Piemonti *et al.* (2000)
Macropinocytosis	↓	Berer *et al.* (2000)
DC maturation markers		
MHC class II and costimulatory molecules (CD40, CD80, CD86)	↓	Berer *et al.* (2000), Gauzzi *et al.* (2005), Pedersen *et al.* (2009), Penna and Adorini (2000), Piemonti *et al.* (2000), Unger *et al.* (2009)
CD83	↓	Gauzzi *et al.* (2005), Pedersen *et al.* (2009), Penna and Adorini (2000), Piemonti *et al.* (2000), Unger *et al.* (2009)
Other DC/monocyte lineage markers		
CD1a	↓	Berer *et al.* (2000), Gauzzi *et al.* (2005), Pedersen *et al.* (2009),
CD14	↑	Penna and Adorini (2000), Piemonti *et al.* (2000), Unger *et al.* (2009)
Chemokine receptors		
CCR7	↓	Pedersen *et al.* (2009) and Unger *et al.* (2009)
CXCR3	↓	Unger *et al.* (2009)
Inhibitory receptors		
ILT3	↑	Manavalan *et al.* (2003), Penna *et al.* (2005, 2007)
PD-L1	↑	Unger *et al.* (2009)
IDO activity	↓	Pedersen *et al.* (2009)

Cytokine secretion		
IL-10	↑	Pedersen *et al.* (2009), Penna and Adorini (2000)
IL-12	↓	Gauzzi *et al.* (2005), Pedersen *et al.* (2009), Penna and Adorini (2000), Piemonti *et al.* (2000), Unger *et al.* (2009)
IL-23	↓	Pedersen *et al.* (2009)
Type I interferons	↓	Gauzzi *et al.* (2005)
TNF-α	↑	Unger *et al.* (2009)
Chemokine secretion		
CCL17	↓	Penna *et al.* (2007)
CCL18	↑	Vulcano *et al.* (2003)
CCL22	↑	Penna *et al.* (2007)
microRNA expression		
miR-155	↓	Pedersen *et al.* (2009)
miR-146a	↓	
Cell death (apoptosis)	↑	Penna and Adorini (2000)
T cell stimulation in vitro		
Allogeneic MLR	↓	Berer *et al.* (2000), Canning *et al.* (2001), Gauzzi *et al.* (2005), Pedersen *et al.* (2009), Penna and Adorini (2000), Piemonti *et al.* (2000), Unger *et al.* (2009)
Antigen-specific T cell responses	↓	Pedersen *et al.* (2009), van Halteren *et al.* (2004)
IFN-γ production by stimulated T cells	↓	Penna *et al.* (2007), Penna and Adorini (2000), van Halteren *et al.* (2004)

surface expression of MHC class II molecules and T cell costimulatory molecules (Berer *et al.*, 2000; Canning *et al.*, 2001; Penna and Adorini, 2000; Piemonti *et al.*, 2000). These modified DCs resist further differentiation into a mature phenotype even when exposed to strong maturation stimuli including proinflammatory cytokines, LPS or CD40L (Pedersen *et al.*, 2009; Penna and Adorini, 2000; Piemonti *et al.*, 2000). In addition, these DCs, just like immature cells, express high levels of mannose receptors and are efficient at taking up antigens (Piemonti *et al.*, 2000) and the DCs retain the cell surface expression of monocyte marker, CD14 (Berer *et al.*, 2000; Canning *et al.*, 2001; Piemonti *et al.*, 2000). While VDR is expressed early on in developing monocyte-derived DCs upon culturing monocyte in the presence of GM-CSF/IL-4 (Szeles *et al.*, 2009), VDR is continuously expressed by differentiating cells and persistent exposure to VD3 during their differentiation is crucial for maximal effect (Pedersen, unpublished data). Indeed, addition of VD3 into already differentiated DCs has only limited effect on DC phenotype (Piemonti *et al.*, 2000). The reduction in antigen presentation and T cell costimulation inarguably contribute to immunomodulation by VD3-modulated DCs by induction of T cell anergy (Morelli and Thomson, 2007).

In addition to suppression of vital receptors for effective stimulation of T cells, some studies demonstrate that VD3-modulated DCs characteristically express higher levels of inhibitory receptors, most notably, immunoglobulin-like transcript 3 (ILT3) (Chang *et al.*, 2002; Manavalan *et al.*, 2003; Penna *et al.*, 2005, 2007). ILT3 belongs to one of the two main families of ILTs, which also include ILT2, ILT4, and ILT5. They are characterized by having a cytoplasmic immunoreceptor tyrosine-based inhibitory motif (ITIM) (Colonna *et al.*, 2000). ILT3 is selectively expressed by APCs, and is involved in negative regulation of APC activation (Cella *et al.*, 1997; Ristich *et al.*, 2005). Although the exact mechanism by which ILT3 exerts its tolerogenic effect is not well understood, it has been shown to be involved in induction of regulatory T cells (Brenk *et al.*, 2009; Penna *et al.*, 2005). Other well-characterized inhibitory receptors on DCs such as programmed cell death ligand 1 (PD-L1) can also be enhanced by VD3 modulation (Unger *et al.*, 2009), which would further contribute to regulation of activated T cells (Keir *et al.*, 2007).

The microenvironment in which DCs regulate subsequent T cell differentiation is largely influenced by the cytokines that are secreted by the DCs. Thus, the impairment in producing the Th1-inducing cytokine IL-12 and the enhanced IL-10 production by VD3-modulated DCs is likely to result in dampened Th1 responses and preferential induction of Th2 responses and/or Treg differentiation (Morelli and Thomson, 2007; Steinman *et al.*, 2003). IL-23, a cytokine that contributes to Th1/Th17 differentiation and maintenance of T cells (Hunter, 2005; Langrish *et al.*, 2004), is produced upon DC maturation, but the VD3 treatment of DCs results in significant reduction of this cytokine (Pedersen *et al.*, 2009). However, the effect of this blockade on T cell function is minimal *in vitro* (Pedersen *et al.*, 2009), and the significance of the reduced IL-23 *in vivo* remains to be determined.

One of the hallmarks of DC biology is their ability to migrate: DCs sample antigens in tissues and migrate to the draining lymph nodes to stimulate T cell responses, and this process is coordinated by chemokines that interact with corresponding receptors on DCs. Circulating monocytes and immature DCs express receptors for inflammatory chemokines, CC-chemokine receptor 1 (CCR1), CCR2, CCR5, and CXC-chemokine receptor 1 (CXCR-1), CXCR2, and CXCR4. DC maturation results in the downregulation of the expression of these chemokine receptors, while the expression of a single lymphoid chemokine receptor, CCR7, is induced (Dieu *et al.*, 1998). Expression of CCR7 switches DC responsiveness to its ligands CCL19 and CCL21 that guide migration to secondary lymphoid organs (Dieu *et al.*, 1998; MartIn-Fontecha *et al.*, 2003). While the expression of chemokine receptor CCR5 on DCs is unaffected by VD3 modulation (Gauzzi *et al.*, 2005; Pedersen *et al.*, 2009), the ability of VD3-modulated DCs to migrate in response to CCL4 is largely abolished (Gauzzi *et al.*, 2005). In contrast, the inflammatory chemokine receptor CXCR3 is enhanced by VD3 (Unger *et al.*, 2009). In addition, CCR7 expression is suppressed by VD3 (Pedersen *et al.*, 2009; Unger *et al.*, 2009), although this does not appear to affect the migration of VD3-treated DCs in response to its ligand CCL21 (Unger *et al.*, 2009). This is in agreement with previous demonstration that partial DC maturation, including the upregulation of expression of MHC, is sufficient to promote DC migration (Lutz and Schuler, 2002).

DCs themselves also contribute to migration of other cell types by secreting chemokines. DCs produce large amounts of inflammatory chemokines upon exposure to maturation inducers, including MIP-1α, MIP-1β, MCP-1, MCP-2, and RANTES (Sallusto *et al.*, 1999). A study in murine mDC showed that the production of inflammatory chemokines such as MIP-1α, MIP-1β, and MCP-1 is enhanced by VD3, which contrasts the effect of another well-characterized tolerance-inducing glucocorticoid (Xing *et al.*, 2002). Interestingly, CCL18 that attracts naïve B and T cells as well as immature DCs is enhanced by VD3-modulated DCs in the absence of maturation signal (Vulcano *et al.*, 2003). Thus, this may contribute to creating microenvironments that favor differentiation of regulatory T cells or induction of T cell anergy. In addition, a number of studies (Penna *et al.*, 2007; Szeles *et al.*, 2009) showed that the production of CCL22 by DCs was enhanced by VD3 modulation. CCL22 is one of the chemokines that specifically attract Treg cells expressing CCR4, and the secretion of this chemokine is enhanced upon maturation of mDCs, thereby illustrating a mechanism to attenuate T cell activation (Iellem *et al.*, 2001; Penna *et al.*, 2007).

One of the main mechanisms underlying DC function in inducing peripheral tolerance involves the expression of indoleamine 2,3-dioxygenase (IDO) (Munn *et al.*, 2002; Penna *et al.*, 2007; Steinman *et al.*, 2003), the rate-limiting enzyme of tryptophan catabolism. The expression of IDO in DCs has been correlated with their suppression of T cell responses in numerous studies (Hwu *et al.*, 2000; Mellor and Munn, 2004; Munn *et al.*, 2002; Penna *et al.*, 2007), although the enhanced IDO activity is not observed in VD3-treated mDCs *in vitro* (Pedersen *et al.*, 2009; Unger *et al.*, 2009). However, IDO activities in VD3-DC might become important after encountering T cells, as activated Treg cells can in turn promote IDO expression in DCs (Fallarino *et al.*, 2003).

Interestingly, this functional modulation by VD3 appears to be restricted to DCs of myeloid lineage (Penna *et al.*, 2007). Direct comparison of mDC and pDC derived from human blood revealed that whereas the surface expression of MHC class II and CCR7 as well as IL-12 production was inhibited by VD3 in mDC, neither the surface molecule expression nor the cytokine/chemokine production was affected in pDC (Penna *et al.*, 2007). This was explained by the selective targeting of NF-κB by VD3 in mDC but not in pDC (Penna *et al.*, 2007). However, pDCs do respond to VDR agonists, as seen by changes in gene expression upon VD3 treatment (Adorini and Penna, 2009), but the tolerogenic function of these cells remains unaltered.

To date, the exact intracellular pathways by which VD3 exerts its phenotype and function-modifying effect on mDCs are not fully understood. However, it is likely to involve a number of pathways including interference with NF-κB signaling leading to inhibition and/or modulation of DC differentiation/maturation processes. For example, the inhibition of IL-12 production by VD3 in mature DCs is mediated by inhibition of NF-κB (D'Ambrosio *et al.*, 1998). A recent work by Szeles *et al.* that examined the impact of VD3 treatment on the transcriptome of differentiating DCs demonstrated that, in contrast to the popular belief that VD3 primarily acts as a general global inhibitor of DC differentiation and maturation, VD3 rather regulates a large set of genes involved in DC tolerogenicity, and suggests that a large part of VD3-induced DC tolerogenicity is mediated by mechanisms that are independent from inhibition of DC differentiation and maturation (Szeles *et al.*, 2009).

Taken together, multiple mechanisms contribute to VD3-DC-mediated tolerogenicity, both by cell–cell contact-dependent receptor-mediated ways and by differential secretion of cytokines and chemokines, all of which together lead to T cell anergy induction, dampening of Th1 responses, and recruitment and differentiation of Treg cells. In addition, VD3 enhances DC apoptosis following exposure to maturation stimuli (LPS) (Penna and Adorini, 2000), which may further contribute to negative regulation of T cell activation.

V. Application of VD3-Modulated DCs in Treatment of Autoimmune Diseases

Due to its immunoregulatory and immunosuppressive role of VD3, there has been increasing clinical interest for the application of VD3 in order to control immune-related disorders, including organ transplantation (Becker *et al.*, 2002; Mathieu and Badenhoop, 2005; van Etten and Mathieu, 2005; VanAmerongen *et al.*, 2004). Indeed, systemic administration of VD3 or its non-calcemic analogs to treat autoimmune diseases such as type 1 diabetes (Gregori *et al.*, 2002; Mathieu *et al.*, 1994), arthritis (Tsuji *et al.*, 1994), and EAE (Cantorna *et al.*, 1996; Mattner *et al.*, 2000; Nashold *et al.*, 2000) has shown promising results in animal models as well as in the control of allergy (Taher *et al.*, 2008) and graft rejection (Gregori *et al.*, 2001; Hullett *et al.*, 1998). Since VDR expression is widespread in the immune system, it is likely that administered VD3 influences the immune system via different cell types, including APCs and T cells, resulting in inhibition of activated autoreactive T cells, induction of tolerogenic DC, and enhanced Treg cell differentiation (reviewed in van Etten and Mathieu, 2005).

However, direct and systemic administration of VD3 also brings about undesired effects, due to high dose of VD3 that needs to be administered in order to achieve beneficial immunoregulatory effects. The side effects include hypercalcemia, hypercalciuria, renal calcification, and increased bone resorption. It is believed that the VD3 toxicity arises when the free concentration of VD3 is inappropriately high, and this depends on the capacity of circulating vitamin D-binding protein (Vieth, 2007). While many studies have described that such limitation can be overcome by a number of strategies, including the use of less calcemic analogs, lowering the VD3 dosage by combined use with synergistic immunosuppressants, or administration of VD3 together with compounds that specifically blocks the side effect (such as bone-resorption inhibitors) (reviewed in van Etten and Mathieu, 2005), a number of safety considerations for clinical use still remain.

In addition, in order to sustain the immunomodulatory effect of VD3, repeated administration might be necessary to reach desired pharmacological effect, which will inevitably be followed by increased side effects. However, to the best our knowledge, no studies so far have demonstrated the direct correlation between serum VD3 concentration and its immunological effects.

In contrast, administration of tolerogenic DCs, such as VD3-modified DCs, offers an attractive alternative approach to benefit from the immunoregulatory effect of VD3. First, treatment therapy with DCs has never been reported with serious side effects, unlike many immunosuppressive or pharmacological drugs. Second, DCs can be loaded with disease-specific antigens and thus a specific targeting of autoreactive T cells is possible, thereby minimizing undesired blockade of immune cell function. In addition, because disease-causing pathological T cells are specifically targeted, this approach has a potential to eradicate the disease, as well as a potential to be used as a prophylactic vaccination. Finally, unlike currently available therapies where frequent and repeated administration is necessary, only a few administrations of tolerogenic DCs might be necessary to establish long-lasting tolerance toward the autoantigens in question. Indeed, the efficacy of VD3-modulated mDCs used as a therapeutic vaccine has been demonstrated in numerous animal models of autoimmune diseases, reviewed extensively elsewhere (Hilkens *et al.*, 2010).

There are other approaches under development that also aim to achieve antigen-specific immunoregulation, most notably the *in vivo* targeting of DCs and adoptive transfer of immunoregulatory T cells. The former approach attempts to induce differentiation of immunoregulatory DCs *in vivo* by means of direct injection of DNA (Liu, 2003) or by the use of carrier molecules, such as liposome (Capini *et al.*, 2009; Zheng *et al.*, 2009), and specific targeting of DC receptors, such as DEC-205 (Tacken *et al.*, 2007; Zheng *et al.*, 2009). While these approaches have an obvious practical advantage of potentially becoming an off-the-shelf medicine, accurate targeting of DCs *in vivo* and ensuring the function of modulated DCs remain difficult to accomplish. In contrast, adoptive transfer of therapeutic T cells, typically achieved by extraction and *in vitro* modulation and/or selection of patients autologous T cells and subsequent administration of T cells back to the patients, has demonstrated some promising data, both in animals and in humans (Correale *et al.*, 2008; Roncarolo and Battaglia, 2007). However, the main hurdle of this technique remains the selective targeting of relevant autoreactive T cells, and as for DC-based vaccines the preparation of this type of therapy is labor-intensive.

VI. Toward Development of Clinically Applicable VD3-DCs

In principle, it should be possible to achieve clinical translation of VD3-modulated DC therapy. The methods to propagate human DCs *in vitro* have been established for over a decade (Romani *et al.*, 1994), and since the initiation of the first clinical exploration of DCs as a strategy for immunotherapeutic intervention in 1995 (Mukherji *et al.*, 1995), the number of such studies is increasing every year (Ridgway, 2003). The DC vaccine trials conducted so far have proven this approach to be safe with minimal side effects (Figdor *et al.*, 2004). In addition, *in vivo* administration of immature myeloid DCs successfully induced antigen-specific T cell tolerance in healthy human volunteers (Dhodapkar *et al.*, 2001). Thus, clinical application of tolerogenic DCs such as VD3-modulated DCs might come to pass in a near future, but some important considerations remain, which are discussed below.

Despite the evidence from animal studies where the efficacy and the safety of VD3-modulated DCs were demonstrated in many disease settings, the main concern over the clinical use of VD3-DCs (or any other form of regulatory DCs) remains the safety and stability of the function of *in vitro* modified DCs injected back into the patient. Because of the versatile function of DCs, identification of their functional phenotype and ensuring the functional stability are extremely crucial prior to administering a DC vaccine to patients. Indeed, there has been an overwhelming interest in the development and establishment of standardized quality control (QC) measure for the application of immunogenic DCs for cancer immunotherapy (Figdor *et al.*, 2004). The provision of such a QC measure, as well as a standardized means to demonstrate the functional consistency of the therapeutics, will be required during the development of clinical trials. However, in contrast to the recent effort in the QC development for immunogenic DCs, such work on clinically applicable tolerogenic DCs is still in its infancy. In fact, the major concerns over the clinical use of these DCs are the absence of clear-cut guidelines for the generation of functionally stable DCs (Xiao *et al.*, 2003) and the lack of information on molecules and markers delineating regulatory DCs.

Although functionally tolerogenic DCs described by many studies show a number of common features, such as the reduced levels of costimulatory molecules and low IL-12 production, many of these features are also shared by unmodified immature DCs which are not stable and prone to differentiate into functionally immunogenic DCs, therefore making them unreliable to use as QC markers. Furthermore, *in vitro* functional assays that can demonstrate the functional tolerogenicity of a given DC population (such as generation of T cells with suppressor activity) are labor-intensive and take several days to perform, and therefore will not be suitable for QC of tolerogenic DCs for clinical use (Petricciani *et al.*, 2007). Thus, we have attempted to find reliable and suitable markers that will be applicable for QC of future VD3-modulated DC therapy. Consistent with previous observations (Penna and Adorini, 2000; Piemonti *et al.*, 2000), VD3-modulated DCs generated from human peripheral blood monocytes exhibited a maturation-resistant phenotype after exposure to proinflammatory cytokine cocktail or LPS, induced T cell hyporesponsiveness and conferred T cells with regulatory function (Pedersen *et al.*, 2009). The functional stability of these DCs and their ability to induce T cell regulatory function were superior in VD3-treated DCs compared with that in DCs treated with IL-10, dexamethasone, or vasoactive intestinal peptides (Pedersen, unpublished data). We were unable to nail down on any single cell surface markers that could clearly distinguish VD3-modified DCs, including PD-L1 and ILT molecules that have been previously described as a marker for VD3-treated DCs (Chang *et al.*, 2002; Manavalan *et al.*, 2003; Penna *et al.*, 2007; Unger *et al.*, 2009). However, there is a set of markers that can be used to distinguish VD3-modified regulatory DCs: VD3-modified regulatory DCs consistently fail to secrete IL-23 or upregulate expression of microRNA-155 (miR-155) upon exposure to maturation stimuli (Pedersen *et al.*, 2009). These markers can be combined with widely accepted means of DC characterization, such as flow cytometry (where VD3-DCs will exhibit immature phenotype together with high CD14 and low CD1a). Importantly, these markers can be analyzed readily with standard laboratory techniques such as ELISA and RT-PCR. We also found that miR-378, whose expression has been demonstrated in a many human cancer cell lines (Jiang *et al.*, 2005) and is also involved in cell growth and survival (Lee *et al.*, 2007), was shown to be enhanced selectively by DCs modulated with VD3, but not by IL-10. However, further studies are required to determine the role of this miRNA and whether the induction of miR-378 is indeed specific for VD3 triggering.

Immunogenic DC vaccines that have been tested in clinical trials are loaded with disease-specific antigens in the form of DNA, RNA, peptides, or protein. Thus, it is interesting to note that many of the animal studies conducted so far that demonstrate the efficacy of tolerogenic DC vaccination in disease settings did not load DCs with any antigens (Creusot *et al.*, 2008; Kim *et al.*, 2001; Machen *et al.*, 2004). It is therefore possible that injected tolerogenic DCs can acquire antigens *in vivo*, resulting in an antigen-specific suppression of autoimmunity. However, administration of unloaded tolerogenic DCs could lead to untargeted tolerance induction, and therefore it is desirable that DCs to be used in human clinical settings are loaded with defined antigens. In addition, there are other variables that still need to be optimized for clinical application of tolerogenic DCs, including the timing of vaccination, frequency and route of administration (discussed further in Hilkens *et al.*, 2010). These questions, however, will remain unanswered until well-designed clinical phase I/II studies in humans are established.

VII. Conclusions

VD3-modified DCs exhibit characteristic features of tolerogenic DCs, which effectively induce immunological tolerance by suppression of T cells and induction of regulatory T cell differentiation. The major advantages of the clinical use of VD3-modified DCs over systemic administration of VD3 are the low toxicity and the ability of DCs to specifically target and tolerize autoantigen-specific T cells. By specific targeting of T cells that are central to immunopathlogy of the autoimmune diseases in question, this approach is likely to result in a more long-lasting, effective immune modulation within treated patients. One of the most important qualities of VD3-modified DCs is their functional stability, and this can be monitored by implementing a standardized QC measure before DCs are released for treatment. Human clinical studies using VD3-modified DCs are about to begin: a group lead of by Prof. Isaacs, University of Newcastle, England (Hilkens *et al.*, 2010) is starting a study in rheumatoid arthritis patients in which VD3-modified DCs (in combination with dexamethasone) will be administered intra-articularly into the affected joint. Such study will, for the first time, reveal the safety of VD3-DC in a clinical application, and will be the stepstone to future studies that examines many other important variables, such as dose and frequency of vaccination.

REFERENCES

Adorini, L., and Penna, G. (2009). Dendritic cell tolerogenicity: A key mechanism in immunomodulation by vitamin D receptor agonists. *Hum. Immunol.* **70,** 345–352.

Adorini, L., Penna, G., Giarratana, N., and Uskokovic, M. (2003). Tolerogenic dendritic cells induced by vitamin D receptor ligands enhance regulatory T cells inhibiting allograft rejection and autoimmune diseases. *J. Cell. Biochem.* **88,** 227–233.

Banchereau, J., and Steinman, R. M. (1998). Dendritic cells and the control of immunity. *Nature* **392,** 245–252.

Becker, B. N., Hullett, D. A., O'Herrin, J. K., Malin, G., Sollinger, H. W., and DeLuca, H. (2002). Vitamin D as immunomodulatory therapy for kidney transplantation. *Transplantation* **74,** 1204–1206.

Berer, A., Stockl, J., Majdic, O., Wagner, T., Kollars, M., Lechner, K., Geissler, K., and Oehler, L. (2000). 1, 25-Dihydroxyvitamin D(3) inhibits dendritic cell differentiation and maturation in vitro. *Exp. Hematol.* **28,** 575–583.

Boonstra, A., Barrat, F. J., Crain, C., Heath, V. L., Savelkoul, H. F., and O'Garra, A. (2001). 1alpha,25-Dihydroxyvitamin d3 has a direct effect on naive CD4(+) T cells to enhance the development of Th2 cells. *J. Immunol.* **167,** 4974–4980.

Brenk, M., Scheler, M., Koch, S., Neumann, J., Takikawa, O., Hacker, G., Bieber, T., and von Bubnoff, D. (2009). Tryptophan deprivation induces inhibitory receptors ILT3 and ILT4 on dendritic cells favoring the induction of human CD4+CD25+ Foxp3+ T regulatory cells. *J. Immunol.* **183,** 145–154.

Canning, M. O., Grotenhuis, K., de Wit, H., Ruwhof, C., and Drexhage, H. A. (2001). 1-alpha,25-Dihydroxyvitamin D3 (1,25(OH)(2)D(3)) hampers the maturation of fully active immature dendritic cells from monocytes. *Eur. J. Endocrinol.* **145,** 351–357.

Cantorna, M. T., Hayes, C. E., and DeLuca, H. F. (1996). 1,25-Dihydroxyvitamin D3 reversibly blocks the progression of relapsing encephalomyelitis, a model of multiple sclerosis. *Proc. Natl. Acad. Sci. USA* **93,** 7861–7864.

Capini, C., Jaturanpinyo, M., Chang, H. I., Mutalik, S., McNally, A., Street, S., Steptoe, R., O'Sullivan, B., Davies, N., and Thomas, R. (2009). Antigen-specific suppression of inflammatory arthritis using liposomes. *J. Immunol.* **182,** 3556–3565.

Cella, M., Dohring, C., Samaridis, J., Dessing, M., Brockhaus, M., Lanzavecchia, A., and Colonna, M. (1997). A novel inhibitory receptor (ILT3) expressed on monocytes, macrophages, and dendritic cells involved in antigen processing. *J. Exp. Med.* **185,** 1743–1751.

Chang, C. C., Ciubotariu, R., Manavalan, J. S., Yuan, J., Colovai, A. I., Piazza, F., Lederman, S., Colonna, M., Cortesini, R., la-Favera, R., and Suciu-Foca, N. (2002). Tolerization of dendritic cells by T(S) cells: The crucial role of inhibitory receptors ILT3 and ILT4. *Nat. Immunol.* **3,** 237–243.

Colonna, M., Nakajima, H., and Cella, M. (2000). A family of inhibitory and activating Ig-like receptors that modulate function of lymphoid and myeloid cells. *Semin. Immunol.* **12,** 121–127.

Colonna, M., Trinchieri, G., and Liu, Y. J. (2004). Plasmacytoid dendritic cells in immunity. *Nat. Immunol.* **5,** 1219–1226.

Correale, J., Farez, M., and Gilmore, W. (2008). Vaccines for multiple sclerosis: Progress to date. *CNS Drugs* **22,** 175–198.

Creusot, R. J., Yaghoubi, S. S., Kodama, K., Dang, D. N., Dang, V. H., Breckpot, K., Thielemans, K., Gambhir, S. S., and Fathman, C. G. (2008). Tissue-targeted therapy of autoimmune diabetes using dendritic cells transduced to express IL-4 in NOD mice. *Clin. Immunol.* **127,** 176–187.

D'Ambrosio, D., Cippitelli, M., Cocciolo, M. G., Mazzeo, D., Di, L. P., Lang, R., Sinigaglia, F., and Panina-Bordignon, P. (1998). Inhibition of IL-12 production by 1, 25-dihydroxyvitamin D3. Involvement of NF-kappaB downregulation in transcriptional repression of the p40 gene. *J. Clin. Invest.* **101,** 252–262.

Decallonne, B., van Etten, E., Overbergh, L., Valckx, D., Bouillon, R., and Mathieu, C. (2005). 1Alpha,25-dihydroxyvitamin D3 restores thymocyte apoptosis sensitivity in non-obese diabetic (NOD) mice through dendritic cells. *J. Autoimmun.* **24,** 281–289.

Dhodapkar, M. V., Steinman, R. M., Krasovsky, J., Munz, C., and Bhardwaj, N. (2001). Antigen-specific inhibition of effector T cell function in humans after injection of immature dendritic cells. *J. Exp. Med.* **193,** 233–238.

Dieu, M. C., Vanbervliet, B., Vicari, A., Bridon, J. M., Oldham, E., Ait-Yahia, S., Briere, F., Zlotnik, A., Lebecque, S., and Caux, C. (1998). Selective recruitment of immature and mature dendritic cells by distinct chemokines expressed in different anatomic sites. *J. Exp. Med.* **188,** 373–386.

Fallarino, F., Grohmann, U., Hwang, K. W., Orabona, C., Vacca, C., Bianchi, R., Belladonna, M. L., Fioretti, M. C., Alegre, M. L., and Puccetti, P. (2003). Modulation of tryptophan catabolism by regulatory T cells. *Nat. Immunol.* **4,** 1206–1212.

Figdor, C. G., de Vries, I. J., Lesterhuis, W. J., and Melief, C. J. (2004). Dendritic cell immunotherapy: Mapping the way. *Nat. Med.* **10,** 475–480.

Gauzzi, M. C., Purificato, C., Donato, K., Jin, Y., Wang, L., Daniel, K. C., Maghazachi, A. A., Belardelli, F., Adorini, L., and Gessani, S. (2005). Suppressive effect of 1alpha,25-dihydroxyvitamin D3 on type I IFN-mediated monocyte differentiation into dendritic cells: Impairment of functional activities and chemotaxis. *J. Immunol.* **174,** 270–276.

Gilliet, M., and Liu, Y. J. (2002). Human plasmacytoid-derived dendritic cells and the induction of T-regulatory cells. *Hum. Immunol.* **63,** 1149–1155.

Gregori, S., Casorati, M., Amuchastegui, S., Smiroldo, S., Davalli, A. M., and Adorini, L. (2001). Regulatory T cells induced by 1 alpha,25-dihydroxyvitamin D3 and mycophenolate mofetil treatment mediate transplantation tolerance. *J. Immunol.* **167,** 1945–1953.

Gregori, S., Giarratana, N., Smiroldo, S., Uskokovic, M., and Adorini, L. (2002). A 1alpha,25-dihydroxyvitamin D(3) analog enhances regulatory T-cells and arrests autoimmune diabetes in NOD mice. *Diabetes* **51,** 1367–1374.

Griffin, M. D., Lutz, W. H., Phan, V. A., Bachman, L. A., McKean, D. J., and Kumar, R. (2000). Potent inhibition of dendritic cell differentiation and maturation by vitamin D analogs. *Biochem. Biophys. Res. Commun.* **270,** 701–708.

Griffin, M. D., Lutz, W., Phan, V. A., Bachman, L. A., McKean, D. J., and Kumar, R. (2001). Dendritic cell modulation by 1alpha,25 dihydroxyvitamin D3 and its analogs: A vitamin D receptor-dependent pathway that promotes a persistent state of immaturity in vitro and in vivo. *Proc. Natl. Acad. Sci. USA* **98,** 6800–6805.

Hewison, M., Freeman, L., Hughes, S. V., Evans, K. N., Bland, R., Eliopoulos, A. G., Kilby, M. D., Moss, P. A., and Chakraverty, R. (2003). Differential regulation of vitamin D receptor and its ligand in human monocyte-derived dendritic cells. *J. Immunol.* **170,** 5382–5390.

Hilkens, C. M., Isaacs, J. D., and Thomson, A. W. (2010). Development of dendritic cell-based immunotherapy for autoimmunity. *Int. Rev. Immunol.* **29,** 156–183.

Hullett, D. A., Cantorna, M. T., Redaelli, C., Humpal-Winter, J., Hayes, C. E., Sollinger, H. W., and DeLuca, H. F. (1998). Prolongation of allograft survival by 1,25-dihydroxyvitamin D3. *Transplantation* **66,** 824–828.

Hunter, C. A. (2005). New IL-12-family members: IL-23 and IL-27, cytokines with divergent functions. *Nat. Rev. Immunol.* **5,** 521–531.

Hwu, P., Du, M. X., Lapointe, R., Do, M., Taylor, M. W., and Young, H. A. (2000). Indoleamine 2,3-dioxygenase production by human dendritic cells results in the inhibition of T cell proliferation. *J. Immunol.* **164,** 3596–3599.

Iellem, A., Mariani, M., Lang, R., Recalde, H., Panina-Bordignon, P., Sinigaglia, F., and D'Ambrosio, D. (2001). Unique chemotactic response profile and specific expression of chemokine receptors CCR4 and CCR8 by CD4(+)CD25(+) regulatory T cells. *J. Exp. Med.* **194,** 847–853.

Jiang, J., Lee, E. J., Gusev, Y., and Schmittgen, T. D. (2005). Real-time expression profiling of microRNA precursors in human cancer cell lines. *Nucleic Acids Res.* **33,** 5394–5403.

Jonuleit, H., Schmitt, E., Schuler, G., Knop, J., and Enk, A. H. (2000). Induction of interleukin 10-producing, nonproliferating CD4(+) T cells with regulatory properties by repetitive stimulation with allogeneic immature human dendritic cells. *J. Exp. Med.* **192,** 1213–1222.

Kadowaki, N., and Liu, Y. J. (2002). Natural type I interferon-producing cells as a link between innate and adaptive immunity. *Hum. Immunol.* **63,** 1126–1132.

Keir, M. E., Francisco, L. M., and Sharpe, A. H. (2007). PD-1 and its ligands in T-cell immunity. *Curr. Opin. Immunol.* **19,** 309–314.

Kim, S. H., Kim, S., Evans, C. H., Ghivizzani, S. C., Oligino, T., and Robbins, P. D. (2001). Effective treatment of established murine collagen-induced arthritis by systemic administration of dendritic cells genetically modified to express IL-4. *J. Immunol.* **166,** 3499–3505.

Langrish, C. L., McKenzie, B. S., Wilson, N. J., de Waal, M. R., Kastelein, R. A., and Cua, D. J. (2004). IL-12 and IL-23: Master regulators of innate and adaptive immunity. *Immunol. Rev.* **202,** 96–105.

Lee, D. Y., Deng, Z., Wang, C. H., and Yang, B. B. (2007). microRNA-378 promotes cell survival, tumor growth, and angiogenesis by targeting SuFu and Fus-1 expression. *Proc. Natl. Acad. Sci. USA* **104,** 20350–20355.

Levings, M. K., Gregori, S., Tresoldi, E., Cazzaniga, S., Bonini, C., and Roncarolo, M. G. (2005). Differentiation of Tr1 cells by immature dendritic cells requires IL-10 but not CD25+CD4+ Tr cells. *Blood* **105,** 1162–1169.

Li, L., Sun, S., Cao, X., Wang, Y., Chang, L., and Yin, X. (2005). Experimental study on induction of tolerance to experimental autoimmune myasthenia gravis by immature dendritic cells. *J. Huazhong. Univ. Sci. Technolog. Med. Sci.* **25,** 215–218.

Liu, M. A. (2003). DNA vaccines: A review. *J. Intern. Med.* **253,** 402–410.

Lu, L., McCaslin, D., Starzl, T. E., and Thomson, A. W. (1995). Bone marrow-derived dendritic cell progenitors (NLDC 145+, MHC class II+, B7-1dim, B7-2−) induce alloantigen-specific hyporesponsiveness in murine T lymphocytes. *Transplantation* **60,** 1539–1545.

Lutz, M. B., and Schuler, G. (2002). Immature, semi-mature and fully mature dendritic cells: Which signals induce tolerance or immunity? *Trends Immunol.* **23,** 445–449.

Lutz, M. B., Suri, R. M., Niimi, M., Ogilvie, A. L., Kukutsch, N. A., Rossner, S., Schuler, G., and Austyn, J. M. (2000). Immature dendritic cells generated with low doses of GM-CSF in the absence of IL-4 are maturation resistant and prolong allograft survival in vivo. *Eur. J. Immunol.* **30,** 1813–1822.

Machen, J., Harnaha, J., Lakomy, R., Styche, A., Trucco, M., and Giannoukakis, N. (2004). Antisense oligonucleotides down-regulating costimulation confer diabetes-preventive properties to nonobese diabetic mouse dendritic cells. *J. Immunol.* **173,** 4331–4341.

Manavalan, J. S., Rossi, P. C., Vlad, G., Piazza, F., Yarilina, A., Cortesini, R., Mancini, D., and Suciu-Foca, N. (2003). High expression of ILT3 and ILT4 is a general feature of tolerogenic dendritic cells. *Transpl. Immunol.* **11,** 245–258.

MartIn-Fontecha, A., Sebastiani, S., Hopken, U. E., Uguccioni, M., Lipp, M., Lanzavecchia, A., and Sallusto, F. (2003). Regulation of dendritic cell migration to the draining lymph node: Impact on T lymphocyte traffic and priming. *J. Exp. Med.* **198,** 615–621.

Mathieu, C., and Badenhoop, K. (2005). Vitamin D and type 1 diabetes mellitus: State of the art. *Trends Endocrinol. Metab.* **16,** 261–266.

Mathieu, C., Waer, M., Laureys, J., Rutgeerts, O., and Bouillon, R. (1994). Prevention of autoimmune diabetes in NOD mice by 1,25 dihydroxyvitamin D3. *Diabetologia* **37,** 552–558.

Mattner, F., Smiroldo, S., Galbiati, F., Muller, M., Di, L. P., Poliani, P. L., Martino, G., Panina-Bordignon, P., and Adorini, L. (2000). Inhibition of Th1 development and treatment of chronic-relapsing experimental allergic encephalomyelitis by a non-hypercalcemic analogue of 1,25-dihydroxyvitamin D(3). *Eur. J. Immunol.* **30,** 498–508.

Mellor, A. L., and Munn, D. H. (2004). IDO expression by dendritic cells: Tolerance and tryptophan catabolism. *Nat. Rev. Immunol.* **4,** 762–774.

Morelli, A. E., and Thomson, A. W. (2007). Tolerogenic dendritic cells and the quest for transplant tolerance. *Nat. Rev. Immunol.* **7,** 610–621.

Moseman, E. A., Liang, X., Dawson, A. J., Panoskaltsis-Mortari, A., Krieg, A. M., Liu, Y. J., Blazar, B. R., and Chen, W. (2004). Human plasmacytoid dendritic cells activated by CpG oligodeoxynucleotides induce the generation of CD4+CD25+ regulatory T cells. *J. Immunol.* **173,** 4433–4442.

Mukherji, B., Chakraborty, N. G., Yamasaki, S., Okino, T., Yamase, H., Sporn, J. R., Kurtzman, S. K., Ergin, M. T., Ozols, J., Meehan, J., *et al.* (1995). Induction of antigen-specific cytolytic T cells in situ in human melanoma by immunization with synthetic peptide-pulsed autologous antigen presenting cells. *Proc. Natl. Acad. Sci. USA* **92,** 8078–8082.

Munn, D. H., Sharma, M. D., Lee, J. R., Jhaver, K. G., Johnson, T. S., Keskin, D. B., Marshall, B., Chandler, P., Antonia, S. J., Burgess, R., Slingluff, C. L., Jr., and Mellor, A. L. (2002). Potential regulatory function of human dendritic cells expressing indoleamine 2,3-dioxygenase. *Science* **297,** 1867–1870.

Nashold, F. E., Miller, D. J., and Hayes, C. E. (2000). 1,25-Dihydroxyvitamin D3 treatment decreases macrophage accumulation in the CNS of mice with experimental autoimmune encephalomyelitis. *J. Neuroimmunol.* **103,** 171–179.

Pedersen, A. W., Holmstrom, K., Jensen, S. S., Fuchs, D., Rasmussen, S., Kvistborg, P., Claesson, M. H., and Zocca, M. B. (2009). Phenotypic and functional markers for

1alpha,25-dihydroxyvitamin D(3)-modified regulatory dendritic cells. *Clin. Exp. Immunol.* **157,** 48–59.
Penna, G., and Adorini, L. (2000). 1 Alpha,25-dihydroxyvitamin D3 inhibits differentiation, maturation, activation, and survival of dendritic cells leading to impaired alloreactive T cell activation. *J. Immunol.* **164,** 2405–2411.
Penna, G., Roncari, A., Amuchastegui, S., Daniel, K. C., Berti, E., Colonna, M., and Adorini, L. (2005). Expression of the inhibitory receptor ILT3 on dendritic cells is dispensable for induction of CD4+Foxp3+ regulatory T cells by 1, 25-dihydroxyvitamin D3. *Blood* **106,** 3490–3497.
Penna, G., Amuchastegui, S., Giarratana, N., Daniel, K. C., Vulcano, M., Sozzani, S., and Adorini, L. (2007). 1,25-Dihydroxyvitamin D3 selectively modulates tolerogenic properties in myeloid but not plasmacytoid dendritic cells. *J. Immunol.* **178,** 145–153.
Petricciani, J., Egan, W., Vicari, G., Furesz, J., and Schild, G. (2007). Potency assays for therapeutic live whole cell cancer vaccines. *Biologicals* **35,** 107–113.
Piemonti, L., Monti, P., Sironi, M., Fraticelli, P., Leone, B. E., Dal Cin, E., Allavena, P., and Di Carlo, V. (2000). Vitamin D3 affects differentiation, maturation, and function of human monocyte-derived dendritic cells. *J. Immunol.* **164,** 4443–4451.
Reichel, H., Koeffler, H. P., Bishop, J. E., and Norman, A. W. (1987). 25-Hydroxyvitamin D3 metabolism by lipopolysaccharide-stimulated normal human macrophages. *J. Clin. Endocrinol. Metab.* **64,** 1–9.
Ridgway, D. (2003). The first 1000 dendritic cell vaccines. *Cancer Invest.* **21,** 873–886.
Rissoan, M. C., Soumelis, V., Kadowaki, N., Grouard, G., Briere, F., de Waal, M. R., and Liu, Y. J. (1999). Reciprocal control of T helper cell and dendritic cell differentiation. *Science* **283,** 1183–1186.
Ristich, V., Liang, S., Zhang, W., Wu, J., and Horuzsko, A. (2005). Tolerization of dendritic cells by HLA-G. *Eur. J. Immunol.* **35,** 1133–1142.
Romani, N., Gruner, S., Brang, D., Kampgen, E., Lenz, A., Trockenbacher, B., Konwalinka, G., Fritsch, P. O., Steinman, R. M., and Schuler, G. (1994). Proliferating dendritic cell progenitors in human blood. *J. Exp. Med.* **180,** 83–93.
Roncarolo, M. G., and Battaglia, M. (2007). Regulatory T-cell immunotherapy for tolerance to self antigens and alloantigens in humans. *Nat. Rev. Immunol.* **7,** 585–598.
Sallusto, F., Palermo, B., Lenig, D., Miettinen, M., Matikainen, S., Julkunen, I., Forster, R., Burgstahler, R., Lipp, M., and Lanzavecchia, A. (1999). Distinct patterns and kinetics of chemokine production regulate dendritic cell function. *Eur. J. Immunol.* **29,** 1617–1625.
Schrader, M., Bendik, I., Becker-Andre, M., and Carlberg, C. (1993). Interaction between retinoic acid and vitamin D signaling pathways. *J. Biol. Chem.* **268,** 17830–17836.
Sigmundsdottir, H., Pan, J., Debes, G. F., Alt, C., Habtezion, A., Soler, D., and Butcher, E. C. (2007). DCs metabolize sunlight-induced vitamin D3 to 'program' T cell attraction to the epidermal chemokine CCL27. *Nat. Immunol.* **8,** 285–293.
Steinman, R. M., and Nussenzweig, M. C. (2002). Avoiding horror autotoxicus: The importance of dendritic cells in peripheral T cell tolerance. *Proc. Natl. Acad. Sci. USA* **99,** 351–358.
Steinman, R. M., Turley, S., Mellman, I., and Inaba, K. (2000). The induction of tolerance by dendritic cells that have captured apoptotic cells. *J. Exp. Med.* **191,** 411–416.
Steinman, R. M., Hawiger, D., and Nussenzweig, M. C. (2003). Tolerogenic dendritic cells. *Annu. Rev. Immunol.* **21,** 685–711.
Steptoe, R. J., Ritchie, J. M., Jones, L. K., and Harrison, L. C. (2005). Autoimmune diabetes is suppressed by transfer of proinsulin-encoding Gr-1+ myeloid progenitor cells that differentiate in vivo into resting dendritic cells. *Diabetes* **54,** 434–442.
Szeles, L., Keresztes, G., Torocsik, D., Balajthy, Z., Krenacs, L., Poliska, S., Steinmeyer, A., Zuegel, U., Pruenster, M., Rot, A., and Nagy, L. (2009). 1,25-Dihydroxyvitamin D3 is

an autonomous regulator of the transcriptional changes leading to a tolerogenic dendritic cell phenotype. *J. Immunol.* **182,** 2074–2083.

Tacken, P. J., de Vries, I. J., Torensma, R., and Figdor, C. G. (2007). Dendritic-cell immunotherapy: From ex vivo loading to in vivo targeting. *Nat. Rev. Immunol.* **7,** 790–802.

Taher, Y. A., van Esch, B. C., Hofman, G. A., Henricks, P. A., and van Oosterhout, A. J. (2008). 1alpha,25-dihydroxyvitamin D3 potentiates the beneficial effects of allergen immunotherapy in a mouse model of allergic asthma: Role for IL-10 and TGF-beta. *J. Immunol.* **180,** 5211–5221.

Takeuchi, A., Reddy, G. S., Kobayashi, T., Okano, T., Park, J., and Sharma, S. (1998). Nuclear factor of activated T cells (NFAT) as a molecular target for 1alpha,25-dihydroxyvitamin D3-mediated effects. *J. Immunol.* **160,** 209–218.

Tsuji, M., Fujii, K., Nakano, T., and Nishii, Y. (1994). 1 Alpha-hydroxyvitamin D3 inhibits type II collagen-induced arthritis in rats. *FEBS Lett.* **337,** 248–250.

Unger, W. W., Laban, S., Kleijwegt, F. S., van der Slik, A. R., and Roep, B. O. (2009). Induction of Treg by monocyte-derived DC modulated by vitamin D3 or dexamethasone: Differential role for PD-L1. *Eur. J. Immunol.* **39,** 3147–3159.

van Etten, E., and Mathieu, C. (2005). Immunoregulation by 1,25-dihydroxyvitamin D3: Basic concepts. *J. Steroid Biochem. Mol. Biol.* **97,** 93–101.

van Halteren, A. G., Tysma, O. M., van Etten, E., Mathieu, C., and Roep, B. O. (2004). 1alpha,25-dihydroxyvitamin D3 or analogue treated dendritic cells modulate human autoreactive T cells via the selective induction of apoptosis. *J. Autoimmun.* **23,** 233–239.

VanAmerongen, B. M., Dijkstra, C. D., Lips, P., and Polman, C. H. (2004). Multiple sclerosis and vitamin D: An update. *Eur. J. Clin. Nutr.* **58,** 1095–1109.

Veldman, C. M., Cantorna, M. T., and DeLuca, H. F. (2000). Expression of 1,25-dihydroxyvitamin D(3) receptor in the immune system. *Arch. Biochem. Biophys.* **374,** 334–338.

Vieth, R. (2007). Vitamin D toxicity, policy, and science. *J. Bone Miner. Res.* **22**(Suppl 2), V64–V68.

Vulcano, M., Struyf, S., Scapini, P., Cassatella, M., Bernasconi, S., Bonecchi, R., Calleri, A., Penna, G., Adorini, L., Luini, W., Mantovani, A., Van Damme, J., *et al.* (2003). Unique regulation of CCL18 production by maturing dendritic cells. *J. Immunol.* **170,** 3843–3849.

Xiao, B. G., Huang, Y. M., and Link, H. (2003). Dendritic cell vaccine design: Strategies for eliciting peripheral tolerance as therapy of autoimmune diseases. *BioDrugs* **17,** 103–111.

Xing, N., ML, L. M., Bachman, L. A., McKean, D. J., Kumar, R., and Griffin, M. D. (2002). Distinctive dendritic cell modulation by vitamin D(3) and glucocorticoid pathways. *Biochem. Biophys. Res. Commun.* **297,** 645–652.

Zella, J. B., and DeLuca, H. F. (2003). Vitamin D and autoimmune diabetes. *J. Cell. Biochem.* **88,** 216–222.

Zheng, X., Vladau, C., Zhang, X., Suzuki, M., Ichim, T. E., Zhang, Z. X., Li, M., Carrier, E., Garcia, B., Jevnikar, A. M., and Min, W. P. (2009). A novel in vivo siRNA delivery system specifically targeting dendritic cells and silencing CD40 genes for immunomodulation. *Blood* **113,** 2646–2654.

CHAPTER FOUR

Retinoic Acid, Immunity, and Inflammation

Chang H. Kim

Contents

Abstract

Vitamin A (also called retinol), absorbed in the intestine and stored mainly in the liver and fat, is normally maintained at significant concentrations in the human blood plasma. Vitamin A is constitutively metabolized at high levels in certain tissues such as the small intestine and eyes. Retinoic acid (RA) produced at high levels in the intestine plays important roles in mucosal immunity and immune tolerance. RA at basal levels is required for immune cell survival and activation. During immune responses, enzymes metabolizing vitamin A are induced in certain types of immune cells such as dendritic cells (DCs) and tissue cells for induced production of RA. As a result, induced gradients of RA are formed during immune responses in the body. RA regulates gene expression, differentiation, and function of diverse immune cells. The cells under the influence of RA in terms of differentiation include myeloid cells such as neutrophils, macrophages, and DCs. Also included

Laboratory of Immunology and Hematopoiesis, Department of Comparative Pathobiology, School of Veterinary Medicine and Center for Cancer Research, Purdue University, West Lafayette, Indiana, USA

Vitamins and Hormones, Volume 86
ISSN 0083-6729, DOI: 10.1016/B978-0-12-386960-9.00004-6

are lymphoid cells such as effector T cells, regulatory T cells, and B cells. Our current understanding of the function of RA in regulation of these immune cells is reviewed in this chapter.

Abbreviations

9cRA	9-*cis* retinoic acid
At-RA	all-*trans* retinoic acid
DC	dendritic cells
GALT	gut-associated lymphoid tissues
IEL	intraepithelial lymphocytes
ILF	isolated lymphoid follicles
LP	lamina propria
LPL	lamina propria lymphocytes
LPS	lipopolysaccharide
M cells	microfold cells
PP	Peyer's patches
RAR	retinoic acid nuclear receptor
SC	secretory component
TLR	toll-like receptor

I. Introduction

Vitamin A is an essential factor in regulation of key biological processes including embryo development, vision, and immune responses (Napoli, 1996b). Vitamin A deficiency (VAD) is associated with defective embryo development, and decreased vision and immunity after birth. This is because vitamin A metabolites serve as ligands for nuclear receptors that play critical roles in gene expression in a broad range of cell types. All-*trans* retinoic acid (At-RA) is a major ligand for retinoic acid nuclear receptors (RARs) and 9-*cis* retinoic acid (9cRA) is a major ligand for retinoid X receptors (RXRs) (Napoli, 1996a). Additionally, 11-*cis*-retinal in rhodopsins serves as the photon receptor in the retina. Recently, we have witnessed a significant progress in the research on the roles of vitamin A and its metabolites in the immune system. Immune cells often adopt different forms depending on the tissue environment of cell differentiation. Vitamin A metabolites are major players in regulating immune cell differentiation. I will discuss the basic features of vitamin A metabolites in the next section and review their detailed functions in the immune system in the rest parts of this chapter.

II. Overview of Vitamin A Metabolism and Function

Retinol is absorbed into epithelial cells after hydrolysis from its precursor form, retinyl ester (Fig. 4.1). β-Carotene, called provitamin A, is converted to retinal by carotene monooxygenase 1 in epithelial cells (Hessel *et al.*, 2007). Retinol is esterified and then packaged into chylomicrons in enterocytes for transportation to the liver. It is esterified again and stored in the liver stellate cells. Retinol is stored also in fat cells. Retinol is metabolized into retinal and then to biologically active retinoic acids (RAs) by sequential action of alcohol dehydrogenases (ADHs) and retinaldehyde dehydrogenase (RALDH1–3)

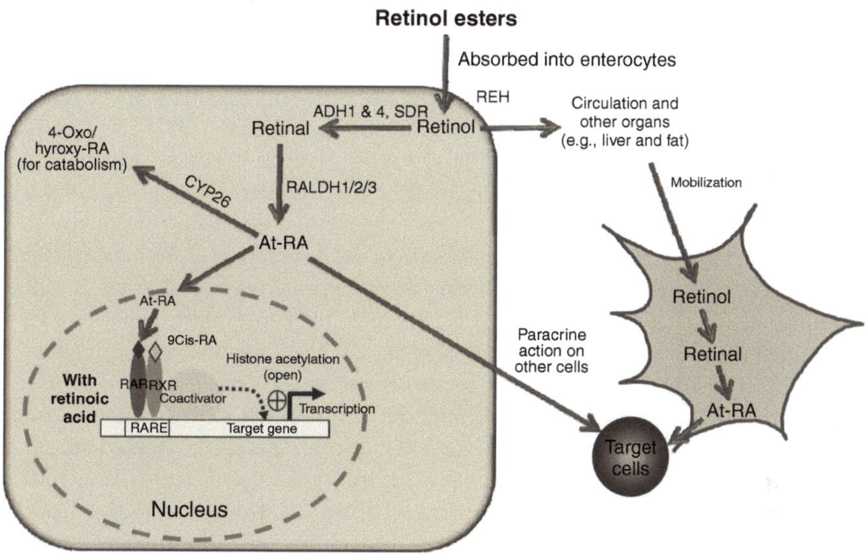

Figure 4.1 *Metabolism and basic action mechanisms of retinoic acid.* Retinol is absorbed into enterocytes and transported into the liver in chylomicrons. Retinols and retinoids in the body are found as complexes with carrier proteins such as retinol binding protein (RBP) in blood and cellular RBP within cells. Retinol is metabolized into retinaldehyde by alcohol dehydrogenase (ADH) or short-chain dehydrogenase/reductase (SDR). Retinaldehyde is metabolized into retinoic acid (At-RA) by retinaldehyde dehydrogenases (RALDH). There are three types of RALDH proteins encoded by different genes (i.e. RALDH1, 2, and 3) and with different patterns of expression. Intestinal epithelial cells and dendritic cells constitutively express RALDH to produce RA. At-RA and its isoform 9-*cis*-RA activate RAR–RXR heterodimers which specifically bind retinoic acid response elements (RAREs) on chromosomes for regulation of gene expression. Receptor activation is necessary to recruit the coactivator and histone acetyltransferase complex to open the chromatin for initiation of gene transcription. RA, produced in certain cell types, can be secreted out of the cells for paracrine action as well as for autocrine action within the same cells. RA can be catabolized into 4-oxo or hydroxy-RA for degradation. (See Color Insert.)

within cells (Duester, 2000). Gut epithelial cells and activated dendritic cells (DCs) are rich with RALDHs and are efficient in production of RA (Duester, 2000; Iwata *et al.*, 2004). It is notable that RA production is induced during immune responses, which is possible through the induction of RALDHs in DCs and tissue cells in response to certain cytokines and toll-like receptor ligands (Elgueta *et al.*, 2008; Manicassamy *et al.*, 2009; Molenaar *et al.*, 2009; Szatmari *et al.*, 2006; Vermot *et al.*, 2000; Yokota *et al.*, 2009). Production of vitamin A metabolites such as At-RA and 9cRA is developmentally regulated in space and time and is critically linked to the initiation of retinoid signal transduction during the embryonic development (Clagett-Dame and DeLuca, 2002; Zile, 1998). They comprehensively regulate the development of the heart, the central nervous system, the circulatory system, the urogenital system, the respiratory system, the skeletal system, and the limbs (Zile, 2001).

Vitamin A deficiency leads insufficient production of rhodopsin, causing night blindness. Another common problem in the eye in vitamin A deficiency is xerophthalmia, with symptoms such as inability to produce tear due to inadequate function of the lacrimal glands and thinning and perforation of the cornea (Sommer, 1998). The disease, caused by RA, but not retinal, deficiency, accompanies keratinization of the tissue and infiltration with inflammatory cells. This suggests that the inflammatory component is an important part of the disease.

It has long been observed that vitamin A deficiency is associated with increased susceptibility to infection at mucosal tissues (Semba, 1994; Stephensen, 2001; West *et al.*, 1989). Vitamin A supplementation has beneficial effects on tissue inflammation (Aukrust *et al.*, 2000; Vladutiu and Cringulescu, 1968). Decreased immunity to pathogens is associated with defective production of the mucosal antibody IgA and defective expression of gut-homing receptors by T and B cells (Iwata *et al.*, 2004; Mora *et al.*, 2006; Tokuyama and Tokuyama, 1993, 1999). RA steers the differentiation of T and B cells in the direction to promote both immunity and immune tolerance (Kim, 2008). Induction of immune tolerance by RA is through several different mechanisms including induction of $FoxP3^+$ T cells (Benson *et al.*, 2007; Coombes *et al.*, 2007; Elias *et al.*, 2008; Jaensson *et al.*, 2008; Kang *et al.*, 2007; Sun *et al.*, 2007). Enhancement of immunity is mediated, in part, through its action on production of phagocytes and regulation of the effector lymphocyte trafficking (Kim, 2008; Mora and von Andrian, 2009; Ongsakul *et al.*, 1985).

III. RA in Regulation of Myeloid Cell Development

RA regulates expression of a number of genes through RAR-α, β, and γ and RXR-α, β, and γ receptors. RAR and RXR form heterodimers which assume the active holoenzyme conformation upon RAR occupancy with

RA (Napoli, 1996a). Retinoid receptor-deficient mice provided useful information regarding the role of RA in differentiation of myeloid cells. In RAR-α/γ double knockout mice, differentiation of bone marrow cells is abnormal in that hematopoietic cells cannot maturate beyond myelocyte/metamyelocyte stages (Labrecque *et al.*, 1998). In RAR-α or γ single knockout mice, however, the differentiation of myeloid cells is apparently normal, suggesting that both isoforms of RARs have redundant roles in the process. In this regard, these receptors are expressed by myeloid cells in the bone marrow. Moreover, a similar defect in myeloid cell differentiation occurs in vitamin A-deficient mice. In vitamin A deficiency, immature GR-1^+ Mac-1^+ myeloid cells are greatly increased in the bone marrow, spleen, and peripheral blood. This abnormal increase in immature myeloid cells can be reversed upon vitamin A supplementation (Kuwata *et al.*, 2000). The fact that many of the GR-1^+ Mac-1^+ myeloid cells in vitamin A-deficient animals undergo spontaneous apoptosis suggests that vitamin A metabolites are required for survival of myeloid cells in the marrow and peripheral tissues. Also, RA controls the cell division of myeloid cells and it was noted that proliferation of myeloid cells is decreased in the presence of RA (Goldman, 1984). Instead, the myeloid cells undergo terminal differentiation into fully mature phagocytes in response to RA. In summary, vitamin A is required for survival and terminal differentiation of myeloid cells. In this regard, At-RA is being used to treat acute promyelocytic leukemia, which is characterized by fusion of promyelocytic leukemia gene (PML) and *RAR*α genes due to chromosomal translocations (Gillard and Solomon, 1993) (Fig. 4.2).

Another phagocyte subset that is profoundly affected by RA is the DC, which is a major subset of antigen presenting cells. Following phagocytosis or infection by pathogens, DCs undergo maturation and migrate to secondary lymphoid tissues for presentation of antigens on major histocompatibility complex (MHC) class I or class II molecules to T cells. DCs originate from monocytes or immature progenitor cells made in the marrow. Myeloid progenitor cells undergo maturation in the periphery to become DCs. DCs are highly heterogeneous in phenotype and function (Banchereau *et al.*, 2003; Gilliet *et al.*, 2008; Ito *et al.*, 2005). DCs are divided largely into myeloid DCs and plasmacytoid DCs. These two DC subsets are different in recognition of microbial pathogens and also in the function to induce innate and adaptive immune responses. Myeloid DCs regulate T cell responses through the production of a number of cytokines and cell surface regulatory molecules. Myeloid DCs produce interleukin (IL)-12, OX40 ligand, inducible costimulator (ICOS) ligand, IL-6, and/or IL-23, and regulate effector (Th1, Th2, and Th17) and suppressor (FoxP3$^+$ cells and Tr1) T cell responses (Penna *et al.*, 2002). Plasmacytoid DCs are highly efficient in production of type I interferons, which is important for antiviral immunity (Naik *et al.*, 2005). RA is known to affect the differentiation of myeloid DCs. The effect of RA on plasmacytoid DCs, however, has not been determined.

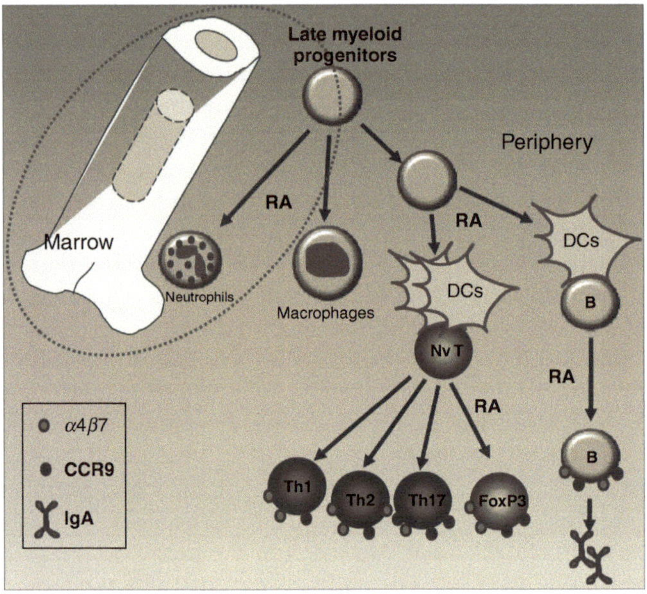

Figure 4.2 *Key functions of retinoic acid in the immune system.* In the bone marrow, RA is required for terminal differentiation of myeloid cells such as neutrophils. Therefore, RA is required to maintain optimal phagocytic activities. Myeloid progenitor cells, migrated out to the periphery, become dendritic cells. RA acts on these differentiating dendritic cells and turn them into FoxP3$^+$ T cell-inducing tolerogenic DCs. When T cells are antigen-primed in the presence of RA at high enough concentrations (~10 nM), T cells become effector T cell such as Th1, Th2, and Th17 cells that express CCR9 and α4β7, the two gut-homing receptors. It requires higher concentrations of RA to upregulate CCR9 than that required for α4β7. These T cells play important roles in formation of immunity in the intestine and potentially other tissues as well. Certain mucosal DCs can produce RA and activate B cells for generation of IgA-producing B cells. RA helps induce both effector and regulatory (suppressive) lymphocytes. This is to assure immune tolerance on one hand and prevention of inflammatory diseases on the other hand. The intestine is a good example of tissues where the RA action is required because commensal bacteria constantly provide stimulatory signals for the immune system and can be inflammatory without appropriate tolerance mechanisms. (See Color Insert.)

Retinoids regulate apoptosis and maturation of DCs (Geissmann *et al.*, 2003). RA promotes DC apoptosis through the RA receptor RARα. In the presence of inflammatory cytokines, RA increases MHC class II and costimulatory molecule expression on DCs and induces their maturation. Interestingly, this maturation of DCs is mediated via an RXR-dependent, but RAR-independent, pathway. Human monocytes-derived DCs, differentiated in the presence of granulocyte/macrophage colony-stimulating factor (GM-CSF) and At-RA, preferentially become IL-12 producers (Mohty *et al.*, 2003). It was demonstrated in a study that At-RA or 9-*cis*-RA in collaboration with GM-CSF promotes the generation of DCs and suppresses their differentiation into granulocytes (Hengesbach and Hoag, 2004). This group noted that MHC class II expression was decreased, whereas the expression of costimulatory molecules such as CD86 was increased by RA. Unlike adult blood cells, At-RA-treated umbilical cord blood monocyte-derived DCs showed a reduced capacity to activate alloreactive T cells compared to control cells with the tendency to induce Th2 cells and decreased secretion of IL-12 and interferon-γ (IFN-γ) but increased production of IL-10 and IL-4 (Tao *et al.*, 2006). It has been reported that 9-*cis*-RA interfered with the differentiation of human monocytes into DCs, and the DCs treated with 9-*cis*-RA preferentially produced IL-10 over IL-12 (Zapata-Gonzalez *et al.*, 2007). In summary, RA profoundly affects the maturation process of DCs, and the exact outcome is determined by the types of progenitor cells and RA and the presence of other factors such as inflammatory cytokines.

In addition to regulation of apoptosis and maturation of DCs, RA induces a specialized DC subset in mucosal tissues. Human monocyte-derived DCs pretreated with At-RA can secrete TGF-β and IL-6. These DCs can induce gut-homing receptors and IgA responses in cocultured B cells (Saurer *et al.*, 2007). The DCs, differentiated in the presence of RA, display the phenotype of certain DCs present in the intestine. These DCs can induce gut-homing receptors such as CCR9 and $\alpha4\beta7$ on T and B cells (Jaensson *et al.*, 2008; Yang *et al.*, 2006). DCs in the small intestine and mesenteric lymph nodes have the ability to produce RA (Iwata *et al.*, 2004). It has been reported that IL-4 can induce retinaldehyde dehydrogenases (RALDHs), the enzymes required for synthesis of RA, in the DCs present in mesenteric lymph nodes (Elgueta *et al.*, 2008). Another notable feature of these DCs is their ability to induce FoxP3$^+$ T cells. The DCs in the lamina propria of small intestine are highly efficient in induction of FoxP3$^+$ T cells, and this induction is dependent on the RA produced by the DCs (Zapata-Gonzalez *et al.*, 2007). The FoxP3 cell induction ability of RA is important to promote immune tolerance in the intestine and other tissues.

Retinoid deficiency induces an unusual subset of DCs in the mesenteric lymph nodes and intestinal lamina propria (Chang *et al.*, 2009). These DCs express langerin (CD207), which is expressed by some DCs in skin-draining lymph nodes and Langerhans cells in the skin epidermis. These DCs have an enhanced ability to induce Th17 cells but a decreased ability to induce FoxP3$^+$ regulatory T cells. Despite their poor ability to induce FoxP3$^+$ T cells, langerin$^+$ DCs induced in vitamin A deficiency appear to contribute to immune tolerance in response to oral antigens. The function of langerin$^+$ DCs in induction of tolerance, however, is disputed because not all langerin$^+$ cells are the DCs induced in vitamin A deficiency and vice versa. Langerin$^+$ DCs are also induced in MLN following topical transcutaneous immunization and involved in the IgA response (Chang *et al.*, 2008). It is unclear if the DCs induced in vitamin A deficiency and following topical transcutaneous immunization are the same or different cell populations. The exact function of these DCs in regulation of immune responses and inflammation remains to be determined.

IV. RA and Effector T Cells

A. Is RA required for the Th1 or Th2 response?

Naïve T cells differentiate into effector T cells such as Th1 cells and Th2 cells in secondary lymphoid tissues in response antigenic stimulation. Th1 cells produce IFN-γ and play important roles in regulation of cell-mediated immunity and certain types of antibody responses required for mounting effective antimicrobial immunity. Th2 cells, however, produce IL-4, IL-5, and IL-13, and regulate IgG4 (in human)/IgE-oriented antibody responses required for effective clearance of helminthes and extracellular pathogens. It has long been observed that the function and differentiation of T cells in response to antigens are altered in VAD (Carman *et al.*, 1989). T cell differentiation into Th1 cells is enhanced, while that to Th2 cells is decreased in vitamin A deficiency. In this regard, it was shown *in vitro* that RA can increase production of IL-4 by T cells (Cantorna *et al.*, 1994; Dawson *et al.*, 2006; Hoag *et al.*, 2002; Iwata *et al.*, 2003; Stephensen *et al.*, 2002). This increased generation of IL-4-producing T cells accompanies a decrease in IFN-γ-producing T cells. The mechanism for this regulation by RA, however, has been unclear but involves RAR or RXR receptors (Grenningloh *et al.*, 2006; Iwata *et al.*, 2003; Stephensen *et al.*, 2002). A mouse strain (pinkie mice) with a mutation in the ligand binding and heterodimerization domain of RXRα resulting in a 90% decline in ligand-inducible transactivation was created (Du *et al.*, 2005). These mice develop progressive alopecia and dermal cysts, and progressive exaggeration of Th1 but loss of Th2 responses. Similar to the mutant mice, mice with a T-cell lineage-specific deficiency of RXRα display a phenotype with increased Th1 cells (Du *et al.*, 2005). These mice do not display alopecia and dermal cysts associated with the RXRα mutant mice, suggesting that the phenotypic abnormality is caused by T cell extrinsic factors. The differences in the pinkie mice and T-cell-specific RXRα KO mice suggest that the increased Th2 cell response is primarily mediated by a T-cell intrinsic factor. A caveat with these studies is that RXR is a subunit of other nuclear hormone receptors such as vitamin D receptor, thyroid hormone receptor, and PPARγ receptor. Other issues include that it is unclear which cell type (Th1 or Th2) would be the direct target of RA and whether indirect regulation through different target cells is involved.

Indeed, indirect mechanisms through other cells are involved in regulation of T cell polarization by RA. As discussed early in this review, RA can regulate antigen presenting cells and other immune cells to indirectly regulate the Th1 and Th2 responses. Similarly, induction of regulatory T cells by RA could decrease the T cell differentiation into Th1 cells. RA or their analogs, when introduced through diets or injections, can decrease the severity of tissue inflammation (Nagai *et al.*, 1999; Racke *et al.*, 1995). The therapeutic effect was observed in an experimental allergic encephalomyelitis (EAE) model and a collagen-induced arthritis model, in which the disease can be induced by not only Th1 but also Th17 cells (Massacesi *et al.*, 1987; Nozaki *et al.*, 2006). The relationship between RA and Th17 cells is discussed in the next section.

B. RA and Th17 cells

Th17 cells are a subset of T helper cells that are defined by their production of IL-17A (Harrington *et al.*, 2006; Stockinger and Veldhoen, 2007; Weaver *et al.*, 2007). In addition, these T cells produce IL-17A, IL-17F, IL-21, and IL-22. Th17 cells play important roles in antimicrobial responses and mediating certain types of tissue inflammation. Th17 cells are induced in a peculiar cytokine condition enriched with TGF-β1, IL-6, and IL-23 (Bettelli *et al.*, 2006). While the impact of IL-6 is direct in upregulation of Th17 cell-inducing transcription factor RORγt, the effect of TGFβ is indirect in that it inhibits the expression of STAT4 (a Th1-inducing factor) and GATA3 (a Th2-inducing factor) (Das *et al.*, 2009). Inhibition of Th1- and Th2-inducing cytokines is important for inducing Th17 cells because Th1 and Th2 cytokines are highly suppressive on induction of Th17 cells.

It was demonstrated *in vitro* that RAs (At-RA and 9-*cis*-RA) and other RAR agonists are effective in suppression of naïve T cell differentiation into Th17 cells (Kang *et al.*, 2007; Mucida *et al.*, 2007; Schambach *et al.*, 2007). In support of this, RAR antagonists can enhance the generation of Th17 cells in response to TGF-β1, IL-6, and IL-23 (Kang *et al.*, 2007; Mucida *et al.*, 2007; Schambach *et al.*, 2007). The intestine is one of the organs that highly produce RA and, therefore, it was expected that few Th17 cells would be found in the intestine. Ironically, Th17 cells are highly enriched in the intestine. This discrepancy between the generation of Th17 cells *in vitro* and *in vivo* may be explained by the use of extremely high concentrations of RA in demonstrating the effect *in vitro* but the production of RA *in vivo* is tightly regulated and would not reach that high to significantly suppress the generation of Th17 cells. It should also be pointed out that the intestine is rich with Th17 cell-inducing commensals (Ivanov *et al.*, 2008, 2009; Niess *et al.*, 2008; Zaph *et al.*, 2008). To support this hypothesis, suppression of Th17 cells by RA readily occurs at high concentrations of RA ($>$30 nM). However, at physiological concentrations ($<$30 nM), the suppression is modest. The Th17 cells, induced in the presence of RA ($>$5 nM), express the gut-homing receptors CCR9 and α4β7 (Wang *et al.*, 2010). These RA-induced Th17 cells are highly efficient in inducing inflammation in the intestine. They are more effective in induction of inflammation than similarly induced Th17 cells generated in the absence of RA. An interesting feature of RA-induced Th17 cells is their tissue tropism. These Th17 cells migrate to the small intestine and cause severe inflammation there (Wang *et al.*, 2010). In contrast, regular Th17 cells induce severe inflammation mainly in the colon (Wang *et al.*, 2010).

V. RA and Regulatory T Cells

$FoxP3^+$ regulatory T cells are a major subset of regulatory T cells that restrain immune responses. $FoxP3^+$ regulatory T cells are made from T cell progenitors in the thymus as naïve type $FoxP3^+$ T cells which migrate to the secondary lymphoid tissues. $FoxP3^+$ regulatory T cells are made also in the periphery from naïve $FoxP3^-$ T cells in response to antigens, and these cells are called induced $FoxP3^+$ T cells. $FoxP3^+$ T cells play essential roles in prevention of autoimmune diseases and maintenance of tolerance. The evidence for the critical role of $FoxP3^+$ T cells includes the multiorgan chronic inflammatory diseases in IPEX (immunodysregulation, polyendocrinopathy, and enteropathy, X-linked) patients and scurfy mice (Bennett *et al.*, 2001; Brunkow *et al.*, 2001; Wildin *et al.*, 2001). Both the diseases in humans and mice are caused by inactivating mutations in the *FoxP3* gene. The FoxP3 protein is a transcription factor/repressor and modulates the function of nuclear factor of activated T cells (NF-AT) and NF-κB (Bettelli *et al.*, 2005; Schubert *et al.*, 2001).

Certain cytokines such as TGF-β1 and IL-2 play crucial roles in induction of $FoxP3^+$ T cells (Chen *et al.*, 2003; Fontenot and Rudensky, 2005; Knoechel *et al.*, 2005; Yu *et al.*, 2009). RA is a potent factor that further enhances the induction of $FoxP3^+$ T cells from naïve T cells during antigenic stimulation (Benson *et al.*, 2007; Coombes *et al.*, 2007; Elias *et al.*, 2008; Kang *et al.*, 2007; Mucida *et al.*, 2007; Schambach *et al.*, 2007; Sun *et al.*, 2007). RA can induce $FoxP3^+$ T cells through direct and indirect mechanisms. As a direct mechanism, RA can regulate the gene expression in T cells. For example, RA can suppress the expression of IL-6R by T cells (Nolting *et al.*, 2009). RAR–RXR nuclear receptors act as transcription factors that can bind RAREs in a number of genes that regulate the expression of the *FoxP3* gene. RA receptors can regulate gene expression also through the regulation of other factors without binding directly to DNA. At-RA and RARα induce histone acetylation at the human FoxP3 promoter (Kang *et al.*, 2007). Another mechanism is through the inhibition of the production of $FoxP3^+$ T-cell suppressing factors. For example, RA acts on effect T cells so that production of inflammatory cytokines, such as IL-6, that suppress the induction of FoxP3$^+$ T cells (Hill *et al.*, 2008). Another mechanism would be induction of antigen presenting cells that are efficient in induction of FoxP3$^+$ T cells. For example, certain DCs such as CD11b$^-$CD103$^+$ DCs can efficiently induce FoxP3$^+$ cells (Coombes *et al.*, 2007; Denning *et al.*, 2007; Jaensson *et al.*, 2008; Jin *et al.*, 2010; Siddiqui and Powrie, 2008; Sun *et al.*, 2007). One of the most interesting features of RA-induced FoxP3$^+$ cells is their expression of two gut-homing receptors CCR9 and $\alpha 4\beta 7$ (Benson *et al.*, 2007; Kang *et al.*, 2007). These T cells migrate efficiently to the intestine, and therefore RA-induced FoxP3$^+$ T cells are believed to be important for immune tolerance particularly in the gut. RA-induced FoxP3$^+$ T cells express granzymes and perforin (Kang *et al.*, 2007), which may be involved in killing target cells (Gondek *et al.*, 2005; Grossman *et al.*, 2004; von Boehmer, 2005). Thus, RA-induced FoxP3$^+$ cells have the potential to suppress target cells via their cytotoxic activity *in vivo*. In addition, these Tregs may use other inhibitory pathways involving TGFβ1, IL-10, and CTLA4/indoleamine 2,3 dioxygenase (IDO) to suppress target cells (Kim, 2007).

VI. RA in Regulation of Antibody Responses

It has been well established that IgA production is defective in vitamin A deficiency. Defective synthesis and transport of IgA antibodies into the bile was observed in vitamin A-deficient rats immunized with *Brucella abortus* or sheep red blood cells directly into the Peyer's patches (PP) (Puengtomwatanakul and Sirisinha, 1986). RA can induce IgA production by LPS-activated murine spleen cells but not the production of other antibody isotypes such as IgM, IgG2a, IgG2b, and IgG3 *in vitro* (Tokuyama and Tokuyama, 1993). Similarly, RA can promote the production of IgA and IgG monoclonal antibodies by hybridoma cells (Aotsuka and Naito, 1991). A potential mechanism for the selective effect of RA on IgA production is through cytokines such as IL-5 and IL-6 (Ballow *et al.*, 1996). IL-6 is known to induce antibody production in B cells, while IL-5 can augment the effect of RA in production of IgA (Tokuyama and Tokuyama, 1996). In contrast, IL-4 has an inhibitory effect on IgA production but has an enhancing effect on production of IgG1 and IgE. IgA is transported from the basal to apical surface of mucosal epithelial cells by the polymeric immunoglobulin receptor (pIgR). pIgR expression is induced by inflammatory cytokines such as IL-4, IFN-γ, and tumor necrosis factor-α (TNF-α) (Denning, 1996; Kvale *et al.*, 1988; Phillips *et al.*, 1990). Importantly, the induction of pIgR expression by these cytokines is blunted in the absence of RA. Thus, vitamin A regulates not only the synthesis but also the transport of IgA across the epithelial cell barrier in mucosal tissues.

Induction of IgA production in B cells by RA appears to be regulated in both direct and indirect ways. Direct action of RA on antibody class switch in B cells is apparent. Additionally, RA can act through non-B cell such as DCs and T cells to promote IgA production. In this regard, RA steers DC differentiation into the cells that can produce RA and cytokines that promote IgA production (Mora *et al.*, 2006; Saurer *et al.*, 2007). Another important function of RA in promotion of IgA production is its effect on migration of helper T cells that provide the help signal for B cells. It is known that $FoxP3^+$ T cells can dampen humoral immune responses (Lim *et al.*, 2005). However, $FoxP3^+$ T cells have been reported to become follicular helper T cells (T-FH cells) in PP (Tsuji *et al.*, 2009). In this regard, RA can make induced $FoxP3^+$ T cells (Coombes *et al.*, 2007; Elias *et al.*, 2008; Kang *et al.*, 2007; Sun *et al.*, 2007) and, thus, could theoretically enhance the IgA response through $FoxP3^+$ T cells and T-FH cells.

VII. RA and Tissue Inflammation

The functions of RA in regulation of differentiation and function of various immune cells and tissue cells suggest that vitamin A intake and levels of retinol and retinoids in the body would have significant impacts on tissue inflammation. VAD can exacerbate or suppress tissue inflammation. Whether VAD worsens or ameliorates tissue inflammation depends on tissue sites. For example, VAD has a beneficial effect on intestinal inflammation through the suppression of the homing of inflammatory T cells into the gut (Kang *et al.*, 2009). This is because T cells require RA for expression of two gut-homing receptors, CCR9 and $\alpha4\beta7$ (Iwata *et al.*, 2004). Moreover, a novel subset of $\alpha E\beta7^+$ $FoxP3^+$ T cells with potent suppressive activity is induced in VAD (Kang *et al.*, 2009). However, tissue inflammation can be worsened in VAD because of decreased RA-dependent generation of tolerogenic DCs and macrophages (Saurer *et al.*, 2007). The integrity of epithelial barriers in various tissues requires normal levels of vitamin A (Filteau *et al.*, 2001; Gorodeski *et al.*, 1997). Mucus-producing epithelial cells can be replaced with atypical nonfunctional epithelial cells in VAD (Rojanapo *et al.*, 1980). Compromised production of mucus and epithelial cell integrity in VAD leads to tissue invasion by bacteria followed by chronic inflammation in mucosal and nonmucosal tissues (Fig. 4.3).

Adequate levels of vitamin A intake can ameliorate inflammation in a mouse model of small intestinal inflammation (Kang *et al.*, 2009). RA promotes the increase of $CCR9^+\alpha4\beta7^+$ $FoxP3^+$ T cells, which preferentially migrate to the intestine and suppress inflammation. RA has been shown to have ameliorating effects on elastase-induced pulmonary emphysema in rats (Massaro and Massaro, 1997). It is thought that the positive and

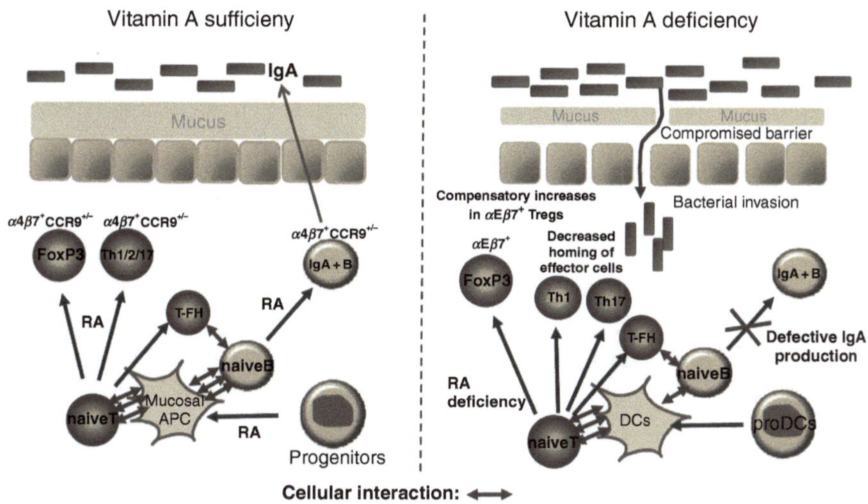

Figure 4.3 *Vitamin A status and mucosal immune system.* When vitamin A intake is sufficient, RA is produced at high levels and promotes formation of epithelial tight junction, secretion of mucus, and expression of pIgR (*trans*-epithelial IgA transporter). Within the lamina propria, RA promotes the production of IgA by B cells, generation of tolerogenic antigen presenting cells, and differentiation of naïve T cells into gut-homing regulatory T cells and effector T cells. Consequently, the gut bacteria are under control by the host immunity and appropriate levels of immune tolerance are achieved at the same time. In vitamin A deficiency, secretion of mucus and integrity of epithelial cells are compromised, allowing the invasion of bacteria into the tissue. Moreover, IgA production and transportation across the epithelial barrier are decreased, resulting in dysregulation of mucosal immunity and potential changes in commensal flora. There is an increased risk for mucosal tissue inflammation in this condition. Interestingly, $FoxP3^+$ Tregs that express $\alpha E\beta 7$ are highly enriched in the body, counteracting the increased risk of tissue inflammation. Another factor that can decrease the tissue inflammation is poor homing of immune cells into the gut due to defective expression of $\alpha 4\beta 7$ and CCR9. Despite the compensatory increase in $\alpha E\beta 7^+$ Tregs, prolonged RA deficiency and decreased immunity lead to the inability to clear bacteria and, then, to chronic tissue inflammation. (See Color Insert.)

negative effects of RA on elastin-production by lung epithelial cells and on the inflammatory cells are likely the mechanisms responsible for the therapeutic effect. RA and its analogs are effective therapeutics for acne vulgaris (Reifen *et al.*, 2002). While the detailed mechanisms remain to be determined, it is thought that RA acts on immune cells and keratinocytes to suppress the inflammation. In the EAE model induced by myelin basic protein-specific T cells, it was reported that RA had a beneficial effect (Racke *et al.*, 1995). The two types of T cells that are important for this type of inflammation are Th1 and Th17 cells. Although it is controversial, RA promotes Th2 but decreases Th1 responses. Generation of Th17 cells is dramatically decreased, while that of $FoxP3^+$ regulatory T cells is greatly increased in the presence of high RA concentrations (>20 nM). Thus, the effects of RA on regulation of T cell polarization would be responsible, in part, for the beneficial effect of RA in this type of inflammation. In a type II collagen-induced arthritis model, RA has been shown to ameliorate inflammation (Nozaki *et al.*, 2006). Similar to the EAE model, Th17 and Th1 cells are the major effector T cells that regulate the tissue inflammation. Thus, the negative effect of RA on the effector T cells is consistent with the ameliorating function of RA on many types of tissue inflammation.

VIII. Conclusions and Remaining Issues

It is becoming clear that vitamin A plays essential roles in the immune system. RA is important for both formation of immunity and prevention of inflammatory diseases. These seemingly paradoxical functions of RA are mediated by different cell types. Promotion of immunity is through terminal differentiation of phagocytes, generation of gut-homing T cells, and induction of IgA-producing B cells. Prevention of inflammation and autoimmunity is mediated through generation of FoxP3$^+$ regulatory T cells and tolerogenic antigen presenting cells or myeloid cells. Regulation of immune responses by RA occurs at multiple stages including cell differentiation, antigen priming, and effector function. More studies are required to determine the regulation of RA synthesis and creation of RA gradients in the mucosal tissues and tissue sites of immune responses. For example, it is thought that the RA concentration is high in the intestine and this helps generate FoxP3$^+$ T cells and gut-homing T and B cells. RA, produced at lower levels in other parts of the body, is still important for regulation of many genes required for normal function of immune cells. Increased RA production occurs following infection and inflammatory responses perhaps to limit excessive immune responses. The exact role of the increased production of RA should be investigated in depth in the future. RA, when injected for therapeutic purposes, could cause a lethal toxic syndrome, which is called "RA syndrome" observed during treatment of acute promyelocytic leukemia. The effective doses for beneficial regulatory effects on inflammatory diseases without the toxic response and any adverse effects on immunity should be determined in animals and humans.

Acknowledgments

This work was supported, in part, from grants from NIH (R01AI074745, R01AI080769 and R01DK076616), the Crohn's and Colitis Foundation of America, and the American Heart Association to C. H. K.

REFERENCES

Aotsuka, Y., and Naito, M. (1991). Enhancing effects of retinoic acid on monoclonal antibody production of human-human hybridomas. *Cell. Immunol.* **133,** 498–505.

Aukrust, P., *et al.* (2000). Decreased vitamin A levels in common variable immunodeficiency: Vitamin A supplementation in vivo enhances immunoglobulin production and downregulates inflammatory responses. *Eur. J. Clin. Invest.* **30,** 252–259.

Ballow, M., *et al.* (1996). The effects of retinoic acid on immunoglobulin synthesis: Role of interleukin 6. *J. Clin. Immunol.* **16,** 171–179.

Banchereau, J., *et al.* (2003). Dendritic cells: Controllers of the immune system and a new promise for immunotherapy. *Ann. N. Y. Acad. Sci.* **987,** 180–187.

Bennett, C. L., *et al.* (2001). The immune dysregulation, polyendocrinopathy, enteropathy, X-linked syndrome (IPEX) is caused by mutations of FOXP3. *Nat. Genet.* **27,** 20–21.

Benson, M. J., *et al.* (2007). All-trans retinoic acid mediates enhanced Treg cell growth, differentiation, and gut homing in the face of high levels of co-stimulation. *J. Exp. Med.* **204,** 1765–1774.

Bettelli, E., *et al.* (2005). Foxp3 interacts with nuclear factor of activated T cells and NF-kappa B to repress cytokine gene expression and effector functions of T helper cells. *Proc. Natl. Acad. Sci. USA* **102,** 5138–5143.

Bettelli, E., *et al.* (2006). Reciprocal developmental pathways for the generation of pathogenic effector TH17 and regulatory T cells. *Nature* **441,** 235–238.

Brunkow, M. E., *et al.* (2001). Disruption of a new forkhead/winged-helix protein, scurfin, results in the fatal lymphoproliferative disorder of the scurfy mouse. *Nat. Genet.* **27,** 68–73.

Cantorna, M. T., *et al.* (1994). In vitamin A deficiency multiple mechanisms establish a regulatory T helper cell imbalance with excess Th1 and insufficient Th2 function. *J. Immunol.* **152,** 1515–1522.

Carman, J. A., *et al.* (1989). Characterization of a helper T lymphocyte defect in vitamin A-deficient mice. *J. Immunol.* **142,** 388–393.

Chang, S. Y., *et al.* (2008). Cutting edge: Langerin+ dendritic cells in the mesenteric lymph node set the stage for skin and gut immune system cross-talk. *J. Immunol.* **180,** 4361–4365.

Chang, S. Y., *et al.* (2009). Lack of retinoic acid leads to increased langerin-expressing dendritic cells in gut-associated lymphoid tissues. *Gastroenterology* **138,** 1468–14781478 e1–1478 e6.

Chen, W., *et al.* (2003). Conversion of peripheral CD4+CD25− naive T cells to CD4+CD25+ regulatory T cells by TGF-beta induction of transcription factor Foxp3. *J. Exp. Med.* **198,** 1875–1886.

Clagett-Dame, M., and DeLuca, H. F. (2002). The role of vitamin A in mammalian reproduction and embryonic development. *Annu. Rev. Nutr.* **22,** 347–381.

Coombes, J. L., *et al.* (2007). A functionally specialized population of mucosal CD103+ DCs induces Foxp3+ regulatory T cells via a TGF-beta and retinoic acid-dependent mechanism. *J. Exp. Med.* **204,** 1757–1764.

Das, J., *et al.* (2009). Transforming growth factor beta is dispensable for the molecular orchestration of Th17 cell differentiation. *J. Exp. Med.* **206,** 2407–2416.

Dawson, H. D., *et al.* (2006). Direct and indirect effects of retinoic acid on human Th2 cytokine and chemokine expression by human T lymphocytes. *BMC Immunol.* **7,** 27.

Denning, G. M. (1996). IL-4 and IFN-gamma synergistically increase total polymeric IgA receptor levels in human intestinal epithelial cells. Role of protein tyrosine kinases. *J. Immunol.* **156,** 4807–4814.

Denning, T. L., *et al.* (2007). Lamina propria macrophages and dendritic cells differentially induce regulatory and interleukin 17-producing T cell responses. *Nat. Immunol.* **8,** 1086–1094.

Du, X., *et al.* (2005). An essential role for Rxr alpha in the development of Th2 responses. *Eur. J. Immunol.* **35,** 3414–3423.

Duester, G. (2000). Families of retinoid dehydrogenases regulating vitamin A function: Production of visual pigment and retinoic acid. *Eur. J. Biochem.* **267,** 4315–4324.

Elgueta, R., *et al.* (2008). Imprinting of CCR9 on CD4 T cells requires IL-4 signaling on mesenteric lymph node dendritic cells. *J. Immunol.* **180,** 6501–6507.

Elias, K. M., *et al.* (2008). Retinoic acid inhibits Th17 polarization and enhances FoxP3 expression through a Stat-3/Stat-5 independent signaling pathway. *Blood* **111,**1013–1020.

Filteau, S. M., *et al.* (2001). The effect of antenatal vitamin A and beta-carotene supplementation on gut integrity of infants of HIV-infected South African women. *J. Pediatr. Gastroenterol. Nutr.* **32,** 464–470.

Fontenot, J. D., and Rudensky, A. Y. (2005). A well adapted regulatory contrivance: Regulatory T cell development and the forkhead family transcription factor Foxp3. *Nat. Immunol.* **6,** 331–337.

Geissmann, F., *et al.* (2003). Retinoids regulate survival and antigen presentation by immature dendritic cells. *J. Exp. Med.* **198,** 623–634.

Gillard, E. F., and Solomon, E. (1993). Acute promyelocytic leukaemia and the t(15;17) translocation. *Semin. Cancer Biol.* **4,** 359–367.

Gilliet, M., *et al.* (2008). Plasmacytoid dendritic cells: Sensing nucleic acids in viral infection and autoimmune diseases. *Nat. Rev. Immunol.* **8,** 594–606.

Goldman, R. (1984). Effect of retinoic acid on the proliferation and phagocytic capability of murine macrophage-like cell lines. *J. Cell. Physiol.* **120,** 91–102.

Gondek, D. C., *et al.* (2005). Cutting edge: Contact-mediated suppression by CD4+CD25+ regulatory cells involves a granzyme B-dependent, perforin-independent mechanism. *J. Immunol.* **174,** 1783–1786.

Gorodeski, G. I., *et al.* (1997). Retinoids regulate tight junctional resistance of cultured human cervical cells. *Am. J. Physiol.* **273,** C1707–C1713.

Grenningloh, R., *et al.* (2006). Cutting edge: Inhibition of the retinoid X receptor (RXR) blocks T helper 2 differentiation and prevents allergic lung inflammation. *J. Immunol.* **176,** 5161–5166.

Grossman, W. J., *et al.* (2004). Human T regulatory cells can use the perforin pathway to cause autologous target cell death. *Immunity* **21,** 589–601.

Harrington, L. E., *et al.* (2006). Expanding the effector CD4 T-cell repertoire: The Th17 lineage. *Curr. Opin. Immunol.* **18,** 349–356.

Hengesbach, L. M., and Hoag, K. A. (2004). Physiological concentrations of retinoic acid favor myeloid dendritic cell development over granulocyte development in cultures of bone marrow cells from mice. *J. Nutr.* **134,** 2653–2659.

Hessel, S., *et al.* (2007). CMO1 deficiency abolishes vitamin A production from beta-carotene and alters lipid metabolism in mice. *J. Biol. Chem.* **282,** 33553–33561.

Hill, J. A., *et al.* (2008). Retinoic acid enhances Foxp3 induction indirectly by relieving inhibition from CD4+CD44hi Cells. *Immunity* **29,** 758–770.

Hoag, K. A., *et al.* (2002). Retinoic acid enhances the T helper 2 cell development that is essential for robust antibody responses through its action on antigen-presenting cells. *J. Nutr.* **132,** 3736–3739.

Ito, T., *et al.* (2005). Functional diversity and plasticity of human dendritic cell subsets. *Int. J. Hematol.* **81,** 188–196.

Ivanov, I. I., *et al.* (2008). Specific microbiota direct the differentiation of IL-17-producing T-helper cells in the mucosa of the small intestine. *Cell Host Microbe* **4,** 337–349.

Ivanov, I. I., *et al.* (2009). Induction of intestinal Th17 cells by segmented filamentous bacteria. *Cell* **139,** 485–498.

Iwata, M., *et al.* (2003). Retinoic acids exert direct effects on T cells to suppress Th1 development and enhance Th2 development via retinoic acid receptors. *Int. Immunol.* **15,** 1017–1025.
Iwata, M., *et al.* (2004). Retinoic acid imprints gut-homing specificity on T cells. *Immunity* **21,** 527–538.
Jaensson, E., *et al.* (2008). Small intestinal CD103+ dendritic cells display unique functional properties that are conserved between mice and humans. *J. Exp. Med.* **205,** 2139–2149.
Jin, C. J., *et al.* (2010). All-trans retinoic acid inhibits the differentiation, maturation, and function of human monocyte-derived dendritic cells. *Leuk. Res.* **34,** 513–520.
Kang, S. G., *et al.* (2007). Vitamin A metabolites induce gut-homing FoxP3+ regulatory T cells. *J. Immunol.* **179,** 3724–3733.
Kang, S. G., *et al.* (2009). High and low vitamin A therapies induce distinct FoxP3+ T-cell subsets and effectively control intestinal inflammation. *Gastroenterology* **137**(1391–402), e1–e6.
Kim, C. H. (2007). Molecular targets of FoxP3+ regulatory T cells. *Mini Rev. Med. Chem.* **7,** 1136–1143.
Kim, C. H. (2008). Roles of retinoic acid in induction of immunity and immune tolerance. *Endocr. Metab. Immune Disord. Drug Targets* **8,** 289–294.
Knoechel, B., *et al.* (2005). Sequential development of interleukin 2-dependent effector and regulatory T cells in response to endogenous systemic antigen. *J. Exp. Med.* **202,** 1375–1386.
Kuwata, T., *et al.* (2000). Vitamin A deficiency in mice causes a systemic expansion of myeloid cells. *Blood* **95,** 3349–3356.
Kvale, D., *et al.* (1988). Tumor necrosis factor-alpha up-regulates expression of secretory component, the epithelial receptor for polymeric Ig. *J. Immunol.* **140,** 3086–3089.
Labrecque, J., *et al.* (1998). Impaired granulocytic differentiation in vitro in hematopoietic cells lacking retinoic acid receptors alpha1 and gamma. *Blood* **92,** 607–615.
Lim, H. W., *et al.* (2004). Regulatory T cells can migrate to follicles upon T cell activation and suppress GC-Th cells and GC-Th cell-driven B cell responses. *J. Clin. Invest.* **114,** 1640–1649.
Lim, H. W., *et al.* (2005). Cutting edge: Direct suppression of B cells by CD4+ CD25+ regulatory T cells. *J. Immunol.* **175,** 4180–4183.
Manicassamy, S., *et al.* (2009). Toll-like receptor 2-dependent induction of vitamin A-metabolizing enzymes in dendritic cells promotes T regulatory responses and inhibits autoimmunity. *Nat. Med.* **15,** 401–409.
Massacesi, L., *et al.* (1987). Suppression of experimental allergic encephalomyelitis by retinoic acid. *J. Neurol. Sci.* **80,** 55–64.
Massaro, G. D., and Massaro, D. (1997). Retinoic acid treatment abrogates elastase-induced pulmonary emphysema in rats. *Nat. Med.* **3,** 675–677.
Mohty, M., *et al.* (2003). All-trans retinoic acid skews monocyte differentiation into interleukin-12-secreting dendritic-like cells. *Br. J. Haematol.* **122,** 829–836.
Molenaar, R., *et al.* (2009). Lymph node stromal cells support dendritic cell-induced gut-homing of T cells. *J. Immunol.* **183,** 6395–6402.
Mora, J. R., and von Andrian, U. H. (2009). Role of retinoic acid in the imprinting of gut-homing IgA-secreting cells. *Semin. Immunol.* **21,** 28–35.
Mora, J. R., *et al.* (2006). Generation of gut-homing IgA-secreting B cells by intestinal dendritic cells. *Science* **314,** 1157–1160.
Mucida, D., *et al.* (2007). Reciprocal TH17 and regulatory T cell differentiation mediated by retinoic acid. *Science* **317,** 256–260.
Nagai, H., *et al.* (1999). Effect of Am-80, a synthetic derivative of retinoid, on experimental arthritis in mice. *Pharmacology* **58,** 101–112.

Naik, S. H., *et al.* (2005). Development of murine plasmacytoid dendritic cell subsets. *Immunol. Cell Biol.* **83,** 563–570.
Napoli, J. L. (1996a). Biochemical pathways of retinoid transport, metabolism, and signal transduction. *Clin. Immunol. Immunopathol.* **80,** S52–S62.
Napoli, J. L. (1996b). Retinoic acid biosynthesis and metabolism. *FASEB J.* **10,** 993–1001.
Niess, J. H., *et al.* (2008). Commensal gut flora drives the expansion of proinflammatory CD4 T cells in the colonic lamina propria under normal and inflammatory conditions. *J. Immunol.* **180,** 559–568.
Nolting, J., *et al.* (2009). Retinoic acid can enhance conversion of naive into regulatory T cells independently of secreted cytokines. *J. Exp. Med.* **206,** 2131–2139.
Nozaki, Y., *et al.* (2006). Anti-inflammatory effect of all-trans-retinoic acid in inflammatory arthritis. *Clin. Immunol.* **119,** 272–279.
Ongsakul, M., *et al.* (1985). Impaired blood clearance of bacteria and phagocytic activity in vitamin A-deficient rats. *Proc. Soc. Exp. Biol. Med.* **178,** 204–208.
Penna, G., *et al.* (2002). Differential migration behavior and chemokine production by myeloid and plasmacytoid dendritic cells. *Hum. Immunol.* **63,** 1164–1171.
Phillips, J. O., *et al.* (1990). Synergistic effect of IL-4 and IFN-gamma on the expression of polymeric Ig receptor (secretory component) and IgA binding by human epithelial cells. *J. Immunol.* **145,** 1740–1744.
Puengtomwatanakul, S., and Sirisinha, S. (1986). Impaired biliary secretion of immunoglobulin A in vitamin A-deficient rats. *Proc. Soc. Exp. Biol. Med.* **182,** 437–442.
Racke, M. K., *et al.* (1995). Retinoid treatment of experimental allergic encephalomyelitis. IL-4 production correlates with improved disease course. *J. Immunol.* **154,** 450–458.
Reifen, R., *et al.* (2002). Vitamin A deficiency exacerbates inflammation in a rat model of colitis through activation of nuclear factor-kappaB and collagen formation. *J. Nutr.* **132,** 2743–2747.
Rojanapo, W., *et al.* (1980). Biochemical and immunological characterization and the synthesis of rat intestinal glycoproteins following the induction of rapid synchronous vitamin A deficiency. *Biochim. Biophys. Acta* **633,** 386–399.
Saurer, L., *et al.* (2007). In vitro induction of mucosa-type dendritic cells by all-trans retinoic acid. *J. Immunol.* **179,** 3504–3514.
Schambach, F., *et al.* (2007). Activation of retinoic acid receptor-alpha favours regulatory T cell induction at the expense of IL-17-secreting T helper cell differentiation. *Eur. J. Immunol.* **37,** 2396–2399.
Schubert, L. A., *et al.* (2001). Scurfin (FOXP3) acts as a repressor of transcription and regulates T cell activation. *J. Biol. Chem.* **276,** 37672–37679.
Semba, R. D. (1994). Vitamin A, immunity, and infection. *Clin. Infect. Dis.* **19,** 489–499.
Siddiqui, K. R., and Powrie, F. (2008). CD103+ GALT DCs promote Foxp3+ regulatory T cells. *Mucosal Immunol.* **1**(Suppl. 1), S34–S38.
Sommer, A. (1998). Xerophthalmia and vitamin A status. *Prog. Retin. Eye Res.* **17,** 9–31.
Stephensen, C. B. (2001). Vitamin A, infection, and immune function. *Annu. Rev. Nutr.* **21,** 167–192.
Stephensen, C. B., *et al.* (2002). Vitamin A enhances in vitro Th2 development via retinoid X receptor pathway. *J. Immunol.* **168,** 4495–4503.
Stockinger, B., and Veldhoen, M. (2007). Differentiation and function of Th17 T cells. *Curr. Opin. Immunol.* **19,** 281–286.
Sun, C. M., *et al.* (2007). Small intestine lamina propria dendritic cells promote de novo generation of Foxp3 T reg cells via retinoic acid. *J. Exp. Med.* **204,** 1775–1785.
Szatmari, I., *et al.* (2006). PPARgamma controls CD1d expression by turning on retinoic acid synthesis in developing human dendritic cells. *J. Exp. Med.* **203,** 2351–2362.

Tao, Y., *et al.* (2006). Effect of all-trans-retinoic acid on the differentiation, maturation and functions of dendritic cells derived from cord blood monocytes. *FEMS Immunol. Med. Microbiol.* **47,** 444–450.
Tokuyama, H., and Tokuyama, Y. (1993). Retinoids enhance IgA production by lipopolysaccharide-stimulated murine spleen cells. *Cell. Immunol.* **150,** 353–363.
Tokuyama, Y., and Tokuyama, H. (1996). Retinoids as Ig isotype-switch modulators. The role of retinoids in directing isotype switching to IgA and IgG1 (IgE) in association with IL-4 and IL-5. *Cell. Immunol.* **170,** 230–234.
Tokuyama, H., and Tokuyama, Y. (1999). The regulatory effects of all-trans-retinoic acid on isotype switching: Retinoic acid induces IgA switch rearrangement in cooperation with IL-5 and inhibits IgG1 switching. *Cell. Immunol.* **192,** 41–47.
Tsuji, M., *et al.* (2009). Preferential generation of follicular B helper T cells from Foxp3+ T cells in gut Peyer's patches. *Science* **323,** 1488–1492.
Vermot, J., *et al.* (2000). Expression of enzymes synthesizing (aldehyde dehydrogenase 1 and reinaldehyde dehydrogenase 2) and metabolizaing (Cyp26) retinoic acid in the mouse female reproductive system. *Endocrinology* **141,** 3638–3645.
Vladutiu, A., and Cringulescu, N. (1968). Suppression of experimental allergic encephalomyelitis by vitamin A. *Experientia* **24,** 718–719.
von Boehmer, H. (2005). Mechanisms of suppression by suppressor T cells. *Nat. Immunol.* **6,** 338–344.
Wang, C. W., *et al.* (2010). Retinoic acid determines the precise tissue tropism of inflammatory Th17 cells in the intestine. *J. Immunol.* **184,** 5519–5526.
Weaver, C. T., *et al.* (2007). IL-17 family cytokines and the expanding diversity of effector T cell lineages. *Annu. Rev. Immunol.* **25,** 821–852.
West, K. P., Jr., *et al.* (1989). Vitamin A and infection: Public health implications. *Annu. Rev. Nutr.* **9,** 63–86.
Wildin, R. S., *et al.* (2001). X-linked neonatal diabetes mellitus, enteropathy and endocrinopathy syndrome is the human equivalent of mouse scurfy. *Nat. Genet.* **27,** 18–20.
Yang, Z. Z., *et al.* (2006). Intratumoral CD4+CD25+ regulatory T-cell-mediated suppression of infiltrating CD4+ T cells in B-cell non-Hodgkin lymphoma. *Blood* **107,** 3639–3646.
Yokota, A., *et al.* (2009). GM-CSF and IL-4 synergistically trigger dendritic cells to acquire retinoic acid-producing capacity. *Int. Immunol.* **21,** 361–377.
Yu, H. Q., *et al.* (2009). sublingual immunotherapy efficacy of dermatophagoides farinae vaccine in a murine asthma model. *Int. Arch. Allergy Immunol.* **152,** 41–48.
Zapata-Gonzalez, F., *et al.* (2007). 9-cis-Retinoic acid (9cRA), a retinoid X receptor (RXR) ligand, exerts immunosuppressive effects on dendritic cells by RXR-dependent activation: Inhibition of peroxisome proliferator-activated receptor gamma blocks some of the 9cRA activities, and precludes them to mature phenotype development. *J. Immunol.* **178,** 6130–6139.
Zaph, C., *et al.* (2008). Commensal-dependent expression of IL-25 regulates the IL-23-IL-17 axis in the intestine. *J. Exp. Med.* **205,** 2191–2198.
Zile, M. H. (1998). Vitamin A and embryonic development: An overview. *J. Nutr.* **128,** 455S–458S.
Zile, M. H. (2001). Function of vitamin A in vertebrate embryonic development. *J. Nutr.* **131,** 705–708.

CHAPTER FIVE

Vitamin A and Retinoic Acid in the Regulation of B-Cell Development and Antibody Production

A. Catharine Ross,*[,†] Qiuyan Chen,* *and* Yifan Ma*

Contents

Abstract

Signaling by vitamin A through its active metabolite retinoic acid (RA) is critical for the normal development and functions of the hematopoietic and immune systems. B cells, as both factories for antibody production and part of the immune regulatory system, are critical to a successful vaccination response. RA is a factor in the development and competence of mature B cells, in B cell proliferation, and in the regulation of transcription factors associated with B cell differentiation, class switch recombination, and the generation of antibody-secreting plasma cells. Emerging evidence suggests that RA can function

* Department of Nutritional Sciences, Pennsylvania State University, University Park, Pennsylvania, USA
† Huck Institute for Life Sciences, Pennsylvania State University, University Park, Pennsylvania, USA

Vitamins and Hormones, Volume 86
ISSN 0083-6729, DOI: 10.1016/B978-0-12-386960-9.00005-8

alone and in combination with other immune system stimuli to augment the formation of germinal centers, leading to increased primary and secondary antibody responses. Taken together, RA could be a useful component in vaccine strategies and/or for immunotherapy.

Abbreviations

APC	antigen-presenting cell(s)
BCR	B-cell receptor
CSR	class switch recombination
DC	dendritic cell(s)
GC	germinal center(s)
Ig	immunoglobulin
LPS	lipopolysaccharide
NF-κB	nuclear factor kappa-light-chain-enhancer of activated B cells
PC	plasma cell(s)
PNA	peanut agglutinin
RA	retinoic acid
RAR	retinoic acid receptor(s)
RXR	retinoid X receptor(s)
SHM	somatic hypermutation
TLR	Toll-like receptor
TNFα	tumor necrosis factor alpha

I. Introduction

Vitamin A has long been implicated as an essential nutritional factor for normal immunity. In the 1920s, vitamin A was named "the anti-infective vitamin," based on observations that vitamin A-deficient animals succumbed to infectious disease, while vitamin A-adequate animals recovered and survived. In humans, vitamin A deficiency is associated with increased mortality in children and pregnant women (Van *et al.*, 2002; West, 2002). Providing vitamin A supplements to vitamin A-deficient children, ages 6–72 months, reduces all-cause mortality by 23%, measles-related mortality by 50%, and diarrheal disease mortality by 33% (WHO/UNICEF, 1998; and previous reviews). The anti-infective effect of vitamin A could be partially attributable to the prevention of VA deficiency. Enhanced immunity may also be involved, due to vitamin A or its active metabolite, retinoic acid (RA), which has gained attention due to its multiple effects on innate and adaptive immunity, including its ability to modulate cytokine production (Ma *et al.*, 2005), promote the development of Th2 cells (Hoag *et al.*, 2002), induce gut-homing T cells (Iwata *et al.*, 2004) and T-regulatory cells (Benson *et al.*, 2007), regulate Th-17 cells (Mucida *et al.*, 2007), stimulate B-cell maturation (Chen and Ross, 2007; Wei *et al.*, 2007), and increase primary and memory antibody responses (DeCicco and Ross, 2000; DeCicco *et al.*, 2000; Ma *et al.*, 2005).

In this chapter, we first discuss vitamin A and RA signaling, which is important in all organ systems, including the hematopoietic and immune systems. We then focus on B cells as a target of retinoid action. B cells are critical to a successful vaccination response, and antibodies are a central hallmark of adaptive immunity. All of the presently licensed vaccines "work" by eliciting antibodies, which recognize and bind to the pathogen and then activate the body's immune system to destroy any of these microorganisms that it later encounters. Hence, understanding the roles of vitamin A in the regulation of B cells and B-cell responses has important implications for vaccine development and effective immunization. B cells are not only important as "factories" for the production of antibodies, but are also one of the types of immune system cell classified as professional antigen-presenting cells (APC). Additionally, B cells may be more multifunctional than previously understood, with recent evident for populations of regulatory B cells (DiLillo *et al.*, 2010). Here, we first discuss RA as a factor in the development and competence of mature B cells, then as a factor in B-cell proliferation, and in the regulation of transcription factors associated with B-cell differentiation, class switch recombination (CSR), and the generation of antibody-secreting plasma cells (PC). We conclude with emerging evidence that RA can function alone and in combination with other immune system stimuli to augment the formation of germinal centers (GC), leading to increased primary and secondary antibody responses. Taken together, the evidence supports the essentiality of vitamin A for normal functions, while suggesting that RA itself could be useful component in vaccine strategies and/or for immunotherapy.

II. The Vitamin A–Retinoic Acid Signaling System

A. Nutritional physiology and functions

Vitamin A is a fat-soluble micronutrient that is required in the diet of all chordates. Although retinol itself has no defined independent activity, it is essential as the precursor for the generation of retinal, a component of rhodopsin, and of all-*trans*-RA, the principal ligand for the nuclear retinoid receptors, RARα, ß, and γ. These class 2 nuclear receptor proteins form a heterodimeric complex with retinoid X receptors (RXR) and together the RAR–RXR function as important transcription factors (Altucci and Gronemeyer, 2001; Bastien and Rochette-Egly, 2004; Wei, 2003). The target DNA sequences in retinoid-regulated target genes to which the RAR–RXR bind, termed RA response elements (RARE), often comprise a direct repeat of the hexanucleotide sequence A(G/A)GTCA with either two or five intervening nucleotides. Current evidence supports a model in which most RAR–RXR proteins are bound to target DNA sequences in an inactive, repressed state in the absence of ligand. The binding of ligand, for example, of physiologically produced all-*trans*-RA, or a suitable exogenous analog, to the RAR triggers a conformational change, specifically a large shift in the position of helix-12 of the RAR protein that, in turn, strengthens the binding of the RAR–RXR to DNA and to coactivator or corepressor molecules that are part of a multiprotein complex that regulates the activity of DNA-dependent RNA polymerase (Altucci and Gronemeyer, 2001; Balmer and Blomhoff, 2002; Bastien and Rochette-Egly, 2004; Wei, 2003). In addition to all-*trans*-RA, numerous synthetic retinoid analogs possess agonistic activity, while other act as antagonistically. Several dozen genes are now considered *bona fide* direct targets of RA (Balmer and Blomhoff, 2002). However, several hundred other genes have been shown to respond in a physiological manner to RA, but direct or indirect mechanisms for these genes have not yet been established. Cell differentiation is often closely controlled by retinoid signaling through the RAR–RXR dimer, making retinoids of great interest in normal biology, as well as in the field of cancer prevention and differentiation therapy (Altucci and Gronemeyer, 2001; Fields *et al.*, 2007; Vitoux *et al.*, 2007). The RXR also form heterodimers with numerous other nuclear receptors including the vitamin D receptor, thyroid hormone receptor, peroxisome proliferator activator receptors (PPARs), lipid-activated receptors (LXR, FXR), and xenobiotic-activated receptors (PXR, CAR; Altucci and Gronemeyer, 2001). Hence, RXR signaling has both a retinoid-specific component mediated by RAR–RXR actions, and a very broad component due to the involvement of RXR with other nuclear receptors.

B. Clinical and experimental uses of RA

Besides being produced *in vivo* in a highly regulated manner (Napoli, 2000; Ross *et al.*, 2001), RA is also used clinically, with applications in the treatment of skin disorders and certain cancers, including leukemias (Fields *et al.*, 2007; Vitoux *et al.*, 2007). It is important to keep in mind that physiologically produced and exogenously administered RA may act differently, due to differences in achieved concentrations or distribution profiles of pharmacological levels of RA (Muindi *et al.*, 1994). Due to its lipophilic nature, RA is readily taken into cells by passive diffusion. In experimental studies, RA is often added directly to cells or organ cultures, sometimes at much higher concentrations than the 10–20 nM level present in normal plasma, or it may be administered to animals by a nonphysiological route, such as via injections (i.p., or s.c., resulting in a "bolus" effect), or in slow-release pellets implanted under the skin, which may deliver low or high doses depending on the retinoid loading and type of pellet. Even orally administered RA is not truly physiological since RA is not present at substantial levels in the diet (Ross, 2010). Despite these caveats, the use of RA administered by these routes may reveal potential mechanisms by which RA can act as a regulator of the immune system. However, it is also possible that the natural, local production of RA is integral to its actual physiological functions, in which case exogenous RA may exert actions that would not normally be observed *in vivo*. As important immunoregulatory roles for RA are further suggested, it will be important to integrate studies of the biological production and catabolism of RA into the larger picture, if a true understanding of the actions of vitamin A and RA in the immune system is to be achieved. Surprisingly, no systematic study has yet been conducted of VA concentrations in the organs of the immune system. However, based on analysis of casual samples, little retinyl ester is stored in the thymus, spleen, or lymph nodes. If this is correct, then immune system tissues depend on plasma retinol, and would be expected to be affected by low plasma levels of vitamin A, such as in situations of marginal or overt vitamin A deficiency. As discussed below, B cells are very sensitive to RA at physiological concentrations, with *in vitro* responses often produced by the addition of 10–20 nM of RA, similar to the physiological concentration of RA in plasma.

III. RA as a Factor in B-Cell Maturation, Activation, and Proliferation

A. Immunocompetence and initial activation

Retinoid signaling is important in all organ systems, including the hematopoietic and immune systems (Ross, 1994). Vitamin A-deficient animals exhibit abnormalities of lymphocyte numbers in plasma and spleen, with reduced T cell and sometimes B-cell populations, and, generally, increases in myeloid cells and especially granulocytes (Kuwata *et al.*, 2000; Zhao and Ross, 1995), whereas RA inhibits granulocyte–macrophage colony-stimulating factor production and granulocyte development (Smeland *et al.*, 1994), and reverses the effects of vitamin A-deficient state *in vivo* (Zhao and Ross, 1995). Animal experiments conducted from several angles have demonstrated that RA signaling plays a critical role in B-lymphoid development. The B cell is the major cell type that mediates the humoral immune response. After lineage development in bone marrow, naive B cells enter the circulation and reside in the secondary lymphoid organs, such as lymph nodes, tonsils, and spleen, and become follicular and marginal zone B cells, depending on location, or they recirculate to the bone marrow to reside in sinuses, where they may receive signal from T cells and/or provide surveillance against the blood-borne antigens. Vitamin A and RA regulate the maturation and differentiation of B cells at multiple levels that, in combination, regulate and often potentiate antibody production overall.

Vitamin A deficiency has been shown to reduce the number of fetal B-cell progenitors, while the pan-RAR antagonist, LE540, inhibited both fetal and adult B lymphopoiesis, as studied *in vitro* (Chen *et al.*, 2009). In another *in vitro* study that used RA at a physiological concentration, although RA inhibited the proliferation of normal B-cell progenitors of both mice and humans (Fahlman *et al.*, 1995), it affected multiple stages of B lymphopoiesis and accelerated the generation of $CD19^{+}sIgM^{+}$ B cells (Chen *et al.*, 2008). These results suggest that RA helps to provide a microenvironment that favors B-cell development and maintains a functional B-cell pool that is essential for the response to antigen (Fig. 5.1).

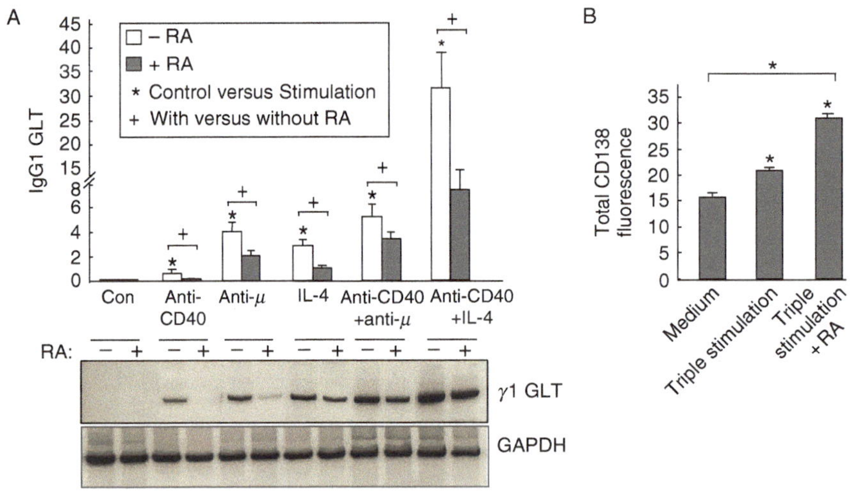

Figure 5.1 Retinoic acid decreased stimulation-induced IgG1 germline transcript expression. B cells were cultured *in vitro* with stimulation as indicated for different times. (A) RA inhibited CD40-ligation-induced γ1 GLT in B cells were variously stimulated with anti-CD40 (1 μg/ml), anti-μ (1 μg/ml), or IL-4 (2 ng/ml) with and without 20 nM RA for 48 h. A representative PCR gel image is showed along with the chart. Data shown were normalized to GAPDH mRNA. (B) RA increased CD138 expression on activated B cells. Flow-sorted CD138-negative B cells were cultured with medium alone or with triple stimulation (anti-μ, anti-CD40, and IL-4) in the presence and absence of 20 nM RA. After 5 days, cells were stained with anti-CD138-PE antibody. Mean ± SEM; $*P < 0.05$. (Figure modified from Chen and Ross, 2007, with permission of Cellular Immunology.)

The majority of mature B cells enter the circulation and reside in the peripheral lymphoid organs. The ligation of the B-cell receptor (BCR) by cognate antigen initiates B-cell activation, which is positively or negatively modulated by the interaction of other signals generated through various receptors present on the surface of the B cell. Several important receptors include CD19, a coreceptor for the BCR (Ishiura *et al.*, 2010); the Toll-like receptors, notably TLR4 which binds lipopolysaccharide (LPS), a well known direct mitogen for B cells; CD40, a receptor for the CD40 ligand expressed by activated T cells, which provides costimulation to B cells; B7 molecules (CD80 and CD86) which interact with CD28 on T cells; and additional molecules such as CD38 and cytokine receptors like the IL-4 receptor. Depending on the nature of stimuli or antigens and the strength of signaling, activated B cells will go through cell proliferation, CSR, and somatic hypermutation (SHM), and eventually become differentiated to antibody-secreting PCs to mount an effective immune response, or, if signaling is either too little or excessive, they will undergo apoptosis. Activation of the BCR triggers B-cell intrinsic signaling by the Src-family kinase, and through the Syk molecule, activating multiple signaling pathways, whereas BAFFR engagement activates the TNF receptor-associated factors. Both signaling pathways stimulate the classical and noncanonical NF-kB pathways, which are critical for B-cell survival, activation, and differentiation (Cancro, 2009; Stadanlick *et al.*, 2008).

B. Proliferation

Cell proliferation is one of the earlier events of B-cell activation, which is necessary to expand the antigen-activated B-cell pool and ensure a sufficient level of immune response. B-cells proliferation can be triggered *in vitro* in multiple ways. The engagement of BCR serves as a primary stimulus but, in addition, several costimulatory molecules or accessory receptors, such as CD38, CD40, and CD19, can directly stimulate B-cell proliferation or reduce the threshold of B-cell activation by antigens (Barrington *et al.*, 2009; Chen and Ross, 2005, 2007). The Toll-like receptor (TLR) agonists, such as LPS and CpG DNA, are multipotent mitogens that stimulate polyclonal B-cell proliferation via TLRs 4 and 9, respectively (Hoshino *et al.*, 1999; Krieg *et al.*, 1995). Recently, it has been shown that a group of glycolipid antigens can stimulate B-cell proliferation through the MHC class I-like molecule CD1d, present on certain B cells (Brigl and Brenner, 2010; Lang *et al.*, 2008), as well as myeloid cells. The prototypical and most often studied antigen for CD1d is alpha-galactosylceramide, a lipid extracted from a marine sponge; however, endogenous glycolipid antigens of mammalian cells also activate CD1d (Zhou *et al.*, 2004).

RA plays various roles to regulate B-cell activation and differentiation through its influences on these intrinsic signaling systems. Several lines of evidence have shown that the regulation of B-cell proliferation by RA depend on the nature of the stimulus encountered. At a physiological level (about 5–20 nM), RA inhibited the rate of proliferation of purified human peripheral blood B cells stimulated by anti-μ antibody (Blomhoff *et al.*, 1992). In murine naïve B cells stimulated with anti-μ to initiate BCR signaling and with anti-CD38 for ligation of the CD38 molecule on the surface of B cells, proliferation was reduced in the population as a whole, but a group of larger sized, less cycling, and more differentiated B cells emerged over time, and these cells expressed more surface(s) Ig, indicative of enhanced progression toward becoming antibody-secreting PCs (Chen and Ross, 2005). In an *in vitro* model of T-cell dependent B-cell activation, RA reduced B-cell proliferation induced by ligation of the BCR and CD40, and by LPS (Chen and Ross, 2005, 2007). The reduction of B-cell proliferation by RA under conditions of various stimuli suggests the involvement of a common pathway resulting in the negative regulation of the cell cycle and growth, when B cells are stimulated by cross-linking of BCR-related receptors and TLR4. Naderi and Blomhoff (1999) showed that the reduction in B-cell proliferation in normal human peripheral B cells was preceded by cell cycle arrest, as evidenced by the altered expression of several cell cycle regulatory factors. A negative regulation of the NF-κB pathway may also contribute to the inhibitory effect of RA on cell proliferation, as NF-κB family members play major roles in controlling B-cell development and proliferation (Chen *et al.*, 2002; Siebenlist *et al.*, 2005). Studies of a B-lymphoid cell line in culture have also demonstrated that RA suppresses proliferation by blocking the ionized calcium channel, which mediates the early calcium response after BCR ligation (Bosma and Sidell, 1988).

In contrast to the inhibitory effect of RA on B-cell proliferation stimulated by BCR ligation and LPS as discussed above, RA increased the proliferation of memory B cells when B cells were stimulated with CpG DNA, which induces cell activation through TLR9 (Ertesvag *et al.*, 2007). The increased rate of B-cell proliferation was accompanied by increased secretion of antibody. In a mechanistic study, Ertesvag *et al.* (2007) demonstrated that the enhanced proliferation and differentiation by RA corresponded to the activation of the p38 MAPK pathway that resulted in retinoblastoma protein phosphorylation and increased the level of cyclin D, factors that stimulate cell cycle progression. We also have also observed that RA increases the proliferation of purified murine spleen B cells stimulated by α-galactosylceramide, a ligand for the CD1d receptor, which was correlated with B-cell differentiation, evidenced by sIgG1 and CD138 expression (Q. Chen, unpublished data), while at the same time RA reduced the proliferation of identical B cells stimulated by LPS.

These contrasting results imply that RA affects B-cell proliferation differentially, in a manner that depends on the B-cell subpopulation as well as the stimulus. Whereas RA inhibits mature B-cell proliferation, which may facilitate their differentiation of the activated B cells toward PCs, RA promotes the expansion of a subset of B cells which undergo further differentiation (Chen and Ross, 2005), both processes leading to the promotion of antibody production. Additionally, whereas physiological levels of RA inhibited B-cell proliferation, RA at the same concentration also prevented spontaneous apoptosis of B lymphocytes (Lomo *et al.*, 1998), further suggesting that although RA inhibits mature B-cell proliferation, it functions to maintain the functional B-cell pool, as required for an effective memory response. Further studies are needed to better define whether it is the stage of B-cell activation *per se* (naïve or memory) or the stimulus itself, or both, that determines whether RA promotes or inhibits B-cell cycling and proliferation.

IV. Transcription Factors, CSR, and B-Cell Differentiation Toward the PC Phenotype

A. Transcription factors promoting B-cell differentiation

Antigens, bacteria products, and T-cell signals can active B cells through engagement of BCR, TLR, and CD40 present on the B-cell surface, which variously trigger multiple pathways that involve activation/inactivation of many transcription factors. The concerted regulation of these factors is necessary to ensure sufficient and specific humoral immunity, while avoiding the generation of self-reactive antibodies. Four key transcription factors that coordinate the B-cell activation and differentiation are the paired box gene 5 (Pax5), B-cell lymphoma 6 (BCL-6), B lymphocyte-induced maturation protein-1 (BLIMP-1, gene *PRDM1*), and X-box binding protein 1 (XBP-1; Iwakoshi *et al.*, 2003). As RA participates in the regulation of B-cell lymphopoiesis as well as B-cell activation, it differentially affects the activity of at least some of these B-cell transcription factors, according to the functional stages of the B cell. A schematic of B-cell development, and the effect of RA on various processes, is shown in Fig. 5.2.

Pax5 is essential for B-cell lineage commitment, and is responsible for sustained B-cell lymphopoiesis and expansion of the B-cell pool (Northrup and Allman, 2008). Pax5, originally known as B-cell-lineage-specific activator protein (BASP), is required for B-cell lineage commitment and development as well as B-cell function through the GC stage (Horcher *et al.*, 2001). Pax5 can activate many B-cell-related genes, including CD19, CD79A, B-cell linker (BLNK), and activation-induced cytidine deaminase (AID), an mRNA deaminase essential for B-cell identity, activation, and the GC reaction (Shapiro-Shelef and Calame, 2005). The major function of AID is to deaminate cytidine residues in the variable or switch regions of the Ig genes, thereby initiating SHM and CSR, respectively (de Yebenes and

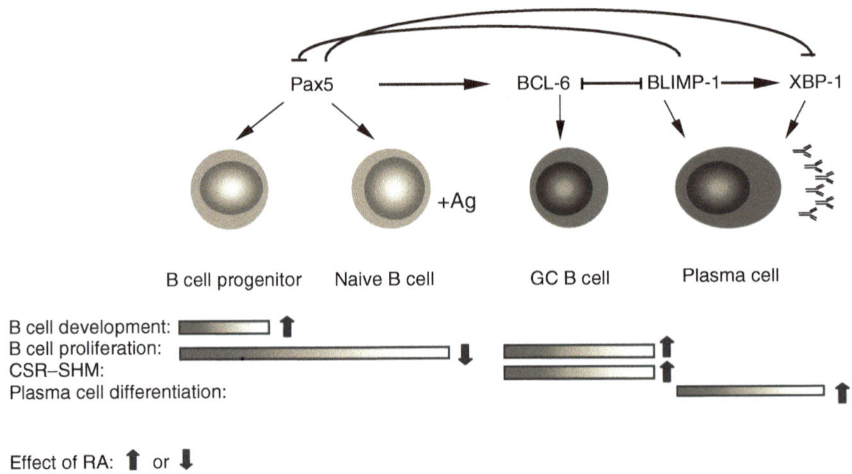

Figure 5.2 Schematic illustration of B-cell maturation/differentiation process under the control of transcriptional factors. Pax5 is indispensable for B-cell lineage development and proliferation, BCL-6 is essential for GC B-cell reaction that includes B-cell proliferation, CSR, and SHM, unselected cells go through apoptosis; BLIMP-1 is critical for plasma cell differentiation, it suppresses Pax5 expression, and together with XBP-1, ensues antibody production. RA regulates the process at multiple steps. As indicated by arrows, RA promotes B-cell lineage development, inhibits the mature B-cell proliferation, enhances CSR and SHM by increasing Aid gene expression, and augments the terminal differentiation of B cells towards plasma cell phenotype.

Ramiro, 2006). In murine B lymphopoiesis, RA markedly increased the Pax5 expression level early in the B-cell development phase (the progenitors), corresponding to promotion of the enrichment of the $CD19^+$ $sIgM^+$ B-cell population (Chen *et al.*, 2008). In contrast, at the mature B-cell phase, the presence of RA decreased the Pax5 expression level, which favors the differentiation of $sIgG1^+$ cells (Chen and Ross, 2005). Pax5 is known to repress genes related to antibody secretion, such as XBP1, IgH, IgL, and the J chain, thereby blocking the development of PCs (Calame *et al.*, 2003). Inhibition of Pax5 downregulates IL-4/LPS-induced Ig class switching (Wakatsuki *et al.*, 1994); in contrast, overexpression of Pax5 stimulates B-cell proliferation but suppresses Ig synthesis in both late B-cell lines and PC lines (Usui *et al.*, 1997). Hence, Pax5 promotes the GC reaction but suppresses PC differentiation. In mouse B cells *in vitro*, RA significantly elevated the mRNA level of AID, suggesting that RA might enhance the isotype switching by inducing the expression of AID (Chen and Ross, 2005).

Oppositely, Blimp-1 is highly expressed in PCs and is known to control many genes that are important for PC differentiation. BLIMP-1 is a 98-kDa transcriptional repressor, expressed in all PCs and a subset of GC B cells, which plays an essential role in PC formation and Ig secretion. Introduction of Blimp-1 into B cells directly repressed genes involved in mature B-cell functions, including the genes for B-cell identity, BCR signaling components, and genes required for Ig class switching (Angelin-Duclos *et al.*, 2000; Calame *et al.*, 2003). Moreover, BLIMP-1 directly inhibited Pax5 and BCL-6, two major transcription factor genes essential for the GC formation. In contrast, BLIMP-1 induced several genes related to PC differentiation and Ig secretion, such as XBP-1 and J chain. Hence, BLIMP-1 functions to terminate the GC reaction, but it promotes plasmacytic cell differentiation by initiating and regulating a cascade of gene expression (Shaffer *et al.*, 2002). BLIMP-1 also regulates XBP-1, which induces formation of the secretory apparatus necessary for the production of antibody, which is crucial for PC differentiation and Ig secretion (Hu *et al.*, 2009). XBP-1 is a basic region leucine zipper protein and a member of the CREB/ATF family of transcription factors. Compared with other immature and mature B cells, the level of XBP-1 is much higher in PC lines. XBP-1 deficiency significantly impairs PC differentiation and severely reduced serum antibody levels, while oppositely, introduction of Xbp1 into B lineage cells initiates PC differentiation (Iwakoshi *et al.*, 2003).

The accepted central concept is that along with B-cell differentiation, stimulation of B cells with antigen releases Blimp-1 from the suppression of BCL-6, increased expression of Blimp-1 suppressed the expression of Pax5 (Lin *et al.*, 2002), leading to cessation of proliferation and, thence, to the terminal differentiation of B cells (Crotty *et al.*, 2010; Tunyaplin *et al.*, 2004). Bcl-6 is expressed predominantly in the GC B cells; however, it is undetectable in antibody-secreting PCs (Cattoretti *et al.*, 1995). Bcl-6 is crucial in the induction of GC B-cell proliferation and the suppression of CSR/SHM; therefore Bcl-6 plays a central role in GC development and inhibition of PC differentiation (Fukuda *et al.*, 1997; Shaffer *et al.*, 2000). Also, for this reason, the elimination of Bcl-6 from PCs is necessary for the terminal differentiation of B cells. Although Bcl-6 mRNA in resting B cells and GC B cells are identical, BCL-6 protein was expressed about three to 34-fold higher in GC B cells than in resting B cells (Allman *et al.*, 1996). The major function of BCL-6 is to inhibit the expression of Blimp-1, a transcription factor inducing PC differentiation, which allows the GC reaction to continue but prevents premature PC differentiation (Shapiro-Shelef and Calame, 2005). At this phase, increased expression of Xbp-1 ensures that the PCs secrete antibody (Hu *et al.*, 2009). Besides the Pax-5/BCL-6/BLIMP-1/XBP-1 axis, another transcription factor, interferon (IFN) regulatory factor 4 (IRF-4) has emerged recently as a critical regulator for B-cell differentiation. A mechanistic study has demonstrated that IRF-4 directly upregulate Blimp-1 transcription to promote PC differentiation (Sciammas *et al.*, 2006). An interesting model was drawn by Sciammas *et al.* (2006) in which a low level of IRF-4 could increase AID expression and promote CSR and SHM, whereas a high level of IRF-4 could increase Blimp-1, that promotes PC differentiation.

Our studies in a model of murine splenic B-cell differentiation have shown that addition of a physiological concentration of RA induces B-cell differentiation after ligation of the BCR, CD38, or CD40. A decreased rate of cell proliferation, located in a population of larger activated B cells, was accompanied by a reduction in Pax5 and an increase in Aid and Blimp-1 expression levels, which led with time in culture to the development of the PC phenotype, with a higher level of sIgG1 expression and CD138 (syndecan-1), known as a hallmark of antibody-secreting cells (Chen and Ross, 2005, 2007). Syndecan-1, also called CD138, is a heparin sulfate-rich proteoglycan present on the plasma membrane. Although it is expressed on several types of cells, the expression of syndecan-1 on B cells is commonly used to identify PCs, as thus serves as a marker of terminally differentiated plasmacytic cells (Sanderson *et al.*, 1989). During normal B-cell differentiation, syndecan-1 is temporarily expressed on pre-B cells, lost on circulating B cells, and then reexpressed on PCs. The onset of syndecan-1 expression on PCs in mice correlates closely with immunoglobulin secretion. In murine B cells in the presence of a physiological concentration of RA, activated spleen B cells expressed a higher level of CD138 that correlated with the increased level of sIgG1 expression, and the cessation of B-cell proliferation, indicating a more differentiated B-cell phenotype.

Although the detailed mechanisms are not yet clear, the involvement of RA in the regulation of multiple signaling pathways, such as NF-κB, MAPK, and cell cycle regulation, may help to explain its regulatory role. It is worthwhile to note that activation of NF-κB is essential for B-cell proliferation through transactivation of cell growth-related genes, but on the other hand, it also activates prmd-1/Blimp-1 gene expression, and is important in PC differentiation (Morgan *et al.*, 2009), suggesting that the spatiotemporal-specific expression of the transcription factors is especially critical.

So far, little is known regarding the regulation by RA of the expression of Xbp-1 and IRF-4. It will be interesting in future studies to further identify the role of RA in this important autoregulatory loop that coordinates the process of PC differentiation.

B. Class switch recombination

After activation by antigen, mature B lymphocytes in the peripheral organs go through CSR and SHM, processes that diversify the immunoglobulin (Ig) genes and increase the affinity of antibody, respectively. Both Ig CSR and SHM are tightly controlled events that are stimulus specific as well as activation stage specific. CSR is a deletional DNA recombination that occurs between two switch (S) regions located upstream of each heavy-chain constant region (C_H). CSR results in replacement of the Cμ gene by one of the downstream C_H genes (Cγ, Cα, or Cε), which consequently leads to the production of IgG, IgA, and IgE (Zhang, 2003). AID, which is expressed at high level mainly in activated mature B cells undergoing CSR and SHM, plays an essential role in both of these processes (de Yebenes and Ramiro, 2006). The expression of AID in B cells can be induced by stimulation with bacterial products, like LPS, cytokines such as IL-4, transforming growth factor-β (TGF-β) and IFN-γ, and the ligand for the costimulatory molecule CD40; all of these stimuli more or less participate in B-cell CSR and SHM to certain levels (Xu *et al.*, 2007). By examining at the promoter of Aid gene, Tran *et al.* (2010) reported a region that is responsible for cytokine or B-cell-specific activator mediated transcription activation of the Aid gene. It is also a region that binds to the transcription factors Pax-5 and E47 to maintain a low level of Aid expression in the steady state. Interestingly, RA increased Aid gene expression in BCR-stimulated B cells, suggesting its positive role in regulation of CSR (Chen and Ross, 2005). Other studies have shown that RA can synergize with TGF-β1 to promote IgA CSR, a process relevant to mucosal immunity (Watanabe *et al.*, 2010). RA also increased the CD40 and IL-4-induced IgG CSR, but inhibited the CD40 and IL-4-induced IgE CSR (Chen and Ross, 2007; Scheffel *et al.*, 2005), indicating that RA can affect the balance of Ig classes produced by antigen-stimulated B cells.

During CSR, the germline transcript (GLT) is first synthesized and then processed to a mature Ig transcript that leads to class-switched Ig production. We have observed that upon stimulation of normal murine naïve B cells, such as by ligation of the BCR, CD38, or CD40 ligation, the stimulated B cells express a higher level of Aid mRNA as well as increased γ1 GLT, which can be detected within 24 h after stimulation. The addition of a physiological concentration of RA (20 nM) increased the Aid mRNA level. However, conversely, RA dramatically decreased the level of γ1GLT and, similarly, the level of Pax5 transcript (Chen and Ross, 2005). After day 3 of stimulation, the surface IgG1 level was increased in the presence of RA regardless of the suppression of γ1 GLT level. This result suggests that, although GLT formation is essential for B cells to undergo class switching, there is not necessarily a direct relationship between the level of γ1 GLT formation and the outcome in terms of IgG1-expressing B cells. Overall, we propose that RA promotes CSR by upregulation of Aid and downregulation of Pax5 gene expression, while the GLT is a temporary product that provides a signal for the initiation of CSR, but is not a quantitatively regulated in a manner that predicts B-cell Ig production. Under the same conditions, RA promotes an increase in syndecan-1 expression, which reflects maturation toward the PC phenotype.

V. RA as a Factor in Germinal Center Formation

To understand the mechanisms regarding RA's effect on the antibody response to T-cell dependent antigens, examination of GC formation is essential. Within the GC, several essential molecular processes take place, such as expansion of B cells, CSR, and SHM, and then the differentiation of memory B cells and PCs, which all are necessary for the evolution of prolonged humoral immunity (Klein and Dalla-Favera, 2008). Upon activation by T-cell dependent antigens (e.g., proteins), some B cells directly go through isotype switching and differentiate into low-affinity PCs. However, many activated B cells migrate into primary follicles, and then rapidly expand to form secondary follicles. About 1 week after antigen priming, the secondary follicle polarizes into the dark zone and the light zone, forming a dynamic structure called the GC, which is primarily comprised of antigen-specific B cells and T-helper cells, follicular dendritic cells (FDC), a type of stromal cell, as well as macrophages (Allen and Cyster, 2008). Histologically, the GC exhibits polarization into two zonal regions termed the dark zone and the light zone. In the dark zone, newly stimulated and still relatively small B cells proliferate rapidly and undergo somatic mutation by the CSR reaction discussed above. The progeny of these B cells, termed centrocytes, migrate into the light zone, where FDC together with antigen-activated Th cells, provide essential signals for B cell survival, CSR, affinity maturation (SHM), and differentiation into long-lived PCs or memory B cells (Benson *et al.*, 2007; Chappell and Jacob, 2007; McHeyzer-Williams *et al.*, 2006; Stavnezer *et al.*, 2008). Hence, the formation of the GC structure and the cellular and molecular processes that occur within the GC are essential for the generation of B cells expressing antibodies of the IgG, IgA, or IgE classes, with high-affinity antigen-combining sites, as well as for the production of memory B cells (McHeyzer-Williams *et al.*, 2006).

The GC reaction and the differentiation of activated B cells into PCs and memory B cells are regulated by the transcription factors described above, that form an autoregulatory loop controlled by Pax5/Bcl-6/Blimp-1. Downregulation of Pax5 and the sequential expression of Bcl-6 and Blimp-1 are required for the induction of PC development. IRF-4 and XBP-1 are also essential to function together with BLIMP-1 in promoting centrocytes to differentiate to PCs (Kallies and Nutt, 2007; Saito *et al.*, 2007). Regarding the role of RA, evidence suggests that RA affects several cell processes that may be expected to facilitate the GC reaction. RA increases CD40 expression on DC that, in turn, enhances the activation of B cells (Park *et al.*, 2004). RA also increases the expression of homing molecules such as the integrin family proteins that promote B-cell migration to the GC (Mora *et al.*, 2006). Moreover, RA affects the FDC to increase the efficiency of antigen presentation and antibody production (Suzuki *et al.*, 2010). Furthermore, as discussed above, RA also regulates the expression of transcription factors that favor the differentiation of PCs and memory B cells (Chen and Ross, 2005). All these processes together may help to explain the enhanced antibody production by RA observed in animal studies in a T-cell dependent antigen immunization model (described below; Ma *et al.*, 2005). In Peyer's patches, the activation of RAR and TLR signaling by the presence of RA with bacteria products activates FDC within GC, and leads to enhanced expression of the chemokine CXCL13 and the survival factor BAFF/April, which then facilitate the secretion of the TGF-ß1, the major cytokine promoting IgA class switching in Peyer's patches. These factors together increase the numbers of GC B cells and promote the generation of IgA (+) B cells within GCs (Suzuki *et al.*, 2010).

Previous studies demonstrated that the combination of RA and polyinosinic acid:polycytidylic acid (PIC), a strong inducer of type I IFN and IFN-γ and other cytokines, significantly enhanced T-cell dependent antibody production in vitamin A-deficient (DeCicco *et al.*, 2000) and vitamin A-adequate rats (DeCicco *et al.*, 2001), and in both adult and neonatal mice immunized with tetanus toxoid (Ma and Ross, 2005; Ma *et al.*, 2005; see Ross *et al.*, 2009 for further review). On one hand, PIC was shown to potentiate the primary antibody response, but have little impact on the memory response (DeCicco *et al.*, 2000). On the other hand, RA enhanced both the primary and secondary responses, but the combination of RA + PIC produced a powerful increase in both the primary and secondary antibody responses (DeCicco *et al.*, 2000, 2001; Ma and Ross, 2005; Ma *et al.*, 2005), although mice were only treated with RA and PIC at the time of priming. From these studies, we proposed that RA both augments and "imprints" the immune response (as shown by Iwata *et al.*, 2004 for gut-homing T cells), whereas PIC through the rapid but transient production of IFNs and other cytokines, affects the initial reactions of APCs and activated T and B cells, but cannot by itself promote the differentiation of memory cells. With these results pointing to the importance of RA and PIC at the time or priming, it was of interest to determine how RA, PIC, and the combination, which produced the strongest impact on antibody production, might affect the GC reaction.

A. Costimulation with RA and PIC enhance antigen-induced GC formation

GC B cells can be identified using two surface markers: B220 and peanut agglutinin (PNA). PNA is a plant lectin that specifically binds to lymphocyte glycoprotein on terminal galactosyl residues (Reichert *et al.*, 1983). PNA was first reported as a surface marker for immature (cortical) thymocytes, which could bind over 90% of thymus cells (Lahvis and Cerny, 1997; Rose *et al.*, 1980). Later studies showed that PNA also selectively bound to

GC cells in peripheral lymphoid organs. Compared with other B cells and T cells, GC B cells bind about 10–30 times more of PNA. Based on these results, PNA is used as a major marker of GC B cells, and GC B cells are defined as $B220^{+}PNA^{Hi}$ cells.

Based on the observations described above that RA and PIC administered at the time of antigen priming promoted a robust primary and secondary antibody response, we hypothesized that RA and PIC alone, and especially in combination, could act as a promising vaccine adjuvant, which might stimulate GC formation. Thus, studies were conducted in normal adult mice that were immunized with tetanus toxoid as a prototypical and clinically relevant T-cell dependent antigen, and treated at the time of priming with RA, PIC, or both in combination (RA + PIC). Immunization with tetanus toxoid alone induced a weak but detectable GC reaction, visualized as relatively small PNA-positive GC, with fewer than 20% of the B-cell follicles containing a visible PNA-positive GC (Fig. 5.3A). However, RA, PIC, and RA+PIC increased the number of GC and elevated the GC-to-B-cell follicle ratio about two- to threefold (Fig. 5.3B), while, in addition, the average size of the GC was increased. The enhanced GC response depended on the antigen challenge, because RA and PIC did not induce the GC formation in naïve mice. These treatments increased the plasma titers of antitetanus IgG1, as expected, and by linear regression analysis the plasma antitetanus IgG1 titers were well correlated with both the fraction of B-cell follicles with a GC ($R^2 = 0.69$; $p < 0.01$; Fig. 5.3C) and the size of GC ($R^2 = 0.51$, $p < 0.05$; see Ma and Ross, 2009). Therefore, RA and PIC alone and especially combined promoted the tetanus toxoid-induced GC response, which may have directly contributed to the enhanced antitetanus IgG response measured in plasma.

B. FDC network formation

Because FDCs, as stromal cells in the GC, play a critical role in the GC response (Cyster *et al.*, 2000), and are particularly important for the positive selection of high-affinity B cells (Park and Choi, 2005), and RA and/or PIC significantly increased antigen-induced GC formation and antitetanus IgG production, we tested their effects on the formation of FDC networks, visualized by staining with anti-mouse FDC-M1, a marker of FDC. The FDC networks were located on the one side of GC (see Fig. 5.3D arrows; RA + PIC treatment), consistent with reports that FDC networks mostly occupy the light zone of the polarized GC (Cozine *et al.*, 2005; MacLennan *et al.*, 1992; Steiniger and Barth, 2000). Although RA and or PIC did not affect FDC number, they enlarged the average area of FDC networks about 30-40%, whereas in the immunized control group, the FDC networks were small and dim (see Fig. 5.3D). After administration of PIC and RA + PIC,

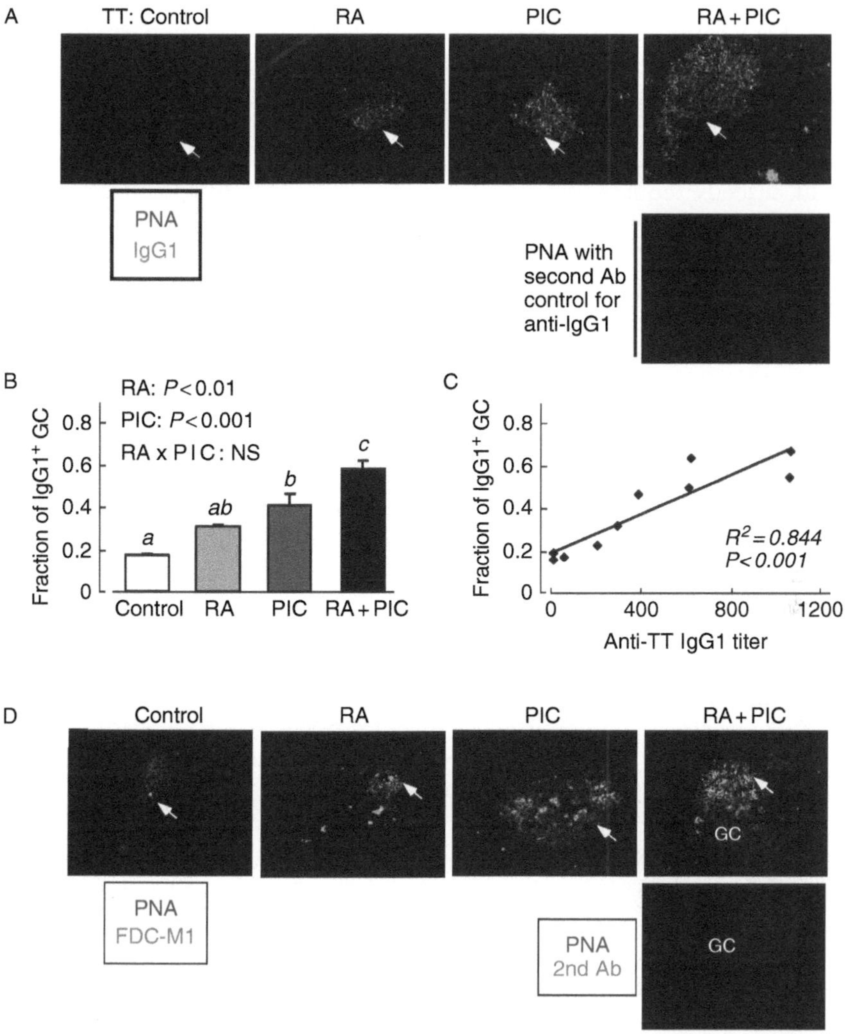

Figure 5.3 RA and PIC promote TT-induced GC formation. Mice were immunized with tetanus toxoid (TT) and treated with RA orally for 5 days and with PIC at the time of antigen priming. (A) On day 10, fixed spleen sections were prepared and 7-μm sections were stained with biotinylated peanut agglutinin (PNA) followed by incubation with Alexa-568-Streptavidin (red) to detect GC, and with FITC-anti-mouse IgD to identify B-cell follicles (green). Results for nonimmunized mice showed no substantial GC formation. (B) The proportion of B-cell follicles containing a GC, determined by microscopic imaging and counting (Ma and Ross, 2009). The number and relative size of GC were determined by imaging a minimum of 20 GC in each spleen. Bars show mean ± SE, $n = 4$ mice/group. Different letters above bars within panels indicate significant differences ($P < 0.05$, $a < b$). Results of two-way ANOVA are also shown in each panel. (C) Linear regression analysis of the plasma anti-TT IgG response versus the proportion of follicles with a GC, determined for the same animals. (D) GC staining of the same spleen samples with biotinylated PNA (red stain), and monoclonal antibody against FDC (FDC-M1, green stain). (Figure modified from (Ma and Ross, 2009), with permission of Clinical and Vaccine Immunology.) (See Color Insert.)

there was a robust enhancement in the formation of FDC networks in GC, as shown by more intense staining and an increase of about 3 times in the average size of the FDC network; these results also correlated well by linear regression with the titers of plasma anti-TT IgG. Therefore, the expansion of FDC networks in GC, mainly influenced by PIC but supported by RA, could directly contribute to the increase in antigen-specific antibody response by modulating GC microarchitecture and promoting the GC response, which is known to enhance the formation of long-lived antibody-secreting cells (Ma and Ross, 2009).

In addition to enhancing the antigen-triggered GC response, RA and/or PIC increased the number of $IgG1^+$ PCs in the periarteriolar lymphoid sheath (PALS) region, a T-cell zone in spleen where naïve B cells are exposed to antigen and become activated. Upon activation, some T-cell dependent antigen-specific B cells remain in the PALS region and differentiate into short-lived PCs (Angelin-Duclos *et al.*, 2000; Jacob *et al.*, 1991). Compared with the long-lived PC, these short-lived PC produce IgM and IgG antibodies with lower affinity and a shorter half-life. Hence, the PCs generated in the PALS region during the primary response contribute to an early adaptive immune response against antigens and pathogens. Thus it was of interest that RA, PIC, and RA plus PIC significantly increased the generation of PCs in the PALS region, suggesting that the treatments also enhanced the early and short-lived antibody production (Ma and Ross, 2009).

C. Future directions

Additional research is needed on the mechanisms by which RA and costimuli to enhance the recruitment of B and T cells to the GC, and/or their expansion through proliferation once recruited. RA plays an essential role in directing T cells to the gut (Iwata *et al.*, 2004), and in promote B-cell migration to the GC (Mora *et al.*, 2006). However, the molecular mechanisms by which RA promotes B- and T-cell homing to lymphoid follicles is presently unknown. Therefore, it will be interesting to determine if RA and stimuli such as PIC regulate GC B- and T-cell recruitment, and which genes and pathways are involved. In addition, the effect of RA and PIC on cell survival and cell death within GCs remains to be determined. Although there is little information on the regulation by RA of the expression of Bcl-6, which is the master regulator of GC reaction, the involvement of a common corepressor has been reported, which also interacted with RAR–RXR transcriptional activity (Dhordain *et al.*, 1997; Yamamoto *et al.*, 2010). While some research has addressed isotype switching through the CSR process, as discussed earlier, essentially nothing is known regarding whether RA affects affinity maturation through the SHM process, and therefore has any effect on the quality of the antibodies produced, through affinity maturation. Given indications as discussed above from studies of isolated B cells that RA can regulate AID (Chen and Ross, 2005, 2007), and that AID also mediates SHM, it would seem reasonable to expect that RA also affects SHM, but direct studies are still necessary. Further studies of AID in the context of GC formation *in vivo* will also be important for better defining the roles of vitamin A and RA in promoting humoral immunity.

Previous studies have shown that RA and PIC cooperatively enhance the secondary antibody response, as well as the primary antibody response in both VA-deficient and VA-sufficient animals (DeCicco *et al.*, 2000, 2001; Ma and Ross, 2005; Ma *et al.*, 2005; Ross *et al.*, 2009). Since GC formation is also important for B memory cell differentiation, further studies are needed to understand how RA and immunomodulatory agents like PIC, even when administered only at the time of priming as in the studies discussed above, can regulate the formation of B-cell memory and generation of long-lived cells that, upon reactivation, mediate the recall response to antigen or pathogen at a later time. Such questions are central to understanding how vitamin A and RA may be used to improve vaccination strategies in the future.

REFERENCES

Allen, C. D., and Cyster, J. G. (2008). Follicular dendritic cell networks of primary follicles and germinal centers: Phenotype and function. *Semin. Immunol.* **20,** 14–25.

Allman, D., Jain, A., Dent, A., Maile, R. R., Selvaggi, T., Kehry, M. R., and Staudt, L. M. (1996). BCL-6 expression during B-cell activation. *Blood* **87,** 5257–5268.

Altucci, L., and Gronemeyer, H. (2001). Nuclear receptors in cell life and death. *Trends Endocrinol. Metab.* **12,** 460–468.

Angelin-Duclos, C., Cattoretti, G., Lin, K. I., and Calame, K. (2000). Commitment of B lymphocytes to a plasma cell fate is associated with Blimp-1 expression in vivo. *J. Immunol.* **165,** 5462–5471.

Balmer, J. E., and Blomhoff, R. (2002). Gene expression regulation by retinoic acid. *J. Lipid Res.* **43,** 1773–1808.

Barrington, R. A., Schneider, T. J., Pitcher, L. A., Mempel, T. R., Ma, M., Barteneva, N. S., and Carroll, M. C. (2009). Uncoupling CD21 and CD19 of the B-cell coreceptor. *Proc. Natl. Acad. Sci. USA* **106,** 14490–14495.

Bastien, J., and Rochette-Egly, C. (2004). Nuclear retinoid receptors and the transcription of retinoid-target genes. *Gene* **328,** 1–16.

Benson, M. J., Pino-Lagos, K., Rosemblatt, M., and Noelle, R. J. (2007). All-trans retinoic acid mediates enhanced T reg cell growth, differentiation, and gut homing in the face of high levels of co-stimulation. *J. Exp. Med.* **204,** 1765–1774.

Blomhoff, H. K., Smeland, E. B., Erikstein, B., Rasmussen, A. M., Skrede, B., Skjonsberg, C., and Blomhoff, R. (1992). Vitamin A is a key regulator for cell growth, cytokine production, and differentiation in normal B cells. *J. Biol. Chem.* **267,** 23988–23992.

Bosma, M., and Sidell, N. (1988). Retinoic acid inhibits Ca2+ currents and cell proliferation in a B-lymphocyte cell line. *J. Cell. Physiol.* **135,** 317–323.

Brigl, M., and Brenner, M. B. (2010). How invariant natural killer T cells respond to infection by recognizing microbial or endogenous lipid antigens. *Semin. Immunol.* **22,** 79–86.
Calame, K. L., Lin, K. I., and Tunyaplin, C. (2003). Regulatory mechanisms that determine the development and function of plasma cells. *Annu. Rev. Immunol.* **21,** 205–230.
Cancro, M. P. (2009). Signalling crosstalk in B cells: Managing worth and need. *Nat. Rev. Immunol.* **9,** 657–661.
Cattoretti, G., Chang, C. C., Cechova, K., Zhang, J., Ye, B. H., Falini, B., Louie, D. C., Offit, K., Chaganti, R. S., and Dalla-Favera, R. (1995). BCL-6 protein is expressed in germinal-center B cells. *Blood* **86,** 45–53.
Chappell, C. P., and Jacob, J. (2007). Germinal-center-derived B-cell memory. *Adv. Exp. Med. Biol.* **590,** 139–148.
Chen, Q., and Ross, A. C. (2005). Vitamin A and immune function: Retinoic acid modulates population dynamics in antigen receptor and CD38-stimulated splenic B cells. *Proc. Natl. Acad. Sci. USA* **102,** 14142–14149.
Chen, Q., and Ross, A. C. (2007). Retinoic acid promotes mouse splenic B cell surface IgG expression and maturation stimulated by CD40 and IL-4. *Cell. Immunol.* **249,** 37–45.
Chen, Q., Ma, Y., and Ross, A. C. (2002). Opposing cytokine-specific effects of all trans-retinoic acid on the activation and expression of signal transducer and activator of transcription (STAT)-1 in THP-1 cells. *Immunology* **107,** 199–208.
Chen, X., Esplin, B. L., Garrett, K. P., Welner, R. S., Webb, C. F., and Kincade, P. W. (2008). Retinoids accelerate B lineage lymphoid differentiation. *J. Immunol.* **180,** 138–145.
Chen, X., Welner, R. S., and Kincade, P. W. (2009). A possible contribution of retinoids to regulation of fetal B lymphopoiesis. *Eur. J. Immunol.* **39,** 2515–2524.
Cozine, C. L., Wolniak, K. L., and Waldschmidt, T. J. (2005). The primary germinal center response in mice. *Curr. Opin. Immunol.* **17,** 298–302.
Crotty, S., Johnston, R. J., and Schoenberger, S. P. (2010). Effectors and memories: Bcl-6 and Blimp-1 in T and B lymphocyte differentiation. *Nat. Immunol.* **11,** 114–120.
Cyster, J. G., Ansel, K. M., Reif, K., Ekland, E. H., Hyman, P. L., Tang, H. L., Luther, S. A., and Ngo, V. N. (2000). Follicular stromal cells and lymphocyte homing to follicles. *Immunol. Rev.* **176,** 181–193.
de Yebenes, V. G., and Ramiro, A. R. (2006). Activation-induced deaminase: Light and dark sides. *Trends Mol. Med.* **12,** 432–439.
DeCicco, K. L., and Ross, A. C. (2000). All-trans-retinoic acid and polyriboinosinoic: polyribocytidylic acid cooperate to elevate anti-tetanus immunoglobulin G and immunoglobulin M responses in vitamin A-deficient Lewis rats and Balb/c mice. *Proc. Nutr. Soc.* **59,** 519–529.
DeCicco, K. L., Zolfaghari, R., Li, N., and Ross, A. C. (2000). Retinoic acid and poly-riboinosinic acid act synergistically to enhance the antibody response to tetanus toxoid during vitamin A deficiency: Possible involvement of interleukin-2 receptor-beta, signal transducer and activator of transcription-1, and interferon regulatory factor-1. *J. Infect. Dis.* **182**(Suppl 1), S29–S36.
DeCicco, K. L., Youngdahl, J. D., and Ross, A. C. (2001). All-trans-retinoic acid and polyriboinosinic:polyribocytidylic acid in combination potentiate specific antibody production and cell-mediated immunity. *Immunology* **104,** 341–348.
Dhordain, P., Albagli, O., Lin, R. J., Ansieau, S., Quief, S., Leutz, A., Kerckaert, J. P., Evans, R. M., and Leprince, D. (1997). Corepressor SMRT binds the BTB/POZ repressing domain of the LAZ3/BCL6 oncoprotein. *Proc. Natl. Acad. Sci. USA* **94,** 10762–10767.
DiLillo, D. J., Matsushita, T., and Tedder, T. F. (2010). B10 cells and regulatory B cells balance immune responses during inflammation, autoimmunity, and cancer. *Ann. N Y Acad. Sci.* **1183,** 38–57.

Ertesvag, A., Aasheim, H. C., Naderi, S., and Blomhoff, H. K. (2007). Vitamin A potentiates CpG-mediated memory B-cell proliferation and differentiation: Involvement of early activation of p38MAPK. *Blood* **109,** 3865–3872.

Fahlman, C., Jacobsen, S. E., Smeland, E. B., Lomo, J., Naess, C. E., Funderud, S., and Blomhoff, H. K. (1995). All-trans- and 9-cis-retinoic acid inhibit growth of normal human and murine B cell precursors. *J. Immunol.* **155,** 58–65.

Fields, A. L., Soprano, D. R., and Soprano, K. J. (2007). Retinoids in biological control and cancer. *J. Cell. Biochem.* **102,** 886–898.

Fukuda, T., Yoshida, T., Okada, S., Hatano, M., Miki, T., Ishibashi, K., Okabe, S., Koseki, H., Hirosawa, S., Taniguchi, M., Miyasaka, N., and Tokuhisa, T. (1997). Disruption of the Bcl6 gene results in an impaired germinal center formation. *J. Exp. Med.* **186,** 439–448.

Hoag, K. A., Nashold, F. E., Goverman, J., and Hayes, C. E. (2002). Retinoic acid enhances the T helper 2 cell development that is essential for robust antibody responses through its action on antigen-presenting cells. *J. Nutr.* **132,** 3736–3739.

Horcher, M., Souabni, A., and Busslinger, M. (2001). Pax5/BSAP maintains the identity of B cells in late B lymphopoiesis. *Immunity* **14,** 779–790.

Hoshino, K., Takeuchi, O., Kawai, T., Sanjo, H., Ogawa, T., Takeda, Y., Takeda, K., and Akira, S. (1999). Cutting edge: Toll-like receptor 4 (TLR4)-deficient mice are hyporesponsive to lipopolysaccharide: Evidence for TLR4 as the Lps gene product. *J. Immunol.* **162,** 3749–3752.

Hu, C. C., Dougan, S. K., McGehee, A. M., Love, J. C., and Ploegh, H. L. (2009). XBP-1 regulates signal transduction, transcription factors and bone marrow colonization in B cells. *EMBO J.* **28,** 1624–1636.

Ishiura, N., Nakashima, H., Watanabe, R., Kuwano, Y., Adachi, T., Takahashi, Y., Tsubata, T., Okochi, H., Tamaki, K., Tedder, T. F., and Fujimoto, M. (2010). Differential phosphorylation of functional tyrosines in CD19 modulates B-lymphocyte activation. *Eur. J. Immunol.* **40,** 1192–1204.

Iwakoshi, N. N., Lee, A. H., and Glimcher, L. H. (2003). The X-box binding protein-1 transcription factor is required for plasma cell differentiation and the unfolded protein response. *Immunol. Rev.* **194,** 29–38.

Iwata, M., Hirakiyama, A., Eshima, Y., Kagechika, H., Kato, C., and Song, S. Y. (2004). Retinoic acid imprints gut-homing specificity on T cells. *Immunity* **21,** 527–538.

Jacob, J., Kassir, R., and Kelsoe, G. (1991). In situ studies of the primary immune response to (4-hydroxy-3-nitrophenyl)acetyl. I. The architecture and dynamics of responding cell populations. *J. Exp. Med.* **173,** 1165–1175.

Kallies, A., and Nutt, S. L. (2007). Terminal differentiation of lymphocytes depends on Blimp-1. *Curr. Opin. Immunol.* **19,** 156–162.

Klein, U., and Dalla-Favera, R. (2008). Germinal centres: Role in B-cell physiology and malignancy. *Nat. Rev. Immunol.* **8,** 22–33.

Krieg, A. M., Yi, A. K., Matson, S., Waldschmidt, T. J., Bishop, G. A., Teasdale, R., Koretzky, G. A., and Klinman, D. M. (1995). CpG motifs in bacterial DNA trigger direct B-cell activation. *Nature* **374,** 546–549.

Kuwata, T., Wang, I.-M., Tamura, T., Ponnamperuma, R. M., Levine, R., Holmes, K. L., Morse, H. C., III, DeLuca, L. M., and Ozato, K. (2000). Vitamin A deficiency in mice causes a systemic expansion of myeloid cells. *Blood* **95,** 3349–3356.

Lahvis, G. P., and Cerny, J. (1997). Induction of germinal center B cell markers in vitro by activated CD4+ T lymphocytes: The role of CD40 ligand, soluble factors, and B cell antigen receptor cross-linking. *J. Immunol.* **159,** 1783–1793.

Lang, G. A., Devera, T. S., and Lang, M. L. (2008). Requirement for CD1d expression by B cells to stimulate NKT cell-enhanced antibody production. *Blood* **111,** 2158–2162.

Lin, K. I., Angelin-Duclos, C., Kuo, T. C., and Calame, K. (2002). Blimp-1-dependent repression of Pax-5 is required for differentiation of B cells to immunoglobulin M-secreting plasma cells. *Mol. Cell. Biol.* **22,** 4771–4780.

Lomo, J., Smeland, E. B., Ulven, S., Natarajan, V., Blomhoff, R., Gandhi, U., Dawson, M. I., and Blomhoff, H. K. (1998). RAR-, not RXR, ligands inhibit cell activation and prevent apoptosis in B-lymphocytes. *J. Cell. Physiol.* **175,** 68–77.

Ma, Y., and Ross, A. C. (2005). The anti-tetanus immune response of neonatal mice is augmented by retinoic acid combined with polyriboinosinic:polyribocytidylic acid. *Proc. Natl. Acad. Sci. USA* **102,** 13556–13561.

Ma, Y., and Ross, A. C. (2009). Toll-like receptor 3 ligand and retinoic acid enhance germinal center formation and increase the tetanus toxoid vaccine response. *Clin. Vaccine Immunol.* **16,** 1476–1484.

Ma, Y., Chen, Q., and Ross, A. C. (2005). Retinoic acid and polyriboinosinic:polyribocytidylic acid stimulate robust anti-tetanus antibody production while differentially regulating type 1/type 2 cytokines and lymphocyte populations. *J. Immunol.* **174,** 7961–7969.

MacLennan, I. C., Liu, Y. J., and Johnson, G. D. (1992). Maturation and dispersal of B-cell clones during T cell-dependent antibody responses. *Immunol. Rev.* **126,** 143–161.

McHeyzer-Williams, L. J., Malherbe, L. P., and McHeyzer-Williams, M. G. (2006). Helper T cell-regulated B cell immunity. *Curr. Top. Microbiol. Immunol.* **311,** 59–83.

Mora, J. R., Iwata, M., Eksteen, B., Song, S. Y., Junt, T., Senman, B., Otipoby, K. L., Yokota, A., Takeuchi, H., Ricciardi-Castagnoli, P., Rajewsky, K., Adams, D. H., *et al.* (2006). Generation of gut-homing IgA-secreting B cells by intestinal dendritic cells. *Science* **314,** 1157–1160.

Morgan, M. A., Magnusdottir, E., Kuo, T. C., Tunyaplin, C., Harper, J., Arnold, S. J., Calame, K., Robertson, E. J., and Bikoff, E. K. (2009). Blimp-1/Prdm1 alternative promoter usage during mouse development and plasma cell differentiation. *Mol. Cell. Biol.* **29,** 5813–5827.

Mucida, D., Park, Y., Kim, G., Turovskaya, O., Scott, I., Kronenberg, M., and Cheroutre, H. (2007). Reciprocal Th-17 and regulatory T cell differentiation mediated by retinoic acid. *Science* **17,** 256–260.

Muindi, J. R. F., Young, C. W., and Warrell, R. P., Jr. (1994). Clinical pharmacology of all-*trans* retinoic acid. *Leukemia* **8,** 1807–1812.

Naderi, S., and Blomhoff, H. K. (1999). Retinoic acid prevents phosphorylation of pRB in normal human B lymphocytes: Regulation of cyclin E, cyclin A, and p21(Cip1). *Blood* **94,** 1348–1358.

Napoli, J. L. (2000). Enzymology and biogenesis of retinoic acid. *In* "Vitamin A and Retinoids: An Update of Biological Aspects and Clinical Applications," (M. A. Livrea, Ed.), pp. 17–27. Birkhèuser Verlag, Basel.

Northrup, D. L., and Allman, D. (2008). Transcriptional regulation of early B cell development. *Immunol. Res.* **42,** 106–117.

Park, C. S., and Choi, Y. S. (2005). How do follicular dendritic cells interact intimately with B cells in the germinal centre? *Immunology* **114,** 2–10.

Park, H. Y., Park, J. Y., Kim, J. W., Lee, M. J., Jang, M. J., Lee, S. Y., Baek, D. W., Park, Y. M., Lee, S. W., Yoon, S., Bae, Y. S., and Kwak, J. Y. (2004). Differential expression of dendritic cell markers by all-trans retinoic acid on human acute promyelocytic leukemic cell line. *Int. Immunopharmacol.* **4,** 1587–1601.

Reichert, R. A., Gallatin, W. M., Weissman, I. L., and Butcher, E. C. (1983). Germinal center B cells lack homing receptors necessary for normal lymphocyte recirculation. *J. Exp. Med.* **157,** 813–827.

Rose, M. L., Birbeck, M. S., Wallis, V. J., Forrester, J. A., and Davies, A. J. (1980). Peanut lectin binding properties of germinal centres of mouse lymphoid tissue. *Nature* **284,** 364–366.

Ross, A. C. (1994). Retinoids and the immune system. The Retinoids: Biology, Chemistry, and Medicine 2nd ed. Raven Press, New York, pp. 521–543.

Ross, A. C. (2010). Diet in vitamin A research. *In* "Retinoids, Methods and Protocols," (H. Sun and G. H. Travis, Eds.), pp. 295–313. Humana Press, Springer, New York.

Ross, A. C., Zolfaghari, R., and Weisz, J. (2001). Vitamin A: Recent advances in the biotransformation, transport, and metabolism of retinoids. *Curr. Opin. Gastroenterol.* **17,** 184–192.

Ross, A. C., Chen, Q., and Ma, Y. (2009). Augmentation of antibody responses by retinoic acid and costimulatory molecules. *Semin. Immunol.* **21,** 42–50.

Saito, M., Gao, J., Basso, K., Kitagawa, Y., Smith, P. M., Bhagat, G., Pernis, A., Pasqualucci, L., and Dalla-Favera, R. (2007). A signaling pathway mediating downregulation of BCL6 in germinal center B cells is blocked by BCL6 gene alterations in B cell lymphoma. *Cancer Cell* **12,** 280–292.

Sanderson, R. D., Lalor, P., and Bernfield, M. (1989). B lymphocytes express and lose syndecan at specific stages of differentiation. *Cell Regul.* **1,** 27–35.

Scheffel, F., Heine, G., Henz, B. M., and Worm, M. (2005). Retinoic acid inhibits CD40 plus IL-4 mediated IgE production through alterations of sCD23, sCD54 and IL-6 production. *Inflamm. Res.* **54,** 113–118.

Sciammas, R., Shaffer, A. L., Schatz, J. H., Zhao, H., Staudt, L. M., and Singh, H. (2006). Graded expression of interferon regulatory factor-4 coordinates isotype switching with plasma cell differentiation. *Immunity* **25,** 225–236.

Shaffer, A. L., Yu, X., He, Y., Boldrick, J., Chan, E. P., and Staudt, L. M. (2000). BCL-6 represses genes that function in lymphocyte differentiation, inflammation, and cell cycle control. *Immunity* **13,** 199–212.

Shaffer, A. L., Lin, K. I., Kuo, T. C., Yu, X., Hurt, E. M., Rosenwald, A., Giltnane, J. M., Yang, L., Zhao, H., Calame, K., and Staudt, L. M. (2002). Blimp-1 orchestrates plasma cell differentiation by extinguishing the mature B cell gene expression program. *Immunity* **17,** 51–62.

Shapiro-Shelef, M., and Calame, K. (2005). Regulation of plasma-cell development. *Nat. Rev. Immunol.* **5,** 230–242.

Siebenlist, U., Brown, K., and Claudio, E. (2005). Control of lymphocyte development by nuclear factor-kappaB. *Nat. Rev. Immunol.* **5,** 435–445.

Smeland, E. B., Rusten, L., Jacobsen, S. E. W., Skrede, B., Blomhoff, R., Wang, M. Y., Funderud, S., Kvalheim, G., and Blomhoff, H. K. (1994). All-*trans* retinoic acid inhibits granulocyte colony-stimulating factor-induced proliferation of CD34 human hematopoietic progenitor cells. *Blood* **9,** 2940–2945.

Stadanlick, J. E., Kaileh, M., Karnell, F. G., Scholz, J. L., Miller, J. P., Quinn, W. J., III, Brezski, R. J., Treml, L. S., Jordan, K. A., Monroe, J. G., Sen, R., and Cancro, M. P. (2008). Tonic B cell antigen receptor signals supply an NF-kappaB substrate for prosurvival BLyS signaling. *Nat. Immunol.* **9,** 1379–1387.

Stavnezer, J., Guikema, J. E., and Schrader, C. E. (2008). Mechanism and regulation of class switch recombination. *Annu. Rev. Immunol.* **26,** 261–292.

Steiniger, B., and Barth, P. (2000). Microanatomy and function of the spleen. *Adv. Anat. Embryol. Cell Biol.* **151**(III–IX), 1–101.

Suzuki, K., Maruya, M., Kawamoto, S., Sitnik, K., Kitamura, H., Agace, W. W., and Fagarasan, S. (2010). The sensing of environmental stimuli by follicular dendritic cells promotes immunoglobulin A generation in the gut. *Immunity* **33,** 71–83.

Tran, T. H., Nakata, M., Suzuki, K., Begum, N. A., Shinkura, R., Fagarasan, S., Honjo, T., and Nagaoka, H. (2010). B cell-specific and stimulation-responsive enhancers derepress Aicda by overcoming the effects of silencers. *Nat. Immunol.* **11,** 148–154.

Tunyaplin, C., Shaffer, A. L., Angelin-Duclos, C. D., Yu, X., Staudt, L. M., and Calame, K. L. (2004). Direct repression of prdm1 by Bcl-6 inhibits plasmacytic differentiation. *J. Immunol.* **173,** 1158–1165.

Usui, T., Wakatsuki, Y., Matsunaga, Y., Kaneko, S., Koseki, H., and Kita, T. (1997). Overexpression of B cell-specific activator protein (BSAP/Pax-5) in a late B cell is sufficient to suppress differentiation to an Ig high producer cell with plasma cell phenotype. *J. Immunol.* **158,** 3197–3204.

Van, D. E., Kulier, R., Gülmezoglu, A. M., and Villar, J. (2002). Vitamin A supplementation during pregnancy. *Cochrane Database Syst. Rev.* **4,** CD001996.

Vitoux, D., Nasr, R., and de The, H. (2007). Acute prmyelocytic leukemia: New issues on pathogenesis and treatment response. *Int. J. Biochem. Cell Biol.* **39,** 1063–1070.

Wakatsuki, Y., Neurath, M. F., Max, E. E., and Strober, W. (1994). The B cell-specific transcription factor BSAP regulates B cell proliferation. *J. Exp. Med.* **179,** 1099–1108.

Watanabe, K., Sugai, M., Nambu, Y., Osato, M., Hayashi, T., Kawaguchi, M., Komori, T., Ito, Y., and Shimizu, A. (2010). Requirement for Runx proteins in IgA class switching acting downstream of TGF-beta 1 and retinoic acid signaling. *J. Immunol.* **184,** 2785–2792.

Wei, L. N. (2003). Retinoid receptors and their coregulators. *Annu. Rev. Pharmacol. Toxicol.* **43,** 47–72.

Wei, D., Yang, Y., and Wang, W. (2007). The expression of retinoic acid receptors in lymph nodes of young children and the effect of all-trans-retinoic acid on the B cells from lymph nodes. *J. Clin. Immunol.* **27,** 88–94.

West, K. P., Jr. (2002). Extent of vitamin A deficiency among preschool children and women of reproductive age. *J. Nutr.* **132,** 2857S–2866S.

WHO/UNICEF (1998). Integration of vitamin A supplementation with immunization: Policy and programme implication. Report of a meeting, 12–13 January 1998, UNICEF, New York, pp. 1–7.

Xu, Z., Pone, E. J., Al-Qahtani, A., Park, S. R., Zan, H., and Casali, P. (2007). Regulation of aicda expression and AID activity: Relevance to somatic hypermutation and class switch DNA recombination. *Crit. Rev. Immunol.* **27,** 367–397.

Yamamoto, Y., Tsuzuki, S., Tsuzuki, M., Handa, K., Inaguma, Y., and Emi, N. (2010). BCOR as a novel fusion partner of retinoic acid receptor alpha in a t(X;17)(p11;q12) variant of acute promyelocytic leukemia. *Blood* **116,** 4274–4283.

Zhang, K. (2003). Accessibility control and machinery of immunoglobulin class switch recombination. *J. Leukoc. Biol.* **73,** 323–332.

Zhao, Z. R., and Ross, A. C. (1995). Retinoic acid repletion restores the number of leukocytes and their subsets and stimulates natural cytotoxicity in vitamin A-deficient rats. *J. Nutr.* **125,** 2064–2073.

Zhou, D., Mattner, J., Cantu, C., III, Schrantz, N., Yin, N., Gao, Y., Sagiv, Y., Hudspeth, K., Wu, Y. P., Yamashita, T., Teneberg, S., Wang, D., *et al.* (2004). Lysosomal glycosphingolipid recognition by NKT cells. *Science* **306,** 1786–1789.

CHAPTER SIX

Retinoic Acid Production by Intestinal Dendritic Cells

Makoto Iwata*,† *and* Aya Yokota*,†

Contents

* Laboratory of Immunology, Faculty of Pharmaceutical Sciences at Kagawa Campus, Tokushima Bunri University, Sanuki-shi, Kagawa, Japan
† Japan Science and Technology Agency, CREST, Chiyoda-ku, Tokyo, Japan

Vitamins and Hormones, Volume 86
ISSN 0083-6729, DOI: 10.1016/B978-0-12-386960-9.00006-X

Abstract

Subpopulations of dendritic cells (DCs) in the small intestine and its related lymphoid organs can produce retinoic acid (RA) from vitamin A (retinol). Through the RA production, these DCs play a pivotal role in imprinting lymphocytes with gut-homing specificity, and contribute to the development of immune tolerance by enhancing the differentiation of Foxp3$^+$ regulatory T cells and inhibiting that of inflammatory Th17 cells. The RA-producing capacity in these DCs mostly depends on the expression of retinal dehydrogenase 2 (RALDH2, ALDH1A2). It is likely that the RALDH2 expression is induced in DCs by the microenvironmental factors in the small intestine and its related lymphoid organs. The major factor responsible for the RALDH2 expression appears to be GM-CSF. RA itself is essential for the GM-CSF-induced RALDH2 expression. IL-4 and IL-13 also enhance RALDH2 expression, but are dispensable. Toll-like receptor-mediated signals can also enhance the GM-CSF-induced RALDH2 expression in immature DCs.

I. Introduction

Food and Agriculture Organization of the United Nations (FAO) estimated that more than one billion people were undernourished worldwide in 2009. Undernutrition is implicated in up to half of all deaths of children under 5 years old. Undernutrition increases susceptibility to infection (Caulfield *et al.*, 2004). The major infectious diseases that cause child deaths are persistent diarrhea, malaria, pneumonia, and measles. In 1986, Sommer and his colleagues reported that vitamin A supplementation significantly decreased the child mortality (Sommer *et al.*, 1986). The effect has been confirmed by other groups as well, and is now considered to be most significant in children under 5 years old. In the middle 1990s, The United Nations Children's Fund (UNICEF) started promoting the vitamin A supplementation program, which may have been saving millions of lives since then. Vitamin A supplementation significantly reduces the severity of diarrhea and complications from measles and deaths by these infectious diseases (Barreto *et al.*, 1994; Daulaire *et al.*, 1992; Glasziou and Mackerras, 1993; Sommer, 1997; Villamor and Fawzi, 2005; Wolfson *et al.*, 2007). In contrast, the effects of vitamin A supplementation on lower respiratory infections have been limited or controversial, and may not be significant except in the presence of complicating measles (Barreto *et al.*, 1994; Daulaire *et al.*, 1992; Glasziou and Mackerras, 1993; Sommer, 1997; Villamor and Fawzi, 2005). Therefore, vitamin A or its derivatives are likely to be critical for gastrointestinal functions and resistance to measles infection.

Vitamin A participates in maintaining the integrity of mucosal epithelia (Rojanapo *et al.*, 1980; Wang *et al.*, 1997), and in enhancing IgA antibody production required for mucosal immunity (Ertesvag *et al.*, 2009; Ross *et al.*, 2009). The beneficial effects of vitamin A supplementation on measles-related outcomes may be partly due to the enhanced T cell-dependent antibody production (Ertesvag *et al.*, 2009; Ross *et al.*, 2009; Villamor and Fawzi, 2005). Vitamin A also plays an essential role in deploying T cells and IgA-producing cells into the small intestinal tissues. In 2004, we found that a population of intestinal dendritic cells (DCs) could produce retinoic acid (RA) from vitamin A (retinol) and imprint naïve T cells with gut-homing specificity upon antigenic stimulation (Iwata *et al.*, 2004). RA-producing DCs imprint gut-homing specificity also on naïve B cells (Mora *et al.*, 2006). Vitamin A deficiency causes severe reduction in lymphocytes in the small intestine, and may thus increase the susceptibility to infection in the gut. Further, RA-producing DCs enhance the differentiation of naïve $CD4^+$ T cells into $Foxp3^+$ inducible regulatory T cells (iTreg), but inhibit that into proinflammatory Th17 cells (Benson *et al.*, 2007; Coombes *et al.*, 2007; Kang *et al.*, 2007; Mucida *et al.*, 2007; Schambach *et al.*, 2007; Sun *et al.*, 2007). RA may contribute to the development of oral tolerance. Therefore, the regulation of RA production in intestinal DCs is critical for the development of immune system as well as the regulation of immune responses.

II. Backgrounds and General Effects of Vitamin A on Host Defense Systems

A. Intestinal epithelia and dietary intakes

Vitamin A contributes to the barrier function of mucosal epithelia partly by facilitating the turnover of epithelial cells (ECs) and keeping up the number of goblet cells that produce mucopolysaccharides (Rojanapo *et al.*, 1980; Wang *et al.*, 1997). Small intestinal enterocytes and goblet cells are derived from multipotent stem cells that are located at or near the base of crypts (Bjerknes and Cheng, 1999). Vitamin A deficiency causes the increased duration of the cell cycle of jejunal crypt cells due mainly to a lengthening of the DNA synthesis phase (Zile *et al.*, 1977). In addition, RA may promote the epithelial barrier function by increasing the expression of genes that are involved in the intercellular tight junction formation (Osanai *et al.*, 2007). Small intestinal ECs are also essential for the absorption of vitamin A. Vitamin A is derived exclusively from the diet under the natural condition. Usually, vitamin A is ingested as precursors such as retinyl esters and provitamin A. A large part of them are hydrolyzed to retinol prior to absorption by ECs. The free retinol is reesterified, incorporated into chylomicrons, which circulate in the intestinal lymph and then move into the general circulation (Blomhoff and Blomhoff, 2006; Harrison, 2005). Vitamin A is eventually stored mainly in the liver as retinyl esters. The stored retinyl esters are hydrolyzed to retinol as needed to keep the serum retinol level almost constant at 1–2 μM. Retinol binds to retinol-binding proteins (RBP) in the blood, and circulates through the body. The cellular retinol-binding proteins (CRBP) participate in the intracellular trafficking of retinol.

B. Retinol and metabolites

1. Retinol

Retinol by itself might support a fundamental process of cell survival. It emerged as an essential cofactor of protein kinase Cδ, without which this enzyme failed to be activated in mitochondria, suggesting that retinol is of importance for energy homeostasis (Acin-Perez *et al.*, 2010). Immune cells might not be exceptional (Buck *et al.*, 1990; Chiu *et al.*, 2008). Retinol is converted into retinal and RA in the cells that express the corresponding enzymes (Fig. 6.1).

2. Retinal (Retinaldehyde)

It is well known that 11-*cis*-retinal is the essential chromophore for the visual pigment rhodopsin. Retinal also plays a role in repressing adipogenesis and diet-induced obesity by antagonizing peroxisome proliferator-activated receptor (PPAR)γ activity in the fat tissue (Ziouzenkova *et al.*, 2007).

3. Retinoic acid

Most of the other effects of vitamin A appear to depend on RA. RA inhibits activation-induced cell death in thymocytes and T cells (Iwata *et al.*, 1992; Yang *et al.*, 1993). Vitamin A deficiency diminishes Th2-dependent responses including IL-4 production and IgG1, IgA, and IgE antibody responses, but enhances some Th1 responses including interferon (IFN)-γ production. On the other hand, RA directly and indirectly inhibits Th1 responses and enhances Th2 responses (Cantorna *et al.*, 1994, 1996; Dawson

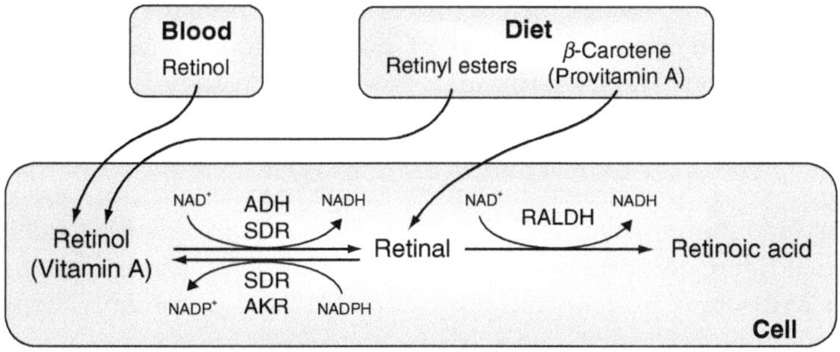

Figure 6.1 *The main pathway of retinoic acid production.* The main pathway to produce retinoic acid (RA) consists of two steps. The first step is the reversible oxidation of retinol to retinal, catalyzed by a subfamily of ADH or that of short-chain dehydrogenase/ reductases (SDR). Retinaldehyde reductase activity has been also found in a subfamily of aldo-keto reductases (AKR). The second step from retinal to RA is catalyzed by RALDH, a subfamily of aldehyde dehydrogenases. RALDH is expressed in limited cell types including DCs in gut-related lymphoid organs and the small intestinal LP.

et al., 2006, 2008; Iwata *et al.*, 2003; Stephensen *et al.*, 2002). Accordingly, Th2 cytokine-dependent IgA responses are enhanced by RA (Ertesvag *et al.*, 2009; Ross *et al.*, 2009). RA also enhances IgA class switching itself (Mora *et al.*, 2006; Tokuyama and Tokuyama, 1999; Watanabe *et al.*, 2010). These findings suggest that RA production by antigen-presenting DCs or bystander DCs may affect Th1/Th2 differentiation. As for measles virus infection, RA may also inhibit the virus replication through upregulating elements of the innate immune response in bystander cells in a type I interferon (IFN)-dependent fashion (Trottier *et al.*, 2009). Further, RA eliminates myeloid-derived suppressor cells (MDSC) that contribute to tumor escape by inducing glutathione synthase and differentiation of these cells into mature myeloid cells (Nefedova *et al.*, 2007).

III. Regulation of Gut-Specific Homing of Lymphocytes by Dendritic Cells

A. Gut-related lymphoid organs

The gut is the largest front line of defense against microorganisms from the outer world, and thus requires the deployment of a large number of immune cells. Naïve lymphocytes that have yet to be activated circulate in the blood, and can occasionally enter lymphoid tissues. They return to the blood circulation via lymphatics if they are not activated. To enter nonlymphoid tissues including intestinal lamina propria (LP) and intraepithelial spaces, they need to be activated with cognate antigen in the secondary lymphoid tissues. The term "homing" is used for the migration of lymphocytes into lymphoid organs or nonlymphoid tissues that are associated with the secondary lymphoid organs where they first encountered cognate antigen. DCs are distributed in almost all the tissues except for the brain, and can trap antigen. DCs that have trapped antigen in the intestinal LP migrate into the draining mesenteric lymph nodes (MLN), and present the processed antigen with MHC molecules. DCs in Peyer's patches (PP) also trap antigen, and present antigen in PP. However, some of them move over to MLN and present antigen there. MLN also contain "lymphoid-tissue-resident" DCs that enter MLN as precursors via the bloodstream (Shortman and Naik, 2007). They may take up and present soluble antigens from the afferent lymphatics (Sixt *et al.*, 2005).

By the way, the Society for Mucosal Immunology recommends that "GALT" (gut-associated lymphoid tissue) comprises PP, the appendix, and isolated lymphoid follicles, but not MLN, as GALTs are considered inductive sites for mucosal B and T cells (Brandtzaeg *et al.*, 2008). Thus, we use "gut-related lymphoid organs" for referring to both MLN and GALT in this review.

B. Gut-homing receptors

Naïve T cells acquire the capacity to migrate into small intestinal tissues upon activation with antigen-presenting DCs in MLN or PP by expressing the gut-homing receptors, integrin $\alpha 4\beta 7$ and chemokine receptor CCR9 (Johansson-Lindbom *et al.*, 2003; Mora *et al.*, 2003; Fig. 6.2). The integrin $\alpha 4\beta 7$ binds to MAdCAM-1 (mucosal addressin cell adhesion molecule-1) that is expressed on the endothelial cells in MLN, PP, and the intestinal LP (Butcher *et al.*, 1999). The CCR9 ligand CCL25 (TECK) is produced by ECs in the small intestine, especially those in the crypt region most closely associated with MAdCAM-1-expressing vessels (Kunkel *et al.*, 2000; Wurbel *et al.*, 2000). For homing to the colon, $\alpha 4\beta 7$ but not CCR9 is required. For Th1 cell homing to the intestinal LP, however, P-selectin glycoprotein ligand 1 (PSGL-1) appears to be a major homing receptor (Haddad *et al.*, 2003).

IV. Imprinting of Gut-Homing Specificity on Lymphocytes by Retinoic Acid

A. Imprinting of homing specificity

Activation of naïve T cells with antibodies to T cell receptor/CD3 and CD28 *in vitro* induces the expression of a part of skin-homing receptors including E-selectin ligands, P-selectin ligands, and the mRNA of CCR4 and α(1,3)fucosyltransferase-VII required for E- and P-selectin ligand

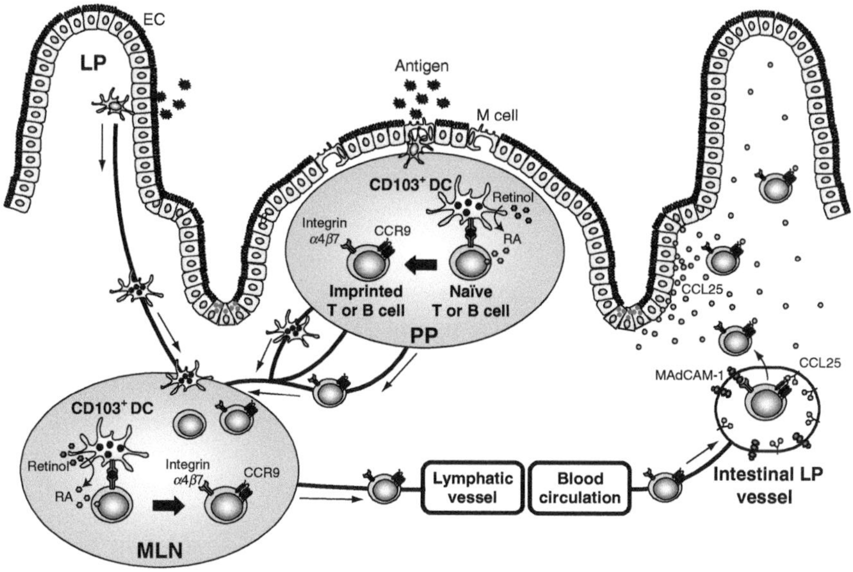

Figure 6.2 DCs in gut-related lymphoid organs imprint T and B cells with gut-homing specificity by providing RA during antigen presentation. Antigen-trapped migratory CD103$^+$ LP-DCs migrate into MLN. MLN-DCs and PP-DCs produce RA from retinol (vitamin A), and imprint gut-homing specificity on T and B cells upon antigenic stimulation. The imprinted T and B cells express both $\alpha4\beta7$ and CCR9, which bind to MAdCAM-1 and CCL25, respectively, and migrate into the small intestinal tissues.

biosynthesis. However, in the presence of the major physiological RA, all-*trans*-RA, even at nanomolar levels, T cells express gut-homing receptors and suppress the skin-homing receptor expression (Iwata *et al.*, 2004). Similar effects can be observed with retinol or retinal only at unphysiologically high concentrations. In vitamin A-deficient mice, $\alpha4\beta7^+$ effector/memory T cells are reduced in the secondary lymphoid organs, and T cells are depleted from the small intestinal LP and intraepithelial spaces (Iwata *et al.*, 2004). In contrast, the vitamin A deficiency does not affect the distribution of CD4$^+$ T cells in the lung tissue (Iwata, 2009; Iwata *et al.*, 2004). During 2–3 months of age under specific pathogen-free (SPF) conditions, few vitamin A-deficient mice show signs of inanition compared with control mice in appearance. In these mice, however, the number of IgA$^+$ cells in the small intestinal LP is also dramatically reduced, whereas the distribution of IgD$^+$ naïve B cells is not affected much in PP (Mora *et al.*, 2006). Similarly, it was reported that IgA$^+$ plasma cells and CD4$^+$ T cells in the ileal LP and CD4$^+$ T cells but not CD8$^+$ T cells in the ileal PP were markedly reduced in vitamin A-deficient rats (Bjersing *et al.*, 2002). These findings collectively suggest that vitamin A is essential for the specific migration of T and B cells into the small intestinal tissues. It is in good accordance with the fact that vitamin A supplementation reduces the severity of diarrhea but not the incidence of acute respiratory infection in children with undernutrition (Barreto *et al.*, 1994; Caulfield *et al.*, 2004; Daulaire *et al.*, 1992; Glasziou and Mackerras, 1993; Sommer, 1997; Villamor and Fawzi, 2005).

B. RAR and RXR

RA exerts its effects mostly via the heterodimer of nuclear receptors, RA receptor (RAR) and retinoid X receptor (RXR). Three isoforms (α, β, and γ) of RAR and three isoforms (α, β, and γ) of RXR have been identified. These receptors are ligand-dependent transcription factors that bind to *cis*-acting DNA sequences, called RA response elements (RARE), located in the promoter region of their target genes. All-*trans*-RA binds to RAR but not RXR at physiological concentrations, while 9-*cis*-RA binds to both RAR and RXR. 9-*cis*-RA also induces α4β7 and CCR9 expression on naïve T cells upon activation (Iwata *et al.*, 2004), although the *in vivo* occurrence of 9-*cis*-RA remains controversial (Wolf, 2006). Am80, a synthetic agonist of RARα and RARβ (Kagechika *et al.*, 1988), but not HX600, a pan-agonist of RXR (Umemiya *et al.*, 1997), also induces α4β7 and CCR9, indicating that RARα or RARβ may be involved in the effect (Iwata *et al.*, 2004). The additive effect of RXR-mediated stimulation was minimal at least on the Am80-induced α4β7 expression. However, the RAR-dependent CCR9 expression can be often enhanced by the RXR-mediated stimulation (Takeuchi *et al.*, 2010). The CCR9 gene expression appears to require the binding of RAR/RXR and NFATc2 to an RA-response element half-site in its promoter (Ohoka *et al.*, 2011).

C. Retinoic acid-producing dendritic cells

Subpopulations of MLN-DCs and PP-DCs but not splenic (SPL)-DCs or PLN-DCs can significantly produce RA, and are responsible for imprinting T cells with gut-homing specificity by providing RA during antigen presentation (Iwata *et al.*, 2004; Fig. 6.2). Indeed, the RARβ and RARα antagonist LE135 (Umemiya *et al.*, 1997) suppressed the capacities of antigen-loaded MLN-DCs and PP-DCs to induce α4β7 expression on T cells. The result indicates further that RARα or RARβ is involved in the imprinting mechanism (Iwata *et al.*, 2004). As we will discuss later, the key enzyme for the RA production by DCs is retinal dehydrogenase (RALDH). The inhibitors of RALDH, citral (3,7-dimethyl-2,6-octadienal; a food and fragrance additive) and DEAB (4-diethylaminobenzaldehyde), also suppressed the capacity of these DCs to induce gut-homing receptors. Conversion of radiolabeled all-*trans*-retinol to all-*trans*-RA was detected in the cell extracts containing MLN-DCs or PP-DCs *in vitro*, although most of retinol-derivatives in the culture supernatants were likely to be more oxidized or degraded by oxygen in the air. To assess RAR-dependent signal levels in T cells, the transgenic DR5-luciferase reporter mice, whose transgene contained RARE motifs from the RAR-β2 promoter might be useful (Svensson *et al.*, 2008).

RA-producing DCs can also imprint B cells with gut-homing specificity in an RAR-dependent fashion (Mora *et al.*, 2006).

V. Regulation of Functional Differentiation of Lymphocytes by Retinoic Acid-Producing Dendritic Cells

A. Regulatory T cells and Th17 cells

In the intestine, although it is crucial to deploy lymphocytes and to elicit immune responses against pathogenic microorganisms, immune responses to food and commensal bacterial antigens should be regulated. Upon antigenic stimulation, naïve T cells differentiate into Foxp3^{+} iTreg in the presence of transforming growth factor (TGF)-β and IL-2, and into proinflammatory Th17 cells in the presence of TGF-β, IL-6, and IL-23. Foxp3^{+} iTreg are different from naturally occurring Foxp3^{+} regulatory T cells (nTreg) that develop in the thymus (Curotto de Lafaille and Lafaille, 2009; Sakaguchi *et al.*, 2008). Th17 cells play an important role also in clearing pathogens during host defense reactions (Korn *et al.*, 2009). When MLN-DCs are employed as antigen-presenting cells, the differentiation of naïve CD4^{+} T cells to Foxp3^{+} iTreg is enhanced in an RA-dependent manner, while that to Th17 cells is suppressed (Benson *et al.*, 2007; Coombes *et al.*, 2007; Kang *et al.*, 2007; Mucida *et al.*, 2007; Schambach *et al.*, 2007; Sun *et al.*, 2007). MLN-DCs obtained from vitamin A-deficient mice have little capacity to produce RA (Yokota *et al.*, 2009), and had higher capacity to induce Th17 cells and lower capacity to induce Foxp3^{+} cells than those obtained from control mice (Chang *et al.*, 2010). However, the development of Th17 cells might also require RA at a low level (Uematsu *et al.*, 2008). Further, specific gut tropism of Th17 cells is also determined by RA (Wang *et al.*, 2010).

Interestingly, RA can not only induce or enhance gut-homing receptor expression in naïve-like CD62L^{high}CD25^{+}CD4^{+} nTreg from normal mice, but also enhance the P-selectin ligand expression unlike in CD4^{+}CD25^{-} T cells (Siewert *et al.*, 2007).

B. Th1 and Th2 cells

RA modulates Th1 and Th2 functions directly or indirectly through the effect on antigen-presenting cells including DCs partly by inhibiting IL-12 production (Grenningloh *et al.*, 2006; Hoag *et al.*, 2002; Kang *et al.*, 2000; Na *et al.*, 1999; Wada *et al.*, 2009). In contrast, Stephensen *et al.* showed that vitamin A-deficient mice had a higher frequency of IL-10-producing Th2 or regulatory T cells and a lower frequency of IFN-γ-producing Th1 cells than did control mice (Stephensen *et al.*, 2004). Further studies might need for clarifying the precise roles of RA in Th1 and Th2 differentiation *in vivo*.

It has become clear that DCs stimulated with thymic stromal lymphopoietin (TSLP) or IL-33 can prime for the differentiation of inflammatory Th2 cells or atypical Th2 cells, respectively (Ito *et al.*, 2005; Rank *et al.*, 2009; Soumelis *et al.*, 2002). On the other hand, expression of Notch ligands including Delta-like-1, Delta-like-4, Jagged-1, and Jagged-2 on DCs regulate Th1 and Th2 differentiation (Amsen *et al.*, 2004; Maekawa *et al.*, 2003). It remains unclear if RA can affect these aspects of the regulation of Th1/Th2 differentiation.

C. Homing specificity of primed T cells

Activation of P-selectin ligand-expressing $CD8^+$ effector/memory T cells from various lymphoid organs in the presence of PP-DCs resulted in enhanced gut-homing receptor expression and reduced E- and P-selectin ligand expression, compared to the cells activated in the presence of peripheral lymph nodes (PLN)-DCs (Mora *et al.*, 2005). Similar results were obtained when $CD8^+$ T cells were primed with PLN-DCs or Langerhans cells, and then restimulated with PP-DCs (Dudda *et al.*, 2005; Mora *et al.*, 2005). It might be possible that RA switched the homing specificity to some extent, especially at "naïve-like" stages as shown in naïve-like nTreg (Siewert *et al.*, 2007).

D. IgA production

RA-producing DCs can also induce IgA production in naïve B cells in a T cell-independent fashion upon activation, partly depending on the production of RA and IL-6 (Mora and von Andrian, 2009; Mora *et al.*, 2006). For IgA production *in vivo*, TNF-α/iNOS-expressing DCs play an important role partly by inducing the receptor for TGF-β (Tezuka *et al.*, 2007). In mice, most of the T cell-independent generation of IgA^+ B cells in the small intestinal LP but not the large intestinal LP may require the presence of TGF-β1 (Fagarasan *et al.*, 2010). Interestingly, topical transcutaneous immunization induces antigen-specific IgA antibody-producing cells that express CCR9 and CCR10 in the small intestine in an RA- and MLN-dependent manner (Chang *et al.*, 2008).

VI. Identification of Retinoic Acid-Producing Dendritic Cells

A. Retinoic acid-producing pathway

The main pathway of RA biosynthesis is dependent on the intracellular oxidative metabolism of retinol via retinal (Duester, 2000; Napoli, 1999; Fig. 6.1). The first step from retinol to retinal is catalyzed by a subfamily of alcohol dehydrogenases (ADH) or by the short-chain dehydrogenase/reductase family, and at least one member of these families is expressed in most cells (Gallego *et al.*, 2006; Liden and Eriksson, 2006). In DC preparations from all of the lymphoid organs tested, the mRNA expression of at least one ADH isoform was detected (Iwata *et al.*, 2004). The second step is an irreversible conversion of retinal to RA, and is catalyzed by RALDH encoded by the *Aldh1a* family, a subfamily of class I aldehyde dehydrogenases (ALDH), which are expressed in limited cell types (Duester, 2000; Napoli, 1999). RALDH mRNA expression was detected in MLN-DC and PP-DC preparations but not significantly in SPL-DC or PLN-DC preparations. MLN-DCs strongly expressed *Aldh1a2* that encodes the RALDH2 isoenzyme (Iwata *et al.*, 2004). Although expression of *Aldh1a1* (encoding RALDH1) was suggested in PP-DCs from mice bred under a conventional condition (Iwata *et al.*, 2004), our recent study on highly purified DCs from naïve SPF mice revealed that *Aldh1a2* expression in PP-DCs, but that no expression of *Aldh1a1*, *Aldh1a3* (encoding RALDH3), *Aldh8a1* (encoding RALDH4) was detectable in DCs or CD11c$^-$ cells from MLN, PP, or SPL (Yokota *et al.*, 2009). Interestingly, low levels of *Aldh1a1* expression were detected in SPL-DCs from BALB/c mice but not in those from B10.D2 mice. The ALDH1A-independent RA-producing enzymes, CYP1B1, and CYP2J6 (Chambers *et al.*, 2007; Zhang *et al.*, 1998), were also undetectable in DCs and CD11c$^-$ cells in the secondary lymphoid organs (Yokota *et al.*, 2009). Therefore, RALDH2 is likely to be the most critical enzyme for RA production by DCs. Among MLN-DCs, it has been shown that CD103$^+$ DCs but not CD103$^-$ DCs express *Aldh1a2* (Coombes *et al.*, 2007).

B. Retinoic acid-producing dendritic cells and ALDEFLUOR assay

We have recently shown that the RALDH2 enzyme activity in each DC could be estimated by flow cytometry with the ALDH-dependent fluorophore, ALDEFLUOR (Yokota *et al.*, 2009). The activity in MLN-DCs was much higher than that in hematopoietic stem or progenitor cells, although ALDEFLUOR was originally manufactured for analyzing the latter cells. Approximately 30% of MLN-DCs and 10% of PP-DCs exhibited the activity in naïve SPF mice. More than 10% of MLN-DCs but only a few PP-DCs (~1%) exhibited high levels of activity. The high activities were found in CD11c^{high}CD4$^{-/low}$CD8α^{intermediate}CD11b$^{-/low}$ F4/80$^{low/intermediate}$CD45RB^{low}CD86^{high}MHC class II^{high}B220^{-}CD103^{+} DCs in both MLN and PP. Therefore, RALDH2 is expressed in a subpopulation of mature CD11c^{high} DCs. No activity was detected in CD103^{-} DCs in PP and MLN. However, CD103 expression levels did not necessarily correspond to the ALDH activity (ALDHact) levels. Unexpectedly, a small number of DCs from skin-draining PLN exhibited the activity. Some of them exhibited high ALDHact levels (Yokota *et al.*, 2009). Interestingly, it was recently shown that these ALDHact^{+} PLN-DCs were CD103-negative, but could induce iTreg (Guilliams *et al.*, 2010). They detected ALDHact^{+} DCs in skin and in the lung.

It has been shown that small intestinal LP-DCs are more potent than MLN-DCs or PP-DCs in their ability to generate α4β7^{+}CCR9^{+}CD8^{+} T cells, and that the proportion of CD103^{+} DCs in LP-DCs is much higher than that in MLN-DCs (Johansson-Lindbom *et al.*, 2005). Thus, the proportion of RA-producing DCs in LP has been presumed to be higher than that in MLN. Indeed, CD103^{+} LP-DCs were found to promote a high level of iTreg conversion in the presence of TGF-β (Sun *et al.*, 2007). Uematsu *et al.* have shown that *Aldh1a2* is expressed in CD11c^{high}CD11b^{high}F4/80^{moderate} LP-DCs (Uematsu *et al.*, 2008). Further, CD11b^{+}CD11c^{-} macrophages in LP have been shown to express *Aldh1a2* and *Aldh1a1* (Denning *et al.*, 2007; Manicassamy and Pulendran, 2009). Human CD14^{+} macrophages bearing the DC marker CD209 in LP also expressed *ALDH1A2* (Kamada *et al.*, 2009).

VII. The Origin of Retinoic Acid-Producing Dendritic Cells

A. Lamina propria-dendritic cell subsets

In the small intestinal LP, CD103^{-} DCs are also present. The two major subsets of LP-DCs are CD103^{+} CX3CR1^{-} DCs derived from common monocyte-DC precursors via DC-committed intermediates and CD103^{-}CD11b^{+}CX3CR1^{+} DCs derived from Ly6C^{high} monocytes (Bogunovic *et al.*, 2009; Iwasaki, 2007; Varol *et al.*, 2009). The former subset is mainly found in the villus of LP, expresses CCR7, and can migrate into MLN upon antigen trapping (Coombes *et al.*, 2007; Jaensson *et al.*, 2008; Jang *et al.*, 2006; Johansson-Lindbom *et al.*, 2005; Schulz *et al.*, 2009). The latter subset is primarily located in the dome region of solitary intestinal lymphoid tissue, and is capable of sampling luminal antigens by extending dendrites through the epithelium (Chieppa *et al.*, 2006; del Rio *et al.*, 2010;

Niess *et al.*, 2005; Rescigno *et al.*, 2001). Both subsets can be induced through Fms-like tyrosine kinase 3 ligand (Flt3L) pathways, but the role of granulocyte-macrophage colony-stimulating factor (GM-CSF) in the induction of each LP-DC subset is controversial (Bogunovic *et al.*, 2009; Varol *et al.*, 2009). CX3CR1$^+$ DCs appear to be less efficient at generating RA compared with CD103$^+$ DCs (Jaensson *et al.*, 2008; Schulz *et al.*, 2009). Therefore, CD103$^+$ DCs containing RALDH2$^+$ DCs may serve as classical DCs to initiate adaptive immune responses in MLN, whereas CX3CR1$^+$ DCs may serve as first line barrier against invading pathogens in the intestine. The precise relationship or collaboration between the two subsets remains unclear.

B. E-cadherin-mediated adhesion

CD103 is also known as integrin αE that binds to integrin β7 to form the heterodimer αEβ7. The main ligand for αEβ7 is E-cadherin, an adhesion molecule. The cell surface E-cadherin also binds homophylically to E-cadherin on another cell. Interestingly, E-cadeherin is implicated in the anchoring of DCs in the intestinal mucosa (Rescigno *et al.*, 2001). Under steady-state conditions without microbial stimulants, DC maturation occurs by disruption of E-cadherin-mediated homophilic adhesion (Jiang *et al.*, 2007). These DCs were suggested to be the elusive steady-state tolerogenic DCs. RA may contribute to the DC migration from the periphery to draining lymph nodes partly by enhancing the production of matrix metalloproteinases (MMPs) and simultaneously suppressing or unaffecting that of tissue inhibitors of MMPs (TIMPs; Darmanin *et al.*, 2007; Lackey *et al.*, 2008). E-cadherin can be cleaved by MMPs. On the other hand, RA may impair CCR7- and CXCR4-dependent DC migration by inhibiting CCR7 and CXCR4 expression (Villablanca *et al.*, 2008). The role of RA in the DC migration remains to be clarified.

C. Mesenteric lymph node-dendritic cells

In MLN, the majority of CD103$^+$ and CD103$^-$ DCs appear to represent tissue-derived migratory and lymphoid-resident populations, respectively (Jaensson *et al.*, 2008). Although CD103$^+$ DCs may migrate in the steady state from LP to MLN (Annacker *et al.*, 2005; Johansson-Lindbom *et al.*, 2005), these DCs may become a major population only after introduction of an inflammatory stimulus (Jakubzick *et al.*, 2008). Steady-state DCs migrating in the lymph from the intestine contribute to induce tolerance to harmless intestinal antigens, but are paradoxically able to induce strong inflammatory responses from naïve T cells (Milling *et al.*, 2009). It might be possible that an additional factor in MLN is required for maintaining or obtaining the tolerogenic capacity of CD103$^+$ MLN-DCs. On the other hand, most of CD103$^-$ MLN-DCs may be maintained through local homeostatic proliferation and through recruitment of blood-derived precursors (Jaensson *et al.*, 2008). It has been suggested that early antigen presentation by lymphoid-resident DCs initiates activation and trapping of antigen-specific T cells in skin-draining lymph nodes, without sufficing for clonal expansion, and that migratory DCs interact with the $CD4^+$ T cells retained in the lymph nodes to induce proliferation (Allenspach *et al.*, 2008). Similar relationship might operate in MLN.

VIII. Induction of Retinoic Acid-Producing Capacity in Dendritic Cells

A. GM-CSF and IL-4

GM-CSF or Flt3L is often used for inducing differentiation of bone marrow (BM) cells or monocytes into DCs (Inaba *et al.*, 1992; McKenna *et al.*, 2000). We found that GM-CSF-generated BM-DCs but not Flt3L-generated BM-DCs expressed *Aldh1a2* (Yokota *et al.*, 2009). GM-CSF potently induced RALDH2 expression in Flt3L-generated BM-DCs and even more potently in SPL-DCs within 1–2 days of culture. IL-4 and IL-13 are also potent inducers of RALDH2 in these DCs (Yokota *et al.*, 2009), and enhances RALDH2 expression in MLN-DCs (Elgueta *et al.*, 2008). GM-CSF and IL-4 synergistically enhanced the RALDH2 expression in BM-DCs and SPL-DCs (Yokota *et al.*, 2009). The levels of ALDH activity and RALDH2 expression induced by the combination of GM-CSF and IL-4 in SPL-DCs *in vitro* were equivalent to those found in the $ALDHact^{high}$ population of MLN-DCs. SPL-DCs treated with GM-CSF and/or IL-4 significantly enhanced $Foxp3^+$ cell induction and suppressed Th17 cell induction. MLN-DCs from mice deficient of GM-CSF receptor (common β subunit) exhibited significantly lower ALDH activities and the capacity to induce gut-homing receptors on naïve T cells than those from wild type (wt) mice. Further, the numbers of T cells in the small intestinal LP and intraepithelial spaces of these mice were much lower than those of wt mice. On the other hand, these changes were not observed in IL-4 receptor α chain-deficient mice, suggesting that IL-4 and IL-13 are dispensable. These results collectively suggest that multiple factors may be involved in the RALDH2 expression in MLN-DCs in naïve wt mice, and that, among the factors, GM-CSF plays a major role (Yokota *et al.*, 2009) (Fig. 6.3).

B. LXR and PPARγ

Ligands of liver X receptor (LXR) and PPARγ may also participate in RALDH expression. Huq *et al.* reported that dietary cholesterol supplementation enhanced *Aldh1a1* and *Aldh1a2* expression and cellular RA

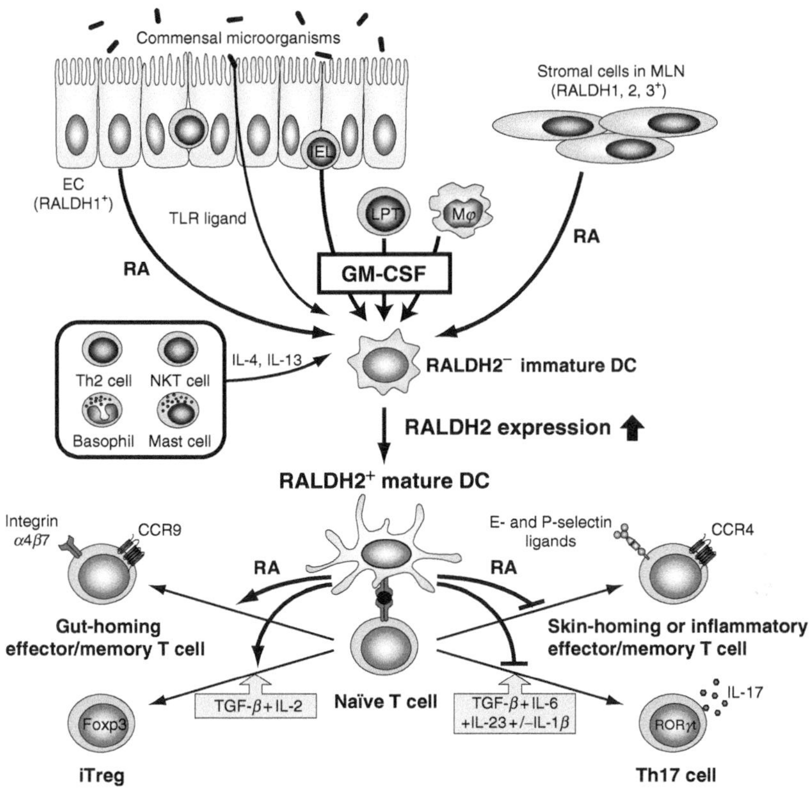

Figure 6.3 The induction mechanism of RA-producing capacity in intestinal DCs. The expression of the major RA-producing enzyme RALDH2 can be induced by multiple factors in the small intestine and MLN. Among the factors, GM-CSF appears to play a pivotal role. RA itself, IL-4, IL-13, and TLR ligands may enhance the induction of RALDH2 expression. The RA-producing DCs not only modulate the homing specificity of T cells but also enhance Foxp3$^+$ iTreg differentiation and inhibit Th17 differentiation.

content in murine organs such as the brain, kidney, liver, and heart, through the activation of LXR and upregulation of sterol regulatory element binding protein-1c (SREBP-1c; Huq *et al.*, 2006). Szatmari *et al.* showed that stimulation of PPARγ-induced RALDH2 expression and RA production in human monocyte-derived DCs (Szatmari *et al.*, 2006). Therefore, some cholesterol metabolites, eicosanoids, and other lipids might participate in the induction. However, ligands or agonists of LXR and PPARγ did not significantly induce RALDH2 expression in mouse Flt3L-generated BM-DCs and in purified SPL-DCs, comparing to the GM-CSF effect (Yokota *et al.*, 2009). The apparent discrepancy remains to be clarified.

C. Retinoic acid as a cofactor

Saurer *et al.* (2007) reported that pretreatment of porcine monocyte-derived DCs with RA induced the capacity of secreting TGF-β and IL-6 and enhancing gut-homing receptor expression and IgA responses in cocultured lymphocytes. Although they proposed a mechanism that DCs might store and carry RA rather than *de novo* synthesis of RA, their results might imply that RA might contribute to RALDH induction in DCs through an autocrine mechanism. We found that GM-CSF-induced RALDH2 expression in Flt3L-generated BM-DCs was suppressed with the RAR antagonist LE540, and that RA significantly enhanced the GM-CSF-induced RALDH2 expression, although RA by itself induced a low level of RALDH2 expression in Flt3L-generated BM-DCs (Yokota *et al.*, 2009). However, GM-CSF-induced RALDH2 expression in SPL-DCs was only moderately affected by LE540 or RA. RA by itself did not significantly induce RALDH2 in SPL-DCs. The results suggest that RA contributes to the RALDH2 expression in DCs as an essential cofactor in an autocrine fashion in immature DCs (Fig. 6.3). The RA requirement might be inversely correlated to the maturity of DCs. However, RA appears to suppress Flt3L-depedent generation of BM-DCs, but enhance GM-CSF-dependent differentiation of BM cells into myeloid lineage DCs (Hengesbach and Hoag, 2004). RA also affects human monocyte differentiation into DCs. RA skews GM-CSF-dependent differentiation into IL-12-secreting DC-like cells, but inhibits their IL-4-dependent differentiation into DCs (de Sousa-Canavez *et al.*, 2009; Mohty *et al.*, 2003).

D. Mesenteric lymph node stromal cells

Hammerschmidt *et al.* (2008) found that stromal MLN cells were essential for the generation of gut-homing T cells *in vivo*, and that MLN but not PLN stromal cells expressed *Aldh1a1*, *Aldh1a2*, and *Aldh1a3*. It was suggested that, in MLN, stromal cells might deliver positive signals including RA, and cooperate with DCs to induce gut-homing receptors on T cells (Hammerschmidt *et al.*, 2008; Molenaar *et al.*, 2009). These findings are in good accord with the fact that the GM-CSF-induced RALDH2 expression in BM-DCs depends on RA or RAR-mediated signals. Initial RA for inducing RALDH2 in DCs might be provided by these stromal cells.

E. Mucosal epithelial cells

Mucosal ECs may also contribute to provide RA to adjacent DCs or T cells, as they strongly express RALDH1 (Frota-Ruchon *et al.*, 2000; Iwata *et al.*, 2004; Westerlund *et al.*, 2007), although the enzymatic activity of RALDH1 is considered to be lower than that of RALDH2 (Grun *et al.*, 2000; Haselbeck *et al.*, 1999). Indeed, it was shown that intestinal ECs drove the differentiation of iTreg-promoting DCs depending on the production of TGF-β and RA but not TSLP (Iliev *et al.*, 2009a,b) or that intestinal ECs could induce iTreg independently of local DCs through direct antigen-presentation to T cells (Westendorf *et al.*, 2009).

F. Toll-like receptor ligands

Intestinal microorganisms may affect the RALDH expression in DCs. The *Aldh1a2* expression in LP-DCs can be enhanced upon Toll-like receptor (TLR)5-mediated stimulation with flagellin (Uematsu *et al.*, 2008). We found that TLR ligands only slightly induced *Aldh1a2* expression, but significantly enhanced the GM-CSF- and/or IL-4-induced *Aldh1a2* expression and $ALDHact^+$ cells in Flt3L-generated BM-DCs (Yokota *et al.*, 2009). TLR ligands enhanced the IL-4- but not GM-CSF-induced *Aldh1a2* expression in SPL-DCs. However, in Flt3L-generated BM-DCs, the ALDH activity levels that were induced synergistically with GM-CSF, IL-4, and a TLR ligand were equivalent to those found in the $ALDHact^{high}$ population of MLN-DCs. The resultant DCs enhanced the expression of gut-homing receptors. Interestingly, Manicassamy *et al.* (2009) reported that TLR2 ligands induced *Aldh1a2* expression in SPL-DCs. These findings suggest that TLR ligands may contribute to the induction or enhancement of RALDH2 expression in DCs (Fig. 6.3). It remains to be clarified if TLR-mediated stimulation is essential for the full expression of RALDH2 in intestinal DCs *in vivo*.

G. Basophils

Mast cell-derived IL-3 induced RALDH2 expression and RA production in human basophils (Spiegl *et al.*, 2008). The produced RA may modulate IL-3-induced gene expression in them in an autocrine fashion and may contribute to the RALDH2 expression in adjacent DCs.

IX. Degradation of Retinoic Acid *In Vivo* and *In Vitro*

As known in the embryonic development, the RA concentration appears to be strictly controlled by its synthesis, degradation, or sequestration *in vivo*. Cytochrome P450 (Cyp26s) and UDP-glucuronosyltransferase may be involved in RA metabolism in the intestine (Czernik *et al.*, 2000; Salyers *et al.*, 1993; Takeuchi *et al.*, 2011; Thatcher and Isoherranen, 2009). However, little is known how DC-derived RA is metabolized. Nonetheless, RA is both light and air sensitive, and easily undergoes oxidative degradation and *cis/trans* isomerism *in vitro*, and thus requires special care for handling (Dell, 2004; Iwata *et al.*, 2003; Napoli, 1986).

X. Conclusions and Future Directions

RA-producing DCs in the intestine play critical roles in the regulation of lymphocyte trafficking and functional differentiation. Multiple microenvironmental factors in the small intestine may contribute to the induction of RALDH expression in DCs. GM-CSF appears to play a major role to induce RALDH2 expression in DCs in the steady-state intestine. RA assists GM-CSF to induce the expression in immature DCs, and may be initially provided by MLN stromal cells or the intestinal ECs. The RALDH2 expression might be also affected by other factors including TLR ligands and IL-4, which could be introduced by microorganisms, ingested foods, or immune responses in the intestine. It remains unclear how the production and the effect of GM-CSF are controlled in the intestine and other tissues. The identity of the RA-producing stromal cells and the molecular mechanism of RALDH2 induction in DCs also remain to be clarified. Disrupted RA signals might be involved in diseases such as inflammatory bowel diseases, type I diabetes, food allergy, and some infectious diarrhea, through altered homing or functional differentiation of lymphocytes. Regulation of local RA production and RA-mediated signals might open up a new way for prevention and treatment of these and other diseases.

Acknowledgments

This work was supported in part by Grants-in-Aid for Scientific Research from MEXT and JSPS, and research grants from JST, CREST, and The Danone Institute of Japan.

References

Acin-Perez, R., Hoyos, B., Zhao, F., Vinogradov, V., Fischman, D. A., Harris, R. A., Leitges, M., Wongsiriroj, N., Blaner, W. S., Manfredi, G., and Hammerling, U. (2010). Control of oxidative phosphorylation by vitamin A illuminates a fundamental role in mitochondrial energy homoeostasis. *FASEB J.* **24,** 627–636.

Allenspach, E. J., Lemos, M. P., Porrett, P. M., Turka, L. A., and Laufer, T. M. (2008). Migratory and lymphoid-resident dendritic cells cooperate to efficiently prime naive CD4 T cells. *Immunity* **29,** 795–806.

Amsen, D., Blander, J. M., Lee, G. R., Tanigaki, K., Honjo, T., and Flavell, R. A. (2004). Instruction of distinct CD4 T helper cell fates by different notch ligands on antigen-presenting cells. *Cell* **117,** 515–526.

Annacker, O., Coombes, J. L., Malmstrom, V., Uhlig, H. H., Bourne, T., Johansson-Lindbom, B., Agace, W. W., Parker, C. M., and Powrie, F. (2005). Essential role for CD103 in the T cell-mediated regulation of experimental colitis. *J. Exp. Med.* **202,** 1051–1061.

Barreto, M. L., Santos, L. M., Assis, A. M., Araujo, M. P., Farenzena, G. G., Santos, P. A., and Fiaccone, R. L. (1994). Effect of vitamin A supplementation on diarrhoea and acute lower-respiratory-tract infections in young children in Brazil. *Lancet* **344,** 228–231.

Benson, M. J., Pino-Lagos, K., Rosemblatt, M., and Noelle, R. J. (2007). All-trans retinoic acid mediates enhanced T reg cell growth, differentiation, and gut homing in the face of high levels of co-stimulation. *J. Exp. Med.* **204,** 1765–1774.

Bjerknes, M., and Cheng, H. (1999). Clonal analysis of mouse intestinal epithelial progenitors. *Gastroenterology* **116,** 7–14.

Bjersing, J. L., Telemo, E., Dahlgren, U., and Hanson, L. A. (2002). Loss of ileal IgA$^+$ plasma cells and of CD4$^+$ lymphocytes in ileal Peyer's patches of vitamin A deficient rats. *Clin. Exp. Immunol.* **130,** 404–408.

Blomhoff, R., and Blomhoff, H. K. (2006). Overview of retinoid metabolism and function. *J. Neurobiol.* **66,** 606–630.

Bogunovic, M., Ginhoux, F., Helft, J., Shang, L., Hashimoto, D., Greter, M., Liu, K., Jakubzick, C., Ingersoll, M. A., Leboeuf, M., *et al.* (2009). Origin of the lamina propria dendritic cell network. *Immunity* **31,** 513–525.

Brandtzaeg, P., Kiyono, H., Pabst, R., and Russell, M. W. (2008). Terminology: Nomenclature of mucosa-associated lymphoid tissue. *Mucosal Immunol.* **1,** 31–37.

Buck, J., Ritter, G., Dannecker, L., Katta, V., Cohen, S. L., Chait, B. T., and Hammerling, U. (1990). Retinol is essential for growth of activated human B cells. *J. Exp. Med.* **171,** 1613–1624.

Butcher, E. C., Williams, M., Youngman, K., Rott, L., and Briskin, M. (1999). Lymphocyte trafficking and regional immunity. *Adv. Immunol.* **72,** 209–253.

Cantorna, M. T., Nashold, F. E., and Hayes, C. E. (1994). In vitamin A deficiency multiple mechanisms establish a regulatory T helper cell imbalance with excess Th1 and insufficient Th2 function. *J. Immunol.* **152,** 1515–1522.

Cantorna, M. T., Nashold, F. E., Chun, T. Y., and Hayes, C. E. (1996). Vitamin A down-regulation of IFN-γ synthesis in cloned mouse Th1 lymphocytes depends on the CD28 costimulatory pathway. *J. Immunol.* **156,** 2674–2679.

Caulfield, L. E., de Onis, M., Blossner, M., and Black, R. E. (2004). Undernutrition as an underlying cause of child deaths associated with diarrhea, pneumonia, malaria, and measles. *Am. J. Clin. Nutr.* **80,** 193–198.

Chambers, D., Wilson, L., Maden, M., and Lumsden, A. (2007). RALDH-independent generation of retinoic acid during vertebrate embryogenesis by CYP1B1. *Development* **134,** 1369–1383.

Chang, S. Y., Cha, H. R., Igarashi, O., Rennert, P. D., Kissenpfennig, A., Malissen, B., Nanno, M., Kiyono, H., and Kweon, M. N. (2008). Cutting edge: Langerin$^+$ dendritic cells in the mesenteric lymph node set the stage for skin and gut immune system cross-talk. *J. Immunol.* **180,** 4361–4365.

Chang, S. Y., Cha, H. R., Chang, J. H., Ko, H. J., Yang, H., Malissen, B., Iwata, M., and Kweon, M. N. (2010). Lack of retinoic acid leads to increased langerin-expressing dendritic cells in gut-associated lymphoid tissues. *Gastroenterology* **138,** 1468–1478.

Chieppa, M., Rescigno, M., Huang, A. Y., and Germain, R. N. (2006). Dynamic imaging of dendritic cell extension into the small bowel lumen in response to epithelial cell TLR engagement. *J. Exp. Med.* **203,** 2841–2852.

Chiu, H. J., Fischman, D. A., and Hammerling, U. (2008). Vitamin A depletion causes oxidative stress, mitochondrial dysfunction, and PARP-1-dependent energy deprivation. *FASEB J.* **22,** 3878–3887.

Coombes, J. L., Siddiqui, K. R., Arancibia-Carcamo, C. V., Hall, J., Sun, C. M., Belkaid, Y., and Powrie, F. (2007). A functionally specialized population of mucosal CD103$^+$ DCs induces Foxp3$^+$ regulatory T cells via a TGF-β and retinoic acid-dependent mechanism. *J. Exp. Med.* **204,** 1757–1764.

Curotto de Lafaille, M. A., and Lafaille, J. J. (2009). Natural and adaptive foxp3$^+$ regulatory T cells: More of the same or a division of labor? *Immunity* **30,** 626–635.

Czernik, P. J., Little, J. M., Barone, G. W., Raufman, J. P., and Radominska-Pandya, A. (2000). Glucuronidation of estrogens and retinoic acid and expression of UDP-glucuronosyltransferase 2B7 in human intestinal mucosa. *Drug Metab. Dispos.* **28,** 1210–1216.

Darmanin, S., Chen, J., Zhao, S., Cui, H., Shirkoohi, R., Kubo, N., Kuge, Y., Tamaki, N., Nakagawa, K., Hamada, J., Moriuchi, T., and Kobayashi, M. (2007). All-*trans* retinoic acid enhances murine dendritic cell migration to draining lymph nodes via the balance of matrix metalloproteinases and their inhibitors. *J. Immunol.* **179,** 4616–4625.

Daulaire, N. M., Starbuck, E. S., Houston, R. M., Church, M. S., Stukel, T. A., and Pandey, M. R. (1992). Childhood mortality after a high dose of vitamin A in a high risk population. *BMJ* **304,** 207–210.

Dawson, H. D., Collins, G., Pyle, R., Key, M., Weeraratna, A., Deep-Dixit, V., Nadal, C. N., and Taub, D. D. (2006). Direct and indirect effects of retinoic acid on human Th2 cytokine and chemokine expression by human T lymphocytes. *BMC Immunol.* **7,** 27.

Dawson, H. D., Collins, G., Pyle, R., Key, M., and Taub, D. D. (2008). The Retinoic Acid Receptor-α mediates human T-cell activation and Th2 cytokine and chemokine production. *BMC Immunol.* **9,** 16.

de Sousa-Canavez, J. M., de Oliveira Massoco, C., de Moraes-Vasconcelos, D., Corneta, E. C., Leite, K. R., and Camara-Lopes, L. H. (2009). Retinoic acid inhibits dendritic cell differentiation driven by interleukin-4. *Cell. Immunol.* **259,** 41–48.

del Rio, M. L., Bernhardt, G., Rodriguez-Barbosa, J. I., and Förster, R. (2010). Development and functional specialization of CD103$^+$ dendritic cells. *Immunol. Rev.* **234,** 268–281.

Dell, D. (2004). Labile metabolite. *Chromatographia* **59,** S139–S148.

Denning, T. L., Wang, Y. C., Patel, S. R., Williams, I. R., and Pulendran, B. (2007). Lamina propria macrophages and dendritic cells differentially induce regulatory and interleukin 17-producing T cell responses. *Nat. Immunol.* **8,** 1086–1094.

Dudda, J. C., Lembo, A., Bachtanian, E., Huehn, J., Siewert, C., Hamann, A., Kremmer, E., Forster, R., and Martin, S. F. (2005). Dendritic cells govern induction and reprogramming of polarized tissue-selective homing receptor patterns of T cells: Important roles for soluble factors and tissue microenvironments. *Eur. J. Immunol.* **35,** 1056–1065.

Duester, G. (2000). Families of retinoid dehydrogenases regulating vitamin A function: Production of visual pigment and retinoic acid. *Eur. J. Biochem.* **267,** 4315–4324.

Elgueta, R., Sepulveda, F. E., Vilches, F., Vargas, L., Mora, J. R., Bono, M. R., and Rosemblatt, M. (2008). Imprinting of CCR9 on CD4 T cells requires IL-4 signaling on mesenteric lymph node dendritic cells. *J. Immunol.* **180,** 6501–6507.

Ertesvag, A., Naderi, S., and Blomhoff, H. K. (2009). Regulation of B cell proliferation and differentiation by retinoic acid. *Semin. Immunol.* **21,** 36–41.

Fagarasan, S., Kawamoto, S., Kanagawa, O., and Suzuki, K. (2010). Adaptive immune regulation in the gut: T cell-dependent and T cell-independent IgA synthesis. *Annu. Rev. Immunol.* **28,** 243–273.

Frota-Ruchon, A., Marcinkiewicz, M., and Bhat, P. V. (2000). Localization of retinal dehydrogenase type 1 in the stomach and intestine. *Cell Tissue Res.* **302,** 397–400.

Gallego, O., Belyaeva, O. V., Porté, S., Ruiz, F. X., Stetsenko, A. V., Shabrova, E. V., Kostereva, N. V., Farrés, J., Pares, X., and Kedishvili, N. Y. (2006). Comparative functional analysis of human medium-chain dehydrogenases, short-chain dehydrogenases/reductases and aldo-keto reductases with retinoids. *Biochem. J.* **399,** 101–109.

Glasziou, P. P., and Mackerras, D. E. (1993). Vitamin A supplementation in infectious diseases: A meta-analysis. *Bmj* **306,** 366–370.

Grenningloh, R., Gho, A., di Lucia, P., Klaus, M., Bollag, W., Ho, I. C., Sinigaglia, F., and Panina-Bordignon, P. (2006). Cutting Edge: Inhibition of the retinoid X receptor (RXR) blocks T helper 2 differentiation and prevents allergic lung inflammation. *J. Immunol.* **176,** 5161–5166.

Grun, F., Hirose, Y., Kawauchi, S., Ogura, T., and Umesono, K. (2000). Aldehyde dehydrogenase 6, a cytosolic retinaldehyde dehydrogenase prominently expressed in sensory neuroepithelia during development. *J. Biol. Chem.* **275,** 41210–41218.

Guilliams, M., Crozat, K., Henri, S., Tamoutounour, S., Grenot, P., Devilard, E., de Bovis, B., Alexopoulou, L., Dalod, M., and Malissen, B. (2010). Skin-draining lymph nodes contain dermis-derived CD103^{-} dendritic cells that constitutively produce retinoic acid and induce Foxp3^{+} regulatory T cells. *Blood* **115,** 1958–1968.

Haddad, W., Cooper, C. J., Zhang, Z., Brown, J. B., Zhu, Y., Issekutz, A., Fuss, I., Lee, H. O., Kansas, G. S., and Barrett, T. A. (2003). P-selectin and P-selectin glycoprotein ligand 1 are major determinants for Th1 cell recruitment to nonlymphoid effector sites in the intestinal lamina propria. *J. Exp. Med.* **198,** 369–377.

Hammerschmidt, S. I., Ahrendt, M., Bode, U., Wahl, B., Kremmer, E., Förster, R., and Pabst, O. (2008). Stromal mesenteric lymph node cells are essential for the generation of gut-homing T cells in vivo. *J. Exp. Med.* **205,** 2483–2490.

Harrison, E. H. (2005). Mechanisms of digestion and absorption of dietary vitamin A. *Annu. Rev. Nutr.* **25,** 87–103.

Haselbeck, R. J., Hoffmann, I., and Duester, G. (1999). Distinct functions for Aldh1 and Raldh2 in the control of ligand production for embryonic retinoid signaling pathways. *Dev. Genet.* **25,** 353–364.

Hengesbach, L. M., and Hoag, K. A. (2004). Physiological concentrations of retinoic acid favor myeloid dendritic cell development over granulocyte development in cultures of bone marrow cells from mice. *J. Nutr.* **134,** 2653–2659.

Hoag, K. A., Nashold, F. E., Goverman, J., and Hayes, C. E. (2002). Retinoic acid enhances the T helper 2 cell development that is essential for robust antibody responses through its action on antigen-presenting cells. *J. Nutr.* **132,** 3736–3739.

Huq, M. D., Tsai, N. P., Gupta, P., and Wei, L. N. (2006). Regulation of retinal dehydrogenases and retinoic acid synthesis by cholesterol metabolites. *EMBO J.* **25,** 3203–3213.

Iliev, I. D., Mileti, E., Matteoli, G., Chieppa, M., and Rescigno, M. (2009a). Intestinal epithelial cells promote colitis-protective regulatory T-cell differentiation through dendritic cell conditioning. *Mucosal Immunol.* **2,** 340–350.

Iliev, I. D., Spadoni, I., Mileti, E., Matteoli, G., Sonzogni, A., Sampietro, G. M., Foschi, D., Caprioli, F., Viale, G., and Rescigno, M. (2009b). Human intestinal epithelial cells promote the differentiation of tolerogenic dendritic cells. *Gut* **58,** 1481–1489.

Inaba, K., Inaba, M., Romani, N., Aya, H., Deguchi, M., Ikehara, S., Muramatsu, S., and Steinman, R. M. (1992). Generation of large numbers of dendritic cells from mouse bone marrow cultures supplemented with granulocyte/macrophage colony-stimulating factor. *J. Exp. Med.* **176,** 1693–1702.

Ito, T., Wang, Y. H., Duramad, O., Hori, T., Delespesse, G. J., Watanabe, N., Qin, F. X., Yao, Z., Cao, W., and Liu, Y. J. (2005). TSLP-activated dendritic cells induce an inflammatory T helper type 2 cell response through OX40 ligand. *J. Exp. Med.* **202,** 1213–1223.

Iwasaki, A. (2007). Mucosal dendritic cells. *Annu. Rev. Immunol.* **25,** 381–418.

Iwata, M. (2009). Retinoic acid production by intestinal dendritic cells and its role in T-cell trafficking. *Semin. Immunol.* **21,** 8–13.

Iwata, M., Mukai, M., Nakai, Y., and Iseki, R. (1992). Retinoic acids inhibit activation-induced apoptosis in T cell hybridomas and thymocytes. *J. Immunol.* **149,** 3302–3308.

Iwata, M., Eshima, Y., and Kagechika, H. (2003). Retinoic acids exert direct effects on T cells to suppress Th1 development and enhance Th2 development via retinoic acid receptors. *Int. Immunol.* **15,** 1017–1025.

Iwata, M., Hirakiyama, A., Eshima, Y., Kagechika, H., Kato, C., and Song, S. Y. (2004). Retinoic acid imprints gut-homing specificity on T cells. *Immunity* **21,** 527–538.

Jaensson, E., Uronen-Hansson, H., Pabst, O., Eksteen, B., Tian, J., Coombes, J. L., Berg, P. L., Davidsson, T., Powrie, F., Johansson-Lindbom, B., and Agace, W. W. (2008). Small intestinal $CD103^+$ dendritic cells display unique functional properties that are conserved between mice and humans. *J. Exp. Med.* **205,** 2139–2149.

Jakubzick, C., Bogunovic, M., Bonito, A. J., Kuan, E. L., Merad, M., and Randolph, G. J. (2008). Lymph-migrating, tissue-derived dendritic cells are minor constituents within steady-state lymph nodes. *J. Exp. Med.* **205,** 2839–2850.

Jang, M. H., Sougawa, N., Tanaka, T., Hirata, T., Hiroi, T., Tohya, K., Guo, Z., Umemoto, E., Ebisuno, Y., Yang, B. G., Seoh, J. Y., Lipp, M., *et al.* (2006). CCR7 is critically important for migration of dendritic cells in intestinal lamina propria to mesenteric lymph nodes. *J. Immunol.* **176,** 803–810.

Jiang, A., Bloom, O., Ono, S., Cui, W., Unternaehrer, J., Jiang, S., Whitney, J. A., Connolly, J., Banchereau, J., and Mellman, I. (2007). Disruption of E-cadherin-mediated adhesion induces a functionally distinct pathway of dendritic cell maturation. *Immunity* **27,** 610–624.

Johansson-Lindbom, B., Svensson, M., Wurbel, M. A., Malissen, B., Márquez, G., and Agace, W. (2003). Selective generation of gut tropic T cells in gut-associated lymphoid tissue (GALT): Requirement for GALT dendritic cells and adjuvant. *J. Exp. Med.* **198,** 963–969.

Johansson-Lindbom, B., Svensson, M., Pabst, O., Palmqvist, C., Marquez, G., Förster, R., and Agace, W. W. (2005). Functional specialization of gut $CD103^+$ dendritic cells in the regulation of tissue-selective T cell homing. *J. Exp. Med.* **202,** 1063–1073.

Kagechika, H., Kawachi, E., Hashimoto, Y., Himi, T., and Shudo, K. (1988). Retinobenzoic acids. 1. Structure-activity relationships of aromatic amides with retinoidal activity. *J. Med. Chem.* **31,** 2182–2192.

Kamada, N., Hisamatsu, T., Honda, H., Kobayashi, T., Chinen, H., Kitazume, M. T., Takayama, T., Okamoto, S., Koganei, K., Sugita, A., Kanai, T., and Hibi, T. (2009). Human $CD14^+$ macrophages in intestinal lamina propria exhibit potent antigen-presenting ability. *J. Immunol.* **183,** 1724–1731.

Kang, B. Y., Chung, S. W., Kim, S. H., Kang, S. N., Choe, Y. K., and Kim, T. S. (2000). Retinoid-mediated inhibition of interleukin-12 production in mouse macrophages suppresses Th1 cytokine profile in $CD4^+$ T cells. *Br. J. Pharmacol.* **130,** 581–586.

Kang, S. G., Lim, H. W., Andrisani, O. M., Broxmeyer, H. E., and Kim, C. H. (2007). Vitamin A metabolites induce gut-homing $FoxP3^+$ regulatory T cells. *J. Immunol.* **179,** 3724–3733.

Korn, T., Bettelli, E., Oukka, M., and Kuchroo, V. K. (2009). IL-17 and Th17 Cells. *Annu. Rev. Immunol.* **27,** 485–517.

Kunkel, E. J., Campbell, J. J., Haraldsen, G., Pan, J., Boisvert, J., Roberts, A. I., Ebert, E. C., Vierra, M. A., Goodman, S. B., Genovese, M. C., Wardlaw, A. J., Greenberg, H. B., *et al.* (2000). Lymphocyte CC chemokine receptor 9 and epithelial thymus-expressed chemokine (TECK) expression distinguish the small intestinal immune compartment: Epithelial expression of tissue-specific chemokines as an organizing principle in regional immunity. *J. Exp. Med.* **192,** 761–768.

Lackey, D. E., Ashley, S. L., Davis, A. L., and Hoag, K. A. (2008). Retinoic acid decreases adherence of murine myeloid dendritic cells and increases production of matrix metalloproteinase-9. *J. Nutr.* **138,** 1512–1519.

Liden, M., and Eriksson, U. (2006). Understanding retinol metabolism: Structure and function of retinol dehydrogenases. *J. Biol. Chem.* **281,** 13001–13004.

Maekawa, Y., Tsukumo, S., Chiba, S., Hirai, H., Hayashi, Y., Okada, H., Kishihara, K., and Yasutomo, K. (2003). Delta1-Notch3 interactions bias the functional differentiation of activated $CD4^+$ T cells. *Immunity* **19,** 549–559.

Manicassamy, S., and Pulendran, B. (2009). Retinoic acid-dependent regulation of immune responses by dendritic cells and macrophages. *Semin. Immunol.* **21,** 22–27.

Manicassamy, S., Ravindran, R., Deng, J., Oluoch, H., Denning, T. L., Kasturi, S. P., Rosenthal, K. M., Evavold, B. D., and Pulendran, B. (2009). Toll-like receptor 2-dependent induction of vitamin A-metabolizing enzymes in dendritic cells promotes T regulatory responses and inhibits autoimmunity. *Nat. Med.* **15,** 401–409.

McKenna, H. J., Stocking, K. L., Miller, R. E., Brasel, K., De Smedt, T., Maraskovsky, E., Maliszewski, C. R., Lynch, D. H., Smith, J., Pulendran, B., Roux, E. R., Teepe, M., *et al.* (2000). Mice lacking flt3 ligand have deficient hematopoiesis affecting hematopoietic progenitor cells, dendritic cells, and natural killer cells. *Blood* **95,** 3489–3497.

Milling, S. W., Jenkins, C. D., Yrlid, U., Cerovic, V., Edmond, H., McDonald, V., Nassar, M., and Macpherson, G. (2009). Steady-state migrating intestinal dendritic cells induce potent inflammatory responses in naive $CD4^+$ T cells. *Mucosal Immunol.* **2,** 156–165.

Mohty, M., Morbelli, S., Isnardon, D., Sainty, D., Arnoulet, C., Gaugler, B., and Olive, D. (2003). All-*trans* retinoic acid skews monocyte differentiation into interleukin-12-secreting dendritic-like cells. *Br. J. Haematol.* **122,** 829–836.

Molenaar, R., Greuter, M., van der Marel, A. P., Roozendaal, R., Martin, S. F., Edele, F., Huehn, J., Forster, R., O'Toole, T., Jansen, W., Eestermans, I. L., Kraal, G., *et al.* (2009). Lymph node stromal cells support dendritic cell-induced gut-homing of T cells. *J. Immunol.* **183,** 6395–6402.

Mora, J. R., and von Andrian, U. H. (2009). Role of retinoic acid in the imprinting of gut-homing IgA-secreting cells. *Semin. Immunol.* **21,** 28–35.

Mora, J. R., Bono, M. R., Manjunath, N., Weninger, W., Cavanagh, L. L., Rosemblatt, M., and Von Andrian, U. H. (2003). Selective imprinting of gut-homing T cells by Peyer's patch dendritic cells. *Nature* **424,** 88–93.

Mora, J. R., Cheng, G., Picarella, D., Briskin, M., Buchanan, N., and von Andrian, U. H. (2005). Reciprocal and dynamic control of CD8 T cell homing by dendritic cells from skin- and gut-associated lymphoid tissues. *J. Exp. Med.* **201,** 303–316.

Mora, J. R., Iwata, M., Eksteen, B., Song, S. Y., Junt, T., Senman, B., Otipoby, K. L., Yokota, A., Takeuchi, H., Ricciardi-Castagnoli, P., Rajewsky, K., Adams, D. H., *et al.* (2006). Generation of gut-homing IgA-secreting B cells by intestinal dendritic cells. *Science* **314,** 1157–1160.

Mucida, D., Park, Y., Kim, G., Turovskaya, O., Scott, I., Kronenberg, M., and Cheroutre, H. (2007). Reciprocal TH17 and regulatory T cell differentiation mediated by retinoic acid. *Science* **317,** 256–260.

Na, S. Y., Kang, B. Y., Chung, S. W., Han, S. J., Ma, X., Trinchieri, G., Im, S. Y., Lee, J. W., and Kim, T. S. (1999). Retinoids inhibit interleukin-12 production in macrophages through physical associations of retinoid X receptor and NFκB. *J. Biol. Chem.* **274,** 7674–7680.

Napoli, J. L. (1986). Quantification of physiological levels of retinoic acid. *Methods Enzymol.* **123,** 112–124.

Napoli, J. L. (1999). Interactions of retinoid binding proteins and enzymes in retinoid metabolism. *Biochim. Biophys. Acta* **1440,** 139–162.

Nefedova, Y., Fishman, M., Sherman, S., Wang, X., Beg, A. A., and Gabrilovich, D. I. (2007). Mechanism of all-*trans* retinoic acid effect on tumor-associated myeloid-derived suppressor cells. *Cancer Res.* **67,** 11021–11028.

Niess, J. H., Brand, S., Gu, X., Landsman, L., Jung, S., McCormick, B. A., Vyas, J. M., Boes, M., Ploegh, H. L., Fox, J. G., Littman, D. R., and Reinecker, H. C. (2005). CX3CR1-mediated dendritic cell access to the intestinal lumen and bacterial clearance. *Science* **307,** 254–258.

Ohoka, Y., Yokota, A., Takeuchi, H., Maeda, N., and Iwata, M. (2011). Retinoic acid-induced CCR9 expression requires transient TCR stimulation and cooperativity between NFATc2 and the retinoic acid receptor/retinoid X receptor complex. *J. Immunol.* **186,** 733–744.

Osanai, M., Nishikiori, N., Murata, M., Chiba, H., Kojima, T., and Sawada, N. (2007). Cellular retinoic acid bioavailability determines epithelial integrity: Role of retinoic acid receptor α agonists in colitis. *Mol. Pharmacol.* **71,** 250–258.

Rank, M. A., Kobayashi, T., Kozaki, H., Bartemes, K. R., Squillace, D. L., and Kita, H. (2009). IL-33-activated dendritic cells induce an atypical TH2-type response. *J. Allergy Clin. Immunol.* **123,** 1047–1054.

Rescigno, M., Urbano, M., Valzasina, B., Francolini, M., Rotta, G., Bonasio, R., Granucci, F., Kraehenbuhl, J. P., and Ricciardi-Castagnoli, P. (2001). Dendritic cells express tight junction proteins and penetrate gut epithelial monolayers to sample bacteria. *Nat. Immunol.* **2,** 361–367.

Rojanapo, W., Lamb, A. J., and Olson, J. A. (1980). The prevalence, metabolism and migration of goblet cells in rat intestine following the induction of rapid, synchronous vitamin A deficiency. *J. Nutr.* **110,** 178–188.

Ross, A. C., Chen, Q., and Ma, Y. (2009). Augmentation of antibody responses by retinoic acid and costimulatory molecules. *Semin. Immunol.* **21,** 42–50.

Sakaguchi, S., Yamaguchi, T., Nomura, T., and Ono, M. (2008). Regulatory T cells and immune tolerance. *Cell* **133,** 775–787.

Salyers, K. L., Cullum, M. E., and Zile, M. H. (1993). Glucuronidation of all-*trans*-retinoic acid in liposomal membranes. *Biochim. Biophys. Acta* **1152,** 328–334.

Saurer, L., McCullough, K. C., and Summerfield, A. (2007). In vitro induction of mucosa-type dendritic cells by all-trans retinoic acid. *J. Immunol.* **179,** 3504–3514.

Schambach, F., Schupp, M., Lazar, M. A., and Reiner, S. L. (2007). Activation of retinoic acid receptor-α favours regulatory T cell induction at the expense of IL-17-secreting T helper cell differentiation. *Eur. J. Immunol.* **37,** 2396–2399.

Schulz, O., Jaensson, E., Persson, E. K., Liu, X., Worbs, T., Agace, W. W., and Pabst, O. (2009). Intestinal CD103$^+$, but not CX3CR1$^+$, antigen sampling cells migrate in lymph and serve classical dendritic cell functions. *J. Exp. Med.* **206,** 3101–3114.

Shortman, K., and Naik, S. H. (2007). Steady-state and inflammatory dendritic-cell development. *Nat. Rev. Immunol.* **7,** 19–30.

Siewert, C., Menning, A., Dudda, J., Siegmund, K., Lauer, U., Floess, S., Campbell, D. J., Hamann, A., and Huehn, J. (2007). Induction of organ-selective CD4$^+$ regulatory T cell homing. *Eur. J. Immunol.* **37,** 978–989.

Sixt, M., Kanazawa, N., Selg, M., Samson, T., Roos, G., Reinhardt, D. P., Pabst, R., Lutz, M. B., and Sorokin, L. (2005). The conduit system transports soluble antigens from the afferent lymph to resident dendritic cells in the T cell area of the lymph node. *Immunity* **22,** 19–29.

Sommer, A. (1997). Vitamin A prophylaxis. *Arch. Dis. Child.* **77,** 191–194.

Sommer, A., Tarwotjo, I., Djunaedi, E., West, K. P., Jr., Loeden, A. A., Tilden, R., and Mele, L. (1986). Impact of vitamin A supplementation on childhood mortality. A randomised controlled community trial. *Lancet* **1,** 1169–1173.

Soumelis, V., Reche, P. A., Kanzler, H., Yuan, W., Edward, G., Homey, B., Gilliet, M., Ho, S., Antonenko, S., Lauerma, A., Smith, K., Gorman, D., *et al.* (2002). Human epithelial cells trigger dendritic cell mediated allergic inflammation by producing TSLP. *Nat. Immunol.* **3,** 673–680.

Spiegl, N., Didichenko, S., McCaffery, P., Langen, H., and Dahinden, C. A. (2008). Human basophils activated by mast cell-derived IL-3 express retinaldehyde dehydrogenase-II and produce the immunoregulatory mediator retinoic acid. *Blood* **112,** 3762–3771.

Stephensen, C. B., Rasooly, R., Jiang, X., Ceddia, M. A., Weaver, C. T., Chandraratna, R. A., and Bucy, R. P. (2002). Vitamin A enhances in vitro Th2 development via retinoid X receptor pathway. *J. Immunol.* **168,** 4495–4503.

Stephensen, C. B., Jiang, X., and Freytag, T. (2004). Vitamin A deficiency increases the in vivo development of IL-10-positive Th2 cells and decreases development of Th1 cells in mice. *J. Nutr.* **134,** 2660–2666.

Sun, C. M., Hall, J. A., Blank, R. B., Bouladoux, N., Oukka, M., Mora, J. R., and Belkaid, Y. (2007). Small intestine lamina propria dendritic cells promote de novo generation of Foxp3 T reg cells via retinoic acid. *J. Exp. Med.* **204,** 1775–1785.

Svensson, M., Johansson-Lindbom, B., Zapata, F., Jaensson, E., Austenaa, L. M., Blomhoff, R., and Agace, W. W. (2008). Retinoic acid receptor signaling levels and antigen dose regulate gut homing receptor expression on $CD8^+$ T cells. *Mucosal Immunol.* **1,** 38–48.

Szatmari, I., Pap, A., Ruhl, R., Ma, J. X., Illarionov, P. A., Besra, G. S., Rajnavolgyi, E., Dezso, B., and Nagy, L. (2006). PPARγ controls CD1d expression by turning on retinoic acid synthesis in developing human dendritic cells. *J. Exp. Med.* **203,** 2351–2362.

Takeuchi, H., Yokota, A., Ohoka, Y., Kagechika, H., Kato, C., Song, S.-Y., and Iwata, M. (2010). Efficient induction of CCR9 on T cells requires coactivation of retinoic acid receptors and retinoid X receptors (RXRs): Exaggerated T cell homing to the intestine by RXR activation with organotins. *J. Immunol.* **185,** 5289–5299.

Takeuchi, H., Yokota, A., Ohoka, Y., and Iwata, M. (2011). Cyp26b1 regulates retinoic acid-dependent signals in T cells and its expression is inhibited by transforming growth factor-β. PLoS ONE 6, e16089.

Tezuka, H., Abe, Y., Iwata, M., Takeuchi, H., Ishikawa, H., Matsushita, M., Shiohara, T., Akira, S., and Ohteki, T. (2007). Regulation of IgA production by naturally occurring TNF/iNOS-producing dendritic cells. *Nature* **448,** 929–933.

Thatcher, J. E., and Isoherranen, N. (2009). The role of CYP26 enzymes in retinoic acid clearance. *Expert Opin. Drug Metab. Toxicol.* **5,** 875–886.

Tokuyama, H., and Tokuyama, Y. (1999). The regulatory effects of all-*trans*-retinoic acid on isotype switching: Retinoic acid induces IgA switch rearrangement in cooperation with IL-5 and inhibits IgG1 switching. *Cell. Immunol.* **192,** 41–47.

Trottier, C., Colombo, M., Mann, K. K., Miller, W. H., Jr., and Ward, B. J. (2009). Retinoids inhibit measles virus through a type I IFN-dependent bystander effect. *FASEB J.* **23,** 3203–3212.

Uematsu, S., Fujimoto, K., Jang, M. H., Yang, B. G., Jung, Y. J., Nishiyama, M., Sato, S., Tsujimura, T., Yamamoto, M., Yokota, Y., Kiyono, H., Miyasaka, M., *et al.* (2008). Regulation of humoral and cellular gut immunity by lamina propria dendritic cells expressing Toll-like receptor 5. *Nat. Immunol.* **9,** 769–776.

Umemiya, H., Fukasawa, H., Ebisawa, M., Eyrolles, L., Kawachi, E., Eisenmann, G., Gronemeyer, H., Hashimoto, Y., Shudo, K., and Kagechika, H. (1997). Regulation of retinoidal actions by diazepinylbenzoic acids. Retinoid synergists which activate the RXR-RAR heterodimers. *J. Med. Chem.* **40,** 4222–4234.

Varol, C., Vallon-Eberhard, A., Elinav, E., Aychek, T., Shapira, Y., Luche, H., Fehling, H. J., Hardt, W. D., Shakhar, G., and Jung, S. (2009). Intestinal lamina propria dendritic cell subsets have different origin and functions. *Immunity* **31,** 502–512.

Villablanca, E. J., Zhou, D., Valentinis, B., Negro, A., Raccosta, L., Mauri, L., Prinetti, A., Sonnino, S., Bordignon, C., Traversari, C., and Russo, V. (2008). Selected natural and synthetic retinoids impair CCR7- and CXCR4-dependent cell migration in vitro and in vivo. *J. Leukoc. Biol.* **84,** 871–879.

Villamor, E., and Fawzi, W. W. (2005). Effects of vitamin a supplementation on immune responses and correlation with clinical outcomes. *Clin. Microbiol. Rev.* **18,** 446–464.

Wada, Y., Hisamatsu, T., Kamada, N., Okamoto, S., and Hibi, T. (2009). Retinoic acid contributes to the induction of IL-12-hypoproducing dendritic cells. *Inflamm. Bowel Dis.* **15,** 1548–1556.

Wang, J. L., Swartz-Basile, D. A., Rubin, D. C., and Levin, M. S. (1997). Retinoic acid stimulates early cellular proliferation in the adapting remnant rat small intestine after partial resection. *J. Nutr.* **127,** 1297–1303.

Wang, C., Kang, S. G., HogenEsch, H., Love, P. E., and Kim, C. H. (2010). Retinoic acid determines the precise tissue tropism of inflammatory Th17 cells in the intestine. *J. Immunol.* **184,** 5519–5526.

Watanabe, K., Sugai, M., Nambu, Y., Osato, M., Hayashi, T., Kawaguchi, M., Komori, T., Ito, Y., and Shimizu, A. (2010). Requirement for Runx proteins in IgA class switching acting downstream of TGF-β1 and retinoic acid signaling. *J. Immunol.* **184,** 2785–2792.

Westendorf, A. M., Fleissner, D., Groebe, L., Jung, S., Gruber, A. D., Hansen, W., and Buer, J. (2009). $CD4^+Foxp3^+$ regulatory T cell expansion induced by antigen-driven interaction with intestinal epithelial cells independent of local dendritic cells. *Gut* **58,** 211–219.

Westerlund, M., Belin, A. C., Felder, M. R., Olson, L., and Galter, D. (2007). High and complementary expression patterns of alcohol and aldehyde dehydrogenases in the gastrointestinal tract: Implications for Parkinson's disease. *FEBS J.* **274,** 1212–1223.

Wolf, G. (2006). Is 9-*cis*-retinoic acid the endogenous ligand for the retinoic acid-X receptor? *Nutr. Rev.* **64,** 532–538.

Wolfson, L. J., Strebel, P. M., Gacic-Dobo, M., Hoekstra, E. J., McFarland, J. W., and Hersh, B. S. (2007). Has the 2005 measles mortality reduction goal been achieved? A natural history modelling study. *Lancet* **369,** 191–200.

Wurbel, M. A., Philippe, J. M., Nguyen, C., Victorero, G., Freeman, T., Wooding, P., Miazek, A., Mattei, M. G., Malissen, M., Jordan, B. R., Malissen, B., Carrier, A., *et al.* (2000). The chemokine TECK is expressed by thymic and intestinal epithelial cells and attracts double- and single-positive thymocytes expressing the TECK receptor CCR9. *Eur. J. Immunol.* **30,** 262–271.

Yang, Y., Vacchio, M. S., and Ashwell, J. D. (1993). 9-*cis*-retinoic acid inhibits activation-driven T-cell apoptosis: Implications for retinoid X receptor involvement in thymocyte development. *Proc. Natl. Acad. Sci. USA* **90,** 6170–6174.

Yokota, A., Takeuchi, H., Maeda, N., Ohoka, Y., Kato, C., Song, S. Y., and Iwata, M. (2009). GM-CSF and IL-4 synergistically trigger dendritic cells to acquire retinoic acid-producing capacity. *Int. Immunol.* **21,** 361–377.

Zhang, Q. Y., Raner, G., Ding, X., Dunbar, D., Coon, M. J., and Kaminsky, L. S. (1998). Characterization of the cytochrome P450 CYP2J4: Expression in rat small intestine and role in retinoic acid biotransformation from retinal. *Arch. Biochem. Biophys.* **353,** 257–264.

Zile, M., Bunge, C., and Deluca, H. F. (1977). Effect of vitamin A deficiency on intestinal cell proliferation in the rat. *J. Nutr.* **107,** 552–560.

Ziouzenkova, O., Orasanu, G., Sharlach, M., Akiyama, T. E., Berger, J. P., Viereck, J., Hamilton, J. A., Tang, G., Dolnikowski, G. G., Vogel, S., *et al.* (2007). Retinaldehyde represses adipogenesis and diet-induced obesity. *Nat. Med.* **13,** 695–702.

CHAPTER SEVEN

Immune Regulator Vitamin A and T Cell Death

Nikolai Engedal

Contents

Abstract

Proper regulation of T cell death is of vital importance for the function of the immune system. Positive and negative selection of developing T cells in the thymus ensures the survival of only those T cells that can recognize peptides presented by self-MHC molecules and at the same time not respond to self-antigens, and thus, T cell death within the thymus is instrumental in shaping the mature T cell repertoire. The death of activated peripheral T cells is crucial for

Centre for Molecular Medicine Norway, Nordic EMBL Partnership, University of Oslo, Oslo, Norway

Vitamins and Hormones, Volume 86
ISSN 0083-6729, DOI: 10.1016/B978-0-12-386960-9.00007-1

processes such as down-modulation of immune responses after clearance of infectious agents, peripheral tolerance, and maintenance of immune-privileged sites. These processes are largely proceeding due to the enhanced susceptibility of activated T cells to spontaneous, activation-, and Fas-induced apoptosis. The active metabolite of the immune regulator vitamin A, retinoic acid, has been reported to influence various types of apoptotic processes in both thymocytes and activated peripheral T cells. This chapter gives an overview of, and discusses the reported effects of vitamin A on spontaneous and activation-induced cell death of thymocytes and mature T cells, as well as on Fas-induced T cell death.

I. Introduction

The immunomodulatory role of vitamin A was recognized already in the 1920s, when it was termed "the anti-infective vitamin" (Green and Mellanby, 1928). Since then, it has become increasingly clear that vitamin A operates at several levels to modulate immune function. Vitamin A is not only involved in maintaining the integrity of mucosal epithelial barriers, but can also directly affect the function of several cell types of the immune system. For reviews on the influence of vitamin A on the immune system, see (Hayes *et al.*, 1999; Semba, 1994; Stephensen, 2001; Villamor and Fawzi, 2005.) An intriguing discovery made over the last two decades has been the demonstration that vitamin A can directly regulate T cell death at multiple stages of T cell development, indicating that this may be one of the mechanisms whereby vitamin A modulates the immune system.

II. Mechanism of Action of Vitamin A

With the exception of night blindness and photoreceptor degeneration, the vitamin A-metabolite retinoic acid (RA) can prevent and eliminate most of the defects caused by a vitamin A-deficient diet in animal models (Chambon, 1994; Dickman *et al.*, 1997; Kastner *et al.*, 1995). Furthermore, mice lacking one or several of the nuclear receptors for RA, retinoic acid receptors (RARs), and retinoid X receptors (RXRs), display many of the defects observed in vitamin A-deficient animals (Kastner *et al.*, 1995; Mark *et al.*, 1999). Thus, it is generally held that RA is the major active metabolite of vitamin A and that most of the biological effects of vitamin A are mediated by RARs and RXRs. In line with this, the immunomodulatory effect of vitamin A also appears to be mediated mainly by RA (Hayes *et al.*, 1999), and the effects of vitamin A described in the current chapter are mostly based on studies of the effect of RA on T cells.

Each of the two RA receptor families consists of three isotypes encoded by separate genes (RAR-α, -β, and -γ and RXR-α, -β, and -γ; Chambon, 1996; Mangelsdorf and Evans, 1995). With respect to RA-induced biological effects, RARs and RXRs function primarily as RAR/RXR heterodimer transcription factors, which are activated by RA ligation (Kastner *et al.*, 1997; Mark *et al.*, 1999; Wei, 2003). The most active natural RA isomers are considered to be all-*trans* and 9-*cis* RA (atRA and 9cRA), of which atRA is by far the most abundantly observed form. In fact, the *in vivo* existence of 9cRA is disputed (Blomhoff and Blomhoff, 2006; Wolf, 2006), and this will be discussed in Section VII, since several of the effects on T cell death described in this chapter are preferentially mediated by 9cRA over atRA. Whereas atRA preferentially binds to and thereby activates RARs, 9cRA has high affinities for both RARs and RXRs (Chambon, 1996; Mangelsdorf and Evans, 1995). RAR- but not RXR-ligation alone is sufficient to activate the RAR/RXR heterodimer, and simultaneous ligation of both RAR and RXR can act synergistically on RAR/RXR transcriptional activity (Bastien and Rochette-Egly, 2004; Gronemeyer and Miturski, 2001). More than 100 genes have been found to be directly regulated by RA-mediated activation of RAR/RXR (Balmer and Blomhoff, 2002). In addition, RA can indirectly, for instance, via RAR/RXR-mediated cross-talk with other transcription factors, regulate the expression of several hundred other genes (Balmer and Blomhoff, 2002).

Vitamin A is mainly stored in the liver in the form of retinyl esters. Upon mobilization, retinyl esters are hydrolyzed to free retinol, which is then complexed to serum retinol-binding protein. Plasma levels of retinol are strictly regulated and normally lie around 2 μM (Blomhoff *et al.*, 1990). One of the major means by which cells obtain active vitamin A metabolites is through uptake of retinol bound to retinol-binding protein, or uptake of lipoproteins containing retinyl esters, retinol, and carotenoids. The major path of intracellular synthesis of active vitamin A metabolites involves the oxidation of all-*trans* retinol to all-*trans* retinal, which in turn is oxidized to atRA. The enzymes required for these oxidation reactions are alcohol dehydrogenases and retinal dehydrogenases, respectively. For a review on the metabolism of vitamin A, see (Blomhoff and Blomhoff, 2006.) Cells can also obtain active vitamin A metabolites, for example, atRA, directly from the plasma. The concentration of atRA in human plasma is normally 5–10 nM (Blomhoff *et al.*, 1990; Napoli, 1994), typically increases two to four times after ingestion of a large amount of vitamin A (Hartmann *et al.*, 2005), and can reach levels of 1–5 μM during therapeutic treatment with atRA (Regazzi *et al.*, 1997). Cells that cannot convert retinol to RA themselves and are not in direct contact with the plasma may still respond to vitamin A by obtaining RA locally from neighboring RA-producing cells. Uptake of RA from plasma and/or from neighboring cells may be relevant for the *in vivo* response of T cells to vitamin A, since thymocytes and mature T cells do not appear to express the set of enzymes necessary for the conversion of retinol to RA (Iwata *et al.*, 2004; Kiss *et al.*, 2008). Such a process of T cell acquisition of RA seems to be operable at least in some parts of the gut, where dendritic cells and possibly also macrophages, are believed to deliver RA to T cells (Manicassamy and Pulendran, 2009).

III. Cell Death Pathways

Physiological cell death occurs to a large extent through an active and ordered process of self-destruction termed apoptosis (Thompson, 1995), and most forms of T cell death (see next section) show apoptotic features. Typically, apoptosis is characterized by cytoplasmic and nuclear shrinkage, chromatin condensation, cleavage of DNA and proteins, and finally, fragmentation of the cell into membrane-enclosed, so-called "apoptotic bodies" that are phagocytosed and subsequently degraded by macrophages or by neighboring cells. The central executors of apoptosis are a family of aspartate-specific cysteine proteases known as caspases (Pop and Salvesen, 2009). Most caspases are expressed in the form of relatively inactive zymogens (procaspases), which are activated upon proteolytic cleavage. By sequentially cleaving and thereby activating each other, caspases can initiate so-called caspase cascades, which begin with the activation of "initiator caspases" (caspase-2, -8, -9, or -10) and conclude with the activation of "effector caspases" (caspase-3, -6, and -7). In general, the signals that lead to apoptosis can be divided into two major pathways that normally converge with the activation of caspases. These are termed the extrinsic (or death receptor) and the intrinsic (or mitochondrial) pathways. The extrinsic pathway is initiated by the ligation of a death receptor, leading to the assembly of a death-inducing signaling complex (DISC) at the cytoplasmic tail of the death receptor. The DISC minimally contains the death receptor (e.g., Fas) and an adaptor protein (e.g., FADD), which recruits an initiator caspase zymogen (e.g., procaspase-8). Within the DISC, the initiator caspase is activated and subsequently initiates a caspase cascade leading to apoptosis. The intrinsic pathway can be initiated by a wide variety of signals, including those originating from conditions of cellular starvation, stress, or DNA damage, culminating in the permeabilization of the outer mitochondrial membrane, the consequent release of proapoptotic factors from the mitochondrial intermembrane space to the cytosol, and typically, the activation of caspase-9. Outer mitochondrial membrane permeabilization and the release of proapoptotic mitochondrial proteins are crucially controlled by proteins of the Bcl-2 family. Thus, in general, the intrinsic, but not the extrinsic apoptotic pathway, can be inhibited by overexpression of antiapoptotic Bcl-2 family members (e.g., Bcl-2, Bcl-X_L, Bcl2-A1, and Mcl-1). Among the proapoptotic Bcl-2 proteins, the "BH3 only" proteins (e.g., Bim, Bad, and Bid) act by either binding to and thereby functionally neutralizing antiapoptotic Bcl-2 proteins, or by aiding Bax-like proteins (Bax, Bak, and Bok) in promoting outer mitochondrial membrane permeabilization (Festjens *et al.*, 2004). The function of Bcl-2 proteins can also be altered by non-Bcl-2 family proteins. This can be exemplified by the orphan nuclear receptor Nur77, which can translocate from the nucleus to the mitochondria to interact with and convert Bcl-2 into a proapoptotic molecule (Lin *et al.*, 2004).

IV. Forms of T Cell Death

A. Death of thymocytes

In the thymus, developing T cells (thymocytes) are carefully screened to select for cells that can engage strongly only with non-self-antigens in the context of presentation by self-MHC molecules. The major driving force for this selection process is cell death. In fact, less than 1% of the thymocytes survive the selection pressure in the thymus (Bettini and Vignali, 2010). In the thymic cortex, double-positive $CD4^+CD8^+$ thymocytes whose T cell receptors (TCRs) display a moderate avidity for self-peptide-filled MHC molecules presented by cortical thymic epithelial cells receive survival signals and are positively selected. Thymocytes bearing TCRs with no or very low avidity for the self-peptide-filled MHC molecules do not receive sufficient survival signals and die in a process often referred to as "death by neglect" or the "default death pathway". The large majority of double-positive thymocytes are believed to die as a result of neglect. This is reflected by the relatively high rate of spontaneous cell death displayed by isolated thymocytes in culture compared to that shown by resting mature T cells. Death by neglect may be facilitated by glucocorticoids and is correlated to the lack of Bcl-2 expression in double-positive thymocytes, as opposed to single-positive thymocytes and peripheral T cells (Ashwell *et al.*, 2000). Apart from this, the molecular details of the default death pathway are poorly characterized. The positively selected thymocytes move to the corticomedullary junction and the medulla. Here, their TCRs are challenged with a whole range of self-antigen peptides effectively presented by medullary thymic epithelial cells and dendritic cells. In this context, thymocytes bearing TCRs that interact with self-antigens are efficiently induced to die, in a process referred to as activation-induced cell death (AICD). Only thymocytes bearing TCRs with low avidity for self-antigens survive. By this negative selection process, the survival of most autoreactive T cells is prevented. For recent reviews concerning positive and negative selection of thymocytes, see (Nitta *et al.*, 2008; Ziegler *et al.*, 2009).

The molecular mechanism responsible for thymocyte AICD is incompletely understood. It does not seem to require Fas (Herron *et al.*, 1993; Newton *et al.*, 1998; Singer and Abbas, 1994), except upon encounter with high doses of antigen (Kishimoto *et al.*, 1998). Rather, it appears that thymocyte AICD is for the most part mediated by an intrinsic pathway involving the induced expression and possibly, the posttranslational modification of proapoptotic proteins such as Bim and Nur77 (Siggs *et al.*, 2006).

B. Death of mature T cells

Mature, resting human T cells are relatively resistant to apoptosis, due to high expression of antiapoptotic Bcl-2 proteins and low expression of death receptors such as Fas (Ashwell *et al.*, 2000; Marrack and Kappler, 2004). However, upon activation, the balance between pro- and antiapoptotic Bcl-2 proteins is altered, the expression of death receptors such as Fas is induced, and other alterations occur, which with time, lead to a greatly enhanced susceptibility of activated T cells toward both intrinsic and extrinsic apoptotic pathways. Three major types of cell death of activated T cells, with relevance to later sections, will be described here: (i) activated T cell autonomous death (ACAD), (ii) AICD, and (iii) Fas-induced cell death.

During an immune response, T cell numbers rapidly increase due to antigen-induced T cell proliferation. When the antigen is cleared, a corresponding decrease in T cell numbers occurs due to rapid apoptosis of the activated T cells (Akbar *et al.*, 1993; Harty and Badovinac, 2002; Kaech *et al.*, 2002). Only a small fraction of the antigen-specific T cells survive, and these may develop into memory T cells (Kaech *et al.*, 2002; Sprent and Surh, 2001). The efficient contraction of clonally expanded T cells is believed to occur as a result of the fading of life-sustaining cytokines at the end of an immune response, leading to a shift in the balance between pro- and antiapoptotic members of the Bcl-2 family, and thus the initiation of an intrinsic apoptotic pathway (Hildeman *et al.*, 2002; Rathmell and Thompson, 2002). This spontaneous death of activated T cells was termed ACAD in order to clearly distinguish it from AICD (Hildeman *et al.*, 2002). In contrast to ACAD, AICD is induced directly by TCR signaling, and occurs in mature T cells upon reactivation of already activated and expanded T cells. AICD most likely functions primarily to eliminate autoreactive T cells and T cells reacting toward a chronic infection (Bouillet and O'Reilly, 2009; Brenner *et al.*, 2008), but might also be expected to limit the clonal expansion of T cells at late stages of an acute immune response and contribute to the initial elimination or effector T cells at the end of an acute immune response. AICD of mature T cells can be mimicked *in vitro* by culturing activated T cells with interleukin-2 (IL-2) for 4–7 days, upon which restimulation induces cell death. A major mechanism for AICD involves the TCR-mediated induction of Fas ligand (FasL) expression and the subsequent extrinsic T cell death mediated by FasL ligation of Fas (Green *et al.*, 2003; Krammer *et al.*, 2007). During the primary activation, the expression of both Fas and FasL is rapidly induced (Peter *et al.*, 1997; Westendorp *et al.*, 1995), but immediate cell death is avoided by simultaneous initiation of antiapoptotic TCR-induced signals (Klas *et al.*, 1993; Peter *et al.*, 1997). During the secondary activation, the antiapoptotic mechanism fails. The lag time required for activated T cells to become sensitive to AICD coincides with the lag time required for them to become sensitive to Fas-induced cell death. At this stage, activated T cells can also die via Fas-induced cell death upon encounter with non-T cells that express FasL at their cell surface, for example, cells of immune-privileged sites, or FasL-expressing cancer cells (Green *et al.*, 2003; Li-Weber and Krammer, 2003). The physiological importance of FasL–Fas interactions in T cells is underscored by the fact that defects in Fas-induced cell death is associated with autoimmune diseases as well as T cell malignancies (Nagata, 1998; Straus *et al.*, 2001; Zhang *et al.*, 2003).

V. Regulation of Thymocyte Cell Death by Vitamin A

A. Effect of vitamin A on death by neglect of thymocytes

The influence of vitamin A on death by neglect has been studied by examining the effect of RA on spontaneous apoptosis of freshly isolated murine thymocytes *in vitro*. Whereas one group showed that both atRA and 9cRA could enhance cell death under these conditions (Fesus *et al.*, 1995; Szondy *et al.*, 1997), another group did not observe any effect of atRA (Iwata *et al.*, 1992). However, both groups found that RA could enhance cell death in the presence of glucocorticoids (Fesus *et al.*, 1995; Iwata *et al.*, 1992), which are known to stimulate the death of neglected thymocytes both *in vitro* and *in vivo* (Ashwell *et al.*, 2000; Herold *et al.*, 2006). The best response to RA was observed in those cultures where the rate of spontaneous apoptosis was highest (Fesus *et al.*, 1995). It was speculated that the differences in the rate of spontaneous apoptosis observed between different animals were due to different endogenous glucocorticoid levels in the animals, and thus that the observed effects of RA might reflect a stimulation of glucocorticoid-mediated enhancement of death by neglect, rather than RA acting by itself (Fesus *et al.*, 1995). Since the rate of spontaneous apoptosis was relatively low (~10–20% after 16–18 h) in the publication where atRA did not show any effect (Iwata *et al.*, 1992), whereas it was markedly higher (~20–25% after 6 h) in the two publications where RA was effective (Fesus *et al.*, 1995; Szondy *et al.*, 1997), this could explain the inconsistencies observed with RA alone. It should be noted, however, that the *in vivo* role of glucocorticoids in thymocyte cell death is disputed (Herold *et al.*, 2006; Sacedón *et al.*, 2007), and thus it might well be that RA is acting in concert with other endogenous components to facilitate the *in vitro* death of neglected thymocytes. It was observed that the required effective concentrations of atRA (0.1–10 μM) were higher than those of 9cRA (0.01–0.3 μM), indicating an involvement of RXR (Fesus *et al.*, 1995; Szondy *et al.*, 1997). RA was shown to directly enhance apoptosis of isolated $CD4^{+}CD8^{+}$ murine thymocytes, which were shown to express RAR-α and -γ, but not RAR-β (Szondy *et al.*, 1997; whereas RXR-α and -β are expressed by most cell types in the body). Furthermore, by using a panel of synthetic RAR and RXR isotype-specific agonists and antagonists, it was indicated that the spontaneous apoptosis of murine thymocytes is induced by RAR-γ/RXR heterodimers in which RAR-γ is ligated. This effect was reported to be antagonized by RAR-α/RXR heterodimers in which RAR-α was ligated. However, the antagonism could be suspended by double-ligated RAR-α/RXR heterodimers (Szondy *et al.*, 1997), explaining why 9cRA (which efficiently ligates both RARs and RXRs) was more effective than atRA (which ligates RAR-α and RAR-γ with similar efficiency) in inducing thymocyte apoptosis. Of note, this conclusion should be taken with some caution, since the *in vivo* specificities of many of the existing synthetic RAR and RXR isotype-specific agonists and antagonists have not been extensively characterized, and the RAR-γ agonist that by far showed the strongest apoptosis-inducing effect in the above-mentioned study, CD437, is known to induce apoptosis independently of RAR-γ in many cell types (Pfahl and Piedrafita, 2003). However, under the assumption that the RAR-βγ antagonist CD2665 acted specifically at 3 μM, a case for RAR-γ in the induction of thymocyte apoptosis was indicated by the ability of CD2665 to completely abolish the effect of CD437, 9cRA, or a combination of atRA and an RXR-α agonist (Szondy *et al.*, 1997). In contrast, however, *in vivo* murine models do not support a specific role for RAR-γ in thymocyte development (Gordy *et al.*, 2009). Thus, further studies are needed to clarify the role of RA and RARs/RXRs on the death of neglected murine thymocytes *in vitro* and *in vivo*. Moreover, the potential effect of RA on the spontaneous death of human thymocytes remains to be investigated.

B. Effect of vitamin A on AICD of thymocytes

The influence of vitamin A on AICD of thymocytes has been studied by examining the effect of RA on murine thymocytes activated by various means. In freshly isolated murine thymocytes, it was reported that atRA could efficiently inhibit AICD induced by either the combination of immobilized anti-CD3 and anti-LFA-1 antibodies, or the combination of phorbol ester (12-*O*-tetradecanoylphorbol 13-acetate (TPA)) and calcium ionophore (ionomycin; Iwata *et al.*, 1992). The effective concentrations of atRA were much lower in the former case (0.01–1 μM) than in the latter (10–20 μM). In another study, AICD was induced in thymocytes from female mice expressing TCR-αβ chains specific for the male H-Y antigen by *in vitro* coculture with murine male thymic antigen presenting cells. Both atRA and 9cRA were shown to efficiently inhibit this specific antigen-driven AICD (Yang *et al.*, 1993). 9cRA was effective at about 10-fold lower concentrations than atRA (0.01–0.1 μM vs. 0.1–1 μM for 9cRA and atRA, respectively), implicating a role for RXR in this process. Another group also found 9cRA to be much more effective than atRA in inhibiting AICD of freshly isolated murine thymocytes induced by the combination of phorbol dibutyrate (PdBu) and the calcium ionophore A23187 (Fesus *et al.*, 1995; Szondy *et al.*, 1998b). Here, the requirement for simultaneous RAR- and RXR-ligation was demonstrated by the observation that if atRA was added together with a low concentration of an RXR-α specific agonist, it was just as effective as 9cRA (Szondy *et al.*, 1998b). Moreover, by using a panel of synthetic RAR and RXR isotype-specific agonists and antagonists, it was indicated that PdBu/A23187-induced AICD of murine thymocytes is inhibited by RAR-α/RXR heterodimers in which RAR-α is ligated. This effect was reportedly antagonized by RAR-γ/RXR heterodimers in which RAR-γ was ligated, and the antagonism could be suspended by RXR coligation (Szondy *et al.*, 1998b). These findings offer an explanation to why 9cRA was more effective than atRA in AICD inhibition, but again some caution should be exerted in conclusions that are based solely on the use of synthetic analogs and extrapolations from their *in vitro* binding capacities. Nevertheless, it is interesting to note that the RAR-α selective agonist, CD336 (also known as AM-580), was shown to protect murine $CD4^+CD8^+$ thymocytes from anti-CD3 antibody-induced cell death *in vivo* (Szondy *et al.*, 1998b). Thus, CD336 could completely reverse the ~50% thymic weight loss that was observed in mice 1 day after injection of anti-CD3 antibodies, and both the anti-CD3-induced decrease in the $CD4^+CD8^+$ subpopulation and the anti-CD3-induced DNA fragmentation in the thymocytes were abolished by CD336 (Szondy *et al.*, 1998b). This finding was followed up by examining the *in vivo* effect of CD336 on thymocyte AICD induced by either specific antigen (injection of pigeon cytochrome *c* (PCC) in TCR-αβ transgenic mice carrying a receptor specific for a fragment of PCC) or the superantigen Staphylococcal enterotoxin A. Whereas CD336 had similar effects on antigen-induced thymocyte AICD as those observed upon injection of anti-CD3 antibodies, it had no effect on superantigen-induced AICD (Szegezdi *et al.*, 2003). This differential effect of CD336 was correlated to the lack of Nur77 and Bim induction in thymocytes from superantigen-treated mice, as opposed to mice treated with anti-CD3 antibodies or PCC. Moreover, CD336 was shown to inhibit anti-CD3- and PCC-induced Bim synthesis and DNA binding of Nur77 in the murine thymocytes, indicating a mechanism for the antiapoptotic effect of CD336 (Szegezdi *et al.*, 2003). It was concluded that engagement of thymocyte TCR by anti-CD3 antibodies or specific antigen stimulates similar, CD336-inhibitable signaling pathways to induce AICD, whereas superantigen initiates separate signals that are not accessible by CD336. An interesting question that remains to be answered is how CD336 mediates its effects in these *in vivo* experimental systems. Although CD336 preferentially binds to RAR-α *in vitro* (K_d = 8 nM), it also shows some affinity for RAR-β (K_d = 131 nM) and RAR-γ (K_d = 450 nM) (Schneider *et al.*, 2000; Szondy *et al.*, 1998b). Moreover, as determined by transcriptional reporter activity assays, the concentrations needed to activate the receptors are much lower, showing 50% activation already at 0.36, 24.6, and 27.9 nM for RAR-α, -β, and -γ, respectively, compared to 6.7, 2.8, and 4.9 nM for atRA (Schneider *et al.*, 2000). Thus, above a certain concentration, CD336 can be anticipated to activate all the three RAR subtypes, and would, in that respect, be expected to behave as atRA. Thus, it is possible that CD336 activated not only RAR-α in the two *in vivo* studies mentioned above (the doses of CD336 used in the two studies were 400 and 50 μg, respectively; Szegezdi *et al.*, 2003; Szondy *et al.*, 1998b). To that end, it would be interesting to test whether atRA could display the same effect as that of CD336 in these *in vivo* experimental systems.

In conclusion, it appears that the effect of RA on thymocyte AICD will depend on the type and/or strength of thymocyte TCR engagement. A role of RXR is generally implicated in the inhibition of thymocyte AICD. However, in certain cases, RAR ligation alone may be sufficient, since atRA was found to be effective already at 10 nM in inhibiting murine thymocyte AICD induced by anti-CD3/anti-LFA-1 (Iwata *et al.*, 1992). Further studies are required to clarify these issues. Moreover, the effect of vitamin A on AICD of human thymocytes has not been investigated.

VI. Regulation of Mature T Cell Death by Vitamin A

A. Effect of vitamin A on death by neglect of mature T cells

Resting mature T cells are relatively resistant to apoptosis, but are thought to require continual low-affinity MHC-interactions and cytokines for their long-term peripheral survival (Marrack *et al.*, 2000). Upon culturing, resting peripheral human T cells show a slow rate of spontaneous cell death, which is not affected by atRA (Engedal *et al.*, 2004) (Fig. 7.1).

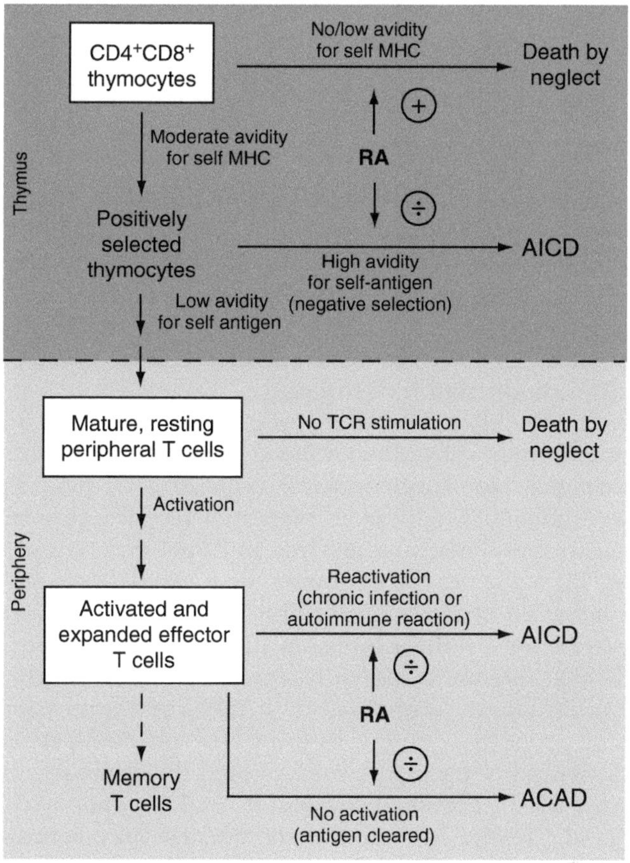

Figure 7.1 Regulation of T cell death by the vitamin A-metabolite retinoic acid (RA). This simplified scheme depicts some of the major cell death pathways of developing T cells in the thymus and mature T cells in the periphery. Effector T cells that escape activation-induced cell death (AICD) and activated T cell autonomous death (ACAD) may develop into memory T cells (indicated by the dotted arrow). Proposed actions of RA, as suggested from the mainly *in vitro* model systems described in the text, are indicated. *Note*: The putative RA-mediated regulation of Fas-induced T cell death downstream of Fas engagement is not shown. See text for further details.

B. Effect of vitamin A on ACAD of mature T cells

Physiological concentrations of atRA can stimulate the proliferation of isolated human T cells by enhancing activation-induced IL-2 production (Engedal *et al.*, 2004; Ertesvag *et al.*, 2002). The most prominent effect of atRA is observed when the phorbol ester TPA is used as an activator (Ertesvag *et al.*, 2002). Considering that cytokines of the IL-2 family have been shown to inhibit ACAD both *in vitro* and *in vivo* (Vella *et al.*, 1998), the effect of RA on the spontaneous apoptosis of TPA-activated peripheral human T cells was examined in order to assess the effect of vitamin A on ACAD (Engedal *et al.*, 2004). atRA was found to inhibit ACAD of TPA-activated T cells at physiological concentrations (10 nM was as efficient as 100 nM) and independently of its action on T cell proliferation (Engedal *et al.*, 2004). The inhibition of ACAD was correlated with the ability of atRA to stimulate IL-2 production and was abolished by neutralizing anti-IL-2 receptor antibodies. Moreover, recombinant IL-2 could fully mimic the effect of atRA, and the use of synthetic RAR-selective agonists and antagonists indicated that the effect of atRA was dependent on RAR. 9cRA and atRA were equally effective in inhibiting ACAD. It was concluded that RA inhibits ACAD of TPA-activated human T cells via a RAR-dependent increase in IL-2 production (Engedal *et al.*, 2004).

This is so far the only published report on the effect of RA on ACAD of T lymphocytes from healthy blood donors. However, studies on the *in vitro* death of peripheral blood mononuclear cells (PBMCs) and T cells from HIV-infected individuals appear to support a role for RA in inhibiting ACAD. Due to the persistence of virus and viral replication throughout the course of HIV disease, the immune system of HIV-infected patients is chronically activated (Fauci, 1993). This includes chronic activation of PBMCs, as reflected by the expression of activation antigens on $CD4^+$ and $CD8^+$ T cells, and increased expression of cytokines and IL-2 receptors (Fauci, 1993). Strikingly, as opposed to T cells from healthy individuals, a relatively large proportion of T cells from HIV-infected patients undergo spontaneous apoptosis upon *in vitro* culture, the intensity of which is correlated to HIV disease progression and lymphocyte activation (Gougeon *et al.*, 1996). It should be noted that only a relatively small number of T cells is actually infected with HIV in patients with AIDS, indicating that direct viral cytopathicity is not a major mechanism for the T cell death observed. Thus, spontaneous *in vitro* cell death of T cells from HIV^+ patients is for the most part likely to be caused by ACAD. Interestingly, oral atRA administration to a small cohort of HIV-infected patients enrolled in a phase I/II clinical trial ($n = 6$) was reported to significantly inhibit the spontaneous *ex vivo* apoptosis of their PBMCs (Yang *et al.*, 1995a). The peak blood level of atRA achieved on the first day of therapy was 1 μM. Apoptosis of PBMCs from HIV-infected individuals could also be inhibited by *in vitro* treatment with 0.1 μM atRA, and the effect of atRA was more pronounced on PBMCs from patients with low $CD4^+$ counts (200–499 $CD4^+$ cells/mm^3, $n = 12$) than on PBMCs from patients with high $CD4^+$ counts (>500 $CD4^+$ cells/mm^3, $n = 9$). It should be noted that the contribution of atRA-mediated inhibition of B cell apoptosis was not assessed in this study. This could be important, since *ex vivo* spontaneous B cell apoptosis constitute between 10% and 35% of the apoptotic PBMC population, and is higher for B cells from HIV^+ patients than for B cells from healthy individuals (Gougeon *et al.*, 1996). Moreover, subsequent studies have reported that atRA can reduce the spontaneous apoptosis of B lymphocytes obtained from either healthy (Lomo *et al.*, 1998) or HIV-infected blood donors (Szondy *et al.*, 1998a). In the latter of these two studies, 0.01–10 μM atRA was shown to reduce spontaneous apoptosis of PBMCs from HIV^+ patients in a dose-dependent manner. Importantly, atRA was shown to also specifically inhibit spontaneous apoptosis of $CD4^+$, but not $CD8^+$, T cells from HIV-infected individuals (Szondy *et al.*, 1998a). Furthermore, in agreement with the above-mentioned observation in PBMCs from HIV^+ patients (Yang *et al.*, 1995a), the ability of atRA to inhibit $CD4^+$ T cell death was found to correlate with disease progression, that is, the effect of atRA was stronger on $CD4^+$ cells from patients with low $CD4^+$ counts ($CD4^+ < 14\%$) than on those from patients with higher $CD4^+$ counts (Szondy *et al.*, 1998a). In conclusion, these studies indicate that atRA inhibits the ACAD of $CD4^+$ T cells from HIV-infected patients. The mechanism involved is unknown. It has been suggested that the Fas pathway may be partly involved in spontaneous apoptosis of T cells from HIV^+ patients with a late-stage disease (Szondy *et al.*, 1998a), and as mentioned above, atRA-mediated stimulation of IL-2 secretion can protect activated T cells from autonomous cell death (Engedal *et al.*, 2004). Thus, future studies should aim to clarify the putative involvement of IL-2 and the Fas pathway in atRA-mediated protection from spontaneous apoptosis of T cells from HIV^+ patients. Furthermore, additional studies are needed to further clarify the role of vitamin A on ACAD of healthy T cells.

C. Effect of vitamin A on AICD of mature T cells

Although RA is generally regarded as an inhibitor of T cell AICD *in vitro*, with the mechanisms involved being at least partly clarified (Li-Weber and Krammer, 2003), it is important to note that the effect of RA on AICD of normal, mature T cells has only been examined in one experiment (Yang *et al.*, 1995a). Here, PBMCs were stimulated with concanavalin A (a plant lectin that stimulates T cells via binding to carbohydrate moieties of TCR–CD3 complexes and costimulatory receptors) for 3 days, followed by expansion with IL-2 for an additional 3 days. Then, the resulting T cell blasts were activated by immobilized anti-CD3 antibodies for 40 h (to induce AICD) in the absence or presence of various concentrations of atRA (0.001–10 μM). As assessed by trypan blue exclusion of quadruplicate cultures, atRA inhibited AICD in a dose-dependent manner, showing half-maximal inhibition already at the physiological concentration of 10 nM (Yang *et al.*, 1995a). The mechanisms involved were not assessed, and the effect of 9cRA was not examined. Thus, at present, clues about the mechanisms that may be involved in RA-mediated inhibition of AICD of normal, mature T cells have to be extrapolated from studies performed on nonnormal T cells. These include for the most part studies on various murine T cell hybridoma cell lines (Bissonnette *et al.*, 1995; Cui *et al.*, 1996; Iwata *et al.*, 1992; Toth *et al.*, 2001; Yang *et al.*, 1993, 1995b,c), but also human leukemic Jurkat T cells (Lee *et al.*, 2002; Toth *et al.*, 2001) and T cells from HIV-infected individuals (Szondy *et al.*, 1998a; Yang *et al.*, 1995a; see below).

Murine hybridoma T cells are usually produced by fusing antigen-primed murine T cell blasts with spontaneously proliferating murine thymic lymphoma cells. The hybridomas behave as already activated T cells, and (as is also the case for thymocytes) a single activation is enough to induce AICD. It was originally thought that T cell hybridomas could be used to study the AICD that occurs in thymocytes during negative selection. However, the AICD of T cell hybridomas was found to resemble more the AICD of mature T cells, in that it is mediated via FasL–Fas interactions (Brunner *et al.*, 1995; Ju *et al.*, 1995), whereas as described earlier, Fas plays only a minor, if any role in thymocyte AICD. The reported effects of RA on AICD in various T cell hybridomas generally agree and complement each other, and in all of these studies, AICD was induced by treatment with anti-CD3 antibodies. From these publications, it is evident that in hybridoma T cells, 9cRA is more potent than atRA in inhibiting anti-CD3-induced AICD, the effective range of 9cRA (0.01–1 μM) being about 10-fold lower than that of atRA (0.1–10 μM) (Bissonnette *et al.*, 1995; Cui *et al.*, 1996; Iwata *et al.*, 1992; Toth *et al.*, 2001; Yang *et al.*, 1993, 1995c). This strongly points to an involvement of RXR, and by overexpressing wild-type or dominant negative forms of RXR-β (Yang *et al.*, 1995c), or by studying the effects of various combinations of RAR- and RXR-selective synthetic agonists (Bissonnette *et al.*, 1995; Yang *et al.*, 1995c), it was demonstrated that simultaneous ligation of both RAR and RXR was necessary for efficient inhibition of AICD. Furthermore, 9cRA, or high concentrations of atRA, was shown to effectively block anti-CD3-mediated induction of FasL mRNA expression (Bissonnette *et al.*, 1995; Cui *et al.*, 1996; Yang *et al.*, 1995b), and as determined by the use of flow cytometry and functional FasL killing assays, activation-mediated induction of cell surface FasL protein expression was strongly reduced by RA (Bissonnette *et al.*, 1995; Cui *et al.*, 1996; Yang *et al.*, 1995b,c). Simultaneous ligation of both RAR and RXR was necessary for efficient inhibition of both FasL mRNA (Bissonnette *et al.*, 1995) and FasL cell surface protein expression (Yang *et al.*, 1995c). RA did not downregulate the expression of Fas mRNA or cell surface Fas proteins (Bissonnette *et al.*, 1995; Cui *et al.*, 1996). Moreover, FasL-expressing effector cells were still able to induce cell death in hybridoma cells that had been cotreated with anti-CD3 antibodies and AICD-inhibitory concentrations of atRA (Cui *et al.*, 1996), strongly indicating that RA does not considerably interfere with the Fas-mediated cell death pathway downstream of Fas engagement. This conclusion was supported by the findings that 9cRA does not interfere with Fas-mediated cell death either in Fas-expressing mouse T leukemia L1210.fas cells cocultured with preactivated FasL-expressing hybridoma T cells (Bissonnette *et al.*, 1995) or in Jurkat cells treated with anti-Fas antibodies (Bissonnette *et al.*, 1995; Engedal *et al.*, 2009).

In summary, these studies collectively demonstrate that 9cRA efficiently inhibits anti-CD3-induced AICD of murine hybridoma T cells by blocking activation-induced FasL cell surface expression, in a manner that requires ligation of both RAR and RXR. The inhibition of FasL cell surface expression is likely to be caused by the strong repression of activation-induced FasL mRNA expression observed upon RA cotreatment. RA-mediated inhibition of FasL mRNA expression has also reported in Jurkat cells stimulated with anti-CD3 antibodies or TPA/ionomycin (Lee *et al.*, 2002; Toth *et al.*, 2001). In the latter case, atRA was effective already at 10 nM, indicating that ligation of RAR alone may be sufficient for repression of FasL expression under some conditions (Lee *et al.*, 2002). Moreover, the same group showed that atRA repressed the transcriptional activity of the FasL promoter, and more specifically that atRA could repress TPA/ionomycin-induced transcriptional activation of a reporter gene driven by the nuclear factor of activated T cell (NFAT) binding motif from the FasL promoter. It was also demonstrated that atRA could repress TPA/ionomycin-induced DNA-binding activity of NFAT in Jurkat cells, with atRA again being effective already at 10 nM (Lee *et al.*, 2002). Thus, it appears that in Jurkat cells, atRA can inhibit FasL expression at the transcriptional level by interfering with the ability of NFAT to bind to the FasL promoter. A possible mechanism was indicated by the finding that TPA/ionomycin-induced translocation of NFAT from the cytoplasm to the nucleus was blocked by atRA in NFAT-overexpressing HeLa cells (Lee *et al.*, 2002). RA has also been reported to interfere with anti-CD3- or TPA/ionomycin-induced activation of Nur77 in Jurkat cells (Kang *et al.*, 2000; Toth *et al.*, 2001), and it was suggested that this might be a mechanism by which RA represses FasL transcription. However, although FasL levels are elevated in Nur77 transgenic mice, and overexpression of dominant negative Nur77 can inhibit TCR-mediated AICD, the potential role of Nur77 in controlling FasL transcription and AICD is unclear, since the FasL promoter does not seem to contain a recognizable Nur77 binding site, and TCR/CD3-mediated AICD is intact in T cells from Nur77 knockout mice (Li-Weber and Krammer, 2003). Finally, although it is generally held that upregulation of FasL cell surface expression during AICD is a direct consequence of elevated FasL mRNA and protein levels, there are examples of hybridoma T cells and Jurkat sublines that contain intracellularly located, preformed FasL, and respond to TCR stimulation by transporting the preformed FasL to the plasma membrane (Toth *et al.*, 1999). Interestingly, in such a T cell hybridoma (the influenza hemagglutinin-specific IP-12-7 cell line) atRA and, more potently so, 9cRA were shown to inhibit anti-CD3-induced FasL cell surface expression and AICD (Toth *et al.*, 2001), indicating that RA may regulate T cell AICD by blocking the intracellular transport of FasL to the plasma membrane. The relevance of this pathway for AICD in normal T cells must be determined before one can conclude further about the importance of this potential action of RA.

AtRA has been reported to inhibit AICD also in T cells from HIV-infected patients (Szondy *et al.*, 1998a; Yang *et al.*, 1995a). Consistent with the T cells of HIV-infected individuals being chronically activated *in vivo* (Fauci, 1993) upon *in vitro* culture, a single activation signal with anti-CD3 antibodies leads to AICD (Gougeon *et al.*, 1996). Oral administration of atRA to six HIV^+ patients was shown to inhibit not only the *ex vivo* spontaneous apoptosis of their PBMCs but also that induced by anti-CD3 antibodies (Yang *et al.*, 1995a). *Ex vivo* atRA treatment could also inhibit anti-CD3-induced apoptosis of PBMCs from HIV^+ patients (Szondy *et al.*, 1998a; Yang *et al.*, 1995a), with some effect noted already with 10 nM atRA, whereas optimal effects were obtained within the range of 0.1–10 μM atRA. In the latter study, it was more specifically found that atRA inhibited AICD of $CD4^+$ and not $CD8^+$ T cells (Szondy *et al.*, 1998a). Furthermore, like in T cell hybridomas, atRA was found to inhibit anti-CD3-induced production of FasL, and not Fas (Szondy *et al.*, 1998a), indicating that atRA inhibits AICD of T cells from HIV^+ patients via repression of TCR-induced FasL expression. This mechanism would fit well with the observation that atRA inhibited AICD of $CD4^+$, and not $CD8^+$ T cells from HIV^+ patients (Szondy *et al.*, 1998a), given the demonstration that AICD of normal mature $CD4^+$ T cells is mainly mediated by FasL, whereas that of normal mature $CD8^+$ T cells is instead mostly mediated by tumor necrosis factor (Zheng *et al.*, 1995). It should be noted that the relative increase in apoptosis observed upon stimulation with anti-CD3 antibodies in the two studies mentioned above (Szondy *et al.*, 1998a; Yang *et al.*, 1995a) was, in general, rather modest compared to another study where T cells from a higher number of blood donors were examined (Gougeon *et al.*, 1996), and also compared to the observed higher rate of spontaneous apoptosis of PBMCs from HIV-infected patients versus that of PBMCs from healthy individuals (Szondy *et al.*, 1998a; Yang *et al.*, 1995a). Thus, and since in many of the experiments, the effect of atRA was only examined in the presence of anti-CD3 antibodies and not alone, the relative contribution of atRA-mediated inhibition of AICD compared to the overall atRA-mediated inhibition of the *ex vivo* apoptosis of T cells from HIV^+ patients (AICD + ACAD) is unclear, and may have been overestimated in these two studies. The effect of 9cRA on T cells from HIV-infected patients has not been examined.

In conclusion, it seems reasonable to assume that RA acts to inhibit AICD in normal mature T cells, at least *in vitro*, and that some of the mechanisms that have been demonstrated in nonnormal T cells are also involved in this process. However, it is important to emphasize that these issues still need to be experimentally tested in normal, mature T cells. Notably, it remains to be more firmly determined at which concentrations atRA is effective in inhibiting AICD of normal T cells, and whether 9cRA is more potent than atRA also in this situation. The observations that atRA can be effective already at 10 nM in normal T cells (Yang *et al.*, 1995a), as well as in T cells from HIV-infected patients (Yang *et al.*, 1995a) and Jurkat cells (Lee *et al.*, 2002), whereas much higher concentrations of atRA are generally needed to inhibit AICD in murine hybridoma T cells, indicate that the requirements for RA-mediated repression of AICD in mature human T cells might differ from those reported in murine hybridoma T cells. In that regard, it is interesting to note that AICD occurs much faster in hybridoma than in normal T cells. Whereas in murine hybridoma T cells AICD is typically initiated within a few hours after TCR stimulation, this can take up to 24 h or more in normal human T cells. Thus, one may reason that RA will have more time to exert its antiapoptotic effects in normal T cells than in the model hybridoma T cells, and further speculate that single ligation of RAR in the RAR/RXR heterodimer (occurring at low concentrations of atRA) may suffice in the former case, whereas double ligation of RAR and RXR (occurring with 9cRA or high concentrations of atRA) is required to mediate fast-enough effects to interfere with the cell death pathway in the latter case.

D. Effect of vitamin A on Fas-induced T cell death downstream of Fas engagement

TCR/CD3-induced antiapoptotic signaling is believed to protect primary activated T cells from the Fas-induced cell death that would otherwise occur due to activation-induced production of both Fas and FasL (Klas *et al.*, 1993; Peter *et al.*, 1997; Westendorp *et al.*, 1995). Using the Jurkat cell line as a model, it has been shown that such antiapoptotic signals may be related to activation of the mitogen-activated protein kinase ERK and the transcription factor NFκB (Engedal and Blomhoff, 2003; Holmstrom *et al.*, 1998; Wilson *et al.*, 1999) and at least in part to a block in FasL-induced DISC assembly (Engedal *et al.*, 2009; Gomez-Angelats and Cidlowski, 2001; Meng *et al.*, 2002). Available data indicate that RA does not directly affect T cell death downstream of Fas receptor engagement (Bissonnette *et al.*, 1995; Cui *et al.*, 1996; Engedal *et al.*, 2009). However, in a recent report, it was shown that RA can reverse mitogen-mediated repression of Fas-induced cell death in Jurkat cells (Engedal *et al.*, 2009). Thus, RA significantly abolished the antiapoptotic effects of concanavalin A or TPA on cell death induced by anti-Fas antibodies or membrane-bound FasL (Engedal *et al.*, 2009). 9cRA was found to be more potent than atRA, showing some effect at 10 nM and maximal effect at 1 μM. Furthermore,

9cRA was shown to act by reversing mitogen-mediated repression of Fas DISC assembly, without interfering with mitogen-induced activation of ERK or NFκB. Thus, TPA-mediated inhibition of Fas-induced recruitment and cleavage of procaspase-8 within the DISC was abolished by 9cRA (Engedal *et al.*, 2009). More work is needed to assess the putative importance of this novel mechanism of action of RA in the regulation of T cell death. For example, it remains to be determined whether this mechanism is restricted to malignant T cells or whether a similar mechanism also operates in normal T cells. Moreover, although it can be envisioned, it is unclear to what degree mitogenic signals are involved in the regulation of Fas-induced cell death under conditions such as activated T cell encounter with FasL-expressing cells of immune-privileged sites or FasL-expressing malignant cells.

VII. Concluding Discussion and Future Perspectives

A. Are the effects observed with 9cRA physiologically relevant?

For many of the reported effects of RA on T cell death, 9cRA has been found to be more potent than atRA. In this regard, it is important to note that although 9cRA can be produced either via isomerization of atRA (Heyman *et al.*, 1992) or via oxidation of 9-*cis* retinol and 9-*cis* retinal in reactions that can be catalyzed by naturally occurring enzymes (Lin *et al.*, 2003), the *in vivo* existence of 9cRA is yet to be conclusively proved, and available data indicate that 9cRA is not likely to be the major physiologic ligand for RXR (Blomhoff and Blomhoff, 2006; Wolf, 2006). Does this imply that the effects of 9cRA on T cell death described in this chapter are without physiological relevance for the effect of vitamin A on T cell death? At least two arguments indicate that this is not necessarily the case. First, it is possible that the lack of definitive proof for endogenous 9cRA is simply due to methodological constraints and/or that detectable and biologically active concentrations of 9cRA are being produced only locally or transiently *in vivo*. Second, naturally occurring RXR-activating ligands other than 9cRA, for example, eicosanoids, phytanic acid, and several types of unsaturated fatty acids, have been described (Blomhoff and Blomhoff, 2006; Wolf, 2006). Thus, the combined presence of atRA and such RXR-activating compounds could lead to simultaneous ligation of RARs and RXRs and might thereby produce the same effects as those observed with 9cRA alone. As an example of this possibility, it is well documented that eicosanoids are produced in the thymus, where they are postulated to be involved in the education of thymocytes (Juzan *et al.*, 1992). Moreover, RAR-stimulating ligands as well as enzymes that are required for RA production are expressed by thymic epithelial cells (Kiss *et al.*, 2008). Thus, it can be envisioned that thymocytes can simultaneously receive compounds that activate both RAR (e.g., atRA or other RAR-stimulating ligands) and RXR (e.g., eicosanoids) *in vivo*, and this could be expected to have the same effect on thymocyte cell death as that observed with 9cRA *in vitro*. Given such a scenario, even if future studies should reveal that 9cRA is not present in the thymus, the reported effects of 9cRA on thymocytes may still be of physiological relevance. Similar scenarios can be envisioned for T cells in other locations in the body. In conclusion, the possibilities and effects of the simultaneous presence of RXR- and RAR-activating ligands in various tissues must be examined before one can draw conclusions on whether the observed effects of 9cRA on T cell death may be of physiologic relevance or not.

B. Physiological implications of the effects of vitamin A on T cell death

If RA stimulates the death of neglected thymocytes and inhibits thymocyte AICD *in vivo*, one would expect vitamin A to be involved in shaping the T cell repertoire at two levels. By enhancing the death of neglected thymocytes, it would help prevent the development of functionally inadequate mature T cells, that is, T cells with too low affinity for self-MHC molecules. However, by inhibiting thymocyte AICD, it would regulate the threshold for negative selection in a manner that could result in the survival and development of potentially autoreactive peripheral T cells. If RA also inhibits peripheral AICD and ACAD *in vivo*, as suggested from *in vitro* studies, potentially autoreactive T cells would stand an even better chance of long-time survival. Together with the observation that RA, unlike glucocorticoids, does not inhibit T cell activation (it can, on the contrary, costimulate T cell proliferation *in vitro*; Engedal *et al.*, 2004, 2006; Ertesvag *et al.*, 2002), it would be expected that vitamin A should promote autoimmunity. However, this seems not to be the case, since no general association between vitamin A and the promotion of autoimmunity has been reported. One possible explanation for this could be that vitamin A-mediated support of suppressive T regulatory (Treg) cells counterbalances its support of autoreactive cells. Recent studies have demonstrated that atRA promotes the development of TGF-β-induced adaptive Treg cells in the gut (Mucida *et al.*, 2009), and vitamin A is therefore implicated in oral tolerance. Prevention of autoimmunity is believed to be predominantly mediated by natural Treg cells rather than by adaptive Treg cells (Curotto de Lafaille and Lafaille, 2009). Since the development of both adaptive and natural Treg cells can be induced by TGF-β, and RA clearly can modulate TGF-β-induced signaling (Mucida *et al.*, 2009), the possibility exists that RA also promotes natural Treg production in the thymus. Future studies should reveal whether this is the case. Another unanswered question is whether vitamin A can regulate Treg cell death. Natural Treg cells are selected by high-avidity TCR–self-peptide–MHC interactions in the thymus, an interaction that leads to AICD in conventional thymocytes (negative selection). It is not completely understood how thymocytes committed to become natural Treg cells escape negative selection. An involvement of vitamin A could be considered, since, as described above, RA can inhibit thymocyte AICD, and RAR-stimulating ligands as well as enzymes that are required for RA production are expressed by murine thymic epithelial cells. Whether RA could regulate the death of Treg cells in the periphery is also an open question.

What may be the net effect of vitamin A-mediated regulation of T cell death on the immune system, provided that the enhanced survival of potentially autoreactive T cells is balanced by vitamin A promoting Treg cell development? One interesting possibility in relation to vitamin A-mediated inhibition of peripheral AICD and ACAD concerns the production of memory T cells. Since memory T cells are believed to originate from the pool of effector T cells, the number of memory cells generated will depend on the number of effector cells that survive the elimination of T cells at the end of an immune response (Sprent and Surh, 2001). Thus, by inhibiting ACAD, and perhaps also by inhibiting peripheral AICD, vitamin A may enhance the number of surviving effector T cells and thereby promote the generation of memory T cells. This could potentially help explain why vitamin A enhances the efficiency of several types of vaccines, for example, diphtheria, measles, and polio type I vaccines (Bahl *et al.*, 2002; Benn *et al.*, 2002; Bhaskaram and Rao, 1997; Rahman *et al.*, 1999).

The recent demonstration that RA can reverse mitogen-mediated repression of Fas-induced apoptosis in T cells (Engedal *et al.*, 2009) adds to the diversity of the mechanisms by which vitamin A may regulate T cell death. Since this effect has been shown only in the leukemic Jurkat T cell line so far, it remains to be determined whether this mechanism of RA is also operable in normal T cells, or whether it may be restricted to malignant T cells or malignant cells in general. Thus, at present, it is too early to speculate on the possible physiological implications of this finding, although in the latter case, it is tempting to hypothesize that this mechanism might be involved in RA/retinoid-mediated anticancer activity (Altucci and Gronemeyer, 2001).

Although more studies are needed, two reports have demonstrated a protective effect of RA on both spontaneous and AICD of T cells from HIV^{+} individuals (Szondy *et al.*, 1998a; Yang *et al.*, 1995a). Controlled clinical trials show that periodic vitamin A supplementation of HIV-infected infants and children reduces all-cause mortality and morbidity associated with the disease (Mehta and Fawzi, 2007). It is conceivable that RA-mediated protection of T cell death may improve T cell immune function in HIV-infected patients and thereby provide one of the explanations for the beneficial effect of vitamin A supplementation of HIV-infected children.

In conclusion, it is clear that vitamin A may affect T cell death at multiple levels to modulate T cell immune function, and this justifies further research on the subject. In particular, much more needs to be learned about the *in vitro* and *in vivo* effects of vitamin A on the death of human thymocytes and normal mature T cells. Moreover, further work in determining the distribution and local production of vitamin A metabolites, as well as ligands for RXR throughout the body, will help in assessing the putative physiological relevance of the reported *in vitro* actions of atRA and 9cRA on T cell death.

REFERENCES

Akbar, A. N., Salmon, M., Savill, J., and Janossy, G. (1993). A possible role for bcl-2 in regulating T-cell memory—A 'balancing act' between cell death and survival. *Immunol. Today* **14,** 526–532.

Altucci, L., and Gronemeyer, H. (2001). The promise of retinoids to fight against cancer. *Nat. Rev. Cancer* **1,** 181–193.

Ashwell, J. D., Lu, F. W., and Vacchio, M. S. (2000). Glucocorticoids in T cell development and function*. *Annu. Rev. Immunol.* **18,** 309–345.

Bahl, R., Bhandari, N., Kant, S., Molbak, K., Ostergaard, E., and Bhan, M. K. (2002). Effect of vitamin A administered at Expanded Program on Immunization contacts on antibody response to oral polio vaccine. *Eur. J. Clin. Nutr.* **56,** 321–325.

Balmer, J. E., and Blomhoff, R. (2002). Gene expression regulation by retinoic acid. *J. Lipid Res.* **43,** 1773–1808.

Bastien, J., and Rochette-Egly, C. (2004). Nuclear retinoid receptors and the transcription of retinoid-target genes. *Gene* **328,** 1–16.

Benn, C. S., Balde, A., George, E., Kidd, M., Whittle, H., Lisse, I. M., and Aaby, P. (2002). Effect of vitamin A supplementation on measles-specific antibody levels in Guinea-Bissau. *Lancet* **359,** 1313–1314.

Bettini, M. L., and Vignali, D. A. (2010). Development of thymically derived natural regulatory T cells. *Ann. NY Acad. Sci.* **1183,** 1–12.

Bhaskaram, P., and Rao, K. V. (1997). Enhancement in seroconversion to measles vaccine with simultaneous administration of vitamin A in 9-months-old Indian infants. *Indian J. Pediatr.* **64,** 503–509.

Bissonnette, R. P., Brunner, T., Lazarchik, S. B., Yoo, N. J., Boehm, M. F., Green, D. R., and Heyman, R. A. (1995). 9-cis Retinoic acid inhibition of activation-induced apoptosis is mediated via regulation of fas ligand and requires retinoic acid receptor and retinoid X receptor activation. *Mol. Cell. Biol.* **15,** 5576–5585.

Blomhoff, R., and Blomhoff, H. K. (2006). Overview of retinoid metabolism and function. *J. Neurobiol.* **66,** 606–630.

Blomhoff, R., Green, M. H., Berg, T., and Norum, K. R. (1990). Transport and storage of vitamin A. *Science* **250,** 399–404.

Bouillet, P., and O'Reilly, L. A. (2009). CD95, BIM and T cell homeostasis. *Nat. Rev. Immunol.* **9,** 514–519.

Brenner, D., Krammer, P. H., and Arnold, R. (2008). Concepts of activated T cell death. *Crit. Rev. Oncol. Hematol.* **66,** 52–64.
Brunner, T., Mogil, R. J., LaFace, D., Yoo, N. J., Mahboubi, A., Echeverri, F., Martin, S. J., Force, W. R., Lynch, D. H., Ware, C. F., and Green, D. R. (1995). Cell-autonomous Fas (CD95)/Fas-ligand interaction mediates activation-induced apoptosis in T-cell hybridomas. *Nature* **373,** 441–444.
Chambon, P. (1994). The retinoid signaling pathway: Molecular and genetic analyses. *Semin. Cell Biol.* **5,** 115–125.
Chambon, P. (1996). A decade of molecular biology of retinoic acid receptors. *FASEB J.* **10,** 940–954.
Cui, H., Sherr, D. H., el-Khatib, M., Matsui, K., Panka, D. J., Marshak-Rothstein, A., and Ju, S. T. (1996). Regulation of T-cell death genes: Selective inhibition of FasL- but not Fas-mediated function. *Cell. Immunol.* **167,** 276–284.
Curotto de Lafaille, M. A., and Lafaille, J. J. (2009). Natural and adaptive foxp3+ regulatory T cells: More of the same or a division of labor? *Immunity* **30,** 626–635.
Dickman, E. D., Thaller, C., and Smith, S. M. (1997). Temporally-regulated retinoic acid depletion produces specific neural crest, ocular and nervous system defects. *Development* **124,** 3111–3121.
Engedal, N., and Blomhoff, H. K. (2003). Combined action of ERK and NF kappa B mediates the protective effect of phorbol ester on Fas-induced apoptosis in Jurkat cells. *J. Biol. Chem.* **278,** 10934–10941.
Engedal, N., Ertesvag, A., and Blomhoff, H. K. (2004). Survival of activated human T lymphocytes is promoted by retinoic acid via induction of IL-2. *Int. Immunol.* **16,** 443–453.
Engedal, N., Gjevik, T., Blomhoff, R., and Blomhoff, H. K. (2006). All-trans retinoic acid stimulates IL-2-mediated proliferation of human T lymphocytes: Early induction of cyclin D3. *J. Immunol.* **177,** 2851–2861.
Engedal, N., Auberger, P., and Blomhoff, H. K. (2009). Retinoic acid regulates Fas-induced apoptosis in Jurkat T cells: Reversal of mitogen-mediated repression of Fas DISC assembly. *J. Leukoc. Biol.* **85,** 469–480.
Ertesvag, A., Engedal, N., Naderi, S., and Blomhoff, H. K. (2002). Retinoic acid stimulates the cell cycle machinery in normal T cells: Involvement of retinoic acid receptor-mediated IL-2 secretion. *J. Immunol.* **169,** 5555–5563.
Fauci, A. S. (1993). Multifactorial nature of human immunodeficiency virus disease: Implications for therapy. *Science* **262,** 1011–1018.
Festjens, N., van Gurp, M., van Loo, G., Saelens, X., and Vandenabeele, P. (2004). Bcl-2 family members as sentinels of cellular integrity and role of mitochondrial intermembrane space proteins in apoptotic cell death. *Acta Haematol.* **111,** 7–27.
Fesus, L., Szondy, Z., and Uray, I. (1995). Probing the molecular program of apoptosis by cancer chemopreventive agents. *J. Cell. Biochem. Suppl.* **22,** 151–161.
Gomez-Angelats, M., and Cidlowski, J. A. (2001). Protein kinase C regulates FADD recruitment and death-inducing signaling complex formation in Fas/CD95-induced apoptosis. *J. Biol. Chem.* **276,** 44944–44952.
Gordy, C., Dzhagalov, I., and He, Y. W. (2009). Regulation of CD8(+) T cell functions by RARgamma. *Semin. Immunol.* **21,** 2–7.
Gougeon, M. L., Lecoeur, H., Dulioust, A., Enouf, M. G., Crouvoiser, M., Goujard, C., Debord, T., and Montagnier, L. (1996). Programmed cell death in peripheral lymphocytes from HIV-infected persons: Increased susceptibility to apoptosis of CD4 and CD8 T cells correlates with lymphocyte activation and with disease progression. *J. Immunol.* **156,** 3509–3520.
Green, H. N., and Mellanby, E. (1928). Vitamin A as an anti-infective agent. *Br. Med. J.* **2,** 691–696.

Green, D. R., Droin, N., and Pinkoski, M. (2003). Activation-induced cell death in T cells. *Immunol. Rev.* **193,** 70–81.

Gronemeyer, H., and Miturski, R. (2001). Molecular mechanisms of retinoid action. *Cell. Mol. Biol. Lett.* **6,** 3–52.

Hartmann, S., Brors, O., Bock, J., Blomhoff, R., Bausch, J., Wiegand, U. W., Hartmann, D., and Hornig, D. H. (2005). Exposure to retinyl esters, retinol, and retinoic acids in non-pregnant women following increasing single and repeated oral doses of vitamin A. *Ann. Nutr. Metab.* **49,** 155–164.

Harty, J. T., and Badovinac, V. P. (2002). Influence of effector molecules on the CD8(+) T cell response to infection. *Curr. Opin. Immunol.* **14,** 360–365.

Hayes, C. E., Nashold, F. E., Enrique Gomez, F., and Hoag, K. A. (1999). Retinoids and immunity. *In* "Retinoids: The Biochemical and Molecular Basis of Vitamin A and Retinoid Action," (H. Nau and W. S. Blaner, Eds.), Vol. 139, pp. 589–610. Springer-Verlag, Berlin.

Herold, M. J., McPherson, K. G., and Reichardt, H. M. (2006). Glucocorticoids in T cell apoptosis and function. *Cell. Mol. Life Sci.* **63,** 60–72.

Herron, L. R., Eisenberg, R. A., Roper, E., Kakkanaiah, V. N., Cohen, P. L., and Kotzin, B. L. (1993). Selection of the T cell receptor repertoire in Lpr mice. *J. Immunol.* **151,** 3450–3459.

Heyman, R. A., Mangelsdorf, D. J., Dyck, J. A., Stein, R. B., Eichele, G., Evans, R. M., and Thaller, C. (1992). 9-cis retinoic acid is a high affinity ligand for the retinoid X receptor. *Cell* **68,** 397–406.

Hildeman, D. A., Zhu, Y., Mitchell, T. C., Kappler, J., and Marrack, P. (2002). Molecular mechanisms of activated T cell death in vivo. *Curr. Opin. Immunol.* **14,** 354–359.

Holmstrom, T. H., Chow, S. C., Elo, I., Coffey, E. T., Orrenius, S., Sistonen, L., and Eriksson, J. E. (1998). Suppression of Fas/APO-1-mediated apoptosis by mitogen-activated kinase signaling. *J. Immunol.* **160,** 2626–2636.

Iwata, M., Mukai, M., Nakai, Y., and Iseki, R. (1992). Retinoic acids inhibit activation-induced apoptosis in T cell hybridomas and thymocytes. *J. Immunol.* **149,** 3302–3308.

Iwata, M., Hirakiyama, A., Eshima, Y., Kagechika, H., Kato, C., and Song, S. Y. (2004). Retinoic acid imprints gut-homing specificity on T cells. *Immunity* **21,** 527–538.

Ju, S. T., Panka, D. J., Cui, H., Ettinger, R., el-Khatib, M., Sherr, D. H., Stanger, B. Z., and Marshak-Rothstein, A. (1995). Fas(CD95)/FasL interactions required for programmed cell death after T-cell activation. *Nature* **373,** 444–448.

Juzan, M., Hostein, I., and Gualde, N. (1992). Role of thymus-eicosanoids in the immune response. *Prostaglandins Leukot. Essent. Fatty Acids* **46,** 247–255.

Kaech, S. M., Wherry, E. J., and Ahmed, R. (2002). Effector and memory T-cell differentiation: Implications for vaccine development. *Nat. Rev. Immunol.* **2,** 251–262.

Kang, H. J., Song, M. R., Lee, S. K., Shin, E. C., Choi, Y. H., Kim, S. J., Lee, J. W., and Lee, M. O. (2000). Retinoic acid and its receptors repress the expression and transactivation functions of Nur77: A possible mechanism for the inhibition of apoptosis by retinoic acid. *Exp. Cell Res.* **256,** 545–554.

Kastner, P., Mark, M., and Chambon, P. (1995). Nonsteroid nuclear receptors: What are genetic studies telling us about their role in real life? *Cell* **83,** 859–869.

Kastner, P., Messaddeq, N., Mark, M., Wendling, O., Grondona, J. M., Ward, S., Ghyselinck, N., and Chambon, P. (1997). Vitamin A deficiency and mutations of RXRalpha, RXRbeta and RARalpha lead to early differentiation of embryonic ventricular cardiomyocytes. *Development* **124,** 4749–4758.

Kishimoto, H., Surh, C. D., and Sprent, J. (1998). A role for Fas in negative selection of thymocytes in vivo. *J. Exp. Med.* **187,** 1427–1438.

Kiss, I., Ruhl, R., Szegezdi, E., Fritzsche, B., Toth, B., Pongracz, J., Perlmann, T., Fesus, L., and Szondy, Z. (2008). Retinoid receptor-activating ligands are produced within the mouse thymus during postnatal development. *Eur. J. Immunol.* **38,** 147–155.
Klas, C., Debatin, K. M., Jonker, R. R., and Krammer, P. H. (1993). Activation interferes with the APO-1 pathway in mature human T cells. *Int. Immunol.* **5,** 625–630.
Krammer, P. H., Arnold, R., and Lavrik, I. N. (2007). Life and death in peripheral T cells. *Nat. Rev. Immunol.* **7,** 532–542.
Lee, M. O., Kang, H. J., Kim, Y. M., Oum, J. H., and Park, J. (2002). Repression of FasL expression by retinoic acid involves a novel mechanism of inhibition of transactivation function of the nuclear factors of activated T-cells. *Eur. J. Biochem.* **269,** 1162–1170.
Lin, M., Zhang, M., Abraham, M., Smith, S. M., and Napoli, J. L. (2003). Mouse retinal dehydrogenase 4 (RALDH4), molecular cloning, cellular expression, and activity in 9-cis-retinoic acid biosynthesis in intact cells. *J. Biol. Chem.* **278,** 9856–9861.
Lin, B., Kolluri, S. K., Lin, F., Liu, W., Han, Y. H., Cao, X., Dawson, M. I., Reed, J. C., and Zhang, X. K. (2004). Conversion of Bcl-2 from protector to killer by interaction with nuclear orphan receptor Nur77/TR3. *Cell* **116,** 527–540.
Li-Weber, M., and Krammer, P. H. (2003). Function and regulation of the CD95 (APO-1/Fas) ligand in the immune system. *Semin. Immunol.* **15,** 145–157.
Lomo, J., Smeland, E. B., Ulven, S., Natarajan, V., Blomhoff, R., Gandhi, U., Dawson, M. I., and Blomhoff, H. K. (1998). RAR-, not RXR, ligands inhibit cell activation and prevent apoptosis in B-lymphocytes. *J. Cell. Physiol.* **175,** 68–77.
Mangelsdorf, D. J., and Evans, R. M. (1995). The RXR heterodimers and orphan receptors. *Cell* **83,** 841–850.
Manicassamy, S., and Pulendran, B. (2009). Retinoic acid-dependent regulation of immune responses by dendritic cells and macrophages. *Semin. Immunol.* **21,** 22–27.
Mark, M., Ghyselinck, N. B., Wendling, O., Dupe, V., Mascrez, B., Kastner, P., and Chambon, P. (1999). A genetic dissection of the retinoid signalling pathway in the mouse. *Proc. Nutr. Soc.* **58,** 609–613.
Marrack, P., and Kappler, J. (2004). Control of T cell viability. *Annu. Rev. Immunol.* **22,** 765–787.
Marrack, P., Bender, J., Hildeman, D., Jordan, M., Mitchell, T., Murakami, M., Sakamoto, A., Schaefer, B. C., Swanson, B., and Kappler, J. (2000). Homeostasis of alpha beta TCR+ T cells. *Nat. Immunol.* **1,** 107–111.
Mehta, S., and Fawzi, W. (2007). Effects of vitamins, including vitamin A, on HIV/AIDS patients. *Vitam. Horm.* **75,** 355–383.
Meng, X. W., Heldebrant, M. P., and Kaufmann, S. H. (2002). Phorbol 12-myristate 13-acetate inhibits death receptor-mediated apoptosis in Jurkat cells by disrupting recruitment of Fas-associated polypeptide with death domain. *J. Biol. Chem.* **277,** 3776–3783.
Mucida, D., Park, Y., and Cheroutre, H. (2009). From the diet to the nucleus: Vitamin A and TGF-beta join efforts at the mucosal interface of the intestine. *Semin. Immunol.* **21,** 14–21.
Nagata, S. (1998). Human autoimmune lymphoproliferative syndrome, a defect in the apoptosis-inducing Fas receptor: A lesson from the mouse model. *J. Hum. Genet.* **43,** 2–8.
Napoli, J. L. (1994). Retinoic acid homeostasis. *In* "Vitamin A in Health and Disease," (R. Blomhoff, Ed.), pp. 135–188. Marcel Dekker, Inc., New York.
Newton, K., Harris, A. W., Bath, M. L., Smith, K. G., and Strasser, A. (1998). A dominant interfering mutant of FADD/MORT1 enhances deletion of autoreactive thymocytes and inhibits proliferation of mature T lymphocytes. *EMBO J.* **17,** 706–718.
Nitta, T., Murata, S., Ueno, T., Tanaka, K., and Takahama, Y. (2008). Thymic micro-environments for T-cell repertoire formation. *Adv. Immunol.* **99,** 59–94.
Peter, M. E., Kischkel, F. C., Scheuerpflug, C. G., Medema, J. P., Debatin, K. M., and Krammer, P. H. (1997). Resistance of cultured peripheral T cells towards activation-

induced cell death involves a lack of recruitment of FLICE (MACH/caspase 8) to the CD95 death-inducing signaling complex. *Eur. J. Immunol.* **27,** 1207–1212.

Pfahl, M., and Piedrafita, F. J. (2003). Retinoid targets for apoptosis induction. *Oncogene* **22,** 9058–9062.

Pop, C., and Salvesen, G. S. (2009). Human caspases: Activation, specificity, and regulation. *J. Biol. Chem.* **284,** 21777–21781.

Rahman, M. M., Mahalanabis, D., Hossain, S., Wahed, M. A., Alvarez, J. O., Siber, G. R., Thompson, C., Santosham, M., and Fuchs, G. J. (1999). Simultaneous vitamin A administration at routine immunization contact enhances antibody response to diphtheria vaccine in infants younger than six months. *J. Nutr.* **129,** 2192–2195.

Rathmell, J. C., and Thompson, C. B. (2002). Pathways of apoptosis in lymphocyte development, homeostasis, and disease. *Cell* **109**(Suppl.), S97–S107.

Regazzi, M. B., Iacona, I., Gervasutti, C., Lazzarino, M., and Toma, S. (1997). Clinical pharmacokinetics of tretinoin. *Clin. Pharmacokinet.* **32,** 382–402.

Sacedón, R., Varas, A., Jiménez, E., Hernández-López, C., Muñoz, J. J., Vicente, A., and Zapata, A. G. (2008). Effects of glucocorticoids on the developing thymus. *In* "The Hypothalamus-Pituitary-Adrenal Axis," (A. del Rey, G. P. Chrousos, and H. O. Besedovsky, Eds.), pp. 169–187. Elsevier, Amsterdam.

Schneider, S. M., Offterdinger, M., Huber, H., and Grunt, T. W. (2000). Activation of retinoic acid receptor alpha is sufficient for full induction of retinoid responses in SK-BR-3 and T47D human breast cancer cells. *Cancer Res.* **60,** 5479–5487.

Semba, R. D. (1994). Vitamin A, immunity, and infection. *Clin. Infect. Dis.* **19,** 489–499.

Siggs, O. M., Makaroff, L. E., and Liston, A. (2006). The why and how of thymocyte negative selection. *Curr. Opin. Immunol.* **18,** 175–183.

Singer, G. G., and Abbas, A. K. (1994). The fas antigen is involved in peripheral but not thymic deletion of T lymphocytes in T cell receptor transgenic mice. *Immunity* **1,** 365–371.

Sprent, J., and Surh, C. D. (2001). Generation and maintenance of memory T cells. *Curr. Opin. Immunol.* **13,** 248–254.

Stephensen, C. B. (2001). Vitamin A, infection, and immune function. *Annu. Rev. Nutr.* **21,** 167–192.

Straus, S. E., Jaffe, E. S., Puck, J. M., Dale, J. K., Elkon, K. B., Rosen-Wolff, A., Peters, A. M., Sneller, M. C., Hallahan, C. W., Wang, J., Fischer, R. E., Jackson, C. M., *et al.* (2001). The development of lymphomas in families with autoimmune lymphoproliferative syndrome with germline Fas mutations and defective lymphocyte apoptosis. *Blood* **98,** 194–200.

Szegezdi, E., Kiss, I., Simon, A., Blasko, B., Reichert, U., Michel, S., Sandor, M., Fesus, L., and Szondy, Z. (2003). Ligation of retinoic acid receptor alpha regulates negative selection of thymocytes by inhibiting both DNA binding of nur77 and synthesis of bim. *J. Immunol.* **170,** 3577–3584.

Szondy, Z., Reichert, U., Bernardon, J. M., Michel, S., Toth, R., Ancian, P., Ajzner, E., and Fesus, L. (1997). Induction of apoptosis by retinoids and retinoic acid receptor gamma-selective compounds in mouse thymocytes through a novel apoptosis pathway. *Mol. Pharmacol.* **51,** 972–982.

Szondy, Z., Lecoeur, H., Fesus, L., and Gougeon, M. L. (1998a). All-trans retinoic acid inhibition of anti-CD3-induced T cell apoptosis in human immunodeficiency virus infection mostly concerns CD4 T lymphocytes and is mediated via regulation of CD95 ligand expression. *J. Infect. Dis.* **178,** 1288–1298.

Szondy, Z., Reichert, U., Bernardon, J. M., Michel, S., Toth, R., Karaszi, E., and Fesus, L. (1998b). Inhibition of activation-induced apoptosis of thymocytes by all-trans- and 9-cis-retinoic acid is mediated via retinoic acid receptor alpha. *Biochem. J.* **331**(Pt 3), 767–774.

Thompson, C. B. (1995). Apoptosis in the pathogenesis and treatment of disease. *Science* **267,** 1456–1462.
Toth, R., Szegezdi, E., Molnar, G., Lord, J. M., Fesus, L., and Szondy, Z. (1999). Regulation of cell surface expression of Fas (CD95) ligand and susceptibility to Fas (CD95)-mediated apoptosis in activation-induced T cell death involves calcineurin and protein kinase C, respectively. *Eur. J. Immunol.* **29,** 383–393.
Toth, R., Szegezdi, E., Reichert, U., Bernardon, J. M., Michel, S., Ancian, P., Kis-Toth, K., Macsari, Z., Fesus, L., and Szondy, Z. (2001). Activation-induced apoptosis and cell surface expression of Fas (CD95) ligand are reciprocally regulated by retinoic acid receptor alpha and gamma and involve nur77 in T cells. *Eur. J. Immunol.* **31,** 1382–1391.
Vella, A. T., Dow, S., Potter, T. A., Kappler, J., and Marrack, P. (1998). Cytokine-induced survival of activated T cells in vitro and in vivo. *Proc. Natl. Acad. Sci. USA* **95,** 3810–3815.
Villamor, E., and Fawzi, W. W. (2005). Effects of vitamin a supplementation on immune responses and correlation with clinical outcomes. *Clin. Microbiol. Rev.* **18,** 446–464.
Wei, L. N. (2003). Retinoid receptors and their coregulators. *Annu. Rev. Pharmacol. Toxicol.* **43,** 47–72.
Westendorp, M. O., Frank, R., Ochsenbauer, C., Stricker, K., Dhein, J., Walczak, H., Debatin, K. M., and Krammer, P. H. (1995). Sensitization of T cells to CD95-mediated apoptosis by HIV-1 Tat and gp120. *Nature* **375,** 497–500.
Wilson, D. J., Alessandrini, A., and Budd, R. C. (1999). MEK1 activation rescues Jurkat T cells from Fas-induced apoptosis. *Cell. Immunol.* **194,** 67–77.
Wolf, G. (2006). Is 9-cis-retinoic acid the endogenous ligand for the retinoic acid-X receptor? *Nutr. Rev.* **64,** 532–538.
Yang, Y., Vacchio, M. S., and Ashwell, J. D. (1993). 9-cis-Retinoic acid inhibits activation-driven T-cell apoptosis: Implications for retinoid X receptor involvement in thymocyte development. *Proc. Natl. Acad. Sci. USA* **90,** 6170–6174.
Yang, Y., Bailey, J., Vacchio, M. S., Yarchoan, R., and Ashwell, J. D. (1995a). Retinoic acid inhibition of ex vivo human immunodeficiency virus-associated apoptosis of peripheral blood cells. *Proc. Natl. Acad. Sci. USA* **92,** 3051–3055.
Yang, Y., Mercep, M., Ware, C. F., and Ashwell, J. D. (1995b). Fas and activation-induced Fas ligand mediate apoptosis of T cell hybridomas: Inhibition of Fas ligand expression by retinoic acid and glucocorticoids. *J. Exp. Med.* **181,** 1673–1682.
Yang, Y., Minucci, S., Ozato, K., Heyman, R. A., and Ashwell, J. D. (1995c). Efficient inhibition of activation-induced Fas ligand up-regulation and T cell apoptosis by retinoids requires occupancy of both retinoid X receptors and retinoic acid receptors. *J. Biol. Chem.* **270,** 18672–18677.
Zhang, Y., Finegold, M. J., Porteu, F., Kanteti, P., and Wu, M. X. (2003). Development of T-cell lymphomas in Emu-IEX-1 mice. *Oncogene* **22,** 6845–6851.
Zheng, L., Fisher, G., Miller, R. E., Peschon, J., Lynch, D. H., and Lenardo, M. J. (1995). Induction of apoptosis in mature T cells by tumour necrosis factor. *Nature* **377,** 348–351.
Ziegler, A., Muller, C. A., Bockmann, R. A., and Uchanska-Ziegler, B. (2009). Low-affinity peptides and T-cell selection. *Trends Immunol.* **30,** 53–60.

CHAPTER EIGHT

Vitamin E and Immunity

Didem Pekmezci

Contents

Abstract

Vitamin E is the most important chain-breaking, lipid-soluble antioxidant present in body tissues of all cells and is considered the first line of defense against lipid peroxidation and it is important for normal function of the immune cells. However, vitamin E deficiency is rare in well-nourished healthy subjects and is not a problem, even among people living on relatively poor diets, both T- and B-cell functions are impaired by vitamin E deficiency. While immune cells are particularly enriched in vitamin E because of their high polyunsaturated fatty acid content, this point puts them at especially high risk for oxidative damage. Besides its immunomodulatory effects, vitamin E also plays an important role in carcinogenesis with its antioxidant properties against cancer, and ischemic heart disease with limiting the progression of atherosclerosis. Supplementation of vitamin E significantly enhances both cell mediated and humoral immune functions in humans, especially in the elderly and animals. © 2011 Elsevier Inc.

Department of Internal Medicine, Faculty of Veterinary Medicine, University of Ondokuz Mayıs, Kurupelit, Samsun, Turkey

Vitamins and Hormones, Volume 86
ISSN 0083-6729, DOI: 10.1016/B978-0-12-386960-9.00008-3

I. Introduction

Research interest in vitamin E began following the discovery of this vitamin by Herbert Evans after the appearance of an unrecognized substance necessary for reproduction that was published in a paper that appeared in 1922 in *Science* (McDowell, 2000). Vitamin E was isolated as α-tocopherol. The name tocopherol is derived from the Greek *tokos* meaning childbirth or offspring, the Greek *pherein* meaning to bring forth, and *ol* to designate an alcohol. Recent research, however, has shown that vitamin E is actually a family of molecules, consisting of the tocopherols and the tocotrienols, all of which are important for defending the body against free radical attack or oxidative stress (Kosowski and Clouatre, 2008). Of the many such dietary components, vitamin E has commanded most interest because of its availability, strong marketing potential, overall health impact, and central role in preventing oxidation at the cellular level (Eitenmiller and Lee, 2004). From the discovery of vitamin E to date, numerous studies have been done, and finally nowadays, science can clearly tell us that this vitamin, with various beneficial effects, is very important for both human and animal beings. The immune system is the most important part of a living organism. Without an enhanced immune system, any living organism could challenge with diseases. In more recent years, vitamin E has been shown to be important against free-radical injury; enhancing the immune response; and playing a role in prevention of cancer, heart disease, cataracts, Parkinson's disease, and a number of other disease conditions (McDowell, 2000). Further, with its potent immunomodulatory effects, this chapter revives deficiency and supplementation of vitamin E on the immune responses in animals and humans and the immunostimulating properties with aging.

II. Definition and Structures of Vitamin E

Vitamin E is a generic description for all tocopherols (α-TOH, β-TOH, γ-TOH, δ-TOH) and tocotrienols (α-T3H, β-T3H, γ-T3H, δ-T3H) that exhibit the biological activity of α-tocopherol (Morrissey and Sheehy, 1999; Neuzil *et al.*, 2004) and refers to a family of related compounds that have hydroxylated aromatic rings (chromanol rings) and isoprenoid side chains (Machlin, 1991). The number of methyl groups and the pattern of methylation of the chromanol ring primarily distinguish the tocopherols and tocotrienols. α-tocopherol and tocotrienol have three methyl groups; β- and γ-tocopherol and tocotrienol have two methyl groups, whereas δ-tocopherol and tocotrienol have one methyl group (Kaempf-Rotzoll *et al.*, 2003). There are eight naturally occurring forms of vitamin E: α-, β-, γ-, and δ-tocopherols and α-, β-, γ-, and δ-tocotrienols. Chemically synthesized α-tocopherol contains eight stereoisomers and is designated all-rac-α-tocopherol (historically and incorrectly called DL-α-tocopherol), while naturally occurring stereoisomer of α-tocopherol is *R,R, R*-α-tocopherol (formerly called D-α-tocopherol) (Traber, 1999). Among the naturally occurring tocopherols, α-tocopherol (*R,R,R*-α-tocopherol) is the most abundant, with the highest biological activity (Machlin, 1991), as compared to the other isomers (β-,γ-,δ-). The *R,R,R*-α-tocopherol is found in the highest concentration in human plasma and accounting for ~90–100% of the vitamin E found in tissue (Budowski and Sklan, 1989), whereas γ-tocopherol is present in at least equally high concentrations in the diet (Parker, 1989; Traber *et al.*, 1993). α-tocopherol is specifically retained in the body by the liver α-tocopherol transfer protein (α-TTP), which has been identified, isolated, and characterized from rat and human liver cytosol (Arita *et al.*, 1995; Catignani and Bieri, 1977; Kuhlenkamp *et al.*, 1993; Sato *et al.*, 1991; Yoshida *et al.*, 1992) reaching an average plasma concentration of 23 μM. The plasma concentration of the other tocopherols and tocotrienols is usually below 2 μM because they are not efficiently retained by the liver, metabolized, and predominantly eliminated (Arita *et al.*, 1995). Therefore, most of the studies with vitamin E have been done with α-tocopherol, and stabilized forms of vitamin E are mainly derived from α-tocopherol (Zingg, 2007). The mechanism by which α-TTP facilitates the transfer of α-tocopherol to the plasma membrane for incorporation into very low-density lipoprotein (VLDL), and/or high-density lipoprotein (HDL), has yet to be elucidated (Mustacich *et al.*, 2007). The biological activities of the β-, γ-, and δ-isoforms of vitamin E are 0.5, 0.25, and 0.01, respectively, compared to α-tocopherol (Steger and Muhlebach, 1998). After 1980, the IU was changed to the USP unit where one USP unit of vitamin E was still defined as having the activity of 1 mg of *all-rac-α-tocopheryl* acetate, 0.67 mg *R,R,R*-α-tocopherol, or 0.74 mg *R,R,R*-α-tocopheryl acetate (USP, 1980).

III. Vitamin E Deficiency

Vitamin E deficiency was first described by Evans and Bishop in 1922 in experimental animals, when it was discovered to be essential for fertility. While vitamin E deficiency is rare in well-nourished healthy subjects (Wu *et al.*, 2006), it is not a problem even among people living on relatively poor diets (Bender, 2003). It was not until 1983 that vitamin E was demonstrated to be a dietary essential for human beings, when Muller *et al.* (1983) described the devastating neurological damage from lack of vitamin E in patients with hereditary abetalipoproteinemia. Indeed, vitamin E deficiency could be classified in two classes in human beings. One of them is physiologically occurs and includes: the pregnancy and neonatal periods, and the second one is generally can be caused by genetic defects. Vitamin E is extremely important during the early stages of life, from the time of conception to the postnatal development of the infant (Debier, 2007). Several key stages such as fertilization, development of early embryos (blastocyst stage), implantation, and placental maturation have been identified for vitamin E needs (Ashworth and Antipatis, 2001; Jishage *et al.*, 2001, 2005; Kaempf-Rotzoll *et al.*, 2002; Wang *et al.*, 2002). Vitamin E is also an essential molecule to protect the fetus from an irreparable oxidative stress (Jishage *et al.*, 2001; Kaempf-Rotzoll *et al.*, 2002). Finally, at birth, an adequate supply of vitamin E to the newborn is of utmost importance to protect the organism against oxygen toxicity and to stimulate the development of its immune system (Babinszky *et al.*, 1991; Ostrea *et al.*, 1986), and obviously seen that newborn or premature infants seem particularly susceptible to vitamin E deficiency, while a wide variety of disorders benefit from supplementation (Oski, 1980; Scott, 1980). However, Vitamin E deficiency in human beings is almost always due to factors other than dietary insufficiency (Eitenmiller and Lee, 2004). Deficiency results from genetic abnormalities in production of the α-TTP, fat malabsorption syndromes, and protein-energy malnutrition (Food and Nutrition Board, and Institute of Medicine, 2000). Patients with congenital abetalipoproteinemia, who are unable to synthesize VLDL, were the first condition reported that confirmed the essentiality of vitamin E in human beings (Muller *et al.*, 1983). Genetic abnormalities in lipoprotein metabolism can produce low levels of chylomicrons, VLDLs, and low-density lipoprotein (LDL) that affect absorption and transport of vitamin E (Rader and Brewer, 1993). Abetalipoproteinemia is an autosomal recessive genetic disorder that leads to mutations in the microsomal triglyceride transfer protein (Gordon, 2001; Rader and Brewer, 1993; Wetterau *et al.*, 1991). The microsomal triglyceride transfer protein is completely absent from the intestines of abetalipoproteinemia patients (Wetterau *et al.*, 1992). Patients that have undetectably low plasma levels of α-tocopherol develop devastating ataxic neuropathy and pigmentary retinopathy (Bender, 2003). Friedreich's ataxia is an autosomal recessive disease characterized by cerebellar ataxia, dysarthria, sensory loss in the lower limbs, and other neurological symptoms (Ben Hamida *et al.*, 1993; Stumpf *et al.*, 1987). Early studies on Friedreich's ataxia identified a variant form characterized by normal fat absorption and very low levels of plasma vitamin E. Neurological symptoms were considered to be due to vitamin E deficiency (Ben Hamida *et al.*, 1993; Stumpf *et al.*, 1987). Humans with a defective α-TTP gene have also severe vitamin E deficiency (Cavalier *et al.*, 1998; Ouahchi *et al.*, 1995) with extremely low plasma, nerve, and adipose tissue α-tocopherol concentrations (Traber *et al.*, 1987). Patients who lack the hepatic tocopherol transfer protein and suffer from what has been called ataxia with vitamin E deficiency (AVED) are unable to export α-tocopherol from the liver in VLDL (Bender, 2003; Ouahchi *et al.*, 1995), and display autosomal recessive inheritance of progressive neurodegenerative symptoms (e.g., ataxia, dysarthria, loss of deep tendon reflexes), coupled with low plasma vitamin E levels ($\leq 3\ \mu M$) (Manor and Morley, 2007). Plasma and tissue levels of other lipids (e.g., cholesterol, triglycerides) are typically unaffected (Manor and Morley, 2007). When deficiency does occur, the cause is usually malabsorption as a result of fat malabsorption or genetic abnormalities in lipoprotein metabolism (Meydani and Beharka, 1998). Therefore, few studies have directly examined the effect of vitamin E deficiency on immunologic parameters in adult humans. Deficiencies in vitamin E have also been reported in Human Immunodeficiency Virus (HIV)-infected individuals (Meydani and Beharka, 1998). Plasma vitamin E levels were detected significantly lower in a study of 200 HIV-positive individuals compared with controls (Passi *et al.*, 1993), and these deficiencies were not appear to be due to inadequate intake of vitamin. Favier *et al.* (1994) observed that patients, who had already developed Acquired Immune Deficiency Syndrome (AIDS), had an inverse relationship between serum vitamin E levels and severity of disease. Vitamin E deficiency, in turn, exacerbates the immune dysfunctions caused by HIV infection, leaving individuals more susceptible to opportunistic infections (Tang and Smit, 1998). Vitamin E deficiency in experimental animals results in a number of different conditions, with considerable differences between different species in their susceptibility to different signs of deficiency (Bender, 2003). Results from animal and human studies indicate that vitamin E deficiency impairs both humoral and cellular immunity (Gebremichael *et al.*, 1984; Kowdley *et al.*, 1992). In addition, Bendich (1988) has also reported that both T- and B-cell functions were impaired by vitamin E deficiency. Vitamin E deficiency and the immune response in several studies are presented in Table 8.1.

IV. Vitamin E Requirements and Reference Ranges

Vitamin E has an estimated average requirement (EAR), recommended dietary allowances (RDAs), and tolerable upper intake level (UL) (Murphy and Barr, 2007). The EAR was based on the amount of 2R-α-tocopherol intake that reversed erythrocyte hemolysis in men who were vitamin E-deficient as a result of consuming a vitamin E-deficient diet for 5 years (Food and Nutrition Board, and Institute of Medicine, 2000). RDAs are designed so that, if met at a population level, almost all individuals would meet their requirements and avoid clinical deficiency symptoms (Morrissey and Sheehy, 1999). The UL is the highest level of daily nutrient intake that

Table 8.1 Vitamin E deficiency and the immune response

Research species	Immune response	References
Mice	↓Plaque-forming cells (PFC), ↓hemagglutination (HA) titer	Tengerdy *et al.* (1973)
Pigs	↓Lymphocyte proliferation (Con A, PHA)	Teige *et al.* (1978)
Dogs	↓Lymphocyte proliferation (Con A, PHA, PWM)	Sheffy and Schultz (1979)
Mice	↓Lymphocyte proliferation (Con A, PHA, LPS)	Corwin and Shloss (1980)
Rats	↓ Chemotactic and phagocytic stimuli of PMN	Harris *et al.* (1980)
Dogs	↓Lymphocyte proliferation (Con A, PHA, PWM)	Langweiler *et al.* (1981)
Calves	↔Total IgG_1, IgG_2, IgM	Cipriano *et al.* (1982)
Mice	↓Lymphocyte proliferation (Con A, PHA)	Corwin and Gordon (1982)
Rats	↓M histocompatibility	Gebremichael *et al.* (1984)
Mice	↓T-cell activity	Sharp and Colston (1984)
Rats	↓Lymphocyte proliferation	Eskew *et al.* (1986)
Pigs	↓Lymphocyte proliferation (Con A, PHA)	Jensen *et al.* (1988)
Rats	↓Cellular immunity	Moriguchi *et al.* (1989)
Lambs	↓Lymphocyte proliferation	Turner and Finch (1990)
Human	↓Lymphocyte proliferation (Con A, PHA), ↓DTH, ↓IL-2	Kowdley *et al.* (1992)
Sow	↓Peripheral blood lymphocytes, ↓Polymorphonuclear cell (PMN)	Wuryastuti *et al.* (1993)
Chickens	↓Lymphocyte proliferation (Con A, PHA)	Chang *et al.* (1994)

Concanavalin A (Con A), Phytohaemagglutinin (PHA), Pokeweed mitogen (PWM), Lipopolysaccharides (LPS), Polymorph nuclear neutrophils (PMN), Delayed-type hypersensitivity (DTH).

is likely to pose no risks of adverse health effects to most individuals in the general population (Yates *et al.*, 1998). The functional criterion for the requirement of vitamin E for most age groups is the prevention of hydrogen peroxide (H_2O_2)-induced hemolysis of red blood cells (Murphy and Barr, 2007). Based on the plasma concentration of α-tocopherol to prevent significant hemolysis *in vitro* (14–16 μmol per L), the US/Canadian EAR is 12 mg/day; RDA for vitamin E is currently set at 15 mg/day of α-tocopherol for adults (ages above 19) (Food and Nutrition Board, and Institute of Medicine, 2000), a 50% increase on the previous RDA (National Research Council, 1989). The EAR of vitamin E in 1–3, 4–8, and 9–13 years aged children are 5, 6, 9 mg α-tocopherol per day, respectively (Eitenmiller and Lee, 2004). On the other hand, RDA levels of 1–3, 4–8, and 9–13 years aged children are 6, 7, 11 mg α-tocopherol per day, respectively (Eitenmiller and Lee, 2004). The tolerable UL was set at 1000 mg/day for vitamin E (any form of supplemental α-tocopherol) (Traber, 2007). This was one of the few UL that was set using data in rats, because sufficient and appropriate quantitative data assessing long-term adverse effects of vitamin E supplements in humans was not available (Traber, 2007). Although vitamin E seems to have very low toxicity and habitual intake of supplements of 200–600 mg/day (compared with an average dietary intake of 8–12 mg seems to be without untoward effect; Shrimpton, 1997), very high intakes may antagonize vitamin K and hence potentiate anticoagulant therapy. This is probably the result of inhibition of the vitamin K quinone reductase, but α-tocopheryl quinone may compete with vitamin K hydroquinone and hence inhibit carboxylation of glutamate in target proteins (Bender, 2003). Animal studies show that vitamin E is not mutagenic, carcinogenic, or teratogenic (Abdo *et al.*, 1986; Dysmsza and Park, 1975; Krasavage and Terhaar, 1977). Adults tolerate relatively high doses without significant toxicity; however, muscle weakness, fatigue, double vision, emotional disturbance, breast soreness, thrombophlebitis, nausea, diarrhea, and flatulence have been reported at tocopherol intakes at 1600–3000 mg/day (Anderson and Reid, 1974; Bendich and Machlin, 1998; Food and Nutrition Board, and Institute of Medicine, 2000; Machlin, 1989; Tsai *et al.*, 1978). The vitamin E requirement for ideal immune function depends on its interactions with other antioxidant and pro-oxidant nutrients, especially with polyunsaturated fatty acids (PUFAs), and on other factors that modulate the immune response, such as age and stress, exercise, infection, and tissue trauma all increase vitamin E requirements (Eskew *et al.*, 1986; Meydani and Tengerdy, 1992; Nockels, 1991). Early reports suggested that vitamin E requirements increase with the intake of PUFAs (Bender, 2003), oxidizing agents, vitamin A, carotenoids, gossypol, or trace minerals and decreased with increasing levels of fat-soluble antioxidants, sulfur amino acids, or Se (Dove and Ewan, 1990; Franklin *et al.*, 1998; Hidiroglou *et al.*, 1992; McDowell *et al.*, 1996). Neither the United

Kingdom (Department of Health, 1991) nor the European Union (Scientific Committee for Food, 1993) set reference intakes for vitamin E, but both suggested that an acceptable intake was 0.4 mg of α-tocopherol equivalent per gram of dietary PUFA (Bender, 2003). Morrissey and Sheehy (1999) report that a consensus about the exact daily intake of vitamin E for optimal health protection has not yet been reached. Some authors believe that the scientific evidence is strong enough already, especially for cardiovascular disease (CVD), to recommend daily intakes of the order of 87–100 mg α-tocopherol per day or more (Horwitt, 1991; Packer, 1992; Weber *et al.*, 1997). Gey (1995) has shown that there is an inverse relationship between plasma α-tocopherol and risk of ischemic heart disease over a range of 2.5–4.0 mmol per mol of cholesterol, and has suggested an optimum or desirable plasma concentration >4 mmol of α-tocopherol per mol of cholesterol (>3.4 μmol per gram of total plasma lipid), which corresponds an intake of 17–40 mg of α-tocopherol equivalents per day. Like the elderly, certain groups of population are at greater risk for inadequate dietary intake of vitamin E (Panemangalore and Lee, 1992; Ryan *et al.*, 1992). Ryan *et al.* (1992) reported that over 40% of elderly (65–98 years) had intakes of vitamin E that were below two-thirds the 1989 RDA. In another study done by Panemangalore and Lee (1992), 37% of elderly subjects (average age of 73 years old) consumed below two-thirds RDA and 12% had low lipid adjusted plasma tocopherol status. In several studies, data have shown that elderly humans, as well as laboratory and farm animals, consuming diets that contain more than five times the RDA of vitamin E for their species had significantly increased humoral and cell-mediated immune responses and increased resistance to infectious diseases compared to nonsupplemented controls (Bendich, 1990; Bendich *et al.*, 1986; Meydani and Blumberg, 1991; Meydani *et al.*, 1993; Moriguchi *et al.*, 1990; Tengerdy, 1989; Tengerdy *et al.*, 1990). The minimum vitamin E requirement of normal animals is ~30 ppm of diet as in humans (McDowell, 2000). Beharka *et al.* (1997a) suggested that conventional methods for determining the RDA, while adequate for arriving at the level of vitamin E required to prevent clinical deficiency symptoms, may not adequately predict the optimal level of vitamin E needed to maintain immunological health.

V. Immunomodulatory Effects of Vitamin E

A. Antioxidant functions of vitamin E

Among the factors that can cause damage during an organism's life-span are the free-radical species (FRS; Serafini, 2000). Free radicals, because of their high potential to damage biological systems, have been proposed as contributing factors to aging (Harman, 1956; Miquel *et al.*, 1980; Sastre *et al.*, 2000). According to the free-radical theory of aging proposed by Harman about 40 years ago (Harman, 1956, 1991), FRS produced during aerobic metabolism in the lifetime cause oxidative stress (Halliwell and Gutteridge, 1989), with a subsequent cumulative cell damage leading to aging and cell death (Serafini, 2000). The immune cell functions are specially linked to reactive oxygen species (ROS) generation, such as that involved in the microbicidal activity of phagocytes, cytotoxic activity, or the lymphoproliferative response to mitogens (Goldstone and Hunt, 1997). However, since the ROS have a pivotal role in the regulation of many cellular processes (Brigelius-Flohé, 2006), an adequate oxidant–antioxidant balance is very important for maintaining cell functions (De la Fuente *et al.*, 2008). The damaging effects of ROS on cellular biomolecules such as proteins, lipids, and nucleic acids are well documented and the consequences of such damage have been implicated in the etiology of a number of human disorders (Brennan *et al.*, 2000). Therefore, it is not surprising that immune cells usually contain higher concentrations of antioxidant compounds than other cells (Coquette *et al.*, 1986). However, their excessive presence have detrimental effects to the organism; ROS have been identified as important intracellular transcription-inducers for a number of early response genes, for example, nuclear transcription factors (NF-κB) (Meyer *et al.*, 1993). FRS is also necessary for certain aspects of cellular response, such as activation of the NF-κB or AP-1 (Pahl and Bauerle, 1994; Schreck *et al.*, 1992b) and they have been known to mediate signaling within T-cells (Schreck *et al.*, 1992a). The history of the relationship between antioxidants and immunology began in the early years of the twentieth century with an appreciation that antioxidant nutrient deficiencies may cause disease (Bendich, 1992) and that antioxidants have an immunostimulating action (Del Rio *et al.*, 1998). Meydani (2000) reports that a potential shift in the oxidant:antioxidant balance because of increased production of free radicals may contribute to the decline of cardiovascular, neuronal, muscular, visual, and immune functions over time. This balance is critical in the cells of the immune system, since these cells synthesize ROS as key agents for their functions (Knight, 2000) and because of the high content of PUFAs in the immune system cell plasma membranes (Meydani *et al.*, 1995), these cells are particularly enriched in vitamin E and sensitive to oxidative stress. Enzymes such as superoxide dismutase (SOD), glutathione peroxidase (GSH-P), catalase (CAT), and nonenzymes such as ceruloplasmin, uric acid, α-tocopherol, ascorbic acid, and stress proteins are the essential defense systems for protecting the potentially damaging effects of ROS (Brennan *et al.*, 2000). *N*-acetylcysteine (NAC) and vitamin E are potent antioxidants, the levels of which decrease during oxidative stress (Porter *et al.*, 1999). Both antioxidants inhibit the activation of the NF-κB produced by oxidative stress (Bellezo *et al.*, 1998), which could result in a decrease of free radicals and proinflammatory cytokine production (Sprong *et al.*, 1998; Víctor *et al.*, 1999). Sies and Murphy (1981) reported that vitamin E is the most important chain-breaking, lipid-soluble antioxidant present in body tissues of all cells and is considered the first line of defense against lipid peroxidation. While immune cells are particularly enriched in vitamin E because of their high PUFA content, this point puts them at especially high risk for oxidative damage (Coquette *et al.*, 1986; Hatam and Kayden, 1979). Vitamin E scavenges the FRS by inhibiting the initiation and chain propagation of lipid peroxidation (Halliwell and Gutteridge, 1989), and contributing to membrane stability (Liebler, 1993), vitamin E also regulates fluidity and protects cellular structures against oxidative stress damage (Halliwell and Gutteridge, 1989). Schraufstätter *et al.* (1988) have shown that, of the spectrum of ROS generated by leucocytes at the site of immune and/or inflammatory responses, the major extracellular species causing DNA damage is H_2O_2. In the intracellular environ, it is clear that it is the hydroxyl radical (OH), a breakdown product of H_2O_2, which directly attacks the DNA of those cells exposed to H_2O_2 (Meneghini and Martins, 1993). Vitamin E prevents lipid peroxidation by breaking the chain of events leading to the formation of these hydroperoxides and inhibits the conversion of nitrites to nitrosamines (Herrera and Barbas, 2001; Niki and Noguchi, 2004). This action should also lead to a reduction in Deoxyribonucleic acid (DNA) damage since the intermediate products of lipid peroxidation include lipid peroxides, which can cause strand breaks in DNA (Cheeseman, 1993). Antioxidant roles for vitamin E are numerous (Kosowski and Clouatre, 2008). Besides its immunomodulatory effects, vitamin E also plays an important role in carcinogenesis with its antioxidant properties against cancer (Pryor, 1986, 1987, 2000), and ischemic heart disease with limiting the progression of atherosclerosis, by stabilizing plaque and preventing its rupture and subsequent clot formation (Diaz *et al.*, 1997) which will be discussed later.

B. Immunologic mechanisms of vitamin E

The immune system fights bacteria, viruses, fungi, protozoans, and reacts against cancer cells and foreign substances or matter such as organ transplants (Wintergerst *et al.*, 2007). The association of poor host nutritional status with increased susceptibility to infectious disease has long been thought to be related to the host immune response (Beck, 2001). Similarly to the nutritional deficiencies, the age-related alterations are referred to as immunosenescence (Globerson and Effros, 2000; Gruver *et al.*, 2007; Linton and Dorshkind, 2004), and has been implicated in the etiology of many of the chronic degenerative diseases of the elderly, including arthritis, cancer, autoimmune diseases, and increased susceptibility to infectious diseases (James *et al.*, 1995). Recent studies also suggest that the status of the immune response could predict mortality in the elderly (Roberts-Thomson *et al.*, 1974; Wayne *et al.*, 1990) and animals (Nagel *et al.*,

1988). Further, studies which have been done by Wu and Meydani (2008) show that understanding of the cellular origins and the molecular mechanisms of age-related inflammation could advance our ability to develop strategies in improving quality of health in the elderly and they advocated that several approaches have been used to change the trajectory of immunosenescence, including lifestyle (diet, exercise) and medical therapy (drugs, hormones/cytokines, cell transfer). Specific nutritional deficiencies (Moriguchi and Muraga, 2000) and age-related immune dysfunction include impaired antibody responses, decreased macrophage activity, and T cell dysfunction. Effect of vitamin E on an age-associated decline in T cell functions' nutritional intervention is a practical approach for modulating immune function (Wu and Meydani, 2008). Vitamin E is considered one of the most effective nutrients for its effect on immune cell functions (Wu and Meydani, 2008). Innate immunity consists of epithelial barriers, a cellular component (macrophages (MF), polymorphonuclear leukocytes, natural killer (NK) cells, and dendritic cells (DCs)) and a noncellular component with recognition molecules (C-reactive protein, serum amyloid protein, mannose-binding protein, complement; Wintergerst *et al.*, 2007). Specific immunity is divided into cell-mediated and antibody-mediated immunity (Wintergerst *et al.*, 2007). The majority of the cells of specific immunity are T lymphocytes that can be identified as helper or suppressor based on their cell surface receptors (Janeway and Travers, 1997) (T-cells originating from bone marrow and maturing in the thymus) and B lymphocytes (B-cells originating and maturing in the bone marrow) (Wintergerst *et al.*, 2007). There are also mast cells, which play an important role in the immune system by interacting directly with B- and T-cells and by releasing several mediators (cytokines, chemokines, growth factors, histamine, and proteases) involved in the activation of other cells (Mecheri and David, 1999; Patella *et al.*, 2000; Schneider *et al.*, 2002). The higher presence of mast cells in tissues that are portals of infections and their ability to phagocytose and to present antigens indicates that they mediate also the host response in innate immunity (Féger *et al.*, 2002; Henz *et al.*, 2001). Hyperreactivity of mast cells and their uncontrolled accumulation in tissues lead to increased release of inflammatory mediators contributing to the pathogenesis of several diseases (Zingg, 2007). In the T cell-mediated immune function, cell co-operation between T-cells and MF is essential (Unanue, 1980). The lymphocyte response to antigens requires the presence of the "professional antigen presenting cells": DCs, MF, and B-cells, specialized to process and deliver activating signals to T-cells (Serafini, 2000). Immature T lymphocytes (CD2+, CD3−), NK cells, and memory T lymphocytes increase during aging (Lesourd and Meaume, 1994; Lesourd *et al.*, 1994; Ligthardt *et al.*, 1986), whereas the number of "naïve" T lymphocytes (Lesourd and Meaume, 1994) decreases during aging. MF as activated phagocytic cells increase production of inflammatory mediators such as proinflammatory cytokines (interleukin (IL)-1, 6, and 12), tumor necrosis factor-α (TNF-α), prostaglandins, leukotrienes (Wintergerst *et al.*, 2007) and release up to 50% of their arachidonic acid (AA) content in the form of oxygenated metabolites (Bonney *et al.*, 1985; Humes *et al.*, 1977). AA is present in membrane phospholipids and released by the hydrolytic action of phospholipase A_2 (Meydani *et al.*, 2005). Prostaglandin E_2 (PGE_2), an AA metabolite among the T-cell suppressive factors produced by MF, is the most prominent and thus most intensively studied (Meydani *et al.*, 2005). PGE_2 has been implicated in age-related changes of cellular immunity as a feedback inhibiting factor of T-cell proliferation in humans (Goodwin and Webb, 1981). T-cells from the elderly are more sensitive to inhibition by PGE_2 than the young (Goodwin, 1982; Goodwin and Messner, 1979). Excessive production of PGE_2 by MF extracted from old mice has been shown to suppress T-cell proliferation, and IL-2 production (Beharka *et al.*, 1997b), which is produced by activated T-cells, is needed for the proliferation of T-cells (Tak Cheung *et al.*, 1983). Like other eicosanoids, biosynthesis of PGE_2 is accomplished in a metabolic cascade starting from its precursor fatty acid (Meydani *et al.*, 2005). Released AA is metabolized to unstable intermediate prostanoids by cyclooxygenase (COX), also called PGH_2 synthase (Meydani *et al.*, 2005). COX has bifunctional catalytic properties that it oxygenates and cyclizes AA to form PGG_2 via its COX function, and this is followed by the reduction of PGG_2 to PGH_2 via its peroxidase function (Meydani *et al.*, 2005). PGH_2 is then converted to PGE_2 by the terminal synthase (Meydani *et al.*, 2005). Meydani *et al.* (2005) investigated the underlying mechanism(s) for age-associated upregulation in PGE_2 synthesis. It is obviously understood from the studies that MF and spleen cells from old mice and peripheral blood mononuclear cells from elderly human subjects synthesize significantly more PGE_2 than their young counterparts (Bartocci *et al.*, 1982; Hayek *et al.*, 1994). Moreover, Serafini (2000) suggested that PGE_2 could have a role in the age-associated decline of T cell-mediated immunity by affecting IL-2 production as well as T-cell proliferation, which is also reported by Rappaport and Dodge (1982) previously. Vitamin E also reduces IL-4 secretion in human peripheral blood T-cells in a dose-dependent manner (Li-Weber *et al.*, 2002). As IL-4 promotes the production of immunoglobulin E (IgE) antibodies by B-cells, it is one of the key cytokines in the development of allergic inflammation (Sausenthaler *et al.*, 2009). In turn, PGE_2 has been implicated in shifting the balance of Th1/Th2 cells and their cytokines towards a Th2 profile (Roper *et al.*, 1995). Indeed, Sausenthaler *et al.* (2009) suggests that vitamin E might be protective against the development of allergic sensitization. As mentioned above, the immunostimulatory effect of vitamin E in both old mice and humans was associated with a reduction in PGE_2 production (Meydani *et al.*, 1986, 1990). Vitamin E has a direct effect on T-cell functions independent of its effect on MF and PGE_2 production (Beharka *et al.*, 1997b). Moreover, vitamin E could act through an effect on these mediators (IL-2 and PGE_2) of immune function by decreasing the MF production (Serafini, 2000). These data indicate that naïve T-cells exhibit the greatest age-related defect and show that supplemental vitamin E has a direct immunoenhancing effect on naïve T-cells from old mice (Meydani *et al.*, 2005). The differential effect of vitamin E on naïve and memory T-cells may be due to an underlying difference in the susceptibility of these cells to oxidative stress-induced damage (Lohmiller *et al.*, 1996). Clearly, these results indicate that vitamin E improves T-cell function in aged by two mechanisms: (i) by directly improving the cell dividing and IL-2 producing capacity of naïve T-cells and (ii) by indirectly reducing the production of T-cell suppressive factor PGE_2 from MF (Han *et al.*, 2004; Meydani *et al.*, 2005). The mechanisms through which vitamin E improves cell-cycle division and IL-2 production are currently under investigation (Meydani *et al.*, 2005). Vitamin E may impact several different steps of the activation and proliferation process such as effective immune synapse formation, free-radical-sensitive signal transduction pathways, or cell-cycle-related molecules (Meydani *et al.*, 2005). In addition, animal studies (Brigelius-Flohé, 2005; Cachia *et al.*, 1998; Chow, 2001) showed that vitamin E also decreased the production and release of inflammatory mediators in mast cells. In many of these studies, vitamin E reduced mast cell degranulation by scavenging free radicals, which suggest that vitamin E might also have a possible beneficial effect in inflammatory and allergic diseases (Zingg, 2007) besides the other age-related immune system problems. Eventually, it is understood that a host nutritional deficiency would lead to an impaired immune response (Beck, 2001) and this impairment in immune function would result in increased vulnerability to infectious (Beck, 2001) and other immune related diseases. Both general malnutrition as well as specific nutritional deficiencies have been reported to be associated with immune dysfunction, including impaired antibody responses, decreased MF activity, and T cell dysfunction (Hayek *et al.*, 1997; Moriguchi and Muraga, 2000). However, challenging with the diseases could be problematic in such conditions; vitamin E with its beneficial effects to immunity could definitely help.

VI. Immunological Use of Vitamin E in Humans

Aging is a normal process characterized by morphological and functional changes, most of which are degenerative, that occur as a living system grows older (Eitenmiller and Lee, 2004). The role of free radicals in the aging process and the ability of vitamin E to delay the overall process have been topics of intense investigation for decades (Eitenmiller and Lee, 2004).

Inflammation has been suggested to be one of the mechanisms underlying the pathogenesis of many chronic diseases such as coronary heart disease, cancer, type 2 diabetes, rheumatoid arthritis, neurological disorders (Alzheimer's and Parkinson's disease), and infectious diseases, which have been associated with the action of free radicals (Di Mascio *et al.*, 1991; Freeman and Crapo, 1982; Heneka and O'Banion, 2007; Hotamisligil, 2006; Libby, 2002, 2006; McInnes and Schett, 2007; Rumin *et al.*, 1993; Scrivo *et al.*, 2007; Shoelson *et al.*, 2007; Tansey *et al.*, 2007). It is generally accepted that oxidative damage at the cellular level is significant to the onset of chronic disease (Eitenmiller and Lee 2004). On the other hand, HIV and opportunistic infections can also generate high levels of free radicals and oxidative stress (Tang and Smit, 1998). These highly reactive free radicals have been associated with more rapid progression to AIDS (Wang and Watson, 1994a). In the past few years, there has been increasing evidence supporting the proposition that age-related immune dysfunction might be partially prevented, or even reversed by dietary intervention (Meydani and Beharka, 1998; Meydani *et al.*, 1990). Since vitamin E is the primary fat-soluble antioxidant in mammalian systems, a logical assumption is that supplementation of the human diet with vitamin E potentially could be significant in prevention and/or slowing of the onset of various chronic disease states (Eitenmiller and Lee, 2004). Unfortunately, the body of data does not provide for a clear conclusion on vitamin E and its overall worth when consumed at levels above the RDA (Eitenmiller and Lee, 2004). The evidence available suggests that the current RDA (Food and Nutrition Board, and Institute of Medicine, 2000) for men and women (15 mg/day) may be inappropriately low for an appropriate immunostimulatory activity in aging, and dietary intake may need to be increased (Serafini, 2000). CVD is the major degenerative disease in much of the world (Kosowski and Clouatre, 2008). Current approaches to reducing morbidity and mortality associated with CVD rely largely on reducing dietary fat and sodium intake (Meydani, 2004). The hypothesis that links vitamin E to the prevention of CVD postulates that the oxidation of unsaturated lipids in the LDL particle, which is considered to be a major causative factor in development of CVD (Food and Nutrition Board, and Institute of Medicine, 2000), initiates a complex sequence of events that leads to the development of atherosclerotic plaque (Pryor, 2000). This theory, proposed by Morel *et al.* (1984), Steinberg and Witztum (1990), and Mitchinson (1994), is now generally accepted and provides a strong biological plausibility for the role of vitamin E in preventing CVD. Vitamin E supplementation also leads to a decrease in platelet aggregability; neither vitamin C nor β-carotene has this effect (Calzada *et al.*, 1997; Mower and Steiner, 1982). Clinical trials have also shown certain benefits of supplemental intake of vitamin E. Hodis *et al.* (1995) reported a significantly retarded progression in coronary lesions among men who had previously undergone coronary artery bypass graft surgery and were supplemented with vitamin E. Through careful selection and incorporation of ingredients containing high amounts of vitamin E into daily meals, one can increase dietary intake of vitamin E to 60 IU/day; however, an intake of 200 IU/day is attainable only by supplementation (Meydani, 2000). One mechanism of cancer onset that has received a great deal of scientific examination has been free-radical damage to DNA and the accumulation of unrepaired mutations as one ages (Food and Nutrition Board, and Institute of Medicine, 2000). Similar to CVD, current general opinion is that overall scientific evidence does not support claims for protection against cancers through elevated intakes of vitamin E (Brown and Crowley, 2005), however, tocopherols and other antioxidants may inhibit colon cancer by decreasing the formation of mutagens arising from the free-radical oxidation of fecal lipids as well as by "nonantioxidant" mechanisms (Kosowski and Clouatre, 2008). Patients and experimental animals with advanced cancer often exhibit a poorly functioning immune system (Kiessling *et al.*, 1996, 1999), constituting a barrier to efficient immunotherapy, and contributing to the spread of the disease and to opportunistic infections (Malmberg and Ljunggren, 2006). This situation can be explained by a multitude of factors, including production of PGE_2 and gangliosides by the tumor cells, Fas FasL interaction inducing T cell apoptosis, production of arginase I by myeloid suppressor cells (Hahne *et al.*, 1996; Ladisch *et al.*, 1992; O'Connell *et al.*, 1996; Rabinowich *et al.*, 1998; Zea *et al.*, 2005), manifested by anergy to skin-test antigens (Young *et al.*, 1972), decreased T-cell proliferation (Alexander *et al.*, 1993), alterations in signal transducing molecules (Bukowski *et al.*, 1998; Ling *et al.*, 1998; Matsuda *et al.*, 1995; Uzzo *et al.*, 1999), reduced CD4:CD8 ratios (Arista *et al.*, 1994; Kandil *et al.*, 2001), and deficient production of T-helper 1 cytokines (Elsasser-Beile *et al.*, 1992; Heriot *et al.*, 2000; Wang *et al.*, 1995). These alterations correlate with the severity of the disease and with poor survival (Kuss *et al.*, 1999; Matsuda *et al.*, 1995). Malmberg *et al.* (2002) suggested that vitamin E may be used as an adjuvant to more specific immunotherapy that is dependent on a functional Th1 response which could explain the possible mechanisms behind the immunostimulatory effect of vitamin E and the role of the Th1 cytokines in tumor immunity. Whether this effect is mediated via influence on the immune system or by other mechanisms is unknown. Malmberg *et al.* (2002) showed that vitamin E promoted both IL-2 and interferon (IFN)-γ production by T-cells, which is supported by other studies that vitamin E supplementation to old mice leads to increased IL-2 production only in naïve T-cells (Adolfsson *et al.*, 2001) and increased CD4:CD8 ratios. While colorectal cancer patients with advanced disease have reduced numbers of CD4+ T-cells leading to a decreased CD4:CD8 ratio (Arista *et al.*, 1994; Malmberg *et al.*, 2002), it is obviously seen that supplementation of vitamin E could reverse these decreases (Malmberg *et al.*, 2002). Malmberg *et al.* (2002) have shown that by restoring the antioxidant status in colorectal cancer patients through supplementation of vitamin E, one may improve the function of NK cells. In any event, other epidemiological studies show that an increased dietary intake of vitamin E, mainly in the form of γ-tocopherol, appears to be protective against breast, cervical, and colon cancers (Giuliano *et al.*, 1997; Goodman *et al.*, 1998; Kushi *et al.*, 1996; Stone and Papas, 1997; Zhang *et al.*, 1999). Hainonen *et al.* (1998) reported a 32% decrease in the incidence of prostate cancer in male smokers receiving 50 mg α-tocopherol per day for clinical prostate cancer but not for latent cancer and they found the mortality rate of prostate cancer was 41% lower in the supplemental group. Hainonen *et al.* (1998) in this study suggested that long-term supplementation with α-tocopherol substantially reduced prostate cancer incidence and mortality rates. In summary, increased Th1 responses and, thus, enhanced antitumor activity by the immune system may be one molecular explanation for a beneficial role of vitamin E as primary prevention against cancer (Malmberg *et al.*, 2002). There is no doubt vitamin E and its relationship between diseases such as type 2 diabetes, rheumatoid arthritis, neurological disorders (Alzheimer's and Parkinson's disease) also need to be searched and discussed because of the potent antioxidant properties of vitamin E on reducing or preventing these diseases. Besides the CVD and cancer, immune-related HIV, atopic dermatitis (AD), and infectious diseases especially in the elderly should also be discussed because of the immunomodulatory functions of vitamin E. AD is a well-known, chronic, pruritic, inflammatory skin disease frequently seen in subjects with a personal and/or family history of atopy, such as asthma and allergic rhinitis (Tsoureli-Nikita *et al.*, 2002). Its etiology and pathogenesis are still unclear, although a possible altered immune regulation, with the development of IgE and IgG antinuclear antibodies (ANA), has recently been demonstrated (Muro, 2001; Tada *et al.*, 1994). Vitamin E can be considered to be a safe and active treatment for murine nasal allergy (Zheng *et al.*, 1999) and can reduce serum levels of IgE in atopic subjects (Fogarty *et al.*, 2000). While great attention has been paid to the antioxidative capacity of vitamin E in the past (Hlúbik and Střítecká, 2004; Krajčovičová-Kudláčková *et al.*, 2004) based on the findings from experimental studies in animals and humans, the potential biological mechanisms of vitamin E on IgE production are mainly those exerted on T helper cell differentiation and on regulatory functions in eicosanoid production. Vitamin E also reduces IL-4 secretion in human peripheral blood T-cells in a dose-dependent manner (Li-Weber *et al.*, 2002). As IL-4 promotes the production of IgE antibodies by B-cells, it is one of the key cytokines in the development of allergic inflammation (Sausenthaler *et al.*, 2009). Both studies done by Tsoureli-Nikita *et al.* (2002) and Sausenthaler *et al.* (2009) suggest that vitamin E may play an important role in IgE-mediated atopic responses in humans by significantly decreasing the serum IgE levels. This leads to an improvement in clinical symptoms, offering patients a better quality of life and dermatologists a safe tool for the treatment of AD (Tsoureli-Nikita *et al.*, 2002). HIV and opportunistic infections can generate high levels of free radicals and oxidative stress (Tang and Smit, 1998). Vitamin E deficiency, in turn, exacerbates the immune dysfunctions caused by HIV infection, leaving individuals more susceptible to opportunistic infections (Tang and Smit, 1998). The potential benefits of dietary supplementation of vitamin E in HIV infection and AIDS have been investigated in mice infected with a murine leukemia retrovirus (Meydani and Beharka, 1998). Vitamin E supplementation also decreased indices of lipid peroxidation and decreased the size and frequency of induced esophageal tumors in retrovirus-infected mice and nonimmunocompromised mice (Odeleye *et al.*, 1992). Meydani and Beharka (1998) reported that in retrovirus-infected mice, vitamin E supplementation significantly restored T cell and B cell proliferation and stimulated NK activity, which had been suppressed by retroviral infection. These researchers concluded that vitamin E can help to normalize retrovirus-induced immune defects during progression of murine AIDS and suggested that vitamin E could be potential nutrient to modify human immune dysfunction caused by HIV infection (Wang *et al.*, 1994). Suzuki and Packer (1993) found that several of the naturally occurring vitamin E derivatives (vitamin E acetate, α-tocopheryl succinate, and PMC [2,2,5,7,8-pentamethyl-6-hydroxychromane]) were successful in inhibiting NF-κB activation in an *in vitro* system. NF-κB is a transcription-enhancing factor, and activation of this factor by free radicals is believed to play a key role in HIV replication (Tang and Smit, 1998). It is hypothesized that if vitamin E could inhibit activation of NF-κ B, this would lead to inhibition of HIV transcription (Tang and Smit, 1998). An age-related decline in immune response may increase the risk of infectious diseases and their complications (Miller, 1996). In elderly men and women, an impairment of immune functions was observed in comparison with the respective adult controls and the intake of vitamin E resulted in a significant enhancement of immune parameters in both elderly men and women, bringing their values close to those in the adults (De La Fuente *et al.*, 2008). The incidence of infectious diseases, particularly respiratory diseases, increases with age and is associated with higher morbidity and mortality rates than in the young (Han and Meydani, 1999). Nutritional status is an important determinant of immune function (Chandra, 1990; Keusch *et al.*, 1983). Nutritional supplementation has been shown to enhance older subjects' immune response (Chandra, 1992; Meydani and Blumberg, 1989). For vitamin E, a higher dose, such as 200 mg/day, has been required to demonstrate an effect (Meydani *et al.*, 1997). Meydani *et al.* (1990) conducted the first double-blind placebo-controlled clinical trial, which is very important, analyzing the effect of vitamin E supplementation on immune response in the elderly (>60 years old) and they suggested that short-term vitamin E supplementation improves immune responsiveness in healthy elderly individuals; this effect appears to be mediated by a decrease in PGE_2 and/or other lipid peroxidation products. In the past few years, there has been increasing evidence supporting the proposition that age-related immune dysfunction might be partially prevented, or even reversed by dietary intervention (Meydani *et al.*, 1990; Meydani and Beharka, 1998). De La Fuente *et al.* (2008) analyzed vitamin E supplementation on immune functions, which is the most widely studied, T-cell proliferation to mitogens, and the IL-2 production, functions that decrease in elderly humans. This fact seems to reflect a progressively decreasing proportion of functional T-cells rather than a uniform decline in function of all cells, which could be due to the excessive apoptosis of those lymphocytes (Spaulding *et al.*, 1999). Most studies have investigated the effect of vitamin E on bacterial infections in which phagocytosis is the chief defensive mechanism (Han and Meydani, 1999). On the other hand, few studies have focused on the effect of vitamin E on viral infections (Han and Meydani, 1999). Further, it appears that vitamin E supplementation plays a beneficial role in restoring the compromised immune response of human elderly subjects (Serafini, 2000). Vitamin E supplementation significantly enhances lymphocyte proliferation, IL-2 production of naïve T-cells (the subpopulation of lymphocytes that decreased more with aging) in old mice, with no effect on memory T-cells (Adolfsson *et al.*, 2001; Meydani *et al.*, 2005) and this effect seems to be mediated by the increase of the percentage of old CD4+ T-cells capable of forming an effective immune synapse (Marko *et al.*, 2007). Vitamin E also enhances delayed-type hypersensitivity skin response and decreases PGE_2 production by affecting COX activity (Serafini, 2000), which is described before, and these effects of vitamin E have been investigated extensively. The immune responses of supplementation of vitamin E trials in humans are listed in Table 8.2. Eventually, several investigations have demonstrated that vitamin E significantly enhances immune functions in humans, especially in the elderly and one can say that vitamin E is associated with reduced risk of acquiring infections, particularly upper respiratory infections, in the elderly.

VII. Immunological Use of Vitamin E in Animals

Nutrition has great importance in the maintenance of immune function (Alvarado *et al.*, 2006); this rule is valid for animals like humans. Accumulating evidence suggests a strong association between diets rich in antioxidant compounds and a decreased incidence of cancer and other age-related diseases, and it has been proposed that the immunomodulatory effect of these diets might account, at least in part, for this (Chandra, 2004; Hughes, 1999; Watson *et al.*, 2005). A compromised immune system will affect animal health as well as in humans and result in reduced animal

Table 8.2 Vitamin E supplementation and the immune response in humans

Ages	Immune Response	References
Adults	↔Lymphocyte proliferation, ↔DTH, ↔Antibody	Goodwin and Garry (1983)
Elderly	Positive DTH response	Chavance *et al.* (1984)
Elderly	Positive DTH response, positive correlation with the T-helper/ T-supressor (CD4/CD8) ratio	Chavance *et al.* (1985)
Adults and Elderly	↔Antibody development to influenza virus	Harman and Miller (1986)
Elderly	↑Total serum protein; α-2 and β-2 globulin fraction	Ziemlanski *et al.* (1986)
Elderly	↑Lymphocyte proliferation, ↑DTH, ↑IL-2	Meydani *et al.* (1989)
Elderly	↑Lymphocyte proliferation, ↑DTH, ↔IL-1, ↑IL-2, ↓PGE_2	Meydani *et al.* (1990)
Elderly	↓IL-2	Payette *et al.* (1990)
Young and Elderly	↓IL-6 secretion	Cannon *et al.* (1991)
Adults	↑Lymphocyte proliferation (Con A)	Kramer *et al.* (1991)
Young	↑NK activity	Adachi *et al.* (1997)
Elderly	↔Lymphocyte proliferation (Con A, PHA), ↔IgG, IgA	De Waart *et al.* (1997)
Elderly	↑DTH and antibody titer to hepatitis B and tetanus, ↑IL-2, ↔Lymphocyte proliferation (Con A), ↓PGE_2	Meydani *et al.* (1997)
Elderly	↑Lymphocyte proliferation (PHA), ↑phagocytic functions of PMN	De la Fuente *et al.* (1998)
Elderly	↑Number of positive DTH response, ↔IL-2 production	Pallast *et al.* (1999)
Adults	↑Lymphocyte proliferation (PHA, LPS)	Lee and Wan (2000)
Elderly	↑Lymphocyte proliferation, ↑IL-2, ↑NK activity, ↑Neutrophil chemotaxis and phagocytosis	De la Fuente *et al.* (2008)

Concanavalin A (Con A), Phytohaemagglutinin (PHA), Lipopolysaccharides (LPS), Polymorph nuclear neutrophils (PMN), Delayed-type hypersensitivity (DTH).

production efficiency through increased susceptibility to diseases, thereby leading to increased animal morbidity and mortality (McDowell, 2000). Macrophages and neutrophils from vitamin E-deficient animals have decreased phagocytic activity (Burkholder and Swecker, 1990). However, vitamin E deficiency is rare in human beings, in animals, deficiencies could be seen more frequently rather in some circumstances. More importantly, this possibility makes them more vulnerable to infectious and other metabolic disorders. Since vitamin E acts as a tissue antioxidant and aids in quenching free radicals produced in the body, any infection or other stress factors may exacerbate depletion of the limited vitamin E stores from various tissues (McDowell, 2000). During stress and disease, there is an increase in production of glucocorticoids, epinephrine, eicosanoids, and phagocytic activity (McDowell, 2000). Eicosanoid and corticoid synthesis and phagocytic respiratory bursts are prominent producers of free radicals that challenge the animal's antioxidant systems (McDowell, 2000). Under stress conditions, increased levels of these compounds by endogenous synthesis or exogenous entry may adversely affect immune cell function (Hadden, 1987). Viral diseases such as infectious bursal disease, hydropericardium syndrome, and chicken virus anemia are immunosuppressive (Balamurugan and Kataria, 2006) and fatal for these animals. Vitamin E improves the immune response by enhancing macrophage phagocytic function, decreasing PGE_2, increasing IL-1 secretion by macrophages, enhancing IL-2 production and T-cell proliferation (Moriguchi *et al.*, 1993). For these reasons, the poultry industry often provides supplemental dietary vitamin E at inclusion rates above the National Research Council (1994) recommendations. Same as poultry, vitamin E supplementation of diets has a considerable potential as a method of conferring increased resistance in the sow and the neonatal pig to enteric diseases such as *Escherichia coli*, which is one of the most common diseases in the neonate and contributes to preweaning mortality (Pharazyn *et al.*, 1990). Previous studies have shown that vitamin E supplementation of sow diets improves the immune response of sows and piglets (Pinelli-Saavedra, 2003). Dietary supplementation with 2–10 times more than the currently recommended level of vitamin E significantly increases humoral and cell-mediated immune responses and phagocytic functions in laboratory and farm animals including pigs and increases their resistance to infectious diseases (Meydani and Tengerdy, 1992). It is known that vitamin E can stimulate the immune defense mechanisms in laboratory animals (Sheffy and Schultz 1979), and such beneficial effects also have been recorded in cattle (Cipriano *et al.*, 1982; Reddy *et al.*, 1986). Vitamin E has been associated with increased immune functions in calves (Reddy *et al.*, 1986, 1987a), especially increased IgG and IgM in newborns (Pekmezci and Cakiroglu, 2009) and in dairy cows (Hogan *et al.*, 1992; Politis *et al.*, 1995). While DL-α-tocopherol acetate is viscous oil that can be emulsified with an aqueous antigen to form a water in oil, oil in water, or double emulsion, it may also be used as adjuvants and in vaccination, such adjuvants may boost the immune response to weakly immunogenic antigens, as is the case with many protein antigens (Nervig *et al.*, 1986). When vitamin E is in the oil phase in such an adjuvant, it is in close contact with antigen-processing cells and accessory cells that are attracted to the sites of injections by chemotaxis (peripheral mononuclear cells, lymphocytes, and macrophages; Pinelli-Saavedra, 2003). This contact with the high local concentration of vitamin E (e.g., ~116 mg α-tocopherol per dose used; Franchini *et al.*, 1991, 1995) at the site of action assures the most favorable immunoenhancing effect of the vitamin, far more effectively than is possible by its dietary administration (Meydani and Tengerdy, 1992). Furthermore, vitamin E injections in chicks showed a significant improvement in antibody titers to Newcastle disease virus and *E. coli* antigens (Franchini *et al.*, 1991, 1995). It has long been suggested that supplementation of laboratory and domestic animals with vitamin E has potentiated their cell-mediated and humoral responses, the studies with their results summarized in Table 8.3. Based on numerous studies even in humans and animals, we can say that vitamin E supplementation can improve the immune response.

VIII. Conclusions and Future Aspects

From the date of discovery of vitamin E to nowadays, high budget studies conducted on numerous beneficial effects on humans as well as animals. These studies make us to recognize the significant affects of vitamin E on even preventing or curing the diseases. It is obviously seen that vitamin E, as a family of related molecules, has a number of functions in the body that are not limited to antioxidant activity. In the past few years, there has been increasing evidence supporting the proposition that age-related immune dysfunction might be partially prevented, or even reversed by dietary intervention (Meydani *et al.*, 1990; Meydani and Beharka, 1998). The evidence available suggests that the current RDA (Food and Nutrition Board, and Institute of Medicine, 2000) for men and women (15 mg/day) may be inappropriately low for an appropriate immunostimulatory activity in aging, and dietary intake may need to be increased (Serafini, 2000). Further, vitamin E supplementation has been shown to enhance immunocompromised or older subjects' immune response in various diseases and conditions. The most important point is that, one should know for a beneficial effect that it is necessary to use the right form and the right dose of vitamin E, and other forms of vitamin E such as tocotrienols are also needed to be search as much as the tocopherols.

Table 8.3 Vitamin E supplementation and the immune response in animals

Research Species	Immune Response	References
Mice	↑Helper T-cell activity	Tanaka *et al.* (1979)
Pigs	↑Lymphocyte proliferation (PHA)	Larsen and Tollersud (1981)
Piglets	↑Antibody titer to a challenge	Peplowski *et al.* (1981)
Old mice (C57BL)	↑Lymphocyte proliferation (Con A, LPS), ↑DTH, ↑IL-2, ↓PGE_2	Meydani *et al.* (1986)
Calves	↑Lymphocyte proliferation (Con A, PHA, PWN, LPS)	Reddy *et al.* (1987b)
Rats	↑Lymphocyte proliferation (Con A, LPS)↑NK activity	Moriguchi *et al.* (1990)
Newborn piglets	↑Lymphocyte proliferation (Con A, PHA), ↔IgG, ↔IgM, ↔IgA	Nemec *et al.* (1994)
Gilt	↔Lymphocyte proliferation (Con A, PHA), ↔IgG, ↔IgM, ↔IgA	Nemec *et al.* (1994)
Mice (C57BL/6)	↑IL-2, ↓IL-4, ↓IL-6, ↓Interferon gamma	Wang and Watson (1994b)
Newborn piglets	↑Antibody titer to Keyhole limpet hemocyanin (KLH)	Hidiroglou *et al.* (1995)
Cattle	↔Lymphocyte proliferation (Con A)	Politis *et al.* (1995)
Rats (Fisher)	↑Lymphocyte proliferation (Con A, PHA), ↑IL-2	Sakai and Moriguchi (1997)
Young and old mice (C57BL)	↑Lymphocyte proliferation in young mice, ↔Lymphocyte proliferation in old mice	Wakikawa *et al.* (1999)
Old mice	↑Lymphocyte proliferation, ↑IL-2	Adolfsson *et al.* (2001)
Newborn calves	↑IgG, ↑IgM	Pekmezci and Cakiroglu (2009)

Concanavalin A (Con A), Phytohaemagglutinin (PHA), Pokeweed mitogen (PWM), Lipopolysaccharides (LPS), Delayed-type hypersensitivity (DTH).

ACKNOWLEDGMENTS

The author appreciates to Ph.D. Gokmen Zafer Pekmezci for his valuable help.

REFERENCES

Abdo, K. M., Rao, G., Montgomery, C. A., Dinowitz, M., and Kanagalingam, K. (1986). Thirteen-week toxicity study of d-alpha-tocopheryl acetate (vitamin E) in Fischer 344 rats. *Food Chem. Toxicol.* **24**(10–11), 1043–1050.

Adachi, N., Migita, M., Ohta, T., Higashi, A., and Matsuda, I. (1997). Depressed natural killer cell activity due to decreased natural killer cell population in a vitamin E-deficient patient with Shwachman syndrome: Reversible natural killer cell abnormality by α-tocopherol supplementation. *Eur. J. Pediatr.* **156**(6), 444–448.

Adolfsson, O., Huber, B. T., and Meydani, S. N. (2001). Vitamin E enhanced IL-2 production in old mice: Naive but not memory T cells show increased cell division cycling and IL-2 producing capacity. *J. Immunol.* **167,** 3809–3817.

Alexander, J. P., Kudoh, S., Melsop, K. A., Hamilton, T. A., Edinger, M. G., Tubbs, R. R., Sica, D., Tuason, L., Klein, E., Bukowski, R. M., and Finke, J. H. (1993). T-cells infiltrating renal cell carcinoma display a poor proliferative response even though they can produce interleukin 2 and Express interleukin 2 receptors. *Cancer Res.* **53**(6), 1380–1387.

Alvarado, C. B., Álvarez, P., Puerto, M., Gausserès, N., Jiménez, L., and De la Fuente, M. (2006). Dietary supplementation with antioxidants improves functions and decreases oxidative stress of leukocytes from prematurely aging mice. *Nutrition* **22**(7), 767–777.

Anderson, T. W., and Reid, D. B. (1974). A double-blind trial of vitamin E in angina pectoris. *Am. J. Clin. Nutr.* **27**(10), 1174–1178.

Arista, M. C., Callopoli, A., De Franceschi, L., Santini, A., Schiratti, M., Conti, L., Di Filippo, F., and Gandolfo, G. M. (1994). Flow cytometric study of lymphocyte subsets in patients at different stages of colorectal carcinoma. *Dis. Colon Rectum* **37**(2), 30–34.

Arita, M., Sato, Y., Miyata, A., Tanabe, T., Takahashi, E., Kayden, H. J., Arai, H., and Inoue, K. (1995). Human alpha-tocopherol transfer protein: cDNA cloning, expression and chromosomal localization. *Biochem. J.* **306**(2), 437–443.

Ashworth, C. J., and Antipatis, C. (2001). Micronutrient programming of development throughout gestation. *Reproduction* **122**(4), 527–535.

Babinszky, L., Langhout, D. J., Verstegen, M. W. A., den Hartog, L. A., Joling, P., and Niewl, M. (1991). Effect of vitamin E and fat source in sows' diets on immune response of suckling and weaned piglets. *J. Anim. Sci.* **69,** 1833–1842.

Balamurugan, V., and Kataria, J. M. (2006). Economically important non-oncogenic immunosuppressive viral diseases of chicken—Current status. *Vet. Res. Commun.* **30**(5), 541–566.

Bartocci, A., Maggi, F. M., Welker, R. D., and Veronese, F. (1982). Age-related immunosuppression: Putative role of prostaglandins. *In* "Prostaglandins and Cancer," (T. J. Powles, R. S. Backman, K. V. Hohn, and P. Ramwell, Eds.), pp. 725–730. Alan Riss, New York.

Beck, M. A. (2001). Antioxidants and viral infections: Host immune response and viral pathogenicity. *J. Am. Coll. Nutr.* **20**(5), 384–388.

Beharka, A. A., Redican, S., Lynette, L., and Meydani, S. N. (1997a). Vitamin E status and immune function. *In* "Methods in Enzymology," (D. B. Mccormick, Ed.), Vol. 282, pp. 247–263. Academic Press.

Beharka, A. A., Wu, D., Han, S. N., and Meydani, S. N. (1997b). Macrophage prostaglandin production contributes to the age-associated decrease in T cell function which is reversed by the dietary anti-oxidant vitamin E. *Mech. Ageing Dev.* **93**(1–3), 59–77.

Bellezo, J. M., Leingang, K. A., Bulla, G. A., Britton, R. S., Bacon, B. R., and Fox, E. S. (1998). Modulation of lipopolysaccharide-mediated activation in rat Kupffer cells by antioxidants. *J. Lab. Clin. Med.* **131**(1), 36–44.

Ben Hamida, M., Belal, S., Sirugo, G., Ben Hamida, C., Panayides, K., Ionannou, P., Beckmann, J., Mandel, J. L., Hentati, F., and Koenig, M. (1993). Friedreich's ataxia phenotype not linked to chromosome 9 and associated with selective autosomal recessive vitamin E deficiency in two inbred Tunisian families. *Neurology* **43**(11), 2179–2183.

Bender, D. A. (2003). Vitamin E: Tocopherols and tocotrienols. *In* "Nutritional Biochemistry of the Vitamins," (D. A. Bender, Ed.), pp. 109–130. Cambridge University Press, New York.

Bendich, A. (1988). Antioxidant vitamins and immune responses. *In* "Nutrition and Immunology," (R. K. Chandra, Ed.), pp. 125–148. A. R. Liss, New York.

Bendich, A. (1990). Antioxidant micronutrients and immune responses. *Ann. N. Y. Acad. Sci.* **587,** 168–180.

Bendich, A. (1992). Vitamins and immunity. *J. Nutr.* **122**(3), 601–603.

Bendich, A., and Machlin, L. J. (1998). Safety of oral intake of vitamin E. *Am. J. Clin. Nutr.* **48**(3), 612–619.

Bendich, A., Gabriel, G. E., and Machlin, L. J. (1986). Dietary vitamin E requirement for optimum immune responses in the rat. *J. Nutr.* **116**(4), 675–681.

Bonney, R. J., Opas, E. E., and Humes, J. L. (1985). Lipoxygenase pathway of macrophages. *Fed. Proc.* **44**(14), 2933–2936.

Brennan, L. A., Morris, G. M., Wasson, G. R., Hannigan, B. M., and Barnett, Y. A. (2000). The effect of vitamin C or vitamin E supplementation on basal and H_2O_2-induced DNA damage in human lymphocytes. *Br. J. Nutr.* **84**(2), 195–202.

Brigelius-Flohé, R. (2005). Induction of drug metabolizing enzymes by vitamin E. *J. Plant Physiol.* **162**(7), 797–802.

Brigelius-Flohé, R. (2006). Glutathione peroxidases and redox-regulated transcription factors. *Biol. Chem.* **387**(10–11), 1329–1335.

Brown, B. G., and Crowley, J. (2005). Is there any hope for vitamin E? *JAMA* **293**(11), 1387–1390.

Budowski, P. D., and Sklan, D. (1989). Vitamins E and A. *In* "The Role of Fats in Human Nutrition," (A. J. Vergroesen and M. Crawford, Eds.), pp. 364–406. Academic Press, London.

Bukowski, R. M., Rayman, P., Uzzo, R., Bloom, T., Sandstrom, K., Peereboom, D., Olencki, T., Budd, G. T., McLain, D., Elson, P., Novick, A., and Finke, J. H. (1998). Signal transduction abnormalities in T lymphocytes from patients with advanced renal carcinoma: Clinical relevance and effects of cytokine therapy. *Clin. Cancer Res.* **4**(10), 2337–2347.

Burkholder, W. J., and Swecker, W. S. (1990). Nutritional influences on immunity. *Semin. Vet. Med. Surg. (Small Anim.)* **5**(3), 154–166.

Cachia, O., Benna, J. E., Pedruzzi, E., Descomps, B., Gougerot-Pocidalo, M. A., and Leger, C. L. (1998). Alpha-tocopherol inhibits the respiratory burst in human monocytes. Attenuation of p47 (phox) membrane translocation and phosphorylation. *J. Biol. Chem.* **273**(49), 32801–32805.

Calzada, C., Bruckdorfer, K. R., and Rice-Evans, C. A. (1997). The influence of antioxidant nutrients on platelet function in healthy volunteers. *Atherosclerosis* **128**(1), 97–105.

Cannon, J. G., Meydani, S. N., Fielding, R. A., Fiatarone, M. A., Meydani, M., Farhangmehr, M., Orencole, S. F., Blumberg, J. B., and Evans, W. J. (1991). Acute phase response in exercise. II. Associations between vitamin E, cytokines, and muscle proteolysis. *Am. J. Physiol.* **260,** 1235–1240.

Catignani, G. L., and Bieri, J. G. (1977). Rat liver alpha-tocopherol binding protein. *Biochim. Biophys. Acta* **497**(2), 349–357.
Cavalier, L., Ouahchi, K., Kayden, H. J., Di Donato, S., Reutenauer, L., Mandel, J. L., and Koenig, M. (1998). Ataxia with isolated vitamin E deficiency: Heterogeneity of mutations and phenotypic variability in a large number of families. *Am. J. Hum. Genet.* **62**(2), 301–310.
Chandra, R. K. (1990). Nutrition is an important determinant of immunity in old age. *Prog. Clin. Biol. Res.* **326,** 321–334.
Chandra, R. K. (1992). Effect of vitamin and trace-element supplementation on immune responses and infection in elderly subjects. *Lancet* **340**(8828), 1124–1127.
Chandra, R. K. (2004). Impact of nutritional status and nutrient supplements on immune responses and incidence of infection in older individuals. *Ageing Res. Rev.* **3**(1), 91–104.
Chang, W. P., Hom, J. S., Dietert, R. R., Combs, G. F. J., and Marsh, J. A. (1994). Effect of dietary vitamin E and selenium deficiency on chicken splenocytes proliferation and cell surface marker expression. *Immunopharmacol. Immunotoxicol.* **16**(2), 203–223.
Chavance, M., Brubacher, G., Herbert, B., Vernhers, G., Mistacki, T., Dete, F., Founier, C., and Janot, C. (1984). Immunological nutritional status among the elderly. *In* "Lymphoid Cell Functions in Aging," (A. L. De Wilk, Ed.), pp. 231–237. Eurage, Paris.
Chavance, M., Brubacher, G., Herbert, B., Vernhers, G., Mistacki, T., Dete, F., Founier, C., and Janot, C. (1985). Immunological and nutritional status among the elderly. *In* "Nutrition, Immunity and Illness in the Elderly," (R. K. Chandra, Ed.), pp. 137–142. Pergamon Press, New York.
Cheeseman, K. H. (1993). Lipid peroxidation and cancer. *In* "DNA and Free Radicals," (B. Halliwell and O. I. Aruoma, Eds.), pp. 211–228. Ellis Horwood Ltd., West Sussex.
Chow, C. K. (2001). Vitamin E regulation of mitochondrial superoxide generation. *Biol. Signals Recept.* **10**(1–2), 112–124.
Cipriano, J. E., Morrill, J. L., and Anderson, N. V. (1982). Effect of dietary vitamin E on immune responses of calves. *J. Dairy Sci.* **65**(12), 2357–2365.
Coquette, A., Vray, B., and Vanderpas, J. (1986). Role of vitamin E in the protection of the resident macrophage membrane against oxidative damage. *Arch. Int. Physiol. Biochim.* **94** (5), 529–534.
Corwin, L. M., and Gordon, R. K. (1982). Vitamin E and immune regulation. *Ann. N. Y. Acad. Sci.* **393,** 437–451.
Corwin, L. M., and Shloss, J. (1980). Influence of vitamin E on the mitogenic response of murine lymphoid cells. *J. Nutr.* **110**(5), 916–923.
De la Fuente, M., Ferrandez, M. D., Burgos, M. S., Soler, A., Prieto, A., and Miquel, J. (1998). Immune function in aged women is improved by ingestion of vitamins C and E. *Can. J. Physiol. Pharmacol.* **76,** 373–380.
De la Fuente, M., Hernanz, A., Guayerbas, N., Victor, V. M., and Arnalich, F. (2008). Vitamin E ingestion improves several immune functions in elderly men and women. *Free Radic. Res.* **42**(3), 272–280.
De Waart, F., Portengen, L., Doekes, G., Verwaal, C. J., and Kok, F. J. (1997). Effect of 3 months vitamin E supplementation on indices of the cellular and humoral immune response in elderly subjects. *Br. J. Nutr.* **78,** 761–774.
Debier, C. (2007). Vitamin E during pre and postnatal periods. *In* "Vitamins and Hormones," (G. Litwack, Ed.), Vol. 76, pp. 357–373. Elsevier Inc., California.
Del Rio, M., Ruedas, G., Medina, S., Victor, V. M., and De la Fuente, M. (1998). Improvement by several antioxidants of macrophage function in vitro. *Life Sci.* **63**(10), 871–881.
Department of Health (1991). Dietary Reference Values for Food Energy and Nutrients for the United Kingdom. Her Majesty's Stationery Office. London.

Di Mascio, P. D., Murphy, M. E., and Sies, H. (1991). Antioxidant defense systems: the role of carotenoids, tocopherols and thiols. *Am. J. Clin. Nutr.* **53**(1), 194–200.
Diaz, M. N., Frei, B., Vita, J. A., and Keaney, J. F. (1997). Antioxidants and atheroslcerotic heart disease. *N. Engl. J. Med.* **337**(6), 408–416.
Dove, C. R., and Ewan, R. C. (1990). Effect of excess dietary copper, iron or zinc on the tocopherol and selenium status of growing pigs. *J. Anim. Sci.* **68**(8), 2407–2413.
Dysmsza, H. A., and Park, J. (1975). Excess dietary vitamin E in rats. *Fed. Am. Soc. Exp. Biol.* **34,** 912–916.
Eitenmiller, R., and Lee, J. (2004). Vitamin E: Food chemistry, composition, and analysis. *In* "Nutrition and Health Implications of Vitamin E," (R. Eitenmiller and J. Lee, Eds.), pp. 39–88. Marcel Dekker Inc., New York.
Elsasser-Beile, U., von Kleist, S., Fischer, R., and Monting, J. S. (1992). Impaired cytokine production in whole blood cell cultures from patients with colorectal carcinomas as compared to benign colorectal tumors and controls. *J. Clin. Lab. Anal.* **6**(5), 311–314.
Eskew, M. L., Scheuchenzuber, W. J., Scholz, R. W., Reddy, C. C., and Zarkower, A. (1986). The effects of ozone inhalation on the immunological response of selenium- and vitamin E-deprived rats. *Environ. Res.* **40**(2), 274–284.
Favier, A., Sappey, C., Leclerc, P., Faure, P., and Micoud, M. (1994). Antioxidant status and lipid peroxidation in patients infected with HIV. *Chem. Biol. Interact.* **91**(2–3), 165–180.
Féger, F., Varadaradjalou, S., Gao, Z., Abraham, S. N., and Arock, M. (2002). The role of mast cells in host defense and their subversion by bacterial pathogens. *Trends Immunol.* **23** (3), 151–158.
Fogarty, A., Lewis, S., Weiss, S., and Britton, J. (2000). Dietary vitamin E, IgE concentrations, and atopy. *Lancet* **356**(9241), 1573–1574.
Food and Nutrition Board, and Institute of Medicine (2000). Vitamin E. *In* "Dietary Reference Intakes for Vitamin C, Vitamin E, Selenium, and Carotenoids," pp. 186–283. National Academy Press, Washington.
Franchini, A., Canti, M., Manfreda, G., and Bertuzzi, S. (1991). Vitamin E as adjuvant in emulsified vaccine for chicks. *Poult. Sci.* **70**(8), 1709–1715.
Franchini, A., Bertuzzi, S., Tosarelli, C., and Manfreda, G. (1995). Vitamin E in viral inactivated vaccines. *Poult. Sci.* **74**(4), 666–671.
Franklin, S. T., Sorenson, C. E., and Hammell, D. C. (1998). Influence of vitamin A supplementation in milk on growth, health, concentrations of vitamins in plasma, and immune parameters of calves. *J. Dairy Sci.* **81**(10), 2623–2632.
Freeman, B. A., and Crapo, J. D. (1982). Biology of disease: Free radicals and tissue injury. *Lab. Invest.* **47**(5), 412–426.
Gebremichael, A., Levy, E. M., and Corwin, L. M. (1984). Adherent cell requirement for the effect of vitamin E on in vitro antibody synthesis. *J. Nutr.* **114**(7), 1297–1305.
Gey, K. F. (1995). Cardiovascular disease and vitamins. Concurrent correction of 'suboptimal' plasma antioxidant levels may, as important part of 'optimal' nutrition, help to prevent early stages of cardiovascular disease and cancer, respectively. *Bibl. Nutr. Dieta* **52,** 75–91.
Giuliano, A. R., Papenfuss, M., Nour, M., Canfield, L. M., Schneider, A., and Hatch, K. (1997). Antioxidant nutrients: Associations with persistent human papillomavirus infection. *Cancer Epidemiol. Biomarkers Prev.* **6**(11), 917–923.
Globerson, A., and Effros, R. B. (2000). Ageing of lymphocytes and lymphocytes in the aged. *Immunol. Today* **21**(10), 515–521.
Goldstone, S. D., and Hunt, N. H. (1997). Redox regulation of the mitogenactivated protein kinase pathway during lymphocyte activation. *Biochim. Biophys. Acta* **1355**(3), 353–360.
Goodman, M. T., Kiviat, N., McDuffie, K., Hankin, J. H., Hernandez, B., Wilkens, L. R., Franke, A., Kuypers, J., Kolonel, L. N., Nakamura, J., Ing, G., Branch, B., *et al.* (1998).

The association of plasma micronutrients with the risk of cervical dysplasia in Hawaii. *Cancer Epidemiol. Biomarkers Prev.* **7**(6), 537–544.

Goodwin, J. S. (1982). Changes in lymphocyte sensitivity to prostaglandin E2, histamine, hydrocortisone, and X irradiation with age: Studies in a healthy elderly population. *Clin. Immunol. Immunopathol.* **25**(2), 243–251.

Goodwin, J. S., and Garry, T. J. (1983). Relationship between megadoses vitamin supplementation and immunological function in a healthy elderly population. *Clin. Exp. Immunol.* **51**(3), 647–653.

Goodwin, J. S., and Messner, R. P. (1979). Sensitivity of lymphocytes to prostaglandin E2 increases in subjects over age 70. *J. Clin. Invest.* **64**(2), 434–439.

Goodwin, J. S., and Webb, D. R. (1981). Regulation of the immune response by prostaglandins: A critical review. *Clin. Immunol. Immunopathol.* **15,** 116–132.

Gordon, N. (2001). Hereditary vitamin E deficiency. *Dev. Med. Child Neurol.* **43**(2), 133–135.

Gruver, A. L., Hudson, L. L., and Sempowski, G. D. (2007). Immunosenescence of ageing. *J. Pathol.* **211**(2), 144–156.

Hadden, J. W. (1987). Neuroendocrine modulation of the thymus-dependent immune system. Agonists and mechanisms. *Ann. N. Y. Acad. Sci.* **496,** 39–48.

Hahne, M., Rimoldi, D., Schroter, M., Romero, P., Schreier, M., French, L. E., Schneider, P., Bornand, T., Fontana, A., Lienard, D., Cerottini, J., and Tschopp, J. (1996). Melanoma cell expression of Fas (Apo-1/CD95) ligand: Implications for tumor immune escape. *Science* **274,** 1363–1366.

Hainonen, O. P., Albanes, D., Virtamo, J., Taylor, P. R., Huttunen, J. K., Hartman, A. M., Haapakoski, J., Malila, N., Rautalahti, M., Ripatti, S., Mäenpää, H., Teerenhovi, L., *et al.* (1998). Prostate cancer and supplementation with alpha-tocopherol and beta-carotene: Incidence and mortality in a controlled trial. *J. Natl. Cancer Inst.* **90**(6), 440–446.

Halliwell, B., and Gutteridge, J. M. C. (1989). Free radicals, ageing, and disease. *In* "Free Radicals in Biology and Medicine," (B. Halliwell and J. M. C. Gutteridge, Eds.), 2nd ed., pp. 416–508. Clarendon Press, Oxford.

Han, S. N., and Meydani, S. N. (1999). Vitamin E and infectious diseases in the aged. *Proc. Nutr. Soc.* **58**(3), 697–705.

Han, S. N., Adolfsson, O., Lee, C. K., Prolla, T. A., Ordovas, J., and Meydani, S. N. (2004). Vitamin E and gene expression in immune cells. *Ann. N. Y. Acad. Sci.* **1031,** 96–101.

Harman, D. (1956). Ageing: A theory based on free radical and radiation chemistry. *J. Gerontol.* **11**(3), 298–300.

Harman, D. (1991). The aging process: Major risk factor for the disease and death. *Proc. Natl. Acad. Sci. USA* **88**(12), 5360–5364.

Harman, D., and Miller, R. W. (1986). Effect of vitamin E on the immune response to influenza virus vaccine and the incidence of infectious disease in man. *Age* **9**(1), 21–23.

Harris, R. E., Boxer, L. A., and Baehner, R. L. (1980). Consequences of vitamin-E deficiency on the phagocytic and oxidative functions of the rat polymorphonuclear leukocyte. *Blood* **55**(2), 338–343.

Hatam, L. J., and Kayden, H. J. (1979). A high-performance liquid chromatographic method for the determination of tocopherol in plasma and cellular elements of the blood. *J. Lipid Res.* **20,** 639–645.

Hayek, M. G., Meydani, S. N., Meydani, M., and Blumberg, J. B. (1994). Age differences in eicosanoid production of mouse splenocytes: Effects on mitogen-induced T-cell proliferation. *J. Gerontol.* **49**(5), 197–207.

Hayek, M. G., Taylor, S. F., Bender, B. S., Han, S. N., Meydani, M., Smith, D. E., Eghtesada, S., and Meydani, S. N. (1997). Vitamin E supplementation decreases lung virus titers in mice infected with influenza. *J. Infect. Dis.* **176**(1), 273–276.

Heneka, M. T., and O'Banion, M. K. (2007). Inflammatory processes in Alzheimer's disease. *J. Neuroimmunol.* **184**(1–2), 69–91.
Henz, B. M., Maurer, M., Lippert, U., Worm, M., and Babina, M. (2001). Mast cells as initiators of immunity and host defense. *Exp. Dermatol.* **10**(1), 1–10.
Heriot, A. G., Marriott, J. B., Cookson, S., Kumar, D., and Dalgleish, A. G. (2000). Reduction in cytokine production in colorectal cancer patients: Association with stage and reversal by resection. *Br. J. Cancer* **82**(5), 1009–1012.
Herrera, E., and Barbas, C. (2001). Vitamin E: Action, metabolism and perspectives. *J. Physiol. Biochem.* **57**(2), 43–56.
Hidiroglou, N., Cave, N., Atwal, A. S., Farnsworth, E. R., and McDowell, L. R. (1992). Comparative vitamin E requirements and metabolism in livestock. *Ann. Rech. Vét.* **23,** 337–359.
Hidiroglou, M., Batra, T. R., Farnworth, E. R., and Markham, F. (1995). Effect of vitamin E supplementation on immune status and α-tocopherol in plasma of piglets. *Reprod. Nutr. Dev.* **35**(4), 443–450.
Hlúbik, P., and Stříteckå, H. (2004). Antioxidants-clinical aspects. *Cent. Eur. J. Public Health* **12,** 28–30.
Hodis, H. N., Mack, W. J., LaBree, L., Cashin-Hemphill, L., Sevanian, A., Johnson, R., and Azen, S. P. (1995). Serial coronary angiographic evidence that antioxidant vitamin intake reduces progression of coronary artery atherosclerosis. *JAMA* **273**(23), 1849–1854.
Hogan, J. S., Weiss, W. P., Todhunter, D. A., Smith, K. L., and Schoenberger, P. S. (1992). Bovine neutrophil responses to parenteral vitamin E. *J. Dairy Sci.* **75**(2), 399–405.
Horwitt, M. K. (1991). Data supporting supplementation of humans with vitamin E. *J. Nutr.* **121,** 424–429.
Hotamisligil, G. S. (2006). Inflammation and metabolic disorders. *Nature* **444**(7127), 860–867.
Hughes, D. A. (1999). Effects of dietary antioxidants on the immune function of middle-aged adults. *Proc. Nutr. Soc.* **58**(1), 79–84.
Humes, J. L., Bonney, R. J., and Pebes, L. (1977). Macrophages synthesize and release prostaglandins in response to inflammatory response. *Nature* **259,** 149–151.
James, J. S., Castle, S. C., and Makinodan, T. (1995). Decline in immune function with age: Interaction with specific nutrient deficiencies. *In* "Geriatric Nutrition," (J. E. Morley, Z. Glick, and L. Z. Rubenstein, Eds.), pp. 153–167. Raven Press Ltd., New York.
Janeway, C. A., and Travers, P. (1997). Basic concepts in immunology. *In* "Immunobiology: The Immune System in Health and Disease," (P. Austin, E. Lawrence, and M. Robertson, Eds.), 3rd ed., pp. 1–33. Garland Publishing, New York.
Jensen, M., Fossum, C., Ederoth, M., and Hakkarainen, R. V. (1988). The effect of vitamin E on the cell-mediated immune response in pigs. *J. Vet. Med.* **35,** 549–555.
Jishage, K., Arita, M., Igarashi, K., Iwata, T., Watanabe, M., Ogawa, M., Ueda, O., Kamada, N., Inoue, K., Arai, H., and Suzuki, H. (2001). α-Tocopherol transfer protein is important for the normal development of placental labyrinthine trophoblasts in mice. *J. Biol. Chem.* **276,** 1669–1672.
Jishage, K., Tachibe, T., Ito, T., Shibata, N., Suzuki, S., Mori, T., Hani, T., Arai, H., and Suzuki, H. (2005). Vitamin E is essential for mouse placentation but not for embryonic development itself. *Biol. Reprod.* **73,** 983–987.
Kaempf-Rotzoll, D. E., Igarashi, K., Aoki, J., Jishage, K., Suzuki, H., Tamai, H., Linderkamp, O., and Arai, H. (2002). α-Tocopherol transfer protein is specifically localized at the implantation site of pregnant mouse uterus. *Biol. Reprod.* **67,** 599–604.
Kaempf-Rotzoll, D. E., Traber, M. G., and Arai, H. (2003). Vitamin E and transfer proteins. *Curr. Opin. Lipidol.* **14**(3), 249–254.

Kandil, A., Bazarbashi, S., and Mourad, W. A. (2001). The correlation of Epstein-Barr virus expression and lymphocyte subsets with the clinical presentation of nodular sclerosing Hodgkin disease. *Cancer* **91**(11), 1957–1963.
Keusch, G. T., Wilson, C. S., and Waksall, S. D. (1983). Nutrition, host defenses and the lymphoid system. *Arch. Host Def. Mech.* **2,** 275–359.
Kiessling, R., Kono, K., Petersson, M., and Wasserman, K. (1996). Immunosuppression in human tumor-host interaction: Role of cytokines and alterations in signal-transducing molecules. *Springer Semin. Immunopathol.* **18**(2), 227–242.
Kiessling, R., Wasserman, K., Horiguchi, S., Kono, K., Sjoberg, J., Pisa, P., and Petersson, M. (1999). Tumor-induced immune dysfunction. *Cancer Immunol. Immunother.* **48**(7), 353–362.
Knight, J. A. (2000). The biochemistry of aging. *Adv. Clin. Chem.* **35,** 1–62.
Kosowski, A., and Clouatre, D. L. (2008). Vitamin E: Natural vs. synthetic. *In* "Tocotrienols Vitamin E Beyond Tocopherols," (R. R. Watson and V. R. Preedy, Eds.), pp. 61–78. CRC Press, Boca Raton.
Kowdley, K. V., Mason, J. B., Meydani, S. N., Cornwall, S., and Grand, R. J. (1992). Vitamin E deficiency and impaired cellular immunity related to intestinal fat malabsorption. *Gastroenterology* **102,** 2139–2142.
Krajčovičová-Kudláčková, M., Pauková, V., Bačeková, M., and Dušinská, M. (2004). Lipid peroxidation in relation to vitamin C and vitamin E levels. *Cent. Eur. J. Public Health* **12** (1), 46–48.
Kramer, T. R., Schoene, N., Douglass, L. W., Judd, J. T., Ballard-Barbash, R., Taylor, P. R., Bhagavan, H. N., and Nair, P. P. (1991). Increased vitamin E intake restores fish-oil-induced suppressed blastogenesis of mitogen-stimulated T lymphocytes. *Am. J. Clin. Nutr.* **54**(5), 890–902.
Krasavage, W. J., and Terhaar, C. J. (1977). D-alpha-tocopheryl poly (ethylene glycol) 1000 succinate: Acute toxicity, subchronic feeding, reproduction, and teratologic studies in the rat. *J. Agric. Food Chem.* **25,** 273–278.
Kuhlenkamp, J., Ronk, M., Yusin, M., Stolz, A., and Kaplowitz, N. (1993). Identification and purification of a human liver cytosolic tocopherol binding protein. *Protein Expr. Purif.* **4,** 382–389.
Kushi, L. H., Fee, R. M., Sellers, T. A., Zheng, W., and Folsom, A. R. (1996). Intake of vitamins A, C, and E and postmenopausal breast cancer. The Iowa Women's Health Study. *Am. J. Epidemiol.* **144**(2), 165–174.
Kuss, I., Saito, T., Johnson, J. T., and Whiteside, T. L. (1999). Clinical significance of decreased ζ chain expression in peripheral blood lymphocytes of patients with head and neck cancer. *Clin. Cancer Res.* **5,** 329–334.
Ladisch, S., Becker, H., and Ulsh, L. (1992). Immunosuppression by human gangliosides: I. Relationship of carbohydrate structure to the inhibition of T cell responses. *Biochim. Biophys. Acta* **1125**(2), 180–188.
Langweiler, M., Schultz, R. D., and Sheffy, B. E. (1981). Effect of vitamin E deficiency on the proliferative response of canine lymphocytes. *Am. J. Vet. Res.* **42**(10), 1681–1685.
Larsen, H. J., and Tollersud, S. (1981). Effect if dietary vitamin E and selenium on the phytohaemagglutinin response of pig lymphocytes. *Res. Vet. Sci.* **31,** 301–305.
Lee, C. Y., and Wan, F. (2000). Vitamin E supplementation improves cell-mediated immunity and oxidative stress of Asian men and women. *J. Nutr.* **130**(12), 2932–2937.
Lesourd, B. M., and Meaume, S. (1994). Cell mediated immunity changes in ageing, relative importance of cell sub population switches and of nutritional factors. *Immunol. Lett.* **40,** 235–242.
Lesourd, B. M., Laisney, C., Salvatore, R., Meaume, S., and Moulias, R. (1994). Decreased maturation of T cell populations in the healthy elderly: Influence of nutritional factors on

the appearance of double negative CD4−, CD8−, CD2+ cells. *Arch. Gerontol. Geriatr.* **19**(1), 139–154.
Libby, P. (2002). Inflammation in atherosclerosis. *Nature* **420**(6917), 868–874.
Libby, P. (2006). Inflammation and cardiovascular disease mechanisms. *Am. J. Clin. Nutr.* **83** (2), 456–460.
Liebler, D. C. (1993). The role of metabolism in the anti-oxidant function of vitamin E. *Crit. Rew. Toxicol.* **23,** 147–169.
Ligthardt, G. J., Van Vlokhoven, P. C., Schuit, H. R. E., and Hijmans, W. (1986). The expanded null cell compartment in ageing: Increase in the number of natural killer cells and changes in T-cell and NK-cell subset in human blood. *Immunology* **59,** 353–357.
Ling, W., Rayman, P., Uzzo, R., Clark, P., Kim, H. J., Tubbs, R., Novick, A., Bukowski, R., Hamilton, T., and Finke, J. (1998). Impaired activation of NFkappaB in T cells from a subset of renal cell carcinoma patients is mediated by inhibition of phosphorylation and degradation of the inhibitor, IkappaBalpha. *Blood* **92**(4), 1334–1341.
Linton, P. J., and Dorshkind, K. (2004). Age-related changes in lymphocyte development and function. *Nat. Immunol.* **5,** 133–139.
Li-Weber, M., Giaisi, M., Treiber, M. K., and Krammer, P. H. (2002). Vitamin E inhibits IL-4 gene expression in peripheral blood T cells. *Eur. J. Immunol.* **32**(9), 2401–2408.
Lohmiller, J. J., Roellich, K. M., Toledano, A., Rabinovitch, P. S., Wolf, N. S., and Grossmann, A. (1996). Aged murine T-lymphocytes are more resistant to oxidative damage due to the predominance of the cells possessing the memory phenotype. *J. Gerontol. A Biol. Sci. Med. Sci.* **51**(2), 132–140.
Machlin, L. J. (1989). Use and safety of elevated dosages of vitamin E in adults. *Int. J. Vitam. Nutr. Res.* **30,** 56–68.
Machlin, L. J. (1991). Vitamin E. *In* "Handbook of Vitamins," (L. J. Machlin, Ed.), 2nd ed., pp. 99–146. Marcel Dekker Inc., New York.
Malmberg, K. J., and Ljunggren, H. G. (2006). Escape from immune-and nonimmune-mediated tumor surveillance. *Semin. Cancer Biol.* **16**(1), 16–31.
Malmberg, K. J., Lenkei, R., Petersson, M., Ohlum, T., Ichihara, F., Glimelius, B., Frodin, J. E., Masucci, G., and Kiessling, R. (2002). A short-term dietary supplementation of high doses of vitamin E increases T helper 1 cytokine production in patients with advanced colorectal cancer. *Clin. Cancer Res.* **8**(6), 1772–1778.
Manor, D., and Morley, S. (2007). The α-tocopherol transfer protein. *In* "Vitamins and Hormones," (G. Litwack, Ed.), Vol. 76, pp. 45–65. Elsevier Inc., California.
Marko, M. G., Ahmed, T., Bunnell, S. C., Wu, D., Chung, H., Huber, B. T., and Meydani, S. N. (2007). Age-associated decline in effective immune synapse formation of CD4 (+) T cell is reversed by vitamin E supplementation. *J. Immunol.* **178,** 1443–1449.
Matsuda, M., Petersson, M., Lenkei, R., Taupin, J. L., Magnusson, I., Mellstedt, H., Anderson, P., and Kiessling, R. (1995). Alterations in the signal-transducing molecules of T cells and NK cells in colorectal tumor-infiltrating, gut mucosal, and peripheral lymphocytes: Correlation with the stage of the disease. *Int. J. Cancer* **61**(6), 765–772.
McDowell, L. R. (2000). Vitamin E. *In* "Vitamins in Animal and Human Nutrition," (L. R. Mcdowell, Ed.), 2nd ed., pp. 155–225. Iowa State University Press.
McDowell, L. R., Williams, S. N., Hidiroglou, N., Njeru, C. A., Hill, G. M., Ochoa, L., and Wilkinson, N. S. (1996). Vitamin E supplementation for the ruminant. *Anim. Feed Sci. Tech.* **60,** 273–296.
McInnes, I. B., and Schett, G. (2007). Cytokines in the pathogenesis of rheumatoid arthritis. *Nat. Rev. Immunol.* **7**(6), 429–442.
Mecheri, S., and David, B. (1999). Functional and ultrastructural insights into the immunobiology of mouse and human mast cells. *Allergy Clin. Immunol. Int.* **11,** 226–233.

Meneghini, R., and Martins, S. (1993). Hydrogen peroxide and DNA damage. *In* "DNA and Free Radicals," (B. Halliwell and O. I. Aruoma, Eds.), pp. 211–228. Ellis Horwood Ltd., West Sussex.
Meydani, M. (2000). Effect of functional food ingredients: Vitamin E modulation of cardiovascular diseases and immune status in the elderly. *Am. J. Clin. Nutr.* **71**(suppl), 1665–1668.
Meydani, M. (2004). Vitamin E modulation of cardiovascular disease. *Ann. N. Y. Acad. Sci.* **1031,** 271–279.
Meydani, S. N., and Beharka, A. A. (1998). Recent developments in vitamin E and immune response. *Nutr. Rev.* **56**(1), 49–56.
Meydani, S. N., and Blumberg, J. B. (1989). Nutrition and the immune function in the elderly. *In* "Human Nutrition: A Comprehensive Treatise," (H. Munro and A. Danforth, Eds.), Vol. VII, pp. 61–87. Plenum Press, New York.
Meydani, S. N., and Blumberg, J. B. (1991). Vitamin E supplementation and enhancement of immune responses in the elderly. *In* "Micronutrients in Health and in Disease Prevention," (A. Bendich and C. E. Butterworth, Eds.), pp. 289–306. Marcel Dekker Inc., New York.
Meydani, S. N., and Tengerdy, R. P. (1992). Vitamin E and immun response. *In* "Vitamin E in Health and Disease: Biochemistry and Clinical Applications," (L. Packer and J. Fuchs, Eds.), 1st ed., pp. 549–562. Marcel Dekker Inc., New York.
Meydani, S. N., Meydani, M., Verdon, C. P., Shapiro, A. C., Blumberg, J. B., and Hayes, K. C. (1986). Vitamin E supplementation suppresses prostaglandin E(1)2 synthesis and enhances the immune response of aged mice. *Mech. Ageing Dev.* **34**(2), 191–201.
Meydani, S. N., Meydani, M., Barklund, P. M., Liu, S., Miller, R. A., Cannon, J. G., Rocklin, R., and Blumberg, J. B. (1989). Effect of vitamin E supplementation on immune responsiveness of the aged. *Ann. N. Y. Acad. Sci.* **570,** 283–290.
Meydani, S. N., Barklund, M. P., Liu, S., Meydani, M., Miller, R. A., Cannon, J. G., Morrow, F. D., Rocklin, R., and Blumberg, J. B. (1990). Vitamin E supplementation enhances cell-mediated immunity in healthy elderly subjects. *Am. J. Clin. Nutr.* **52**(3), 557–563.
Meydani, M., Meydani, S. N., Leka, L., Gong, J., and Blumberg, J. B. (1993). Effect of long-term vitamin E supplementation on lipid peroxidation and immune responses of young and old subjects. *FASEB J.* **7,** 415.
Meydani, S. N., Wu, D., Santos, M. S., and Hayek, M. (1995). Antioxidants and immune response in aged persons: Overview of present evidence. *Am. J. Clin. Nutr.* **62,** 1462–1476.
Meydani, S. N., Meydani, M., Blumberg, J. B., Leka, L. S., Siber, G., Loszewski, R., Thompson, C., Pedrosa, M. C., Diamond, R. D., and Stollar, B. D. (1997). Vitamin E supplementation and in vivo immune response in healthy elderly subjects. A randomized controlled trial. *JAMA* **277**(17), 1380–1386.
Meydani, S. N., Han, S. N., and Wu, D. (2005). Vitamin E and immune response in the aged: Molecular mechanisms and clinical implications. *Immunol. Rev.* **205,** 269–284.
Meyer, M., Schreck, R., and Baeuerle, P. A. (1993). H_2O_2 and antioxidants have opposite effects on activation of NF-kB and AP-1 in intact cells: AP-1 as secondary antioxidant-responsive. *EMBO J.* **12,** 2005–2015.
Miller, R. A. (1996). The aging immune system: Primer and prospectus. *Science* **273**(5271), 70–74.
Miquel, J., Economos, A. C., Fleming, J. E., and Johnson, J. E. (1980). Mitochondrial role in cell aging. *Exp. Gerontol.* **15,** 575–591.
Mitchinson, M. J. (1994). The new face of atherosclerosis. *Br. J. Clin. Pract.* **48**(3), 149–151.

Morel, D. W., DiCorleto, P. E., and Chisolm, G. M. (1984). Endothelial and smooth muscle cells alter low density lipoprotein in vitro by free radical oxidation. *Arteriosclerosis* **4**(4), 357–364.

Moriguchi, S., and Muraga, M. (2000). Vitamin E and immunity. *In* "Vitamins and Hormones," (G. Litwack, Ed.), Vol. 59, pp. 305–336. Academic Press.

Moriguchi, S., Kobayashi, N., and Kishino, Y. (1989). Effects of vitamin E deficiency on the functions of splenic lymphocytes and alveolar macrophages. *J. Nutr. Sci. Vitaminol.* **35,** 419–430.

Moriguchi, S., Kobayashi, N., and Kishino, Y. (1990). High dietary intakes of vitamin E and cellular immune functions in rats. *J. Nutr.* **120**(9), 1096–1102.

Moriguchi, S., Miwa, H., Okamura, M., Maekawa, K., Kishino, Y., and Maeda, K. (1993). Vitamin E is an important factor in T cell differentiation in thymus of F344 rats. *J. Nutr. Sci. Vitaminol.* **39**(5), 451–463.

Morrissey, P. A., and Sheehy, P. J. A. (1999). Optimal nutrition: Vitamin E. *Proc. Nutr. Soc.* **58,** 459–468.

Mower, R., and Steiner, M. (1982). Synthetic byproducts of tocopherol oxidation as inhibitors of platelet function. *Prostaglandins* **24**(2), 137–147.

Muller, D. P., Lloyd, J. K., and Wolff, O. H. (1983). Vitamin E and neurological function. *Lancet* **1,** 225–228.

Muro, Y. (2001). Autoantibodies in atopic dermatitis. *J. Dermatol. Sci.* **25**(3), 171–179.

Murphy, S. P., and Barr, S. I. (2007). Dietary reference intakes for vitamins. *In* "Handbook of Vitamins," (J. Zempleni, R. B. Rucker, D. B. McCormick, and J. W. Suttie, Eds.), 4th ed., pp. 559–570. CRC Press.

Mustacich, D. J., Bruno, R. S., and Traber, M. G. (2007). Vitamin E. *In* "Vitamins and Hormones," (G. Litwack, Ed.), 76pp. 1–21. Elsevier Inc., California.

Nagel, J. E., Chopra, R. K., Chrest, F. J., McCoy, M. T., Schneider, E. L., Holbrook, N. J., and Adler, W. H. (1988). Decreased proliferation, interleukin 2 synthesis, and interleukin 2 receptor expression are accompanied by decreased mRNA expression in phytohemagglutinin stimulated cells from elderly donors. *J. Clin. Invest.* **81**(4), 1096–1102.

National Research Council (1989). Fat-soluble vitamins. *In* "Recommended Dietary Allowances" 10th ed., pp. 78–114. National Academy Press, Washington.

National Research Council (1994). Components of poultry diets. *In* "Nutrient Requirements of Poultry" 9th. Rev. ed., pp. 3–18. National Academy Press, Washington.

Nemec, M., Butler, G., Hidiroglou, M., Farnworth, E. R., and Nielsen, K. (1994). Effect of supplementing gilts' diets with different levels of vitamin E and different fats on the humoral and cellular immunity of gilts and their progeney. *J. Anim. Sci.* **72,** 665–676.

Nervig, R. M., Gough, P. M., Kaeberle, M. L., and Whetstone, C. (1986). Advances in Carriers and Adjuvants for Veterinary Biologic. Iowa State University.

Neuzil, J., Tomasetti, M., Mellick, A. S., Alleva, R., Salvatore, B. A., Birringer, M., and Fariss, M. W. (2004). Vitamin E analogues: A new class of inducers of apoptosis with selective anti-cancer effects. *Curr. Cancer Drug Targets* **4**(4), 355–372.

Niki, E., and Noguchi, N. (2004). Dynamics of antioxidant action of vitamin E. *Acc. Chem. Res.* **37**(1), 45–51.

Nockels, C. F. (1991). Vitamin E requirement of beef cattle: Influencing factors. BASF Technical Symposium Bloomington, Minnesota, pp. 40.

O'Connell, J., O'Sullivan, G. C., Collins, J. K., and Shanahan, F. (1996). The Fas counterattack: Fas mediated T cell killing by colon cancer cells expressing Fas ligand. *J. Exp. Med.* **184**(3), 1075–1082.

Odeleye, O. E., Eskelson, C. D., Mufti, S. I., and Watson, R. R. (1992). Vitamin E protection against nitrosamine-induced esophageal tumor incidence in mice immunocompromised by retroviral infection. *Carcinogenesis* **13**(10), 1811–1816.

Oski, F. A. (1980). Anemia in infancy: Iron deficiency and vitamin E deficiency. *Pediatr. Rev.* **1,** 247–253.

Ostrea, E. M., Balun, J. E., Winkler, R., and Porter, T. (1986). Influence of breast-feeding on the restoration of the low serum concentration of vitamin E and b-carotene in the newborn infant. *Am. J. Obstet. Gynecol.* **154,** 1014–1017.

Ouahchi, K., Arita, M., Kayden, H., Hentati, F., Ben Hamida, M., Sokol, R., Arai, H., Inoue, K., Mandel, J. L., and Koenig, M. (1995). Ataxia with isolated vitamin E deficiency is caused by mutations in the α-tocopherol transfer protein. *Nat. Genet.* **9,** 141–145.

Packer, L. (1992). Vitamin E, biological activity and health benefits: Overview. *In* "Vitamin E in Health and Disease: Biochemistry and Clinical Applications," (L. Packer and J. Fuchs, Eds.), 1st ed., pp. 977–982. Marcel Dekker Inc., New York.

Pahl, H. L., and Bauerle, P. A. (1994). Oxygen and the control of gene expression. *Bioessays* **16**(7), 497–502.

Pallast, E. G., Schouten, E. G., de Waart, F. G., Fonk, H. C., Doekes, G., von Blomberg, B. M., and Kok, F. J. (1999). Effect of 50- and 100-mg vitamin E supplements on cellular immune function in noninstitutionalized elderly persons. *Am. J. Clin. Nutr.* **69** (6), 1273–1281.

Panemangalore, M., and Lee, C. J. (1992). Evaluation of the indices of retinol and alpha-tocopherol status in free-living elderly. *J. Gerontol.* **47,** 98–104.

Parker, R. S. (1989). Dietary and biochemical aspects of vitamin E. *Adv. Food Nutr. Res.* **33,** 157–232.

Passi, S., Picardo, M., Morrone, A., De Luca, C., Ippolito, F., Rossi, L., and Rotilio, G. (1993). Study on plasma polyunsaturared phospholipids and vitamin E, and on erythrocyte glutathione peroxidase in high risk HIV infection categories and AIDS patients. *Clin. Chem. Enzym. Commun.* **5,** 169–177.

Patella, V., Florio, G., Giuliano, A., Oriente, A., Spadaro, G., Forte, V., Genovese, A., and Marone, G. (2000). Human mast cells and basophils in immune responses to infectious agents. *In* "Mast Cells and Basophils," (G. Marone, L. M. Lichtenstein, and S. J. Galli, Eds.), pp. 397–418. Academic Press, London.

Payette, H., Rola-Pleszczynski, M., and Ghadirian, P. (1990). Nutrition factors in relation to cellular and regulatory immune variables in a free-living elderly population. *Am. J. Clin. Nutr.* **52**(5), 927–932.

Pekmezci, D., and Cakiroglu, D. (2009). Investigation of immunmodulatory effects of levamisole and vitamin E on immunity and some blood parameters in newborn Jersey calves. *Vet. Res. Comm.* **33**(7), 711–721.

Peplowski, M. A., Mahan, D. C., Murray, F. A., Moxon, A. L., Cantor, A. H., and Ekstron, K. E. (1981). Effect of dietary and selenium in weanling swine antigenically challenged with sheep red blood cells. *J. Anim. Sci.* **51,** 344–351.

Pharazyn, A., Den Hartog, L. A., and Aherne, F. X. (1990). Vitamin E and its role in the nutrition of the gilt and sow: A review. *Livest. Prod. Sci.* **24**(1), 1–13.

Pinelli-Saavedra, A. (2003). Vitamin E in immunity and reproductive performance in pigs. *Reprod. Nutr. Dev.* **43**(5), 397–408.

Politis, H., Hidiroglou, M., Batra, T. R., Gilmore, J. A., Gorewit, R. C., and Scherf, H. (1995). Effects of vitamin E on immune function in dairy cows. *Am. J. Vet. Res.* **56,** 179–184.

Porter, J. M., Ivatury, R. R., Azimuddin, K., and Swami, R. (1999). Antioxidant therapy in the prevention of organ dysfunction syndrome and infectious complications after trauma: Early results of a prospective randomized study. *Am. Surg.* **65,** 478–483.

Pryor, W. A. (1986). Cancer and free radicals. *Basic Life Sci.* **39,** 45–59.

Pryor, W. A. (1987). Cigarette smoke and the involvement of free radical reactions in chemical carcinogenesis. *Br. J. Cancer* **55**(Suppl. VIII), 19–23.

Pryor, W. A. (2000). Vitamin E and heart disease: Basic science to clinical intervention trials. *Free Radic. Biol. Med.* **28**(1), 141–164.
Rabinowich, H., Reichert, T. E., Kashii, Y., Gastman, B. R., Bell, M. C., and Whiteside, T. L. (1998). Lymphocyte apoptosis induced by Fas ligand-expressing ovarian carcinoma cells. Implications for altered expression of T cell receptor in tumor-associated lymphocytes. *J. Clin. Invest.* **101**(11), 2579–2588.
Rader, D. J., and Brewer, H. B. (1993). Abetalipoproteinemia-new insights into lipoprotein assembly and vitamin E metabolism from a rare genetic disease. *JAMA* **270,** 865–869.
Rappaport, R. S., and Dodge, G. R. (1982). Prostaglandin E inhibits the production of human interleukin 2. *J. Exp. Med.* **155**(3), 943–948.
Reddy, P. G., Morrill, J. L., Minocha, H. C., Morrill, M. B., Dayton, A. D., and Frey, R. A. (1986). Effect of supplemental vitamin E on the immune system of calves. *J. Dairy Sci.* **69** (1), 164–171.
Reddy, P. G., Morrill, J. L., and Frey, R. A. (1987a). Vitamin E requirements of dairy calves. *J. Dairy Sci.* **70**(1), 123–129.
Reddy, P. G., Morrill, J. L., Minocha, H. C., and Stevenson, J. S. (1987b). Vitamin E is immunostimulatory in calves. *J. Dairy Sci.* **70,** 993–999.
Roberts-Thomson, I. C., Whittingham, S., Youngchaiyud, U., and Mackay, I. R. (1974). Ageing, immune response, and mortality. *Lancet* **2,** 368–370.
Roper, R. L., Brown, D. M., and Phipps, R. P. (1995). Prostaglandin E_2 promotes B lymphocyte Ig isotype switching to IgE. *J. Immunol.* **154**(1), 162–170.
Rumin, E. B., Stampfer, M. J., Ascherio, A., Giovannucci, E., Colditz, G. A., and Willett, W. C. (1993). Vitamin E consumption and the risk of coronary heart disease in men. *N. Engl. J. Med.* **328**(20), 1450–1456.
Ryan, A., Craig, L. D., and Finn, S. C. (1992). Nutrient intakes and dietary patterns of older Americans: A national survey. *J. Gerontol.* **47,** 145–150.
Sakai, S., and Moriguchi, S. (1997). Long-term feeding of high vitamin E diet improves the decreased mitogen response of rat splenic lymphocytes with aging. *J. Nutr. Sci. Vitaminol.* **43,** 113–122.
Sastre, J., Pallardo, F. V., Garcia de lá Asuncion, J., and Vina, J. (2000). Mitochondria, oxidative stress and aging. *Free Radic. Res.* **32,** 189–198.
Sato, Y., Hayiwara, K., Arai, H., and Inoue, K. (1991). Purification and characterization of the alpha-tocopherol transfer protein from rat liver. *FEBS Lett.* **288,** 41–45.
Sausenthaler, S., Loebel, T., Linseisen, J., Nagel, G., Magnussen, H., and Heinrich, J. (2009). Vitamin E intake in relation to allergic sensitization and IgE serum concentration. *Cent. Eur. J. Public Health* **17**(2), 79–85.
Schneider, E., Rolli-Derkinderen, M., Arock, M., and Dy, M. (2002). Trends in histamine research: New functions during immune responses and hematopoiesis. *Trends Immunol.* **23**(5), 255–263.
Schraufstätter, I., Hyslop, P. A., Jackson, J. H., and Cochrane, C. G. (1988). Oxidant-induced DNA damage of target cells. *J. Clin. Invest.* **82,** 1040–1250.
Schreck, R., Reiber, P., and Baeuerle, P. A. (1992a). Reactive oxygen intermediates as apparently widely used messengers in the activation of the NFkB transcription factor and HIV-1. *EMBO J.* **10,** 2247–2258.
Schreck, R., Albermann, K., and Baeuerle, P. A. (1992b). Nuclear factor kappa B: an oxidative stress-responsive transcription factor of eukaryotic cells. *Free Radic. Res. Commun.* **17,** 221–237(a review).
Scientific Committee for Food (1993). Nutrient and Energy Intakes for the European Community. Commission of the European Communities. Luxemburg.
Scott, M. L. (1980). Advances in our understanding of vitamin E. *Fed. Proc.* **39,** 2736–2739.
Scrivo, R., Di Franco, M., Spadaro, A., and Valesini, G. (2007). The immunology of rheumatoid arthritis. *Ann. N. Y. Acad. Sci.* **1108**(1), 312–322.

Serafini, M. (2000). Dietary vitamin E and T cell-mediated function in the elderly: Effectiveness and mechanism of action. *Int. J. Dev. Neurosci.* **18**(4–5), 401–410.

Sharp, A. K., and Colston, M. J. (1984). Elevated macrophage activity in nude mice. *Exp. Cell Biol.* **52,** 44–47.

Sheffy, B. E., and Schultz, R. D. (1979). Influence of vitamin E and selenium on immune response mechanism. *Fed. Proc.* **38,** 2139–2143.

Shoelson, S. E., Herrero, L., and Naaz, A. (2007). Obesity, inflammation, and insulin resistance. *Gastroenterology* **132**(6), 2169–2180.

Shrimpton, D. (1997). Vitamins and Minerals: A Scientific Evaluation of the Range of Safe Intakes. European Federation of Health Product Manufacturers Associations, Thames Ditton, UK.

Sies, H., and Murphy, M. E. (1981). Role of tocopherols in the protection of biological systems against oxidative damage. *J. Photochem. Photobiol. B* **8,** 211–224.

Spaulding, C., Guo, W., and Effros, R. B. (1999). Resistance to apoptosis in human CD8+ T cells that reach replicative senescence after multiple rounds of antigen-specific proliferation. *Exp. Gerontol.* **34**(5), 633–644.

Sprong, R. C., Winkelhuyzen-Janssen, A. M., Aarsman, C. J., van Oirschot, J. F., van der Bruggen, T., and van Asbeck, B. S. (1998). Low-dose N-acetylcysteine protects rats against endotoxin-mediated oxidative stress, but high dose increases mortality. *Am. J. Respir. Crit. Care Med.* **157,** 1283–1293.

Steger, P. J., and Muhlebach, S. F. (1998). Lipid peroxidation of i.v. lipid emulsions in TPN bags: The influence of tocopherols. *Nutrition* **14,** 179–185.

Steinberg, D., and Witztum, J. L. (1990). Lipoproteins and atherogenesis: Current concepts. *J. Am. Med. Assoc.* **264**(23), 3047–3052.

Stone, W. L., and Papas, A. M. (1997). Tocopherols and the etiology of colon cancer. *J. Natl. Cancer Inst.* **89**(14), 1006–1014.

Stumpf, D. A., Sokol, R., Bettis, D., Neville, H., Ringel, S., Angelini, C., and Bell, R. (1987). Friedreich's disease: V. Variant form with vitamin E deficiency and normal fat absorption. *Neurology* **37,** 68–74.

Suzuki, Y. J., and Packer, L. (1993). Inhibition of NF-kappa B activation by vitamin E derivatives. *Biochem. Biophys. Res. Commun.* **193**(1), 277–283.

Tada, J., Toi, Y., Yoshioka, T., Fujiwara, H., and Arata, J. (1994). Antinuclear antibodies in patients with atopic dermatitis and severe skin facial lesions. *Dermatology* **189**(1), 38–40.

Tak Cheung, H., Twu, J. S., and Richardson, A. (1983). Mechanism of the age-related decline in lymphocyte proliferation: role of IL-2 production and protein synthesis. *Exp. Gerontol.* **18**(6), 451–460.

Tanaka, J., Fujiwara, H., and Torisu, M. (1979). Vitamin E and immune response, enhancement of helper T-cell activity by dietary supplementation of vitamin E in mice. *Immunology* **38,** 727–734.

Tang, A. M., and Smit, E. (1998). Selected vitamins in HIV infection: A review. *AIDS Patient Care STDs* **12**(4), 263–273.

Tansey, M. G., McCoy, M. K., and Frank-Cannon, T. C. (2007). Neuroinflammatory mechanisms in Parkinson's disease: Potential environmental triggers, pathways, and targets for early therapeutic intervention. *Exp. Neurol.* **208**(1), 1–25.

Teige, J., Saxegaard, F., and Froslie, A. (1978). Influence of diet on experimental swine dysentery. *Acta Vet. Scand.* **19,** 133–146.

Tengerdy, R. P. (1989). Immunity and disease resistance in farm animals fed vitamin e supplement. *In* "Antioxidant Nutrients and the Immune Response," (A. Bendich, M. Phillips, and R. Tengerdy, Eds.), pp. 103–110. Plenum Press, New York.

Tengerdy, R. P., Heinzerling, R. H., Brown, G. L., and Mathias, M. M. (1973). Enhancement of the humoral immune response by vitamin E. *Inter. Arch. Allergy Immunol.* **44,** 221–232.

Tengerdy, R. P., Lacetera, N. G., and Nockels, C. F. (1990). Effect of beta carotene on disease protection and humoral immunity in chickens. *Avian Dis.* **34**(4), 848–854.

Traber, M. G. (1999). Vitamin E. *In* "Modern Nutrition in Health and Disease," (M. E. Shils, J. A. Olson, M. Shike, and A. C. Ross, Eds.), pp. 347–362. Williams & Wilkins, Baltimore.

Traber, M. G. (2007). Vitamin E. *In* "Handbook of Vitamins," (J. Zempleni, R. B. Rucker, D. B. McCormick, and J. W. Suttie, Eds.), 4th ed., pp. 153–174. CRC Press.

Traber, M. G., Sokol, R. J., Ringel, S. P., Neville, H. E., Thellman, C. A., and Kayden, H. J. (1987). Lack of tocopherol in peripheral nerves of vitamin E-deficient patients with peripheral neuropathy. *N. Engl. J. Med.* **317,** 262–265.

Traber, M. G., Carpentier, Y. A., Kayden, H. J., Richelle, M., Galeano, N. F., and Deckelbaum, R. J. (1993). Alterations in plasma alpha- and gammatocopherol concentrations in response to intravenous infusion of lipid emulsions in humans. *Metabolism* **42,** 701–709.

Tsai, A. C., Kelley, J. J., Peng, B., and Cook, N. (1978). Study on the effect of megavitamin E supplementation in man. *Am. J. Clin. Nutr.* **31,** 831–837.

Tsoureli-Nikita, E., Hercogova, J., Lotti, T., and Menchini, G. (2002). Evaluation of dietary intake of vitamin E in the treatment of atopic dermatitis: A study of the clinical course and evaluation of the immunoglobulin E serum levels. *Int. J. Dermatol.* **41**(3), 146–150.

Turner, R., and Finch, J. (1990). Immunological malfunctions associated with low selenium-vitamin E diets in lambs. *J. Comp. Pathol.* **102,** 99–109.

Unanue, E. R. (1980). Cooperation between mononuclear phagocytes and lymphocytes in immunity. *N. Engl. J. Med.* **303**(17), 977–985.

USP (1980). The United States Pharmacopeia. National Formulary. United States Pharmacopeial Convention, Rockville, MD.

Uzzo, R. G., Clark, P. E., Rayman, P., Bloom, T., Rybicki, L., Novick, A. C., Bukowski, R. M., and Finke, J. H. (1999). Alterations in NFkappaB activation in T lymphocytes of patients with renal cell carcinoma. *J. Natl. Cancer Inst.* **91**(8), 718–721.

Víctor, V. M., Guayerbas, N., Garrote, D., Del Río, M., and De la Fuente, M. (1999). Modulation of murine macrophage function by N-acetylcysteine in a model of endotoxic shock. *Biofactors* **10**(4), 347–357.

Wakikawa, A., Utsuyama, M., Wakabayashi, A., Kitagawa, M., and Hirokawa, K. (1999). Vitamin E enhances the immune functions of young but not old mice under restraint stress. *Exp. Gerontol.* **34,** 853–862.

Wang, Y., and Watson, R. R. (1994a). Potential therapeutics of vitamin E (tocopherol) in AIDS and HIV. *Drugs* **48**(3), 327–333.

Wang, Y., and Watson, R. R. (1994b). Vitamin E supplementation at various levels alters cytokine production by thymocytes during retrovirus infection causing murine AIDS. *Thymus* **22**(3), 153–165.

Wang, Y., Huang, D. S., Eskelson, C. D., and Watson, R. R. (1994). Long-term dietary vitamin E retards development of retrovirus-induced disregulation in cytokine production. *Clin. Immunol. Immunopathol.* **72**(1), 70–75.

Wang, Q., Redovan, C., Tubbs, R., Olencki, T., Klein, E., Kudoh, S., Finke, J., and Bukowski, R. M. (1995). Selective cytokine gene expression in renal cell carcinoma tumor cells and tumor-infiltrating lymphocytes. *Int. J. Cancer* **61**(6), 780–785.

Wang, X., Falcone, T., Attaran, M. D., Goldberg, J. M., Agarwal, A., and Sharma, R. K. (2002). Vitamin C and vitamin E supplementation reduce oxidative stres-induced embryo toxicity and improve the blastocyst development rate. *Fertil. Steril.* **78,** 1272–1277.

Watson, R. R., Zibadi, S., Vazquez, R., and Larson, D. (2005). Nutritional regulation of immunosenescence for heart health. *J. Nutr. Biochem.* **16**(2), 85–87.

Wayne, S. J., Rhyne, R. L., Garry, P. J., and Goodwin, J. S. (1990). Cell-mediated immunity as a predictor of morbidity and mortality in subjects over 60. *J. Gerontol.* **45**(2), 45–48.

Weber, P., Bendich, A., and Machlin, L. J. (1997). Vitamin E and human health: Rationale for determining recommended intake levels. *Nutrition* **13,** 450–460.

Wetterau, J. R., Aggerbeck, L. P., Laplaud, P. M., and McLean, L. R. (1991). Structural properties of the microsomal triglyceride-transfer protein complex. *Biochemistry* **30,** 4406–4412.

Wetterau, J. R., Aggerbeck, L. P., Bouma, M. E., Eisenberg, C., Munck, A., Hermier, M., Schmitz, J., Gay, G., Rader, D. J., and Gregg, R. E. (1992). Absence of microsomal triglyceride transfer protein in individuals with abetalipoproteinemia. *Science* **258,** 999–1001.

Wintergerst, E. S., Maggini, S., and Hornig, D. H. (2007). Contribution of selected vitamins and trace elements to immune function. *Ann. Nutr. Metab.* **51,** 301–323.

Wu, D., and Meydani, S. N. (2008). Age-associated changes in immune and inflammatory responses: Impact of vitamin E intervention. *J. Leukoc. Biol.* **84**(4), 900–914.

Wu, D., Han Sung, N., Meydani, M., and Meydani, S. N. (2006). Effect of concomitant consumption of fish oil and vitamin E on T cell mediated function in the elderly: A randomized double-blind trial. *J. Am. Coll. Nutr.* **25**(4), 300–306.

Wuryastuti, H., Stowe, H. D., Bull, R. W., and Miller, E. R. (1993). Effects of vitamin E and selenium on immune responses of peripheral blood, colostrum, and milk leukocytes of sows. *J. Anim. Sci.* **71**(9), 2464–2472.

Yates, A. A., Schlicker, S. A., and Suitor, C. W. (1998). Dietary reference intakes the new basis for recommendations for calcium and related nutrients, B vitamins, and choline. *J. Am. Diet. Assoc.* **98**(6), 699–706.

Yoshida, H., Yusin, M., Ren, I., Kuhlenkamp, J., Hirano, T., Stolz, A., and Kaplowitz, N. (1992). Identification, purification and immunochemical characterization of a tocopherol-binding protein in rat liver cytosol. *J. Lipid Res.* **33,** 343–350.

Young, R. C., Corder, M. P., Haynes, H. A., and DeVita, V. T. (1972). Delayed hypersensitivity in Hodgkin's disease. A study of 103 untreated patients. *Am. J. Med.* **52**(1), 63–72.

Zea, A. H., Rodriguez, P. C., Atkins, M. B., Hernandez, C., Signoretti, S., Zabaleta, J., McDermott, D., Quiceno, D., Youmans, A., O'Neill, A., Mier, J., and Ochoa, A. C. (2005). Arginase-producing myeloid suppressor cells in renal cell carcinoma patients: A mechanism of tumor evasion. *Cancer Res.* **65**(8), 3044–3048.

Zhang, S., Hunter, D. J., Forman, M. R., Rosner, B. A., Speizer, F. E., Colditz, G. A., Manson, J. E., Hankinson, S. E., and Willett, W. C. (1999). Dietary carotenoids and vitamins A, C, and E and risk of breast cancer. *J. Natl. Cancer Inst.* **91**(6), 547–556.

Zheng, K., Adjei, A. A., Shinjo, M., Shinjo, S., Todoriki, H., and Ariizumi, M. (1999). Effect of dietary vitamin E supplementation on murine nasal allergy. *Am. J. Med. Sci.* **318**(1), 49–54.

Ziemlanski, S., Wartanowicz, M., Klos, A., Raczka, A., and Klos, M. (1986). The effect of ascorbic acid and alpha-tocopherol supplementation on serum proteins and immunoglobulin concentration in the elderly. *Nutr. Int.* **2,** 1–5.

Zingg, J. M. (2007). Vitamin E and mast cells. *In* "Vitamins and Hormones," (G. Litwack, Ed.), Vol. 76, pp. 393–418. Elsevier Inc., California.

CHAPTER NINE

Vitamin D Effects on Lung Immunity and Respiratory Diseases

Sif Hansdottir *and* Martha M. Monick

Contents

Abstract

Our understanding of vitamin D metabolism and biological effects has grown exponentially in recent years and it has become clear that vitamin D has extensive immunomodulatory effects. The active vitamin D generating enzyme, 1α-hydroxylase, is expressed by the airway epithelium, alveolar macrophages, dendritic cells, and lymphocytes indicating that active vitamin D can be produced locally within the lungs. Vitamin D generated in tissues is responsible for many of the immunomodulatory actions of vitamin D. The effects of vitamin D within the lungs include increased secretion of the antimicrobial peptide cathelicidin, decreased chemokine production, inhibition of dendritic cell activation, and alteration of T-cell activation. These cellular effects are important for host responses against infection and the development of allergic lung diseases like

Department of Medicine, University of Iowa Carver College of Medicine and Veterans Administration Medical Center, Iowa City, Iowa, USA

Vitamins and Hormones, Volume 86
ISSN 0083-6729, DOI: 10.1016/B978-0-12-386960-9.00009-5

asthma. Epidemiological studies do suggest that vitamin D deficiency predisposes to viral respiratory tract infections and mycobacterial infections and that vitamin D may play a role in the development and treatment of asthma. Randomized, placebo-controlled trials are lacking but ongoing.

I. Introduction

Emerging information on vitamin D physiology has revealed that vitamin D is not merely a micronutrient that plays a role in calcium homeostasis but a pluripotent hormone with extensive immunomodulatory functions. Studies have shown that the enzyme 1α-hydroxylase, which catalyzes the last and rate limiting step in the synthesis of active 1,25-dihydroxyvitamin D_3 (1,25D), and the vitamin D receptor (VDR), which mediates the actions of vitamin D, are expressed widely in the body, including the lungs and cells of the immune system. These observations have led to a surge of epidemiological and basic research studies examining the effects of vitamin D on immune responses, lung infections, and the development of lung diseases. Vitamin D insufficiency has been linked to increased risk of infections, in particular, viral respiratory tract infections (Cannell *et al.*, 2006, 2008; Ginde *et al.*, 2009b; Laaksi *et al.*, 2007; Wayse *et al.*, 2004) and tuberculosis (Bornman *et al.*, 2004; Liu *et al.*, 2007b; Martineau *et al.*, 2007a,b; Roth *et al.*, 2004, 2008; Wilkinson *et al.*, 2000). Vitamin D may also play a role in the development of obstructive lung diseases like asthma and COPD (Brehm *et al.*, 2010; Janssens *et al.*, 2009; Sutherland *et al.*, 2010). This chapter focuses on lung-specific vitamin D metabolism, immune effects of vitamin D, and the potential role of vitamin D in the development and treatment of lung diseases.

II. Lung Immune Functions

The respiratory tract has a surface area of $\sim$70 m^2 and is in direct and continuous contact with the surrounding environment. Despite continuous exposure to potential pathogens only rarely do the lungs become colonized or infected. A local defense system with components of both innate and adaptive immunity has evolved to discriminate between nonpathogenic antigens and potential pathogens and to clear pathogens.

The innate immune system involves a rapid, nonspecific, recognition of and response to almost any pathogen. Only those antigens that penetrate the innate immune responses evoke the more specific adaptive immune responses. The main players in innate immunity in the lungs include the airway epithelium itself, alveolar macrophages, and dendritic cells. They all express pattern recognition receptors (PRRs) and ligand engagement results in activation of intracellular signaling pathways that mobilize antimicrobial defenses, inflammation, and adaptive immune responses (Basu and Fenton, 2004). The airway epithelium is the first line of defense and functions as a physical barrier to prevent the entry of inhaled pathogens. When the airway epithelium recognizes the presence of a pathogen it responds by releasing antimicrobials, chemokines, and cytokines. Alveolar macrophages (AMs) recognize, phagocytose, and remove inhaled material. They are activated either in response to pathogens or through an autocrine/paracrine response to cytokines. Activation leads to enhanced phagocytosis and killing of pathogens as well as coordination of both innate and adaptive immune responses. The third major innate immune effector cells in the lung are dendritic cells. Dendritic cells use PRR's to monitor the local environment for pathogens. When a pathogen is encountered, it is ingested and its proteins are processed into peptides which are then presented at the surface of the dendritic cell. Activated dendritic cells produce chemokines and migrate to local lymph nodes where they present the antigenic peptides bound to major histocompatibility complex (MHC) molecules to naïve T-cells (CD4+ T-helper cells and CD8+ T-cytotoxic cells) and induce their activation and differentiation. Dendritic cells thus serve as a link between innate and adaptive immune responses. Vitamin D can influence all three innate immune effectors in the lungs and thus may play an important role in how the lung recognizes and responds to pathogens.

Activation of the innate immune system drives activation of the long-term adaptive immune system (Iwasaki and Medzhitov, 2010). Adaptive immune responses involve the ability of T- and B-lymphocytes to produce cytokines and immunoglobulins, respectively. All phases of the adaptive immune response are specific to unique antigen, from recognition of the antigen by antibody (humoral) or T-lymphocyte (cell-mediated) through lymphocyte activation, to effector function (elimination of antigen) and the development of immunologic memory (Mak and Saunders, 2005). Upon activation, memory T-cells downregulate lymphoid-tissue-homing receptors and upregulate tissue-specific-adhesion molecules and can now migrate to nonlymphoid tissues like the lungs (Holt *et al.*, 2008). Further, once activated, T_H (CD4+) cells differentiate into T_H1, T_H2, or T_H17 effector cells. The effector cells are characterized by the production of distinct set of cytokines (Medzhitov, 2007). Activation of B-cells and their differentiation into antibody-secreting plasma cells can be triggered directly by antigen but usually requires helper T-cells. Last, regulatory T-cells (T_{Regs}) are important for the control of peripheral T-cell responses. In relation to the lungs, they are believed to have key roles in the protection against the inflammatory sequela of airway infections and in the protection against the induction and expression of atopic disease (Holt *et al.*, 2008). There is data to support both indirect (dendritic cells) and direct (T- and B-lymphocytes) effects of vitamin D on adaptive immune responses.

The respiratory tract is continuously exposed to antigens, some of which are pathogenic and some of which are not. A specialized lung immune system has evolved that can recognize and respond to potential pathogens but does not get activated by nonpathogenic antigens which would result in chronic inflammation and tissue damage. The following chapters will focus on how vitamin D may affect cells involved in lung immune responses at all levels, that is, airway epithelium, alveolar macrophages, dendritic cells, and T- and B-cells and thus can have significant overall immunomodulatory effects in the lungs.

III. 1,25-Dihydroxyvitamin D is Generated Locally in the Lungs

Humans get vitamin D through synthesis in the skin following UVB exposure and to a lesser extent from limited dietary sources. Vitamin D from the skin or diet is metabolized primarily in the liver to 25-hydroxyvitamin D_3 (25D; Ponchon *et al.*, 1969). 25D is the "storage form" of vitamin D and is used to determine the vitamin D status of individuals. The last and rate limiting step in the synthesis of "active" 1,25D is catalyzed by the mitochondrial enzyme 1α-hydroxylase and is conventionally known to take place in the kidneys. Renal 1α-hydroxylase activity is under stringent regulation by parathyroid hormone, calcium, calcitonin, phosphorus, and 1,25D itself (Zehnder *et al.*, 1999). Vitamin D is inactivated by the ubiquitous enzyme, 24-hydroxylase, whose expression is inducible by 1,25D, thus creating a negative feedback loop (Holick, 2007). The biological effects of vitamin D are achieved through the regulation of gene expression mediated by VDR Baker *et al.*, 1988). Active vitamin D binds to VDR, and upon ligand binding, the receptor dimerizes with the retinoic X receptor (RXR; MacDonald *et al.*, 1993). The VDR/RXR complex binds to vitamin D responsive elements (VDREs) within the promoter regions of vitamin D-regulated genes (Sutton and MacDonald, 2003).

It is increasingly recognized that localized synthesis of 1,25D rather than systemic production is responsible for many of the immune effects of vitamin D. Extra-renal expression of 1α-hydroxylase has been found in various cells of the immune system including AMs (Adams *et al.*, 1983; Reichel *et al.*, 1987a,b), dendritic cells (Fritsche *et al.*, 2003; Hewison *et al.*, 2003; Sigmundsdottir *et al.*, 2007), and lymphocytes (Chen *et al.*, 2007; Sigmundsdottir *et al.*, 2007) as well as in airway epithelia (Hansdottir *et al.*, 2008; Table 9.1). Locally formed 1,25D acts in an autocrine or paracrine

Table 9.1 Local production and effects of 1,25D in the respiratory tract

Cell type	Conversion of 25D → 1,25D	1,25D effects	References
Airway epithelium	Constitutive	Increases CD14 and cathelicidin; dampens IFN-β and chemokine response during viral infection	Hansdottir *et al.* (2008, 2010)
Alveolar macrophages	Upon activation	Increases the antimicrobial peptide cathelicidin	Liu *et al.* (2006, 2007a,b)
Dendritic cells	Increases with differentiation	Inhibits dendritic cell differentiation, maturation, and function; decreases IL-12 and increases IL-10; alters T-cell activation	Fritsche *et al.* (2003), Sigmundsdottir *et al.* (2007), Piemonti *et al.* (2000), Penna *et al.* (2005)
T-lymphocytes	At least when activated	Inhibits proliferation; modulates cytokine production—inhibits Th1 and Th17 cytokines but induces T_{Regs}	Sigmundsdottir *et al.* (2007), Lemire *et al.* (1995), Daniel *et al.* (2008), Mora *et al.* (2008), Penna *et al.* (2005)
B-lymphocytes	Unclear	Inhibits proliferation of activated B-cells and generation of plasma cells	Chen *et al.* (2007)

fashion to modulate cell proliferation, cell differentiation, and immune function (Bell, 1998; Hewison *et al.*, 2007; White, 2008).

A. Airway epithelium

Defense systems have evolved to clear and inactivate inhaled pathogens so that despite continual exposure to potential antigens, the lung is generally maintained in a quiescent, noninflamed state (Kohlmeier and Woodland, 2008). The airway epithelium is constantly exposed to potentially pathogenic microorganisms. Recognition of pathogens by airway epithelial cells results in activation of intracellular signaling pathways and the end result is transcription of genes for a variety of effector molecules, including antimicrobials, type I interferons, and proinflammatory cytokines and chemokines (Bartlett *et al.*, 2008).

Recent work has found that airway epithelium exposed to the "storage" form of vitamin D is able to generate "active" vitamin D, potentially creating localized areas with higher 1,25D levels than are seen in serum (Hansdottir *et al.*, 2008). Primary human airway epithelial cells express relatively high mRNA levels of 1α-hydroxylase and lower levels of the inactivating 24-hydroxylase at baseline. Unlike alveolar macrophages, which need to be stimulated to convert 25D to 1,25D, airway epithelial cells constitutively generate 1,25D. Not only do airway epithelial cells produce active vitamin D at baseline, they also respond to pathogens by increasing the machinery needed to convert 25D to 1,25D. Viral infection induces expression of 1α-hydroxylase and increases conversion of 25D to 1,25D, which may be of benefit to the host response against the virus (Hansdottir *et al.*, 2008).

Local generation of active vitamin D in the lung potentially regulates pulmonary immune responses. Active vitamin D, generated by airway epithelium, directly increases expression of VDR-regulated genes that are involved in recognition and killing of pathogens, including the TLR co-receptor CD14 and the antimicrobial peptide cathelicidin (Hansdottir *et al.*, 2008). When airway epithelium is infected with a virus, 1,25D modulates the expression of inflammatory chemokines and cytokines in response to the virus (Hansdottir *et al.*, 2010). This will be discussed further in the Section IV.B.

B. Alveolar macrophages

Like airway epithelium, AMs can also generate active vitamin D. In contrast to the constitutive activity of 1α-hydroxylase in airway epithelium, AMs need to be stimulated before converting inactive to active vitamin D. The first description of extrarenal 1α-hydroxylase was in patients with the granulomatous disease, sarcoidosis. It had been noted that some patients with sarcoidosis had hypercalcemia and high vitamin D levels (Barbour *et al.*, 1981; Papapoulos *et al.*, 1979). Subsequently, Adams *et al.* (1983) showed that AMs from patients with sarcoidosis converted 25D to 1,25D whereas AMs from patients with idiopathic pulmonary fibrosis did not. It has since been shown that AMs from normal subjects do not constitutively express 1α-hydroxylase and convert 25D to 1,25D but can do so if activated with TLR 2/1 ligands, IFNγ or LPS (Liu *et al.*, 2006; Reichel *et al.*, 1987a,b). This is different from renal 1α-hydroxylase, which is mainly regulated by mediators of calcium and bone homeostasis. Moreover, activated macrophages lack negative feedback by 25D and 1,25D (Dusso *et al.*, 1997). A nonfunctional alternatively spliced form of 24-hydroxylase has been found in the cytoplasm of macrophages that may be responsible for impeding the access of 25D and 1,25D to the enzyme and preventing their catabolism (Ren *et al.*, 2005). The lack of a negative feedback system contributes to the increased serum vitamin D levels in patients with granulomatous diseases.

Expression of 1α-hydroxylase by stimulated alveolar macrophages, production of 1,25D, and lack of active 24-hydroxylase cannot only have beneficial effects on host defense but also have pathological implications. However, TLR 2/1 ligands (mycobacterial antigen) activate alveolar macrophages, induce 1α-hydroxylase and increase 1,25D which leads to an increase in the vitamin D-regulated antimicrobial peptide cathelicidin. Cathelicidin facilitates killing of *Mycobacterium tuberculosis* (Liu *et al.*, 2006). However, overproduction of 1,25D in macrophages in sarcoidosis, tuberculosis, and various other granulomatous conditions can result in hypercalcemia (Adams *et al.*, 1983). Epidemiological data suggests that low vitamin D is associated with susceptibility to tuberculosis and severity of disease (Gao *et al.*, 2010). Available studies on vitamin D and tuberculosis will be reviewed in the following Section IV.A.

C. Dendritic cells

Dendritic cells play a key role in the initiation and regulation of adaptive immune responses to inhaled antigens. Dendritic cells form a contiguous network throughout the airway epithelium. In the steady state, dendritic cells are specialized for uptake and processing of environmental antigens but lack the capacity for efficient antigen presentation (Holt *et al.*, 2008). If dendritic cells sense an abnormal state, they mature. Maturation is characterized by migration to regional lymph nodes, downregulation of antigen uptake, and an enhanced capacity to activate naïve T-cells. This process of dendritic cell maturation involves changes in the expression of chemokine receptors and is associated with upregulation of costimulatory molecules and markers of dendritic cell activation (Upham, 2003).

Human blood monocytes can be differentiated to dendritic cells by *in vitro* culture with GM-CSF, IL-4, or IL-13. Monocyte-derived dendritic cells constitutively express 1α-hydroxylase. Following terminal differentiation induced by TNFα, IFNγ, polyI:C, or LPS, there is marked increase in expression and function of 1α-hydroxylase (Fritsche *et al.*, 2003; Hewison *et al.*, 2003). Further, dendritic cells metabolize vitamin D precursors to active 1,25D (Fritsche *et al.*, 2003; Hewison *et al.*, 2003; Sigmundsdottir *et al.*, 2007). In contrast, VDR expression may be downregulated during the maturation process (Hewison *et al.*, 2003). 1,25D generated by the dendritic cells themselves and exogenous 1,25D inhibit dendritic cell differentiation, maturation, and function by decreasing the expression of MHC class II and costimulatory molecules, decreasing production of IL-12, and increasing secretion of IL-10 (D'Ambrosio *et al.*, 1998; Mora *et al.*, 2008; Penna and Adorini, 2000; Piemonti *et al.*, 2000). By modulating dendritic cell activation, 1,25D alters T-cell activation favoring the induction of regulatory T-cells and leads to T-cell hyporesponsiveness (Penna and Adorini, 2000; Penna *et al.*, 2005). It has been postulated that inhibition of dendritic cell maturation and T-cell hyporesponsiveness may explain some of the immunosuppressive activities of 1,25D including control of autoimmune diseases and transplantation tolerance (Adorini and Penna, 2008; Gregori *et al.*, 2001; Griffin *et al.*, 2001).

D. Lymphocytes

Vitamin D not only affects lymphocytes indirectly via its effects on dendritic cells as described above but also has direct effects on T-cells and likely B-cells. Activated T-lymphocytes and B-lymphocytes have been found to express VDR and 1α-hydroxylase and to convert 25D to 1,25D (Bhalla *et al.*, 1983; Chen *et al.*, 2007; Provvedini *et al.*, 1986; Sigmundsdottir *et al.*, 2007).

Antigen-mediated activation of naïve T-helper (T_H) cells results in the generation of pluripotent T_H0 lymphocytes that synthesize a broad spectrum of cytokines (IL-2, IL-4, IL-10, and IFNγ) (Adams and Hewison, 2008). Proliferating T_H0 lymphocytes are then able to differentiate into T_H1 (IL-2, IFNγ, TNF), T_H2 (IL-3, IL-4, IL-5, and IL-10), or T_H17 (IL-17) lymphocytes with a more distinct cytokine profile. Vitamin D suppresses the production of T_H1 and T_H17 (Daniel *et al.*, 2008; Lemire *et al.*, 1995; Mora *et al.*, 2008) cytokines but its effects on the production of T_H2 cytokines is less clear. Early studies suggested that 1,25D enhanced the development of T_H2 cells (Boonstra *et al.*, 2001) but subsequent studies indicate that 1,25D does not favor the T_H2 phenotype (Pichler *et al.*, 2002; Staeva-Vieira and Freedman, 2002). Recent studies have shown that the effects of vitamin D are complex and include the generation of IL-10 producing T-regulatory lymphocytes (previously known as suppressor T-cells; Penna *et al.*, 2005). IL-10 is a major anti-inflammatory and immunosuppressive cytokine that inhibits both T_H1 and T_H2 immune responses (Moore *et al.*, 2001). In general, the immunomodulatory effects of vitamin D on T-cell-mediated immunity may be beneficial for conditions in which the immune system is directed at self, that is, autoimmune diseases and graft rejection in transplantation (Barrat *et al.*, 2002; Bikle, 2009; Gregori *et al.*, 2001). In direct relation to the lungs, there is evidence that T_{Reg} function is impaired in allergic and asthmatic disease (Lloyd and Hawrylowicz, 2009). Vitamin D has been shown to reverse steroid resistance, through induction of IL-10 secreting T-cells, in patients with asthma (Xystrakis *et al.*, 2006). The role of vitamin D in asthma pathogenesis and treatment will be discussed in the Section V.

The actions of 1,25D on B-cells are not well studied. A recent study found that 1,25D suppresses immunoglobulin production and B-cell proliferation and differentiation (Chen *et al.*, 2007). This study also found that patients with systemic lupus erythematosus have low vitamin levels and hypothesized that low vitamin D levels may contribute to the B-cell hyperactivity that is seen in this disease.

IV. Vitamin D and Lung Infections

A. Mycobacteria

It was first noted over one century ago that UV light seemed to help in the treatment of mycobacterial infections. The 1903 Nobel Prize in Medicine was awarded to Niels Finsen for demonstrating that UV light is beneficial to patients with lupus vulgaris (tuberculosis of the skin). In the late nineteenth century, Hermann Brehmer built the first sanatorium for the treatment of tuberculosis (Liu *et al.*, 2007a). Patients were exposed to plentiful amounts of high altitude, fresh air, and good nutrition. It has since been speculated that patients with tuberculosis benefitted from sanatoriums because of UV light exposure and increased production of vitamin D precursors in the skin. The first *in vitro* studies looking at vitamin D and *M. tuberculosis* were published in the 1980s. These studies demonstrated that adding 1,25D to *M. tuberculosis*-infected human monocytes and macrophages reduced the intracellular bacterial load (Crowle *et al.*, 1987; Rook *et al.*, 1986). This observation has been followed by a series of observational studies suggesting that individuals with low 25D levels are more susceptible to *M. tuberculosis* infection and often have a more severe course of disease (Gibney *et al.*, 2008; Nnoaham and Clarke, 2008; Ustianowski *et al.*, 2005; Wilkinson *et al.*, 2000). Case-control studies have also found an association between VDR polymorphisms and susceptibility to tuberculosis, in particular, in individuals with low 25D levels (Bornman *et al.*, 2004; Lewis *et al.*, 2005; Roth *et al.*, 2004; Wilkinson *et al.*, 2000).

Several different mechanisms have been proposed for how vitamin D may increase antimicrobial actions of monocytes and macrophages. A multiplicity of studies has been published recently indicating that a vitamin D-induced antimicrobial peptide, cathelicidin, plays a key role. The first study was a translational study published in 2006, showing that adequate 25D levels are required for TLR2/1 activation (by a mycobacterial ligand) and subsequent 1α-hydroxylase and VDR-dependent expression of cathelicidin. This study also revealed increased killing of mycobacteria by macrophages in the presence of 25D (Liu *et al.*, 2006). In a subsequent study of peripheral blood monocytes infected with recombinant mycobacteria, vitamin D strongly induced cathelicidin mRNA and reduced the growth of mycobacteria in a dose-dependent fashion (Martineau *et al.*, 2007a,b). Another study showed a direct correlation between serum 25D levels and monocyte expression of cathelicidin following treatment with TLR 2/1 and TLR 4 ligands. In the same study, *in vivo* supplementation of vitamin D enhanced *ex vivo* innate immune responses by rescuing TLR-mediated suppression of cathelicidin expression (Adams *et al.*, 2009). Last, a study using human monocytic cells found that siRNA knockdown of 1,25D induced cathelicidin resulting in complete loss of antimicrobial activity (Liu *et al.*, 2007b; Fig. 9.1). Alternative mechanisms that have been proposed for the effects of vitamin D include 1,25D induction of superoxide burst and enhancement of phagolysosome fusion both of which are mediated through the phosphatidylinositol 3-kinase pathway (Hmama *et al.*, 2004; Sly *et al.*, 2001).

Human trials looking at vitamin D for prevention or treatment of tuberculosis have been performed. In a double-blinded randomized controlled trial, 192 healthy adult TB contacts were randomized to receive a single oral dose of vitamin D (2.5 mg = 100,000 IU) or placebo. Six weeks later, a functional whole blood assay to assess growth of recombinant reporter mycobacteria *in vitro* (BCG-*lux* assay) was performed. IFN-γ responses to *M. tuberculosis* antigens were also determined. The investigators found that vitamin D significantly enhanced the ability of participants' whole blood to restrict growth of the reporter mycobacteria but did not affect antigen-stimulated IFN-γ secretion (Martineau *et al.*, 2007a,b). Two small randomized studies have looked at adding vitamin D to treatment regimens for tuberculosis and showed faster resolution of symptoms and earlier sputum conversion to culture negativity in patients given vitamin D (Morcos *et al.*, 1998; Nursyam *et al.*, 2006). A larger randomized, double-blind, placebo control trial included 365 patients with TB starting treatment and gave 100,000 IU of vitamin D at inclusion and again 5 and 8 months after the start of treatment. No differences were found in a clinical severity score (TB score), sputum conversion, or 12-month mortality between patients treated with vitamin D or placebo (Wejse *et al.*, 2009). Of note is that 25D levels in the two groups were similar when measured at 2 and 8 months, suggesting that perhaps the dose of vitamin D used was insufficient.

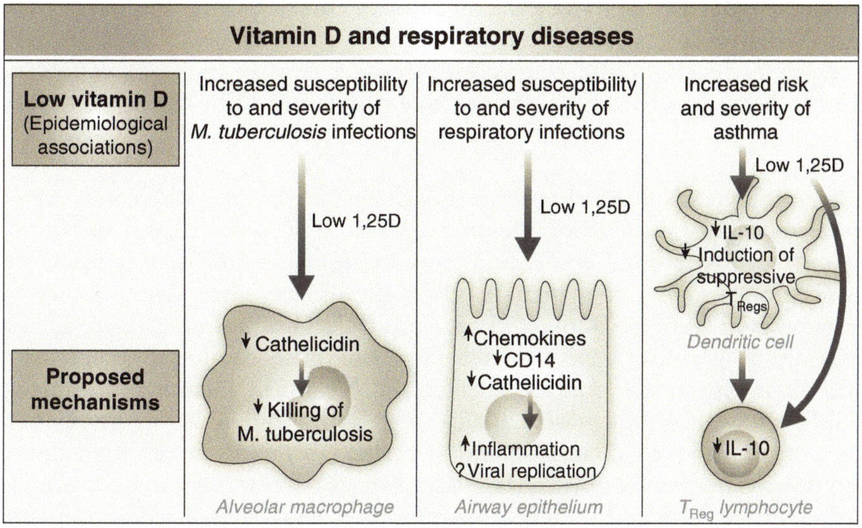

Figure 9.1 *Epidemiological associations between vitamin D deficiency and lung diseases and proposed mechanisms.* Vitamin D deficiency appears to increase susceptibility to TB infections due to lack of induction of the cathelicidin antimicrobial peptide. Vitamin D deficient individuals also report more frequent respiratory tract infections perhaps due to less production of cathelicidin and/or increased production of chemokines leading to uncontrolled inflammatory response. Lastly, vitamin D deficiency has been associated with higher prevalence of asthma and a more severe course of this disease. Two mechanisms have been proposed: (i) Increased risk of respiratory viral infection. (ii) Lack of vitamin D suppressive effects on adaptive immunity, in particular dendritic cells and T regulatory cells.

To date there is ample evidence that vitamin D inhibits growth of mycobacteria *in vivo*. Epidemiological studies suggest that low vitamin D levels increase the susceptibility to and severity of tuberculosis. Clinical trials looking at vitamin D for the treatment of tuberculosis have provided conflicting results and it remains unclear whether vitamin D supplementation is beneficial. Several clinical trials are ongoing that are investigating the impact of vitamin D supplementation on response to treatment of *M. tuberculosis* (www.clinicaltrials.gov).

B. Respiratory infections

Seasonal variation in the incidence of communicable diseases, in particular, respiratory tract infections, is among the oldest observations in population biology, dating back to ancient Greece (Lipsitch and Viboud, 2009). Several mechanisms have been hypothesized to explain this observation, one of which is seasonal variation in vitamin D levels. It has been noted that the peak incidence of respiratory tract infections coincides with the time of the year when there is insufficient UVB light to produce vitamin D, and vitamin D levels in the population are at a low (Cannell *et al.*, 2006, 2008). As our understanding of the role of vitamin D in innate immunity has increased, this hypothesis has gained increased popularity. Further, circumstantial evidence supporting the role of vitamin D comes from epidemiological studies that have shown that children with rickets are at increased risk of respiratory infections (Muhe *et al.*, 1997; Rehman, 1994). More recently, several epidemiological studies have consistently found an association between low vitamin D levels and increased susceptibility to respiratory infections (Aloia and Li-Ng, 2007; Ginde *et al.*, 2009b; Laaksi *et al.*, 2007; Wayse *et al.*, 2004). The largest of those studies was a secondary analysis of the Third National Health and Nutrition Examination Survey (NHANES-III; Ginde *et al.*, 2009b). This study looked at the association between 25D levels of nearly 19,000 participants and self-reported upper respiratory tract infections. After adjusting for demographic and clinical characteristics, lower 25D levels were independently associated with recent respiratory tract infections. Preliminary evidence also suggests an association between VDR polymorphisms and acute lower respiratory tract infection in children. A study of 56 children hospitalized with lower respiratory tract infection (predominantly viral bronchiolitis) found that the odds of infection were higher in children with the *Fok*I *ff* VDR genotype (Roth *et al.*, 2008) when compared with the *Fok*I *FF* genotype (Roth *et al.*, 2008).

At the basic science level, we have recently shown that airway epithelium converts 25D to 1,25D which raises the possibility of higher levels of 1,25D locally in the lungs than are seen in serum (Hansdottir *et al.*, 2008). We have also shown that viral infection increases the amount of 1,25D generated by the airway epithelium. We believe that the increase in local 1,25D in airways will contribute to decreased tissue damage, while maintaining viral clearance. The studies supporting this conclusion are described below.

When examining the role of vitamin D in airway antiviral responses, the transcription factor, nuclear factor-κB (NF-κB) is a potential regulatory point. NF-κB is a well established key player in multiple physiological processes including innate- and adaptive-immune responses and inflammation (Holt *et al.*, 2008). IκBα inhibits the NF-κB pathway by binding to NF-κB subunits in the cytoplasm and inhibiting translocation to the nucleus (Li and Verma, 2002). Relevant to vitamin D control of airway epithelial cell immune responses, we have shown that vitamin D induces IκBα in airway epithelium, leading to less induction of NF-κB-driven genes during viral infection. The end result is decreased secretion of inflammatory chemokines but no change in viral clearance (Hansdottir *et al.*, 2010). While vitamin D dampens expression of inflammatory chemokines, we have also shown that it increases expression of CD14 and cathelicidin which serve a role in recognizing and eliminating pathogens, including viruses.

Combined, these results suggest that vitamin D may potentiate innate immunity while controlling the potentially harmful inflammatory response (Hansdottir *et al.*, 2008, 2010; Fig. 9.1).

Two randomized placebo-controlled trials looking at vitamin D supplementation on respiratory tract infections were recently published. In the former study, 162 adults were given 2000 IU units of vitamin D daily or placebo for 12 weeks. A questionnaire was administered biweekly to record the incidence and severity of upper respiratory tract infection symptoms. This study found no difference in the incidence or severity between the groups (Li-Ng *et al.*, 2009). The second randomized trial looked at the incidence of influenza A in school children treated with 1200 IU vitamin D daily or placebo. In this study, influence A occurred in 18/167 (10.8%) of children in the vitamin D group compared with 31/167 (18.6) in the placebo group (relative risk 0.58; 95% CI 0.34–0.99; $P = 0.04$).

More rigorously designed randomized, placebo-controlled, clinical trials are warranted to further explore and establish the role of vitamin D in preventing and/or treating respiratory tract infections. A trial of vitamin D supplementation for the prevention of influenza and other respiratory infections is ongoing (www.clinicaltrials.gov).

V. Vitamin D and Obstructive Lung Diseases

A. Asthma

Asthma is a chronic inflammatory disorder that causes an increase in airways hyperresponsiveness leading to recurrent episodes of wheezing and shortness of breath. The prevailing consensus is that the immunological bases of allergic disease like asthma results from inappropriate T_H2 responses to common, harmless, airborne antigens. These reactions are normally suppressed by T_{Regs} which maintain airway tolerance (Lloyd and Hawrylowicz, 2009). There is increasing evidence that one mechanism for the development of asthma is imbalance between regulatory and effector T-cells and that the ability to enhance regulatory function may represent an effective treatment for asthma (Lloyd and Hawrylowicz, 2009; Robinson, 2009).

The prevalence of asthma has been steadily increasing over the past several decades and over the same period of time vitamin D insufficiency has also been on the rise. The prevalence of both conditions has been linked to African American race, obesity, and immigration to westernized countries (Litonjua and Weiss, 2007). These observations have prompted the hypothesis that vitamin D deficiency is an important contributor to the asthma epidemic. Epidemiological studies have found that vitamin D insufficiency is common in asthmatics and is associated with increased asthma severity and hospitalizations (Brehm *et al.*, 2009, 2010; Freishtat *et al.*, 2010;

Sutherland *et al.*, 2010). If such an association exists, it may be mediated through increased risk of respiratory viral infection in vitamin D-deficient individuals or by the effects of vitamin D on adaptive immunity, in particular, T-regulatory cells (Litonjua, 2009).

Vitamin D modulates adaptive immunity both indirectly via inhibition of dendritic cell maturation and directly via its effects on T_{Regs}. Regulatory T-cells can either develop as a normal part of the immune system (naturally occurring T_{Regs}) or in response to particular antigenic exposure (induced/adaptive T_{Regs}; Xystrakis *et al.*, 2007). Naturally occurring T_{Regs} are characterized by the expression of the forkhead winged transcription factor FoxP3, whereas induced T_{Regs} may be FoxP3+ or FoxP3− (Dimeloe *et al.*, 2010). Pretreatment of dendritic cells with vitamin D and subsequent coculture with CD4+ cells leads to induction of CD4+FoxP3+ T_{Regs} with suppressive activity (Penna *et al.*, 2005). 1,25D also acts directly on CD4+ T-cells and promotes an IL-10 secreting T_{Reg} population (Barrat *et al.*, 2002; Fig. 9.1). IL-10 inhibits many functions relevant to asthma and has been proposed to play a role in maintaining immune homoeostasis in the airways (Hawrylowicz and O'Garra, 2005). An inverse correlation exists between the presence of IL-10 and the incidence and severity of asthma.

Glucocorticosteroids are the principal controller therapy for patients with persistent asthma but there is a significant variability in the response to this treatment and a proportion of patients do not achieve optimal asthma control despite high doses (Sutherland *et al.*, 2010). Glucocorticosteroids increase T_{Regs} and IL-10 synthesis (Karagiannidis *et al.*, 2004) and the induction may be enhanced by 1,25D (Barrat *et al.*, 2002; Xystrakis *et al.*, 2006, 2007). CD4+ T-cells from steroid-resistant asthmatics fail to demonstrate increased IL-10 synthesis following stimulation in the presence of a glucocorticosteroid (Hawrylowicz *et al.*, 2002). This defect in steroid induced IL-10 can be overcome by the addition of 1,25D to the T-cell culture (Xystrakis *et al.*, 2006). Epidemiological evidence supports a role for vitamin D on the effects of glucocorticosteroids. Low vitamin D levels have been associated with increased use of corticosteroids and reduced *in vitro* glucocorticoid response (Brehm *et al.*, 2009; Searing *et al.*, 2010; Sutherland *et al.*, 2010).

To summarize, vitamin D deficiency is common in asthmatic patients and vitamin D supplementation may result in improvement in asthma severity and treatment response to corticosteroids, likely via induction of T_{Regs} and secretion of IL-10. It should be noted that not all the data support a positive role for vitamin D on the development of asthma. The hypothesis that vitamin D may cause asthma because of inhibition of T_H1 responses also exists (Gale *et al.*, 2008; Hypponen *et al.*, 2004). Several clinical trials are ongoing that are looking at vitamin D and asthma, ranging from maternal supplementation during pregnancy and prevention of childhood asthma to the use of vitamin D as a treatment in individuals with asthma (www.clinicaltrials.gov).

B. Chronic obstructive pulmonary disease

Chronic obstructive pulmonary disease (COPD) is characterized by airflow limitation that is not fully reversible. The airflow limitation is progressive and associated with an abnormal inflammatory response of the lungs to noxious stimulus or gases, like cigarette smoke. In addition to slow progressive loss of lung function, patients with COPD can have acute exacerbations that lead to a faster decline in FEV_1. Exacerbations are most often triggered by viral or bacterial infection. (Papi *et al.*, 2006). Vitamin D deficiency is highly prevalent in COPD and correlates with the severity of COPD (Janssens *et al.*, 2010). In line with new insights into the immunomodulatory effects of vitamin D, including anti-inflammatory and possibly antimicrobial effects, it has been postulated that vitamin D may affect the pathogenesis of COPD (Janssens *et al.*, 2009). Epidemiological studies in healthy subjects and patients with COPD have suggested a dose-dependent association between serum 25D levels and lung function (FVC and FEV_1; Black and Scragg, 2005; Janssens *et al.*, 2010). It is unclear at this time how vitamin D may affect lung function but variants in the vitamin D-binding gene have been linked to vitamin D deficiency and COPD risk (Janssens *et al.*, 2010). These population-based studies do not prove that there is an association between vitamin D deficiency and lung function but they do provide preliminary data and justification for randomized controlled trials of vitamin D supplementation in COPD. A randomized, multicentre, double-blind, placebo-controlled trial of vitamin D supplementation in COPD is currently underway (www.clinicaltrials.gov).

VI. Conclusions and Future Directions

Vitamin D deficiency is on the rise in western countries including the US (Ginde *et al.*, 2009a). Our understanding of vitamin D metabolism and function has grown exponentially over the past decade. It has become clear that vitamin D is not only important for bone and muscle health but has a wide spectrum of biological actions including significant immunomodulatory effects (Holick, 2007). The enzyme 1α-hydroxylase is expressed by a variety of cells and the 1,25D that is produced locally in tissues may have direct effects on nearby cells and be responsible for the broad actions of vitamin D.

Epidemiological studies suggest an association between low vitamin D levels and mycobacterial infections, respiratory viral infections, and asthma (Fig. 9.1). The enzyme 1α-hydroxylase is expressed by airway epithelium, macrophages, dendritic cells, and lymphocytes in the respiratory tract indicating that active vitamin D may be produced locally within the lungs

(Table 9.1). Mechanistic studies have found the 1,25D influences cellular mechanisms that are important for recognition and killing of pathogens, inflammation, and control of adaptive immune functions within the lungs (Fig. 9.1).

Epidemiological and mechanistic studies indicate that vitamin D may play an important role in the development of respiratory diseases but many questions remain. Important clinical trials are ongoing looking at the effects of vitamin D supplementation on mycobacterial infections, respiratory tract infections, asthma, and COPD.

ACKNOWLEDGMENT

This work was supported by National Institutes of Health Grant KL2 RR024980.

REFERENCES

Adams, J. S., and Hewison, M. (2008). Unexpected actions of vitamin D: New perspectives on the regulation of innate and adaptive immunity. *Nat. Clin. Pract. Endocrinol. Metab.* **4** (2), 80–90.

Adams, J. S., Sharma, O. P., *et al.* (1983). Metabolism of 25-hydroxyvitamin D3 by cultured pulmonary alveolar macrophages in sarcoidosis. *J. Clin. Invest.* **72**(5), 1856–1860.

Adams, J. S., Ren, S., *et al.* (2009). Vitamin D-directed rheostatic regulation of monocyte antibacterial responses. *J. Immunol.* **182**(7), 4289–4295.

Adorini, L., and Penna, G. (2008). Control of autoimmune diseases by the vitamin D endocrine system. *Nat. Clin. Pract. Rheumatol.* **4**(8), 404–412.

Aloia, J. F., and Li-Ng, M. (2007). Re: Epidemic influenza and vitamin D. *Epidemiol. Infect.* **135**(7), 1095–1096, (author reply 1097–1098).

Baker, A. R., McDonnell, D. P., *et al.* (1988). Cloning and expression of full-length cDNA encoding human vitamin D receptor. *Proc. Natl. Acad. Sci. USA* **85**(10), 3294–3298.

Barbour, G. L., Coburn, J. W., *et al.* (1981). Hypercalcemia in an anephric patient with sarcoidosis: Evidence for extrarenal generation of 1, 25-dihydroxyvitamin D. *N. Engl. J. Med.* **305**(8), 440–443.

Barrat, F. J., Cua, D. J., *et al.* (2002). In vitro generation of interleukin 10-producing regulatory CD4(+) T cells is induced by immunosuppressive drugs and inhibited by T helper type 1 (Th1)- and Th2-inducing cytokines. *J. Exp. Med.* **195**(5), 603–616.

Bartlett, J. A., Fischer, A. J., *et al.* (2008). Innate immune functions of the airway epithelium. *Contrib. Microbiol.* **15,** 147–163.

Basu, S., and Fenton, M. J. (2004). Toll-like receptors: Function and roles in lung disease. *Am. J. Physiol. Lung Cell. Mol. Physiol.* **286**(5), L887–L892.

Bell, N. H. (1998). Renal and nonrenal 25-hydroxyvitamin D-1alpha-hydroxylases and their clinical significance. *J. Bone Miner. Res.* **13**(3), 350–353.

Bhalla, A. K., Amento, E. P., *et al.* (1983). Specific high-affinity receptors for 1, 25-dihydroxyvitamin D3 in human peripheral blood mononuclear cells: Presence in monocytes and induction in T lymphocytes following activation. *J. Clin. Endocrinol. Metab.* **57** (6), 1308–1310.

Bikle, D. (2009). Nonclassic actions of vitamin D. *J. Clin. Endocrinol. Metab.* **94**(1), 26–34.

Black, P. N., and Scragg, R. (2005). Relationship between serum 25-hydroxyvitamin d and pulmonary function in the third national health and nutrition examination survey. *Chest* **128**(6), 3792–3798.

Boonstra, A., Barrat, F. J., *et al.* (2001). 1alpha, 25-Dihydroxyvitamin d3 has a direct effect on naive CD4(+) T cells to enhance the development of Th2 cells. *J. Immunol.* **167**(9), 4974–4980.

Bornman, L., Campbell, S. J., *et al.* (2004). Vitamin D receptor polymorphisms and susceptibility to tuberculosis in West Africa: A case-control and family study. *J. Infect. Dis.* **190**(9), 1631–1641.

Brehm, J. M., Celedon, J. C., *et al.* (2009). Serum vitamin D levels and markers of severity of childhood asthma in Costa Rica. *Am. J. Respir. Crit. Care Med.* **179**(9), 765–771.

Brehm, J. M., Schuemann, B., *et al.* (2010). Serum vitamin D levels and severe asthma exacerbations in the Childhood Asthma Management Program study. *J Allergy Clin. Immunol.* **126,** 52–58.

Cannell, J. J., Vieth, R., *et al.* (2006). Epidemic influenza and vitamin D. *Epidemiol. Infect.* **134**(6), 1129–1140.

Cannell, J. J., Zasloff, M., *et al.* (2008). On the epidemiology of influenza. *Virol. J.* **5,** 29.

Chen, S., Sims, G. P., *et al.* (2007). Modulatory effects of 1, 25-dihydroxyvitamin D3 on human B cell differentiation. *J. Immunol.* **179**(3), 1634–1647.

Crowle, A. J., Ross, E. J., *et al.* (1987). Inhibition by 1, 25(OH)2-vitamin D3 of the multiplication of virulent tubercle bacilli in cultured human macrophages. *Infect. Immun.* **55**(12), 2945–2950.

D'Ambrosio, D., Cippitelli, M., *et al.* (1998). Inhibition of IL-12 production by 1, 25-dihydroxyvitamin D3. Involvement of NF-kappaB downregulation in transcriptional repression of the p40 gene. *J. Clin. Invest.* **101**(1), 252–262.

Daniel, C., Sartory, N. A., *et al.* (2008). Immune modulatory treatment of trinitrobenzene sulfonic acid colitis with calcitriol is associated with a change of a T helper (Th) 1/Th17 to a Th2 and regulatory T cell profile. *J. Pharmacol. Exp. Ther.* **324**(1), 23–33.

Dimeloe, S., Nanzer, A., *et al.* (2010). Regulatory T cells, inflammation and the allergic response-The role of glucocorticoids and Vitamin D. *J. Steroid Biochem. Mol. Biol.* **120** (2–3), 86–95.

Dusso, A. S., Kamimura, S., *et al.* (1997). gamma-Interferon-induced resistance to 1, 25-(OH)2 D3 in human monocytes and macrophages: A mechanism for the hypercalcemia of various granulomatoses. *J. Clin. Endocrinol. Metab.* **82**(7), 2222–2232.

Freishtat, R. J., Iqbal, S. F., *et al.* (2010). High prevalence of vitamin D deficiency among inner-city African American youth with asthma in Washington, DC. *J. Pediatr.* **156**(6), 948–952.

Fritsche, J., Mondal, K., *et al.* (2003). Regulation of 25-hydroxyvitamin D3–1 alpha-hydroxylase and production of 1 alpha, 25-dihydroxyvitamin D3 by human dendritic cells. *Blood* **102**(9), 3314–3316.

Gale, C. R., Robinson, S. M., *et al.* (2008). Maternal vitamin D status during pregnancy and child outcomes. *Eur. J. Clin. Nutr.* **62**(1), 68–77.

Gao, L., Tao, Y., *et al.* (2010). Vitamin D receptor genetic polymorphisms and tuberculosis: Updated systematic review and meta-analysis. *Int. J. Tuberc. Lung Dis.* **14**(1), 15–23.

Gibney, K. B., MacGregor, L., *et al.* (2008). Vitamin D deficiency is associated with tuberculosis and latent tuberculosis infection in immigrants from sub-Saharan Africa. *Clin. Infect. Dis.* **46**(3), 443–446.

Ginde, A. A., Liu, M. C., *et al.* (2009a). Demographic differences and trends of vitamin D insufficiency in the US population, 1988-2004. *Arch. Intern. Med.* **169**(6), 626–632.

Ginde, A. A., Mansbach, J. M., *et al.* (2009b). Association between serum 25-hydroxyvitamin D level and upper respiratory tract infection in the Third National Health and Nutrition Examination Survey. *Arch. Intern. Med.* **169**(4), 384–390.

Gregori, S., Casorati, M., *et al.* (2001). Regulatory T cells induced by 1 alpha, 25-dihydroxyvitamin D3 and mycophenolate mofetil treatment mediate transplantation tolerance. *J. Immunol.* **167**(4), 1945–1953.
Griffin, M. D., Lutz, W., *et al.* (2001). Dendritic cell modulation by 1alpha, 25 dihydroxyvitamin D3 and its analogs: A vitamin D receptor-dependent pathway that promotes a persistent state of immaturity in vitro and in vivo. *Proc. Natl. Acad. Sci. USA* **98**(12), 6800–6805.
Hansdottir, S., Monick, M. M., *et al.* (2008). Respiratory epithelial cells convert inactive vitamin D to its active form: Potential effects on host defense. *J. Immunol.* **181**(10), 7090–7099.
Hansdottir, S., Monick, M. M., *et al.* (2010). Vitamin D decreases respiratory syncytial virus induction of NF-kappaB-linked chemokines and cytokines in airway epithelium while maintaining the antiviral state. *J. Immunol.* **184**(2), 965–974.
Hawrylowicz, C. M., and O'Garra, A. (2005). Potential role of interleukin-10-secreting regulatory T cells in allergy and asthma. *Nat. Rev. Immunol.* **5**(4), 271–283.
Hawrylowicz, C., Richards, D., *et al.* (2002). A defect in corticosteroid-induced IL-10 production in T lymphocytes from corticosteroid-resistant asthmatic patients. *J. Allergy Clin. Immunol.* **109**(2), 369–370.
Hewison, M., Freeman, L., *et al.* (2003). Differential regulation of vitamin D receptor and its ligand in human monocyte-derived dendritic cells. *J. Immunol.* **170**(11), 5382–5390.
Hewison, M., Burke, F., *et al.* (2007). Extra-renal 25-hydroxyvitamin D3-1alpha-hydroxylase in human health and disease. *J. Steroid Biochem. Mol. Biol.* **103**(3–5), 316–321.
Hmama, Z., Sendide, K., *et al.* (2004). Quantitative analysis of phagolysosome fusion in intact cells: Inhibition by mycobacterial lipoarabinomannan and rescue by an 1alpha, 25-dihydroxyvitamin D3-phosphoinositide 3-kinase pathway. *J. Cell Sci.* **117**(Pt 10), 2131–2140.
Holick, M. F. (2007). Vitamin D deficiency. *N. Engl. J. Med.* **357**(3), 266–281.
Holt, P. G., Strickland, D. H., *et al.* (2008). Regulation of immunological homeostasis in the respiratory tract. *Nat. Rev. Immunol.* **8**(2), 142–152.
Hypponen, E., Sovio, U., *et al.* (2004). Infant vitamin d supplementation and allergic conditions in adulthood: Northern Finland birth cohort 1966. *Ann. NY Acad. Sci.* **1037,** 84–95.
Iwasaki, A., and Medzhitov, R. (2010). Regulation of adaptive immunity by the innate immune system. *Science* **327**(5963), 291–295.
Janssens, W., Lehouck, A., *et al.* (2009). Vitamin D beyond bones in chronic obstructive pulmonary disease: Time to act. *Am. J. Respir. Crit. Care Med.* **179**(8), 630–636.
Janssens, W., Bouillon, R., *et al.* (2010). Vitamin D deficiency is highly prevalent in COPD and correlates with variants in the vitamin D-binding gene. *Thorax* **65**(3), 215–220.
Karagiannidis, C., Akdis, M., *et al.* (2004). Glucocorticoids upregulate FOXP3 expression and regulatory T cells in asthma. *J. Allergy Clin. Immunol.* **114**(6), 1425–1433.
Kohlmeier, J. E., and Woodland, D. L. (2008). Immunity to Respiratory Viruses. *Annu. Rev. Immunol.* **27,** 61–82.
Laaksi, I., Ruohola, J. P., *et al.* (2007). An association of serum vitamin D concentrations <40 nmol/L with acute respiratory tract infection in young Finnish men. *Am. J. Clin. Nutr.* **86**(3), 714–717.
Lemire, J. M., Archer, D. C., *et al.* (1995). Immunosuppressive actions of 1, 25-dihydroxyvitamin D3: Preferential inhibition of Th1 functions. *J. Nutr.* **125**(6 Suppl.), 1704S–1708S.
Lewis, S. J., Baker, I., *et al.* (2005). Meta-analysis of vitamin D receptor polymorphisms and pulmonary tuberculosis risk. *Int. J. Tuberc. Lung Dis.* **9**(10), 1174–1177.
Li, Q., and Verma, I. M. (2002). NF-kappaB regulation in the immune system. *Nat. Rev. Immunol.* **2**(10), 725–734.

Li-Ng, M., Aloia, J. F., *et al.* (2009). A randomized controlled trial of vitamin D3 supplementation for the prevention of symptomatic upper respiratory tract infections. *Epidemiol. Infect.* **137**(10), 1396–1404.

Lipsitch, M., and Viboud, C. (2009). Influenza seasonality: Lifting the fog. *Proc. Natl. Acad. Sci. USA* **106**(10), 3645–3646.

Litonjua, A. A. (2009). Childhood asthma may be a consequence of vitamin D deficiency. *Curr. Opin. Allergy Clin. Immunol.* **9**(3), 202–207.

Litonjua, A. A., and Weiss, S. T. (2007). Is vitamin D deficiency to blame for the asthma epidemic? *J. Allergy Clin. Immunol.* **120**(5), 1031–1035.

Liu, P. T., Stenger, S., *et al.* (2006). Toll-like receptor triggering of a vitamin D-mediated human antimicrobial response. *Science* **311**(5768), 1770–1773.

Liu, P. T., Krutzik, S. R., *et al.* (2007a). Therapeutic implications of the TLR and VDR partnership. *Trends Mol. Med.* **13**(3), 117–124.

Liu, P. T., Stenger, S., *et al.* (2007b). Cutting edge: Vitamin D-mediated human antimicrobial activity against Mycobacterium tuberculosis is dependent on the induction of cathelicidin. *J. Immunol.* **179**(4), 2060–2063.

Lloyd, C. M., and Hawrylowicz, C. M. (2009). Regulatory T cells in asthma. *Immunity* **31** (3), 438–449.

MacDonald, P. N., Dowd, D. R., *et al.* (1993). Retinoid X receptors stimulate and 9-cis retinoic acid inhibits 1, 25-dihydroxyvitamin D3-activated expression of the rat osteocalcin gene. *Mol. Cell. Biol.* **13**(9), 5907–5917.

Mak, T. W., and Saunders, M. E. (2005). The immune response: Basic and clinical principles. Elsevier/Academic, New York.

Martineau, A. R., Wilkinson, K. A., *et al.* (2007a). IFN-gamma- and TNF-independent vitamin D-inducible human suppression of mycobacteria: The role of cathelicidin LL-37. *J. Immunol.* **178**(11), 7190–7198.

Martineau, A. R., Wilkinson, R. J., *et al.* (2007b). A single dose of vitamin D enhances immunity to mycobacteria. *Am. J. Respir. Crit. Care Med.* **176**(2), 208–213.

Medzhitov, R. (2007). Recognition of microorganisms and activation of the immune response. *Nature* **449**(7164), 819–826.

Moore, K. W., de Waal Malefyt, R., *et al.* (2001). Interleukin-10 and the interleukin-10 receptor. *Annu. Rev. Immunol.* **19,** 683–765.

Mora, J. R., Iwata, M., *et al.* (2008). Vitamin effects on the immune system: Vitamins A and D take centre stage. *Nat. Rev. Immunol.* **8,** 685–698.

Morcos, M. M., Gabr, A. A., *et al.* (1998). Vitamin D administration to tuberculous children and its value. *Boll. Chim. Farm.* **137**(5), 157–164.

Muhe, L., Lulseged, S., *et al.* (1997). Case-control study of the role of nutritional rickets in the risk of developing pneumonia in Ethiopian children. *Lancet* **349**(9068), 1801–1804.

Nnoaham, K. E., and Clarke, A. (2008). Low serum vitamin D levels and tuberculosis: A systematic review and meta-analysis. *Int. J. Epidemiol.* **37**(1), 113–119.

Nursyam, E. W., Amin, Z., *et al.* (2006). The effect of vitamin D as supplementary treatment in patients with moderately advanced pulmonary tuberculous lesion. *Acta Med. Indones.* **38**(1), 3–5.

Papapoulos, S. E., Clemens, T. L., *et al.* (1979). 1, 25-dihydroxycholecalciferol in the pathogenesis of the hypercalcaemia of sarcoidosis. *Lancet* **1**(8117), 627–630.

Papi, A., Bellettato, C. M., *et al.* (2006). Infections and airway inflammation in chronic obstructive pulmonary disease severe exacerbations. *Am. J. Respir. Crit. Care Med.* **173** (10), 1114–1121.

Penna, G., and Adorini, L. (2000). 1 Alpha, 25-dihydroxyvitamin D3 inhibits differentiation, maturation, activation, and survival of dendritic cells leading to impaired alloreactive T cell activation. *J. Immunol.* **164**(5), 2405–2411.

Penna, G., Roncari, A., *et al.* (2005). Expression of the inhibitory receptor ILT3 on dendritic cells is dispensable for induction of CD4+Foxp3+ regulatory T cells by 1, 25-dihydroxyvitamin D3. *Blood* **106**(10), 3490–3497.

Pichler, J., Gerstmayr, M., *et al.* (2002). 1 alpha, 25(OH)2D3 inhibits not only Th1 but also Th2 differentiation in human cord blood T cells. *Pediatr. Res.* **52**(1), 12–18.

Piemonti, L., Monti, P., *et al.* (2000). Vitamin D3 affects differentiation, maturation, and function of human monocyte-derived dendritic cells. *J. Immunol.* **164**(9), 4443–4451.

Ponchon, G., Kennan, A. L., *et al.* (1969). "Activation" of vitamin D by the liver. *J. Clin. Invest.* **48**(11), 2032–2037.

Provvedini, D. M., Tsoukas, C. D., *et al.* (1986). 1 alpha, 25-Dihydroxyvitamin D3-binding macromolecules in human B lymphocytes: Effects on immunoglobulin production. *J. Immunol.* **136**(8), 2734–2740.

Rehman, P. K. (1994). Sub-clinical rickets and recurrent infection. *J. Trop. Pediatr.* **40**(1), 58.

Reichel, H., Koeffler, H. P., *et al.* (1987a). Regulation of 1, 25-dihydroxyvitamin D3 production by cultured alveolar macrophages from normal human donors and from patients with pulmonary sarcoidosis. *J. Clin. Endocrinol. Metab.* **65**(6), 1201–1209.

Reichel, H., Koeffler, H. P., *et al.* (1987b). Synthesis in vitro of 1, 25-dihydroxyvitamin D3 and 24, 25-dihydroxyvitamin D3 by interferon-gamma-stimulated normal human bone marrow and alveolar macrophages. *J. Biol. Chem.* **262**(23), 10931–10937.

Ren, S., Nguyen, L., *et al.* (2005). Alternative splicing of vitamin D-24-hydroxylase: A novel mechanism for the regulation of extrarenal 1, 25-dihydroxyvitamin D synthesis. *J. Biol. Chem.* **280**(21), 20604–20611.

Robinson, D. S. (2009). Regulatory T cells and asthma. *Clin. Exp. Allergy* **39**(9), 1314–1323.

Rook, G. A., Steele, J., *et al.* (1986). Vitamin D3, gamma interferon, and control of proliferation of Mycobacterium tuberculosis by human monocytes. *Immunology* **57**(1), 159–163.

Roth, D. E., Soto, G., *et al.* (2004). Association between vitamin D receptor gene polymorphisms and response to treatment of pulmonary tuberculosis. *J. Infect. Dis.* **190**(5), 920–927.

Roth, D. E., Jones, A. B., *et al.* (2008). Vitamin D receptor polymorphisms and the risk of acute lower respiratory tract infection in early childhood. *J. Infect. Dis.* **197**(5), 676–680.

Searing, D. A., Zhang, Y., *et al.* (2010). Decreased serum vitamin D levels in children with asthma are associated with increased corticosteroid use. *J. Allergy Clin. Immunol.* **125**(5), 995–1000.

Sigmundsdottir, H., Pan, J., *et al.* (2007). DCs metabolize sunlight-induced vitamin D3 to 'program' T cell attraction to the epidermal chemokine CCL27. *Nat. Immunol.* **8**(3), 285–293.

Sly, L. M., Lopez, M., *et al.* (2001). 1alpha, 25-Dihydroxyvitamin D3-induced monocyte antimycobacterial activity is regulated by phosphatidylinositol 3-kinase and mediated by the NADPH-dependent phagocyte oxidase. *J. Biol. Chem.* **276**(38), 35482–35493.

Staeva-Vieira, T. P., and Freedman, L. P. (2002). 1, 25-dihydroxyvitamin D3 inhibits IFN-gamma and IL-4 levels during in vitro polarization of primary murine CD4+ T cells. *J. Immunol.* **168**(3), 1181–1189.

Sutherland, E. R., Goleva, E., *et al.* (2010). Vitamin D levels, lung function, and steroid response in adult asthma. *Am. J. Respir. Crit. Care Med.* **181**(7), 699–704.

Sutton, A. L., and MacDonald, P. N. (2003). Vitamin D: More than a "bone-a-fide" hormone. *Mol. Endocrinol.* **17**(5), 777–791.

Upham, J. W. (2003). The role of dendritic cells in immune regulation and allergic airway inflammation. *Respirology* **8**(2), 140–148.

Ustianowski, A., Shaffer, R., *et al.* (2005). Prevalence and associations of vitamin D deficiency in foreign-born persons with tuberculosis in London. *J. Infect.* **50**(5), 432–437.

Wayse, V., Yousafzai, A., *et al.* (2004). Association of subclinical vitamin D deficiency with severe acute lower respiratory infection in Indian children under 5 y. *Eur. J. Clin. Nutr.* **58**(4), 563–567.

Wejse, C., Gomes, V. F., *et al.* (2009). Vitamin D as supplementary treatment for tuberculosis: A double-blind, randomized, placebo-controlled trial. *Am. J. Respir. Crit. Care Med.* **179**(9), 843–850.

White, J. H. (2008). Vitamin D signaling, infectious diseases, and regulation of innate immunity. *Infect. Immun.* **76**(9), 3837–3843.

Wilkinson, R. J., Llewelyn, M., *et al.* (2000). Influence of vitamin D deficiency and vitamin D receptor polymorphisms on tuberculosis among Gujarati Asians in west London: A case-control study. *Lancet* **355**(9204), 618–621.

Xystrakis, E., Kusumakar, S., *et al.* (2006). Reversing the defective induction of IL-10-secreting regulatory T cells in glucocorticoid-resistant asthma patients. *J. Clin. Invest.* **116** (1), 146–155.

Xystrakis, E., Urry, Z., *et al.* (2007). Regulatory T cell therapy as individualized medicine for asthma and allergy. *Curr. Opin. Allergy Clin. Immunol.* **7**(6), 535–541.

Zehnder, D., Bland, R., *et al.* (1999). Expression of 25-Hydroxyvitamin D3-1{alpha}-Hydroxylase in the human kidney. *J. Am. Soc. Nephrol.* **10**(12), 2465–2473.

CHAPTER TEN

Maternal Vitamin D During Pregnancy and Its Relation to Immune-Mediated Diseases in the Offspring

Erkkola Maijaliisa,* Nwaru I. Bright,† *and* Viljakainen T. Heli‡

Contents

Abstract

Vitamin D deficiency during pregnancy is fairly common in many parts of the world. However, currently there is no consensus on the optimal vitamin D intake during pregnancy. Vitamin D is known to be of great importance for the homeostatic functions within the immune system. Maternal vitamin D status during

* Division of Nutrition, Department of Food and Environmental Sciences, University of Helsinki, Finland
† Tampere School of Public Health, University of Tampere, Finland
‡ Hospital for Children and Adolescents, HUS, Finland

Vitamins and Hormones, Volume 86
ISSN 0083-6729, DOI: 10.1016/B978-0-12-386960-9.00010-1

pregnancy may therefore affect the developing immune system of the fetus, thus contributing to the later development of immune-mediated diseases. This chapter introduces the basics of vitamin D during pregnancy and discusses the role of maternal vitamin D intake in the development of asthma, allergic diseases, autoimmune diseases, cancer, and infections in the offspring. So far, the strongest observational evidence underlines the potential of maternal vitamin D intake during pregnancy to influence the likelihood of asthma and allergic outcomes in the offspring. Somewhat conflicting findings imply that there might be critical time windows of exposure to adequate vitamin D levels during pregnancy. More research is needed in order to fully understand the contribution of maternal vitamin D status during pregnancy to the progress of immune-mediated diseases.

I. Introduction

Fetal nutrition and its impact on childhood immune responses is a highly active field of research. Heightened susceptibility to immunological disorders may originate in early life, with long-lasting structural or functional changes to the developing organs or organ systems (Burlingham, 2009). Nutrients act as cofactors and activators for the developing immune system (Cunningham-Rundles *et al.*, 2009), and early education of the immune system seems to already begin *in utero* (e.g., Calder *et al.*, 2006). Pregnancy is a time when maternal nutrition may play an important role in the development of the fetus. Today, the appreciation of the immunological properties of vitamin D has been extended to understand its role in the development of several childhood diseases as a result of *in utero* vitamin D exposure. Consequently, it has been suggested that maternal vitamin D status during pregnancy may play a possible etiological role in the development of several immunological disorders in the offspring during childhood (Lucas *et al.*, 2008; Zittermann and Gummert, 2010). However, at the same time, there is no consensus on either the optimal level of vitamin D intake during pregnancy, or levels that might be unsafe (Hollis and Wagner, 2004; Kovacs, 2008; Prentice, 2008; Specker, 2004; Vieth, 2006).

The present overview starts by briefly describing vitamin D metabolism and functions, which is followed by a discussion on maternal vitamin D status, dietary guidelines, and assessment methods during pregnancy. Finally, we present the current evidence on the possible etiological role of maternal vitamin D intake/status in the development of several immune-mediated diseases in the offspring. Considering the extensive work that has been carried out in the area of skeletal outcomes, we now focus solely on nonskeletal outcomes in the offspring. A PubMed search was conducted in February, 2010, using the following search terms: vitamin D, pregnancy, immune system, asthma, allergy, autoimmune diseases, cancer, and infection.

We included all original studies (published in English), in which the explanatory variable was either the intake and/or a biomarker of vitamin D or exposure to sunlight during pregnancy, and the response variable was one of the following: asthma, allergic rhinitis, atopic eczema, allergic sensitization, autoimmune disease, cancer, or infectious disease. The summary of the studies that were included can be found in Table 10.1. In the introduction to the basics of vitamin D, in order to avoid a potentially excessive reference list, we refer to the comprehensive reviews, wherever it is possible.

II. Vitamin D

A. Forms and sources of vitamin D

Globally, the most important source of vitamin D is sunlight UVB radiation. However, season, latitude, time of day, time spent outdoors, ageing, use of sunscreen, skin pigmentation, and clothing influence the amount of vitamin D produced in the skin (Holick, 2004). Although serum-25-hydroxy vitamin D (S-25-OHD) concentration, a surrogate for vitamin D status, increases with increasing latitude (Kuchuk *et al.*, 2009), factors related to affluence such as dietary supplement use or holidays in sunny resorts may confound this. The human diet contains two predominant forms of vitamin D, namely D_2 and D_3. Vitamin D_2 originates from the algae, ergosterol, while vitamin D_3 is derived from 7-dehydrocholesterol, a precursor of cholesterol. Biologically, D_2 and D_3 are not equivalent (Houghton and Vieth, 2006). D_2 is metabolized faster in the body than D_3. Furthermore, the effects of D_2 on calcium metabolism are not as well studied. However, many supplements still contain D_2, probably due to its better availability.

B. Vitamin D metabolism

Vitamin D from skin or diet accumulates in the liver within a few hours. In the liver, vitamin D undergoes hydroxylation to 25-hydroxy vitamin D (25-OHD) which is rapidly released into circulation bound to its specific carrier, vitamin D binding protein, (DBP; Fig. 10.1). S-25-OHD is the most abundant vitamin D form in the body and a novel indicator of both cumulative exposure to sunlight and dietary vitamin D intake, making it a reliable marker of the overall vitamin D status. 25-OHD has also been found to be associated with chronic disease risk. Its half-life varies from 1 to 2 months (Vieth, 1999). A single assessment of 25-OHD is hardly enough to describe the lifelong variation in vitamin D status.

However, S-25-OHD is still a prehormone requiring further hydroxylation to become the potent steroid hormone calcitriol. Calcitriol (1,25 $(OH)_2D$) produced in the kidneys regulates calcium metabolism, whereas

Table 10.1 Summary of evidence of the role of maternal vitamin D during pregnancy on immune-mediated outcomes in the offspring

Study and country	Design	Number of subjects	Assessment of vitamin D	Main findings
Asthma and allergic outcomes				
Nwaru *et al.* (2010), Finland	Prospective cohort study with 5-year follow-up	931 mother–child pairs	Validated food frequency questionnaire (FFQ) during the eighth month of pregnancy	Increasing maternal intake of vitamin D from foods decreased the risk of IgE-based sensitization to food allergens
Erkkola *et al.* (2009), Finland	Prospective cohort study with 5-year follow-up	1669 mother–child pairs	Validated FFQ during the eighth month of pregnancy	Increasing maternal intake of total vitamin D, and vitamin D from foods was inversely associated with asthma and allergic rhinitis
Miyake *et al.* (2009), Japan	Prospective cohort study	763 mother–child pairs	A diet history questionnaire	Maternal daily intake of ≥ 4.309 µg of vitamin D was associated with reduced risk of wheeze and eczema
Gale *et al.* (2008), United Kingdom	Prospective cohort study	440 mother–child pairs at 9 months and 178 at 9 years	Serum 25-OHD during 28–42 weeks gestation	High maternal concentration of 25-OHD was positively associated with atopic eczema at 9 months and asthma at 9 years
Camargo *et al.* (2007), United States	Prospective cohort study with 3-year follow-up	1194 mother–child pairs	Validated FFQ during the third trimester of pregnancy	High maternal intake of vitamin D from foods and supplements was inversely associated with wheeze
Devereux *et al.* (2007), United Kingdom	Prospective cohort study with 5-year follow-up	1212 mother–child pairs	Validated FFQ during the 32-week of pregnancy	High maternal intake of vitamin D decreased the risk of ever wheeze, wheeze in the previous year, and persistent wheeze
Autoimmune diseases				
Salzer *et al.* (2010), Sweden	Case-control study	9361 multiple sclerosis (MS) cases and 12,116,853 controls	Sunlight exposure: each month of birth separately compared with birth during the other 11 months	More cases of MS were born during the month of June than other months, indicating that decreased exposure to sunlight during pregnancy in the winter months maybe a possible explanation

Fernandes de Abreu *et al.* (2009), France	Descriptive study	583 trios; patient and both parents	Medical files and DNA samples	Fewer of those born during the month of November were diagnosed with multiple sclerosis, which may be a result of increased exposure to sunlight in the summer months
Brekke and Ludvigsson (2007), Sweden	Prospective cohort study	8694 mother–child pairs at year 1 and 7766 at year 2.5	FFQ assessing supplemental vitamin D during pregnancy	Maternal supplemental vitamin D intake was associated with decreased risk of diabetes-related autoimmunity at year 1 but not at year 2.5
Fronczak *et al.* (2003), United States	Prospective cohort study	233 mother–child pairs	Validated FFQ during the third trimester of pregnancy	Maternal intake of vitamin D from foods but not from supplements decreased the risk of appearance of islet diabetes-related autoimmunity
Stene *et al.* (2000), Norway	Population-based case-control study	85 T1D cases and 1070 controls	Mailed questionnaire to assess the use of cod liver oil and supplements during pregnancy	Maternal intake of cod liver oil was associated with lower risk of type 1 diabetes
Infectious diseases				
Karatekin *et al.* (2009), Turkey	Hospital-based case-control study	25 cases of acute lower respiratory infection (ALRI) and 15 controls	Serum 25-OHD	Mean serum 25-OHD concentrations were lower in cases and their mothers than in the control group, indicating that newborns with subclinical vitamin D deficiency may have increased risk of ALRI
Gale *et al.* (2008), United Kingdom	Prospective cohort study	440 mother–child pairs (at 9 months) and 178 (at 9 years)	Serum 25-OHD during 28–42 weeks gestation	High maternal concentration of serum 25-OHD was associated with pneumonia and diarrhea at 9 months
Camargo *et al.* (2007), United States	Prospective cohort study with 3-year follow-up	1194 mother–child pairs	Validated FFQ during the third trimester of pregnancy	No association was found between maternal intake of vitamin D and respiratory infections in the offspring

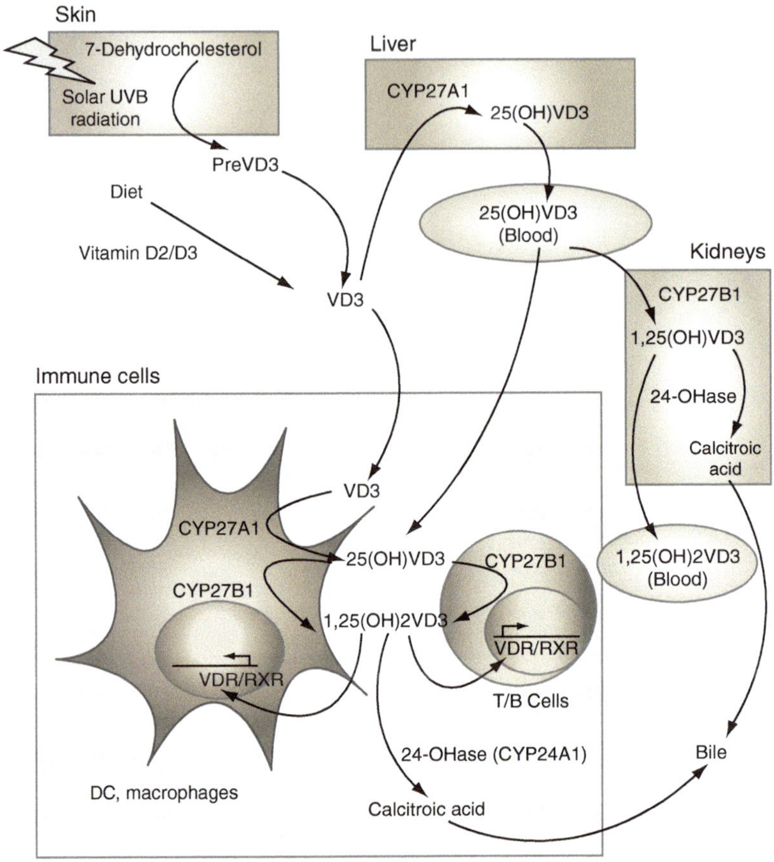

Figure 10.1 Overview of vitamin D metabolism. Vitamin D_3 (VD3) is acquired in the diet or synthesized in the skin and hydroxylated in the liver to 25(OH)VD3, the main circulating form. 25(OH)VD3 is then hydroxylated in the kidneys by the cytochrome P450 protein CYP27B1 to become 1,25(OH)2VD3, the physiologically most active metabolite, which then reaches the blood where it has multiple systemic effects. Cells of the immune system, including macrophages, dendritic cells (DCs), T and B cells express the enzymes CYP27A1 and/or CYP27B1, and therefore can also hydroxylate 25(OH)VD3 to 1,25(OH)2VD3. 1,25(OH)2VD3 acts on immune cells in an autocrine or paracrine manner by binding to the vitamin D receptor (VDR). 24-hydroxylase (CYP24A1) catabolizes 1,25(OH)2VD3 to its inactive metabolite, calcitroic acid, which is excreted in the bile. Reprinted by permission from Macmillan Publishers Ltd: Nature Reviews Immunology (Mora *et al.*, 2008), copyright 2008.

the extrarenal production of calcitriol occurring in at least 10 tissues explains its other biological functions (Norman *et al.*, 2007). Target organs presenting vitamin D receptor (VDR) have been identified in 37 tissues (Norman *et al.*, 2007). Membrane-bound VDR induces rapid signaling such as opening an ion channel or activating enzymes, while nuclear receptor regulates gene expression. Since the VDRs are targeted mainly to calcitriol, circulating 25-OHD bound to DBP needs to form a complex with specific cell membrane proteins when entering the cell. After cytosolic 1-hydroxylation, it is able to manage genomic actions. Rapid actions cross talk with genomic actions delicately modifies the functions in cells (Norman *et al.*, 2004).

Parathyroid glands monitor serum calcium and phosphate concentrations. Parathyroid hormone (PTH), estrogens, growth hormones, and prolactin work together to enhance the production of calcitriol in the kidney (Norman *et al.*, 2007). The production of calcitriol is tightly regulated by various negative feedback systems. Calcitriol also activates an alternative pathway by producing $24{,}25(OH)_2D$ in the kidney. $24{,}25(OH)_2D$ is related to a different set of biological functions than calcitriol (Norman, 2008), and it is more susceptible excreted to urine as a calcitronic acid (Zhou *et al.*, 2010).

C. Functions in the body

The main function of vitamin D is to maintain serum calcium and phosphorus concentrations within the normal range by enhancing calcium absorption from the intestine. If dietary calcium intake is insufficient to meet the body's calcium requirements, calcitriol working together with PTH mobilizes calcium from the bone by activating bone remodeling. Conversely, when the calcium balance in the body becomes positive, vitamin D allows calcium accretion in the bone. In addition, vitamin D directly stimulates osteoblastogenesis (Zhou *et al.*, 2010).

The importance of vitamin D for skeletal development has long been recognized. In infancy and childhood, severe vitamin D deficiency results in poor skeletal growth and has been linked to rickets whereas osteomalacia and myopathy are consequences of deficiency in adulthood. There is convincing evidence that vitamin D decreases falls and fracture in the elderly (Bischoff-Ferrari *et al.*, 2009a,c). Based on animal data and limited human data, fetuses are thought to be protected from adverse skeletal effects of maternal vitamin D deficiency during pregnancy (Kovacs, 2008). Maternal and fetal adaptations seem to provide the necessary calcium relatively independently of the maternal vitamin D status. However, recent results have been contradictory, and suggest that maternal vitamin D status does affect bone mineral accrual and bone size in the fetus during the intrauterine period (Viljakainen *et al.*, 2010).

Beyond the impact on the skeletal development, vitamin D has also been associated with various physiologic systems, for example, in the brain, the pancreas, the heart and cardiovascular system, the immune system, and the development of cancer (Norman *et al.*, 2007). Poor vitamin D status during pregnancy has been associated with increased risk of preeclampsia, gestational diabetes, and preterm birth (Bodnar and Simhan, 2010; Lapillonne, 2010). Mounting data link vitamin D deficiency to increased risk of many common chronic diseases (Lucas *et al.*, 2008; Zittermann and Gummert, 2010). However, the exact mechanisms of vitamin D in each disease are not yet fully elucidated.

D. Immunological functions

Vitamin D plays a very important role in the homeostasis of the immune system (Fig. 10.1). The widespread presence of VDR in the immune system and the expression of the enzymes responsible for the synthesis of the active calcitriol regulated by specific immune signals suggest a paracrine immunomodulatory role for calcitriol (Baeke *et al.*, 2008). Vitamin D has been suggested to modulate innate immunity; epithelial cells, macrophages, monocytes, and granulocytes are able to produce antimicrobial peptides, such as cathelidicin and defencin (Liu *et al.*, 2006). The synthesis of antimicrobial peptides is vitamin D dependent and cells contain 1-α-hydroxylase to activate their production locally. Antimicrobial peptides are responsible for rapid defense against pathogens in epithelial tissues such as the epidermis, mucosa, bladder, and lungs. Infectious pathogens activating toll-like receptors are killed by antimicrobial peptides and oxygen reactants. Vitamin D is shown to decrease chemokine and interferon release in virus-infected epithelial cells, while not affecting viral replication (Hansdottir *et al.*, 2010; Jeffery *et al.*, 2009). This explains the lower inflammatory response and decreased disease severity in humans with superior vitamin D status (Laaksi *et al.*, 2006; McNally *et al.*, 2009; Yamshchikov *et al.*, 2009).

Perinatal exposure to vitamin D acts as an immunoregulatory hormone on the maturation of the immune system by interfering with cytokine production of monocytes and lymphocytes, including those involved in the development of IgE-mediated allergy (Pichler *et al.*, 2002). Vitamin D selectively suppresses Th1, but not Th2 or CD8+ cell activity (Mora *et al.*, 2008). However, in cord blood (naïve) T cells, calcitriol appears to inhibit both Th-1 and Th-2 differentiation (Pichler *et al.*, 2002). The contradictory findings on the role of vitamin D in allergies may be explained by the fact that the effects of vitamin D might differ between naive T cells and the more mature cells. Furthermore, the timing of exposure of the cells to vitamin D (i.e., prenatal vs. postnatal) seems to be of importance. It is also possible that lower vitamin D intakes have different consequences than relatively high-dose supplementation, an excess of potentially toxic vitamin D possibly causing totally opposite effects. However, the role of vitamin D in fetal and early postnatal immunity is not well understood and merits further investigation.

E. Methods for assessing S-25-OHD

Currently, there are six methods to assess S-25-OHD concentration in humans. Care must be taken when comparing study results in the literature as these are produced by different methods that vary in their specificity for 25-OHD_3 and 25-OHD_2. In addition, the available commercial kits have changed over time as their antibodies have been developed and assays recalibrated (Carter, 2009; Looker *et al.*, 2008), which complicates the comparison even further.

High-performance liquid chromatography (HPLC) and liquid chromatography-mass spectrometry (LC-MS/MS) are direct methods for detecting 25-OHD and have greater accuracy than immunoassays. However, these higher-technology methods are demanding and require skilful and experienced analysts. Since we are still lacking a reference measurement procedure for 25-OHD, most of the direct measurements are in-house methods with different protocols (Carter *et al.*, 2010). The bottom line in 25-OHD measurements is still adhering to the vitamin D quality assessment scheme and comparing one's own method with others to ensure that the level of results is maintained. The most commonly used methods are DiaSorin radioimmunoassay and Immunodiagnostic Systems (IDS) enzyme immunoassay. As discussed by Binkley *et al.* (2009), the use of different methods has let the debate on thresholds for vitamin D status to continue for decades.

III. Vitamin D Status During Pregnancy

The S-25-OHD concentrations of pregnant women are similar to that of nonpregnant women in that they fluctuate according to season and are affected by dietary intake. While the S-25-OHD status of pregnant women is either inferior or similar to nonpregnant women, the concentration of calcitriol is elevated (Kovacs, 2008; Lucas *et al.*, 2008). This illustrates efficient vitamin D metabolism, and is possibly due to the increased requirement. 25-OHD crosses the placenta and similar 25-OHD concentrations are observed both in mothers and their newborn (Greer, 2008; Nicolaidou *et al.*, 2006). Circulating concentrations of calcitriol double or triple from early to late pregnancy, and have been shown to be higher in pregnant compared to nonpregnant women (Kovacs, 2008). No studies have yet addressed whether the ideal concentration of 25-OHD during pregnancy should differ from the concentration considered sufficient for nonpregnant women. Currently, S-25-OHD below 50 nmol/l is considered deficient, between 50 and 80 nmol/l insufficient, and above 80 nmol/l sufficient (Bischoff-Ferrari *et al.*, 2009b; Lips *et al.*, 2009). The only way to achieve a 25-OHD concentration of above 80 nmol/l without vitamin D supplementation is to spend time in the sun (Vieth, 2006).

Relatively few countries have nationally representative data on either the vitamin D status of their population or the risk of vitamin D deficiency, as estimated by S-25-OHD concentration (Prentice, 2008). However, vitamin D deficiency during pregnancy is a common problem worldwide (Holmes *et al.*, 2009; Nicolaidou *et al.*, 2006; Sahu *et al.* 2009; Viljakainen *et al.* 2010). There has been increasing recognition of a high prevalence of severe vitamin D deficiency (<25 nmol/l; 10 ng/ml), especially among pregnant women from ethnic minority groups in Northern Europe, Australasia, and the United States, suggesting a high risk of vitamin D deficiency diseases (Prentice, 2008).

IV. Dietary Guidelines and Maternal Vitamin D Intake

A. Dietary guidelines during pregnancy

Vitamin D requirements during pregnancy must be met through dietary intake, dietary supplements, and sun exposure (Hollis and Wagner, 2004; Kovacs, 2008; Specker, 2004). Internationally, the recommendations for vitamin D intake during pregnancy vary widely, as much as 10-fold (Lucas *et al.*, 2008). The appropriate dose of vitamin D during pregnancy is still unknown, although it is thought to be higher than the current dietary reference intake of 200–400 IU/day (5–10 μg/day). The scientific basis for this recommendation is not well defined, and the recommended dose has been criticized as having little or no effect in women (Hollis and Wagner, 2004; Vieth, 1999). Several studies have indicated that doses exceeding 25 μg (1000 IU) vitamin D/day are required during pregnancy to achieve a robust normal concentration of circulating 25-OHD (Hollis and Wagner, 2004; Vieth, 1999). Studies reviewed by Vieth (1999) support the belief that total-body sun exposure can easily provide the equivalent of 250 μg (10,000 IU) vitamin D/day, suggesting that this is a physiologic limit.

Vitamin D is potentially toxic though the exact amount of vitamin D required to induce toxicity is unknown in humans. However, intake of >25 μg (1000 IU)/day has not been recommended. There is no evidence of adverse effects on S-25-OHD concentrations, which do not exceed 140 nmol/l; to exceed this level is thought to require a total vitamin supply of 250 μg (10,000 IU; Vieth, 1999). In comparison to the toxic amounts in animal models, millions of units of vitamin D would have to be ingested to achieve the similar toxicity in humans. Dosing recommendations for mothers during pregnancy should be aimed at preventing any health problems in neonates and infants, and a vitamin D dose sufficient for the mother during pregnancy should produce normal cord blood 25-OHD concentrations at birth (Kovacs, 2008). It could also be argued whether the same dietary recommendations apply to such a heterogeneous group as pregnant women in general. Additional recommendations, specially focused on some subgroups of pregnant women, could be beneficial.

B. Maternal vitamin D intake from food and supplements

Vitamin D intake from diet varies from one country to another depending on dietary habits, the use of dietary supplements, and the extent to which the national food supply is fortified with vitamin D. Naturally, vitamin D is found only in a limited number of foods such as fish, egg yolk, and some wild mushrooms (Holick, 1994). In many countries, specific foods, namely margarine, breakfast cereals, and milk products, are fortified with vitamin D. A considerable leap in vitamin D intake from food sources in pregnant women has been illustrated as a consequence of food fortification with vitamin D (Prasad *et al.*, 2010). Populations at risk of vitamin D deficiency are those for which, for environmental, cultural, or medical reasons, exposure to sunlight is poor and the dietary intake of vitamin D is low. Studies in developed countries have indicated that vitamin D is one of the most critical nutrients in terms of deficiencies during pregnancy (Holmes *et al.*, 2009; Nicolaidou *et al.*, 2006; Prasad *et al.*, 2010; Sahu *et al.*, 2009). Studies conducted in Europe during the past two decades have shown that the prevalence of low vitamin D status is higher in the countries of the Mediterranean and Central Europe than in Scandinavia and other northern regions reflecting the higher vitamin D intakes in Northern European countries coupled with differences in skin exposure to UVB sunlight (Prentice, 2008). Accordingly, differences are due to different skin types; the response to solar exposure in fair skin is more efficient than in dark skin (Clemens *et al.*, 1982).

Intake of vitamin D from dietary supplements is of particular importance in countries located furthest north, thus vitamin D supplementation in winter months (between October and March) is recommended during pregnancy (Nordic Nutrition Recommendations, 2004). However, it appears that less than half of the pregnant women adhere to these recommendations (Arkkola *et al.*, 2006). The use of dietary supplements is influenced by socio-demographic factors: those belonging to older age groups, having longer education, and normal weight before pregnancy favoring more frequent supplement use (Arkkola *et al.*, 2006). Few intervention studies during pregnancy have successfully improved vitamin D status of both the mothers and their newborn (Brooke *et al.*, 1980; Mallet *et al.*, 1986). However, women who report taking multivitamin supplements during pregnancy might have higher vitamin D status, but may still remain vitamin D insufficient (Bodnar *et al.*, 2007; Holmes *et al.*, 2009).

C. Dietary assessment during pregnancy

Pregnant women are more conscious about their diet, and their food choices are more strongly driven by safety concerns, when compared to nonpregnant women (Verbeke and De Bourdeaudhuij, 2007). Differences in food choice mainly relate to the claimed avoidance of specific foods (Verbeke and De Bourdeaudhuij, 2007), and more frequent use of dietary supplements during pregnancy (Arkkola *et al.*, 2006). The result of measurements of dietary intake and status of pregnant women is influenced by the timing of the assessment. Appetite fluctuations, nausea, vomiting, and heartburn are the most common symptoms experienced in pregnancy, and they may influence results of long-term diet reports (Jewell and Young,

2003; Richter, 2003; Wirfält, 1998). Diet during pregnancy is recalled with similar accuracy or perhaps slightly lower accuracy than adult diet in general (Bunin *et al.*, 2001).

In most of the studies that are reviewed in the present chapter (Table 10.1), the dietary information was collected retrospectively by a food frequency questionnaire (FFQ). The FFQ is often considered as the primary dietary assessment method in nutritional epidemiology (Willett, 1998). Although FFQs are not considered appropriate for estimating actual nutrient intakes, they can be used for categorizing individuals accurately according to relative intake, and for identifying subjects at the extremes of intakes. The FFQ method typically leads to overestimation of nutrient intake (Erkkola *et al.*, 2001). However, overestimation does not necessarily produce problems in epidemiological studies if the ranking of the persons according to their dietary intake is valid (Willett, 1998). Since the mothers fill in the FFQs retrospectively, the influence of the current diet is a possible source of bias (Bunin *et al.*, 2001). However, changes in food intake during pregnancy tend to be relatively small and, hence, difficult to detect by using this rather imprecise dietary assessment method (King, 2000).

Getting the maximum insight into the relationship between nutrient intake and disease risk requires examining the intake from both foods and supplements. Pregnancy seems to act as an additional motivator for taking dietary supplements, thus their use is widespread among pregnant women (e.g., Arkkola *et al.*, 2006). Therefore, ranking subjects according to nutrient intake exclusively from diet could lead to serious misclassification. Inclusion of dietary supplement intake is of particular importance in northern countries where vitamin D supplementation is recommended during pregnancy. However, with the continuous renewal of dietary supplements available in the market, maintaining a valid database is challenging and requires frequent updating

V. Maternal Vitamin D During Pregnancy and Disease Outcomes in the Offspring

A. Allergic diseases and asthma

Although the immunological processes related to the development of allergic diseases and asthma are not very clearly understood (Michail, 2009), current evidence suggests that the process may be the result of an induced shift in the balance between the Th1 and Th2 cytokines that favors Th2 dominance (Kay, 2001). The activities of vitamin D are believed to support the above proposition (Litonjua and Weiss, 2007). However, it has also been suggested that vitamin D may play a dual effect by both enhancing, whilst at the same time suppressing, Th2 allergy-associated responses

(Litonjua, 2009). These suggested contradictory effects are, however, believed to be due to the timing and chronicity of vitamin D administration (Ginde *et al.*, 2009; Litonjua, 2009).

So far, the only empirical evidence linking maternal vitamin D status or intake to allergic diseases and asthma in the offspring has come from some recent observational epidemiological studies. The most recent one is a prospective Finnish birth cohort study, in which maternal intake of vitamin D from foods (assessed by means of a validated FFQ) during pregnancy, was inversely associated with IgE-based sensitization to food allergens in 931 children followed for 5 years (Nwaru *et al.*, 2010). In a different subject series of the same Finnish cohort ($n = 1669$), increasing maternal intake of total vitamin D from foods during pregnancy was inversely associated with asthma, allergic rhinitis, but not with atopic eczema in 5-year-old children (Erkkola *et al.*, 2009). High maternal intake of vitamin D from foods assessed by means of a dietary history questionnaire during pregnancy has been associated with a reduced risk of wheeze and eczema in Japanese infants aged 16–24 months (Miyake *et al.*, 2009). Similar observations have been reported in two earlier prospective cohort studies from the U.S. (Camargo *et al.*, 2007) and UK (Devereux *et al.*, 2007). In the American study, which was FFQ based, high maternal vitamin D intake from foods and supplements was inversely associated with wheeze but not with eczema in 3-year-old children, while the UK study reported a decreased risk of wheezing but not atopic sensitization in children aged 5 years.

Contrary to the findings from the above-mentioned studies, which may be limited by the questionnaire-based assessment of maternal vitamin D status, another UK study with a 9-year follow-up reported an association between high maternal concentration of vitamin D (25-OHD) during pregnancy and increased risk of atopic eczema at the age of 9 months, and asthma at age of 9 years (Gale *et al.*, 2008). However, this study was subject to a number of shortcomings, including substantial loss to follow-up, especially at 9 years of age, as well as the lack of adjustment for potential confounders. Overall, at present, the observational evidence linking low maternal vitamin D status during pregnancy with increase in the risk of allergies and asthma in the offspring seems stronger. The next step to elucidate this hypothesis would be a clinical trial, and at the moment, one ongoing prenatal vitamin D supplementation is reported in the U.S. (Litonjua, 2009).

B. Autoimmune diseases

The processes that initiate the development of autoimmune diseases are not yet clearly understood (Chaudhuri, 2005; Harris, 2005; Knip *et al.*, 2010; Zipitis and Akobeng, 2008). Here we discuss the two most common autoimmune diseases in children—type 1 diabetes and multiple sclerosis.

Type 1 diabetes is generally considered to be a chronic, immune-mediated disease with a subclinical prodrome during which β cell autoimmunity develops into a clinical manifestation at a variable rate in genetically susceptible individuals (Knip *et al.*, 2010). Accumulated evidence supports a critical role for environmental factors in the disease development, and prospective birth cohort studies have shown that the first signs of β cell autoimmunity may be initiated during the first year of life. The etiology of multiple sclerosis is still strongly debated (Behan *et al.*, 2002), although there is evidence suggesting that it may be related to geographic location and seasonality (Chaudhuri, 2005). In this regard, some studies have proposed that sunlight exposure and seasonal fluctuation in vitamin D concentration may be associated with multiple sclerosis (Chaudhuri, 2005).

Vitamin D deficiency has been shown to be associated with an increased risk of Th1-mediated autoimmune diseases, such as multiple sclerosis and type 1 diabetes, suggesting that vitamin D deficiency leads to a decreased suppression of pathologic Th1-polarized immune responses (Baeke *et al.*, 2008). The preventive role of vitamin D against the incidence of type 1 diabetes has been indicated in animal models in which active vitamin D has modified T-cell differentiation, dendritic cell action, and induced cytokine secretion, resulting in a shift of balance to regulatory T cells (Mathieu and Badenhoop, 2005).

In a recent large Swedish registry-based case-control study, the relationship between birth season and multiple sclerosis incidence was examined by comparing each month of birth separately to birth during the other 11 months of the year. More multiple sclerosis subjects were born during June compared to those born during the other months. The authors concluded that their findings support the previous suggestions of an association between multiple sclerosis and season of birth. However, a more likely explanation for these findings may be the decreased exposure to sunlight during the winter period, which leads to low vitamin D concentration during pregnancy for births taking place after winter (Salzer *et al.*, 2010). Fernandes de Abreu *et al.* (2009) investigated whether it was the season of birth, or VDR polymorphisms or the combination of a high risk month of birth and VDR polymorphisms that is associated with multiple sclerosis. Medical files and DNA samples from 583 French multiple sclerosis patients and both of their parents were used. They reported a decrease in the number of children born during November with multiple sclerosis with no association observed between the VDR polymorphisms and multiple sclerosis. The study concluded that high levels of vitamin D during the third trimester of pregnancy (i.e., during the summer month for births occurring during winter) could be a protective factor for multiple sclerosis. The results from the above studies favor the suggested immunosuppressive effects of ultraviolent radiation, which has been shown by the latitudinal variations in the occurrence of multiple sclerosis (McMichael and Hall, 1997). However, this proposal has also been debated, and it has been advocated that actual routine supplementation of vitamin D during pregnancy may be favorable in preventing multiple sclerosis in the offspring, both from the public health perspective and in economic terms (Chaudhuri, 2005).

A Norwegian case-control study that evaluated the effect of cod liver oil and multivitamin supplementation during pregnancy on type 1 diabetes in the offspring associated maternal consumption of cod liver oil with a lower risk of type 1 diabetes (Stene *et al.*, 2000). Multivitamin supplementation during pregnancy, however, was not associated with the risk of type 1 diabetes. Since cod liver oil is rich both in vitamin D and omega-3 fatty acids, the authors concluded that the protective effect of maternal cod liver oil intake may be due to either vitamin D or omega-3 fatty acids, or a combination of both. A study from the U.S. (Fronczak *et al.*, 2003) and another from Sweden (Brekke and Ludvigsson, 2007) prospectively examined the effects of maternal vitamin D intake during pregnancy on the appearance of diabetes-related autoimmunity in the offspring. The U.S. study followed the subjects for 4 years and observed a decreased risk of islet autoimmunity with maternal intake of vitamin D from food but not from supplements. Conversely, the Swedish study observed a decreased risk of diabetes-related autoimmunity in the children at the age of 1 year with maternal vitamin D intake from supplements. In addition to these ambiguous findings, the use of islet autoimmunity as an endpoint in the above studies makes it more difficult to draw a valid conclusion on the effect of maternal pregnancy vitamin D on type 1 diabetes in the offspring. Some previous studies have reported a similar protective effect of intake of vitamin D supplements during infancy and later type 1 diabetes (Hyppönen *et al.*, 2001; The EURODIAB Substudy 2 Study Group, 1999). However, no significant differences were observed between the circulating vitamin D concentrations of pregnant women from Russian Karelia and Finland, the former having a low incidence and the latter an extremely high incidence of type 1 diabetes (Viskari *et al.*, 2006). This finding speaks against a critical role of vitamin D deficiency in the development of β cell autoimmunity and type 1 diabetes.

C. Infectious diseases

The role of vitamin D in preventing infections has long been recognized (Martineau *et al.*, 2007). For instance, from the 1930s until the introduction of anti-infective chemotherapy in the 1950s, vitamin D_3, which was isolated from cod liver oil, was widely used for the treatment of tuberculosis (Martineau *et al.*, 2007). It has been shown that vitamin D can help in enhancing innate immunity by stimulating the synthesis of an antimicrobial peptide cathelicidin in human skin cells (Schauber *et al.*, 2008). Of recent, some epidemiological studies have demonstrated a protective role for vitamin D in respiratory tract infections (Ginde *et al.*, 2009; Laaksi *et al.*, 2007; Urashima *et al.*, 2010). A recent case-control study showed that newborns with subclinical vitamin D deficiency, as a result of low maternal S-25-OHD concentrations during pregnancy, may be at increased risk of acute lower respiratory infection (Karatekin *et al.*, 2009). However, in an earlier prospective cohort study, maternal intake of vitamin D during pregnancy was not associated with any respiratory infection in the offspring at 3 years of age (Camargo *et al.*, 2007). Moreover, Gale *et al.* (2008) reported an increased risk of pneumonia and diarrhea at 9 months with high maternal concentrations of S-25-OHD during pregnancy, in another prospective cohort study. Since no consensus can be found in the above studies, the role of maternal vitamin D status during pregnancy in preventing infectious diseases in the offspring remains inconclusive; thus, more rigorous randomized controlled trials would be required to decipher the putative effect of vitamin D.

D. Cancer

Recent evidence suggests that VDRs, which have been found on melanoma cell lines and tissues, are possibly associated with a decreased risk of cancers through vitamin D actions on cell proliferation, differentiation, cell death, and angiogenesis (Egan, 2009; Eisman *et al.*, 1980). 1,25-hydroxy vitamin D has also been identified to promote cell survival and inhibit the invasion and metastasis of tumor cells (Osborne and Hutchinson, 2002). To our knowledge, no study has so far investigated the association between maternal vitamin D during pregnancy and cancers in the offspring. However, a recent Finnish population-based case-control study focusing on the association between maternal S-25-OHD levels measured during the first trimester of pregnancy and breast cancer and pregnancy-associated breast cancer, reported an association between vitamin D and an increased risk of pregnancy-associated breast cancer but not with breast cancer (Agborsangaya *et al.*, 2010). Another case-control study derived from the same cohort reported a null association between S-25-OHD and the risk of ovarian cancer in the women (Toriola *et al.*, 2010).

VI. Conclusions

Vitamin D deficiency during pregnancy is prevalent in many parts of the world, a fact that goes hand in hand with the observed increase in the incidence of immune-mediated diseases in the offspring. Maternal vitamin D status during pregnancy is a key determinant of the vitamin D status of the infant. S-25-OHD concentration presents a useful marker of the risk of clinical deficiency, despite limitations caused by the lack of methodological standardization. There is general agreement that the appropriate dose of vitamin D during pregnancy is likely higher than the current dietary reference intake for the pregnant women with only modest UVB-exposure. If the advice to avoid UVB light is followed, the goal of raising 25-OHD concentrations can be achieved efficiently only by providing vitamin D through dietary supplementation.

The observations from birth cohort studies indicate a beneficial association for higher maternal vitamin D intake during pregnancy against childhood asthma and allergic diseases in the offspring. However, some conflicting findings do suggest that the timing of exposure to lower or higher vitamin D levels is of importance. Further work is required to define the critical windows of exposure to adequate vitamin D levels during pregnancy. The effect of maternal vitamin D on type 1 diabetes, multiple sclerosis, and infectious diseases remains inconclusive. More research is required to confirm the contribution of maternal dietary factors to the development of immune-mediated diseases.

We lack the knowledge on the mechanisms by which vitamin D influences fetal development. The complex relationship between maternal nutrition and birth outcomes emphasizes the need for consistent and thorough assessment of women's diets throughout the duration of pregnancy. Researchers in this field are also faced with the methodological challenges of eliminating biases and adequately adjusting for potentially important confounding factors. More evidence is needed to better understand the net risks and benefits of maternal and early postnatal vitamin D status in relation to a range of immunologic and other diseases. There is a call for clinical trials and large birth cohorts where there are valid measures of maternal and fetal vitamin D intake and long-term health outcomes.

REFERENCES

Agborsangaya, C., Surcel, H. M., Toriola, A. T., Pukkala, E., Parkkila, S., Tuohimaa, P., Lukanova, A., and Lehtinen, M. (2010). Serum 25-hydroxyvitamin D at pregnancy and risk of breast cancer in a prospective cohort study. *Eur. J. Cancer* **46,** 467–470.

Arkkola, T., Räsänen, M., Metsälä, J., Kronberg-Kippilä, C., Erkkola, M., Knip, M., Ovaskainen, M.-L., and Virtanen, S. M. (2006). Food consumption and nutrient intake of Finnish pregnant women. *Br. J. Nutr.* **96,** 913–920.

Baeke, F., van Etten, E., Gysemans, C., Overbergh, L., and Mathieu, C. (2008). Vitamin D signalling in immune-mediated disorders: Evolving insights and therapeutic opportunities. *Mol. Aspects Med.* **29,** 376–387.

Behan, P. O., Chaudhuri, A., and Roep, B. O. (2002). The pathogenesis of multiple sclerosis revisited. *J. R. Coll. Physicians Edinb.* **32,** 244–265.

Binkley, N., Krueger, D., and Lensmeyer, G. (2009). 25-hydroxyvitamin D measurement, 2009: A review for clinicians. *J. Clin. Densitom.* **12,** 417–427.

Bischoff-Ferrari, H. A., Dawson-Hughes, B., Staehelin, H. B., Orav, J. E., Stuc, A. E., Theiler, R., Wong, J. B., Egli, A., Kiel, D. P., and Henschkowski, J. (2009a). Fall prevention with supplemental and active forms of vitamin D: A meta-analysis of randomised controlled trials. *Br. Med. J.* **399,** b3692.

Bischoff-Ferrari, H. A., Shao, A., Dawson-Hughes, B., Hathcock, J., Giovannucci, E., and Willett, W. C. (2009b). Benefit-risk assessment of vitamin D supplementation. *Osteoporos. Int.* **21,** 1121–1132.

Bischoff-Ferrari, H. A., Willett, W. C., Wong, J. B., Stuck, A. E., Staehelin, H. B., Orav, E. J., Thoma, A., Kiel, D. P., and Henschkowski, J. (2009c). Prevention of nonvertebral fractures with oral vitamin D and dose dependency: A meta-analysis of randomized controlled trials. *Arch. Intern. Med.* **23,** 551–561.

Bodnar, L. M., and Simhan, H. N. (2010). Vitamin D may be a link to black-white disparities in adverse birth outcomes. *Obstet. Gynecol. Surv.* **65,** 273–284.

Bodnar, L. M., Simhan, H. N., Powers, R. W., Frank, M. P., Cooperstein, E., and Roberts, J. M. (2007). High prevalence of vitamin D insufficiency in black and white pregnant women residing in the northern United States and their neonates. *J. Nutr.* **137,** 447–452.

Brekke, H. K., and Ludvigsson, J. (2007). Vitamin D supplementation and diabetes-related autoimmunity in the ABIS study. *Pediatr. Diabetes* **8,** 11–14.

Brooke, O. G., Brown, I. R., Bone, C. D., Carter, N. D., Cleeve, H. J., Maxwell, J. D., Robinson, V. P., and Winder, S. M. (1980). Vitamin D supplements in pregnant Asian women: Effects on calcium status and fetal growth. *Br. Med. J.* **15,** 751–754.

Bunin, G. R., Gyllstrom, M. E., Brown, J. E., Kahn, E. B., and Kushi, L. H. (2001). Recall of diet during a past pregnancy. *Am. J. Epidemiol.* **154,** 1136–1142.

Burlingham, W. J. (2009). A lesson in tolerance—Maternal instruction to fetal cells. *N. Engl. J. Med.* **360,** 1355–1357.

Calder, P. C., Krauss-Etschmann, S., de Jong, E. C., Dupont, C., Frick, J. S., Frokiaer, H., Heinrich, J., Garn, H., Koletzko, S., Lack, G., Mattelio, G., Renz, H., *et al.* (2006). Early nutrition and immunity—Progress and perspectives. *Br. J. Nutr.* **96,** 774–790.

Camargo, C. A., Rifas-Shiman, S. L., Litonjua, A. A., Rich-Edwards, J. W., Weiss, S. T., Godl, D. R., Kleinman, K., and Gillman, M. W. (2007). Maternal intake of vitamin D during pregnancy and risk of recurrent wheeze in children at 3 y of age. *Am. J. Clin. Nutr.* **85,** 788–795.

Carter, G. D. (2009). 25-Hydroxyvitamin D assays: The quest for accuracy. *Clin. Chem.* **55,** 1300–1302.

Carter, G. D., Berry, J. L., Gunter, E., Jones, G., Jones, J. C., Makin, H. L., Sufi, S., and Wheeler, M. J. (2010). Proficiency testing of 25-Hydroxyvitamin D (25-OHD) assays. *J. Steroid Biochem. Mol. Biol.* **121,** 176–179.

Chaudhuri, A. (2005). Why we should offer routine vitamin D supplementation in pregnancy and childhood to prevent multiple sclerosis. *Med. Hypotheses* **64,** 608–618.

Clemens, T. L., Adams, J. S., Henderson, S. L., and Holick, M. F. (1982). Increased skin pigment reduces the capacity of skin to synthesizes vitamin D3. *Lancet* **319,** 74–76.

Cunningham-Rundles, S., Ling, H., Ho-Lin, D., Dnistrian, A., Cassileth, B. R., and Perlman, J. M. (2009). Role of nutrients in the development of neonatal immune responses. *Nutr. Rev.* **67,** 152S–163S.

Devereux, G., Litonjua, A. A., Turner, S. W., Craig, L. C., McNeill, G., Martindale, S., Helms, P. J., Seaton, A., and Weiss, S. T. (2007). Maternal vitamin D intake during pregnancy and early childhood wheezing. *Am. J. Clin. Nutr.* **85,** 853–859.

Egan, K. M. (2009). Vitamin D and melanoma. *Ann. Epidemiol.* **19,** 455–461.

Eisman, J. A., Martin, T. J., MacIntyre, I., Frampton, R. J., Moseley, J. M., and Witehead, R. (1980). 1, 25-Dihydroxyvitamin D3 receptor in a cultured human breast cancer cell line (MCF 7 cells). *Biochem. Biophys. Res. Commun.* **93,** 9–15.

Erkkola, M., Karppinen, M., Javanainen, J., Räsänen, L., Knip, M., and Virtanen, S. M. (2001). Validity and reproducibility of a food frequency questionnaire for pregnant Finnish women. *Am. J. Epidemiol.* **154,** 466–476.

Erkkola, M., Kaila, M., Nwaru, B. I., Kronberg-Kippilä, C., Ahonen, S., Nevalainen, J., Pekkanen, J., Ilonen, J., Simell, O., Knip, M., and Virtanen, S. M. (2009). Maternal vitamin D intake during pregnancy is inversely associated with asthma and allergic rhinitis in 5-year-old children. *Clin. Exp. Allergy* **39,** 875–882.

Fernandes de Abreu, D. A., Babron, M. C., Rebeix, I., Fontenille, C., Yaouanq, J., Brassat, D., Fontaine, B., Clerget-Darpoux, F., Jehan, F., and Feron, F. (2009). Season of birth and not vitamin D receptor promoter polymorphisms is a risk factor for multiple sclerosis. *Mult. Scler.* **15,** 1146–1152.

Fronczak, C. M., Barón, A. E., Chase, H. P., Ross, C., Brady, H. L., Hoffman, M., Eisenbarth, G. S., Rewers, M., and Norris, J. M. (2003). In utero dietary exposures and risk of islet autoimmunity in children. *Diab. Care* **26,** 3237–3242.

Gale, C. R., Robinson, S. M., Harvey, N. C., Javaid, M. K., Jiang, B., Martyn, C. N., Godfrey, K. M., and Cooper, C. (2008). The Princess Anne Hospital Study Group. Maternal vitamin D status during pregnancy and child outcomes. *Eur. J. Clin. Nutr.* **62,** 68–77.

Ginde, A. A., Mansbach, J. M., and Camargo, C. A. (2009). Association between serum 25-hydroxyvitamin D level and upper respiratory tract infection in the Third National Health and Nutrition Examination Survey. *Arch. Intern. Med.* **23,** 384–390.

Greer, F. R. (2008). 25-Hydroxyvitamin D: Functional outcomes in infants and young children. *Am. J. Clin. Nutr.* **88,** 529S–533S.

Hansdottir, S., Monick, M. M., Lovan, N., Powers, L., Gerke, A., and Hunninghake, G. W. (2010). Vitamin D decreases respiratory syncytial virus induction of NF-kappaB-linked chemokines and cytokines in airway epithelium while maintaining the antiviral state. *J. Immunol.* **15,** 965–974.

Harris, S. S. (2005). Vitamin D in type 1 diabetes prevention. *J. Nutr.* **135,** 323–325.

Holick, M. F. (1994). McCollum Award Lecture, 1994: Vitamin D—New horizons for the 21st century. *Am. J. Clin. Nutr.* **60,** 619–630.

Holick, M. F. (2004). Sunlight and vitamin D for bone health and prevention of autoimmune diseases, cancers, and cardiovascular disease. *Am. J. Clin. Nutr.* **80,** 1678S–1688S.

Hollis, B. W., and Wagner, C. L. (2004). Assessment of dietary vitamin D requirements during pregnancy and lactation. *Am. J. Clin. Nutr.* **79,** 717–726.

Holmes, V. A., Barnes, M. S., Alexander, H. D., McFaul, P., and Wallace, J. M. (2009). Vitamin D deficiency and insufficiency in pregnant women: A longitudinal study. *Br. J. Nutr.* **102,** 876–881.

Houghton, L. A., and Vieth, R. (2006). The case against ergocalciferol (vitamin D2) as a vitamin supplement. *Am. J. Clin. Nutr.* **84,** 694–697.

Hyppönen, E., Läärä, E., Reunanen, A., Järvelin, M. R., and Virtanen, S. M. (2001). Intake of vitamin D and risk of type 1 diabetes: A birth-cohort study. *Lancet* **358,** 1500–1503.

Jeffery, L. E., Burke, F., Mura, M., Zheng, Y., Qureshi, O. S., Hewison, M., Walker, L. S., Lammas, D. A., Raza, K., and Sansom, D. M. (2009). 1, 25-Dihydroxyvitamin D3 and IL-2 combine to inhibit T cell production of inflammatory cytokines and promote development of regulatory T cells expressing CTLA-4 and FoxP3. *J. Immunol.* **183,** 5458–5467.

Jewell, D., and Young, G. (2003). Interventions for nausea and vomiting in early pregnancy. *Cochrane Database Syst. Rev.* **4,** CD000145.

Karatekin, G., Kaya, A., Salihoglu, O., Balci, H., and Nuhoglu, A. (2009). Association of subclinical vitamin D deficiency in newborns with acute lower respiratory infection and their mothers. *Eur. J. Clin. Nutr.* **63,** 473–477.

Kay, A. B. (2001). Allergy and allergic diseases: First of two parts. *N. Engl. J. Med.* **344,** 30–37.
King, J. C. (2000). Physiology of pregnancy and nutrient metabolism. *Am. J. Clin. Nutr.* **71,** 1218S–1225S.
Knip, M., Virtanen, S. M., and Åkerblom, H. K. (2010). Infant feeding and the risk of type 1 diabetes. *Am. J. Clin. Nutr.* **91,** 1506S–1513S.
Kovacs, C. S. (2008). Vitamin D in pregnancy and lactation: Maternal, fetal, and neonatal outcomes from human and animal studies. *Am. J. Clin. Nutr.* **88,** 520S–528S.
Kuchuk, N. O., van Schoor, N. M., Pluijm, S. M., Chines, A., and Lips, P. (2009). Vitamin D status, parathyroid function, bone turnover, and BMD in postmenopausal women with osteoporosis: Global perspective. *J. Bone Miner. Res.* **24,** 693–701.
Laaksi, I., Ruohola, J. P., Tuohimaa, P., Auvinen, A., Haataja, R., Pihlajamäki, H., and Ylikomi, T. (2007). An association of serum vitamin D concentrations < 40 nmol/L with acute respiratory tract infection in young Finnish men. *Am. J. Clin. Nutr.* **86,** 714–717.
Lapillonne, A. (2010). Vitamin D deficiency during pregnancy may impair maternal and fetal outcomes. *Med. Hypotheses* **74,** 71–75.
Lips, P., Bouillon, R., van Schoor, N. M., Vanderschueren, D., Verschueren, S., Kuchuk, N., Milisen, K., and Boonen, S. (2009). Reducing fracture risk with calcium and vitamin D. *Clin. Endocrinol. (Oxf)* **73,** 277–285.
Litonjua, A. A. (2009). Childhood asthma may be a consequence of vitamin D deficiency. *Curr. Opin. Allergy Clin. Immunol.* **9,** 202–207.
Litonjua, A. A., and Weiss, S. T. (2007). Is vitamin D deficiency to blame for the asthma epidemic? *J. Allergy Clin. Immunol.* **120,** 1031–1035.
Liu, P. T., Stenger, S., Li, H., Wenzel, L., Tan, B. H., Krutzik, S. R., Ochoa, M. T., Schauber, J., Wu, K., Meinken, C., Kamen, D. L., Wagner, M., *et al.* (2006). Toll-like receptor triggering of a vitamin D-mediated human antimicrobial response. *Science* **24,** 1770–1773.
Looker, A. C., Pfeiffer, C. M., Lacher, D. A., Schleicher, R. L., Picciano, M. F., and Yetley, E. A. (2008). Serum 25-hydroxyvitamin D status of the US population: 1988–1994 compared with 2000–2004. *Am. J. Clin. Nutr.* **88,** 1519–1527.
Lucas, R. M., Ponsonby, A., Pasco, J. A., and Morley, R. (2008). Future health implications of prenatal and early-life vitamin D status. *Nutr. Rev.* **66,** 710–720.
Mallet, E., Gügi, B., Brunelle, P., Hénocq, A., Basuyau, J. P., and Lemeur, H. (1986). Vitamin D supplementation in pregnancy: A controlled trial of two methods. *Obstet. Gynecol.* **68,** 300–304.
Martineau, A. R., Honecker, F. U., Wilkinson, R. J., and Griffiths, C. J. (2007). Vitamin D in the treatment of pulmonary tuberculosis. *J. Steroid Biochem. Mol. Biol.* **103,** 793–798.
Mathieu, C., and Badenhoop, K. (2005). Vitamin D and type 1 diabetes mellitus: State of the art. *Trends Endocrinol. Metab.* **16,** 261–266.
McMichael, A. J., and Hall, A. J. (1997). Does immunosuppressive ultraviolent radiation explain the latitude gradient for multiple sclerosis? *Epidemiology* **8,** 642–645.
McNally, J. D., Leis, K., Matheson, L. A., Karuananyake, C., Sankaran, K., and Rosenberg, A. M. (2009). Vitamin D deficiency in young children with severe acute lower respiratory infection. *Pediatr. Pulmonol.* **44,** 981–988.
Michail, S. (2009). The role of probiotics in allergic diseases. *Allergy Asthma Clin. Immunol.* **5,** 5.
Miyake, Y., Sasaki, S., Tanaka, K., and Hirota, Y. (2009). Dairy food, calcium, and vitamin D in take in pregnancy and wheeze and eczema in infants. *Eur. Respir. J.* **35,** 1228–1234.
Mora, J. R., Iwata, M., and von Andriano, U. H. (2008). Vitamin effects on the immune system: Vitamins A and D take centre stage. *Nat. Rev. Immunol.* **8,** 685–698.
Nicolaidou, P., Hatzistamatiou, Z., Papadopoulou, A., Kaleyias, J., Floropoulou, E., Lagona, E., Tsagris, V., Costalos, C., and Antsaklis, A. (2006). Low vitamin D status in mother-newborn pairs in Greece. *Calcif. Tissue Int.* **78,** 337–342.

Nordic Nutrition Recommendations (2004). Integrating Nutrition and Physical Activity, 4th ed. Nordic Council of Ministers, Copenhagen, Nord 2004:13.
Norman, A. W. (2008). A vitamin D nutritional cornucopia: New insights concerning the serum 25-hydroxyvitamin D status of the US population. *Am. J. Clin. Nutr.* **88,** 1455–1456.
Norman, A. W., Mizwicki, M. T., and Norman, D. P. (2004). Steroid-hormone rapid actions, membrane receptors and a conformational ensemble model. *Nat. Rev. Drug Discov.* **3,** 27–41.
Norman, A. W., Bouillon, R., Whiting, S. J., Vieth, R., and Lips, P. (2007). 13th Workshop consensus for vitamin D nutritional guidelines. *J. Steroid Biochem. Mol. Biol.* **103,** 204–205.
Nwaru, B. I., Ahonen, S., Kaila, M., Erkkola, M., Haapala, A.-M., Kronberg-Kippilä, C., Veijola, R., Ilonen, J., Simell, O., Knip, M., and Virtanen, S. M. (2010). Maternal diet during pregnancy and allergic sensitization in the offspring by 5 years of age: A prospective cohort study. *Pediatr. Allergy Immunol.* **21,** 29–37.
Osborne, J. E., and Hutchinson, P. E. (2002). Vitamin D and systemic cancer: Is this relevant to malignant melanoma? *Br. J. Dermatol.* **147,** 197–213.
Pichler, J., Gerstmayr, M., Szépfalusi, Z., Urbanek, R., Peterlik, M., and Willheim, M. (2002). 1 alpha, 25(OH)2D3 inhibits not only Th1 but also Th2 differentiation in human cord blood T cells. *Pediatr. Res.* **52,** 12–18.
Prasad, M., Lumia, M., Erkkola, M., Tapanainen, H., Kronberg-Kippilä, C., Tuokkola, J., Uusitalo, U., Simell, O., Veijola, R., Knip, M., Ovaskainen, M.-L., and Virtanen, S. M. (2010). Diet composition of pregnant Finnish women: Changes over time and across seasons. *Public Health Nutr.* **13,** 939–946.
Prentice, A. (2008). Vitamin D deficiency: A global perspective. *Nutr. Rev.* **66,** 153S–164S.
Richter, J. E. (2003). Gastroesophageal reflux disease during pregnancy. *Gastroenterol. Clin. North Am.* **32,** 235–261.
Sahu, M., Bhatia, V., Aggarwal, A., Rawat, V., Saxena, P., Pandey, A., and Das, V. (2009). Vitamin D deficiency in rural girls and pregnant women despite abundant sunshine in northern India. *Clin. Endocrinol. (Oxf)* **70,** 680–684.
Salzer, J., Svenningsson, A., and Sundström, P. (2010). Season of birth and multiple sclerosis in Sweden. *Acta Neurol. Scand.* **121,** 20–23.
Schauber, J., Dorschner, R. A., Coda, A. B., Büchau, A. S., Liu, P. T., Kiken, D., Helfrich, Y. R., Kang, S., Elalieh, H. Z., Steinmeyer, A., Zügel, U., Bikle, D. D., *et al.* (2008). Injury enhances TLR2 function and antimicrobial peptide expression through a vitamin D-dependent mechanism. *J. Clin. Investig.* **117,** 803–811.
Specker, B. (2004). Vitamin D requirements during pregnancy. *Am. J. Clin. Nutr.* **80,** 1740S–1747S.
Stene, L. C., Ulriksen, J., Magnus, P., and Joner, G. (2000). Use of cod liver oil during pregnancy associated with Type 1 diabetes in the offspring. *Diabetologia* **43,** 1093–1098.
The EURODIAB Substudy 2 Study Group (1999). Vitamin D supplement in early childhood and risk for type I (insulin-dependent) diabetes mellitus. *Diabetologia* **42,** 51–54.
Toriola, A. T., Surcel, H. M., Agborsangaya, C., Grankvist, K., Tuohimaa, P., Toniolo, P., Lukanova, A., Pukkala, E., and Lehtinen, M. (2010). Serum 25-hydroxyvitamin D and the risk of ovarian cancer. *Eur. J. Cancer* **46,** 364–369.
Urashima, M., Segawa, T., Okazaki, M., Kurihara, M., Wada, Y., and Ida, H. (2010). Randomized trial of vitamin D supplementation to prevent seasonal influenza A in schoolchildren. *Am. J. Clin. Nutr.* **91,** 1255–1260.
Verbeke, W., and De Bourdeaudhuij, I. (2007). Dietary behaviour of pregnant versus non-pregnant women. *Appetite* **48,** 78–86.
Vieth, R. (1999). Vitamin D supplementation, 25-hydroxyvitamin D concentrations, and safety. *Am. J. Clin. Nutr.* **69,** 842–856.

Vieth, R. (2006). What is the optimal vitamin D status for health? *Prog. Biophys. Mol. Biol.* **92,** 26–32.
Viljakainen, H. T., Saarnio, E., Hytinantti, T., Miettinen, M., Surcel, H., Mäkitie, O., Andersson, S., Laitinen, K., and Lamberg-Allardt, C. (2010). Maternal vitamin D status determines bone variables in the newborn. *J. Clin. Endocrinol. Metab.* **95,** 1749–1757.
Viskari, H., Kondrashova, A., Koskela, P., Knip, M., and Hyöty, H. (2006). Circulating vitamin D concentrations in two neighboring populations with markedly different incidence of type 1 diabetes. *Diab. Care* **29,** 1458–1459.
Willett, W. (1998). Nutritional Epidemiology. 2nd ed. Oxford University Press, New York.
Wirfält, E. (1998). Cognitive aspects of dietary assessment. *Scand. J. Nutr.* **42,** 56–59.
Yamshchikov, A. V., Desai, N. S., Blumberg, H. M., Ziegler, T. R., and Tangpricha, V. (2009). Vitamin D for treatment and prevention of infectious diseases: A systematic review of randomized controlled trials. *Endocr. Pract.* **15,** 438–449.
Zhou, S., LeBoff, M. S., and Glowacki, J. (2010). Vitamin D metabolism and action in human bone marrow stromal cells. *Endocrinology* **151,** 14–22.
Zipitis, C. S., and Akobeng, A. K. (2008). Vitamin D supplementation in early childhood and risk of type 1 diabetes: A systematic review and meta-analysis. *Arch. Dis. Child.* **93,** 512–517.
Zittermann, A., and Gummert, J. F. (2010). Sun, vitamin D, and cardiovascular disease. *J. Photochem. Photobiol. B* **101,** 124–129.

CHAPTER ELEVEN

Vitamin D Deficiency and Connective Tissue Disease

Eva Zold, Zsolt Barta, *and* Edit Bodolay

Contents

Abstract

Recently, the evidence linking vitamin D status as a potential environmental factor affecting autoimmune disease prevalence continues to accumulate. Beyond that the traditional known metabolic activities, vitamin D has been shown to modulate the immune system and has anti-inflammatory properties. The immune-regulatory role of vitamin D affects both the innate and adaptive immune responses contributing to the immune-tolerance of self-structures. Vitamin D deficiency skews the immunologic response towards loss of tolerance.

Serum levels of vitamin D have been found to be significantly lower in several autoimmune or immune-mediated diseases than in the healthy population. Experimental animal models and clinical studies show that 1,25-dihydroxyvitamin D3 or vitamin D receptor (VDR) agonists can either prevent or suppress symptoms of type 1 diabetes, experimental autoimmune encephalomyelitis, rheumatoid arthritis, systemic lupus erthyematosus and inflammatory bowel disease.

Division of Clinical Immunology, 3rd Department of Medicine, Medical and Health Science Center, University of Debrecen, Debrecen, Hungary

Vitamins and Hormones, Volume 86
ISSN 0083-6729, DOI: 10.1016/B978-0-12-386960-9.00011-3

The heading aims at reviewing the complex immune-regulatory role of vitamin D from the cellular and humoral level through animal models of autoimmune rheumatic diseases and representing the known contribution of vitamin D in the pathogenesis of connective tissue diseases. Increased vitamin D intakes might reduce the incidence and severity of autoimmune disorders besides reducing the rate of osteoporotic bone fracture.

I. Introduction

Environmental factors play an important role in the development and progression of systemic autoimmune diseases, as does a susceptible genetic and hormonal background. Since the 1990s, an increasing number of observations support the idea that impaired vitamin D homeostasis contributes to autoimmune processes. The first clinical description of vitamin D-related disease, rickets, was made by Glisson in 1651, and the association between lack of sunshine and rickets was first recognized in the beginning of the twentieth century (Holick, 1994).

As a nutrient, Vitamin D is unique in that it can be obtained both from dietary sources and the action of sunlight on skin. The term "vitamin D" refers to several different forms of this vitamin, two of which are important in humans: vitamin D_2 (ergocalciferol) and vitamin D_3 (cholecalciferol). Vitamin D_2 is synthesized by plants, while vitamin D_3 is synthesized by humans in the skin when it is exposed to ultraviolet-B (UVB) rays from sunlight. Foods may contain vitamin D_2 or D_3. In humans, the primary source of vitamin D precursors is the skin; dietary intake can provide only 20% of the body's daily requirements of vitamin D (Cutolo *et al.*, 2009). In the skin, the cutaneous exposure to UVB light results in the photolytic conversion of 7-dehydrocholesterol to previtamin-D_3 followed by thermal isomerization to vitamin D_3. Further exposure of previtamin-D_3 to UVB results in the formation of inactive vitamin D compounds. This process serves as a protective mechanism against vitamin D toxicity. Subsequently, thermal isomerization, a two-step activation process, occurs with hepatic hydroxylation to form 25-hydroxyvitamin D_3 (25(OH)D) and further, with renal hydroxylation, to form 1,25-dihydroxyvitamin D_3 ($1,25(OH)_2D_3$). 25-hydroxylation is poorly regulated, with levels of 25(OH)D increasing proportionately with increases in dietary vitamin D intake and cutaneous production (Dusso *et al.*, 2005). Renal hydroxylation is highly regulated by dietary calcium and phosphate, circulating levels of $1,25(OH)_2D_3$ metabolite, and parathormone (PTH). Vitamin D metabolites are bound in the blood circulation to vitamin D binding protein, which has a high homology to albumin. The active metabolite $1,25(OH)_2D_3$ enters the target cell from the blood circulation and binds to a vitamin D receptor (VDR) in the cytoplasm which then enters the nucleus and heterodimerizes with the retinoid

X receptor (RXR). The $1,25(OH)_2D_3$-RXR-VDR complex then binds to vitamin D response elements (VDRE) located on DNA. This is followed by transcription and translation and the formation of proteins, such as calcium binding protein and osteocalcin.

All biologic responses ascribed to vitamin D are now known to arise primarily due to the active metabolite of vitamin D, namely $1,25(OH)_2D_3$, the molecule of which is known to have multiple functions. $1,25(OH)_2D_3$ was originally described as an essential hormone for bone and mineral homeostasis. The discovery of VDR in the cells of the immune system suggests that vitamin D could have immunoregulatory properties (Fritsche *et al.*, 2003). VDR is constitutively expressed by antigen-presenting cells (APCs) such as macrophages and dendritic cells (DCs) and inductibly expressed by lymphocytes following activation. The recognition that extra-renal 1-α hydroxylation of 25(OH)D occurs in many different tissues represents a further advance in understanding the diverse actions of vitamin D.

II. The Immune-Regulative Role of Vitamin D

In the immune system, active vitamin D is generated mainly locally as the synthetic product of the CYP27B1-hydroxylase gene and acts locally on both macrophages and lymphocytes in the inflammatory microenvironment (Adams *et al.*, 1983). These local immunoregulatory effects of active vitamin D metabolite are below the limit of our detection clinically. On the other hand, in granulomatous diseases such as sarcoidosis and tuberculosis, vitamin D metabolite also provides at least part of the molecular basis for the excessive production of $1,25(OH)_2D_3$ by macrophages that results in hypercalcemia (Iannuzzi *et al.*, 2007). In contrast to the systemic endocrine system, the macrophage CYP27B1-hydroxylase is stimulated by the Toll-like receptor (TLR)4 ligand lipopolysaccharide (LPS) and the tuberculosis TLR2/1 ligand and by the monokine interferon (IFN)-γ. The activity of CYP27B1-hydroxylase enzyme is associated with the inflammatory index of the underlying disease and is driven by endogenously synthesized nitric oxide (NO).

III. Effect of Vitamin D on Innate Immunity

The innate immune cells have key direct functions in immune response: rapid detection of microbes, phagocytosis of those microbes, and antimicrobial activity. Vitamin D has been shown to act on innate immune cells to inhibit their inflammatory activity and capacity to prime adaptive immune responses, promoting direct antimicrobial function. The VDR promotes antigen processing, phagocytosis, superoxide synthesis, interleukin 1-beta, and tumor necrosis factor (TNF)-α production. $1,25(OH)_2D_3$ increases the level of acid phosphatese and augments oxidative burst.

TLRs recognize nonspecific pathogen-associated molecular patterns and are important for the induction of early inflammatory immuneresponses. Many microarray studies found that signaling through human macrophage TLR1/2 toll-like receptor heterodimers stimulated with bacterial lipopeptides and induced expression of both CYP27B1 and VDR (Liu *et al.*, 2006). In addition, *in vitro* treatment of human monocytes with VDR ligand inhibits their expression of the TLRs (Oberg *et al.*, 1993; Sadeghi *et al.*, 2006; Scherberich *et al.*, 2005). *In vivo*, treating human monocytes with $1,25(OH)_2D_3$ suppressed expression of both TLR2 and TLR4 mRNA and protein in a time- and dose-dependent manner (Thomas *et al.*, 1998). Downregulation of monocyte TLR expression led to reduced production of the pro-inflammatory cytokine TNF-α.

Furthermore, vitamin D promotes synthesis of antimicrobial peptide products, such as cathelicidin, cationic peptides, and defensine, which are endogenous antibiotics and have a direct microbe damaging function, particularly in the mucosal immune system. The antimicrobial peptides CAMP (cathelicidin antimicrobial peptide, hCAP18, LL37) and DEFB2 (DEFB4, β-defensin 2) contain promoter-proximal consensus natural DR3-type response elements (VDREs) (Wang *et al.*, 2004). Dimeloe *et al.* found lower levels of vitamin D in patients with sepsis than in healthy controls (Dimeloe *et al.*, 2010). In these patients, the serum 25(OH)D level correlated with serum LL-37, which is a active cationic peptide, suggesting that the systemic level of LL-37 may be regulated by vitamin D status. *In vitro*, the induction of cathelicidin in human monocytes and neutrophiles via vitamin D analogue treatment increased antimicrobia activity against some respiratory pathogens (Martineau *et al.*, 2007; Wang *et al.*, 2004; Yim *et al.*, 2007).

In vitro, calprotectin and S100-proteins, important regulators of the innate immune system, have been described as increasing in response to vitamin D in human cancer cell lines (Kuruto-Niwa *et al.*, 1998).

The association between vitamin D physiology and infectious disease is also supported by genetic studies implicating polymorphisms in the gene that encodes the VDR in disease susceptibility (Uitterlinden *et al.*, 2004). These studies show the link between VDR polymorphisms and a number of infectious diseases, including susceptibility to *Mycobacterium tuberculosis* and *Mycobacterium leprae* infection and treatment outcome. That TLR-activated macrophages can convert vitamin D to produce antimicrobial peptides could be a possible mechanism by which supplementation of patients with inactive vitamin D leads to a positive therapeutic outcome. Well-documented clinical observations show that, compared to lightly pigmented individuals, darkly pigmented black individuals are more susceptible to virulent infections of tuberculosis and have lower circulating serum 25 (OH)D levels because of their relatively diminished capacity to synthesize vitamin D in their skin during sunlight exposure.

IV. Modulation of Adaptive Immunity

A. Vitamin D and monocytes/dendritic cells

APCs, such as monocytes/macrophages, and DCs represent an important component of the adaptive immune system. DCs, the professional APCs that have an essential role in the initiation and maintenance of T-cell-dependent immune responses, are recognized as central targets for $1,25(OH)_2D_3$ (Baeke *et al.*, 2007). During DC differentiation, these APCs downregulate the monocyte marker CD14 while upregulating the DC marker CD1. $1,25(OH)_2D_3$ has been shown to effectively inhibit DC maturation and differentiation to monocytes using a VDR-dependent mechanism (Penna and Adorini, 2000; van Halteren, 2002). Adding active vitamin D completely inhibits the differentiation of CD1a+ DC cells while sustaining the expression of monocytic markers (Berer *et al.*, 2000). It should be noted that the final 1-α-hydroxilation step of active vitamin D synthesis has been demonstrated in activated macrophages and DC cells, enabling them to synthesize and secrete $1,25(OH)_2D_3$ in a regulated fashion.

Physiologic levels of $1,25(OH)_2D_3$ reduce the major histocompatibility complex (MHC) class II expression of costimulatory receptors (such as CD40, CD80, and CD86) and other maturation-induced surface markers (e.g., CD83), determining the ability of APCs to present secondary signals necessary for full T-cell activation (Fig. 11.1) (Gauzzi *et al.*, 2005; Pedersen *et al.*, 2009). APCs secretion of cytokines, which are central to recruit and activate T lymphocytes, is also controlled by $1,25(OH)_2D_3$. Active vitamin D inhibits the production of immunostimulatory cytokines IL-12 and IL-23 (known as major cytokines driving T helper 1 (Th1) differentiation and Th17 differentiation, respectively) and enhances the release of immunosuppressive cytokine IL-10 and chemokine MIP-3α (also known as CCL22, a chemokine involved in the recruitment of CCR4-expressing regulatory T-cells (Tregs; Mosser and Zhang, 2008; Penna and Adorini, 2000; van Halteren, 2002; Zhu and Paul, 2008)). Depending on the differentiation and maturation status of monocytes and macrophages, $1,25(OH)_2D_3$ also modulates the inflammatory cytokine TNF-α. Prostaglandin E2, a suppressive cytokine, is also stimulated by active vitamin D, while suppressing the granulocyte-macrophage colony stimulating factor (GM-CSF) (Koren *et al.*, 1986).

$1,25(OH)_2D_3$- mediated modulation of DC-derived cytokines alters the Th balance by limiting inflammatory Th1 and Th17 response, while skewing the T-cell response toward a Th2 phenotype. $1,25(OH)_2D_3$ has a major impact on adaptive immune responses, as demonstrated by its ability to regulate T-cell responses. In contrast to these effects, the chemotactic and phagocytic capacity of monocytes and macrophages, which is necessary for antimicrobacterial activity and tumor cell cytotoxicity, is augmented by exposure to $1,25(OH)_2D_3$.

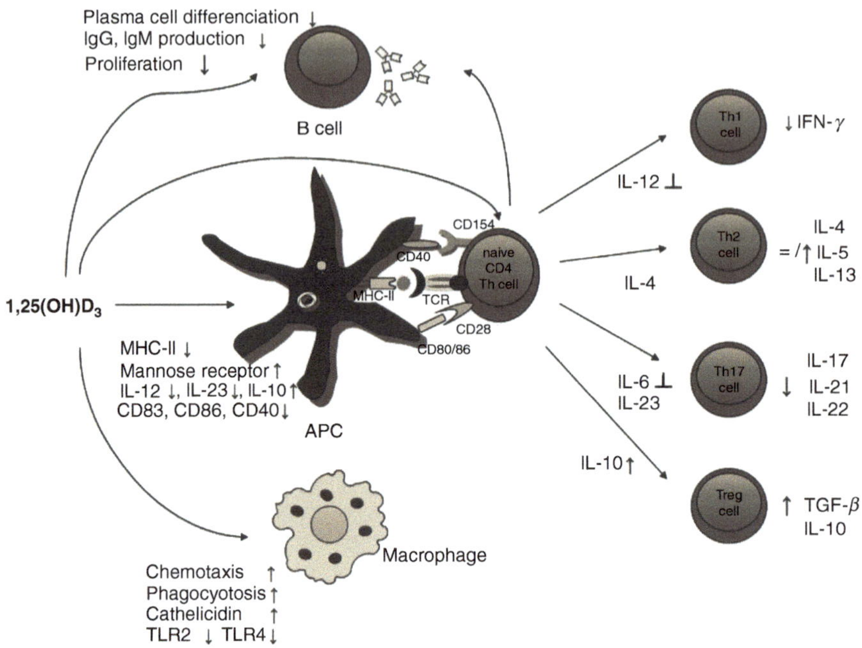

Figure 11.1 Vitamin D and adaptive immune cells: molecular actions—modulation of immunity. (See Color Insert.)

V. Lymphocytes as Direct Targets for $1,25(OH)_2D_3$

It seems that the vitamin D is a physiological regulator of T-cell development. *In vitro*, $1,25(OH)_2D_3$ has been shown to be a differentiation factor for monocytes and other cell types, such as tumor cells (DeLuca, 1988). In T-cells, $1,25(OH)_2D_3$ seems to primarily downregulate Th1 cells both by decreasing proliferation and cytokine secretion (Lemire, 1995). Vitamin D receptors are found in the nuclease of these cells and, when bound to the VDR ligand, they regulate transcription of targeted genes (Ross *et al.*, 1994). Vitamin D might act as a transcriptional regulator of Th cell cytokine synthesis and the factors to regulate Th cell differentiation. The transcription of several key cytokines of Th1 cells, such as interferon (IFN)-γ, interleukin-(IL)2, and IL-12, is a direct target of $1,25(OH)_2D_3$. By inhibiting IFN-γ transcription, the important positive feedback signal for

APCs, the inhibition of antigen presentation prevents the further recruitment of T-cells. In addition, $1,25(OH)_2D_3$ promotes IL-5 and IL-10 production, which further tilts T-cell response towards Th2 dominance. The effect of $1,25(OH)_2D_3$ on Th17 cells has recently been discovered: active vitamin D can inhibit Th17 development and function (Daniel *et al.*, 2008; Nakae *et al.*, 2003). Th17 is a special subset of Th cells and produces IL-17. Th17 cells are distinct from Th1 and Th2; excessive numbers of these cells are thought to play a pivotal role in maintaining inflammation and mediating tissue destruction; however, they serve an important function in antimicrobial immunity at the epithelium and mucosal barriers. Therefore, a severe lack of Th17 cells may leave the host susceptible to opportunistic infections. In human cells, IL-6, IL-21, and IL-23, and TGF-β in combination promote the differentiation of pathogenic Th17 effector cells (Bettelli *et al.*, 2006, 2007; Chen and O'Shea, 2008). *In vitro*, post-vitamin D analogue treatment showed that the initial downregulation of IL-6 cytokines decreased Th17 development and allowed TGF-β to induce Foxp3+ T regulatory cells, thereby promoting immune tolerance (Bettelli *et al.*, 2006, 2007). The Foxp3+ T regulatory cells (Tregs) cells have an essential regulatory-suppressor function and play a key role in maintaining immune system homeostasis and tolerance to self-antigens. There is an important dichotomy between Tregs and Th17 cells, and the balance between these two types of T-cells is crucial for determining the outcome of an immune response. As a result of these processes, the absence of $1,25(OH)_2D_3$ may contribute to the development of autoimmune diseases, such as systemic lupus erythematosus (SLE), rheumatoid arthritis (RA), insulin-dependent diabetes mellitus (IDDM), or multiple sclerosis (MS). In the presence of active vitamin D the induction of Tregs is facilitated, and Tregs are also able to suppress Th17 cells (Bettelli *et al.*, 2007; Gregori *et al.*, 2001; Penna *et al.*, 2005).

The exact role of $1,25(OH)_2D_3$ vitamin on Th2 cells is not fully known. IL-4 is a Th2-associated cytokine whose production has been shown to be upregulated *in vivo* by $1,25(OH)_2D_3$ treatment. However, other observations have shown inhibition of both Th1 and Th2 cell cytokine production, including inhibition of IL-4 (Cantorna *et al.*, 1998; Staeva-Vieira and Freedman, 2002).

Regarding humoral immune response, vitamin D directly affects B cells (Lemire *et al.*, 1984). Exposing B cells to $1,25(OH)_2D_3$ inhibits their proliferation, plasma cell differentiation, immunoglobulin secretion (IgG and IgM), and memory B cell generation, and induces B cell apoptosis (Chen *et al.*, 2007). *In vitro*, adding vitamin D to the peripheral mononuclear cells from SLE patients significantly reduced both polyclonal antibody and anti-dsDNA autoantibody production (Linker-Israeli *et al.*, 2001).

VI. Low Level of Vitamin D and Autoimmune Diseases

Experimental and clinical studies provide evidence that vitamin D status influences cancer rates and infectious and cardiovascular diseases (Schwalfenberg, 2007). Vitamin D is one of several environmental factors, which by modulating the immune system, affect the prevalence of autoimmune syndromes; in addition, vitamin D deficiency may play a role in the pathogenesis of systemic autoimmune diseases. Vitamin D status is influenced by skin exposure to sunlight. Very little vitamin D is produced in areas beyond a latitude of 35° from October to March and synthesis depends on skin pigmentation, sun protection, age, and clothing coverage (Holick and Chen, 2008; Matsuoka *et al.*, 1992). Moreover, sex, lifestyle, and vitamin D supplementation are also important determinants of vitamin D levels. In countries with temperate climates, serum vitamin D concentrations rise and fall throughout the year, in parallel with the sun exposure (Rucker *et al.*, 2002; Steingrimsdottir *et al.*, 2005; Vieth *et al.*, 2001). It has been demonstrated that the prevalence of vitamin D deficiency is much higher in Europe than in Asia, Australia, or the United States.

At the same time, it has been observed that several autoimmune conditions develop in special distribution proportionally with north–south gradients (Adorini, 2003; Brown, 2006; Lim *et al.*, 2005). The correlation is clear between the frequency of IDDM, MS, RA, SLE, and inflammatory bowel disease (IBD) and the north–south latitude, sun exposure, and vitamin D levels. MS, IDDM, and RA are more prevalent in temperate high latitudes than at the equatorial latitude. MS and IBD are prevalent in Canada, the northern parts of the US, and Europe. Seasonal variation in MS has proven that its incidence and severity is affected by serum vitamin D level and sun exposure. Higher levels of vitamin D intake, regardless of sunlight exposure, are associated with reduced risk of developing IDDM, RA, and MS. Because of the short half-life and strict regulation of $1,25(OH)_2D_3$, the serum 25(OH) D level is the best indicator of true vitamin D status.

However, there is no uniform definition of vitamin D status; vitamin D deficiency is commonly defined as circulating 25(OH)D levels of less than 20 ng/ml (50 nM) (Bischoff-Ferrari *et al.*, 2006; Holick, 2006, 2007; Malabanan *et al.*, 1998; Thomas *et al.*, 1998). Vitamin D is generally considered to be sufficient if the circulating 25(OH)D concentration is greater than 30–32 ng/ml (75–80 nM) (Chapuy *et al.*, 1997; Holick, 2005). In healthy person, the daily requirement for vitamin D for those 51–70 and over 71 is 400 and 600 IU, respectively, while children and young adults need at least about 600 IU. Limited work has been done on response to different dosing regimens and routes of administration in autoimmune diseases.

Nevertheless, vitamin D supplementation may reduce the prevalence of some autoimmune disease and may also modulate disease activity.

VII. Causes of Vitamin D Deficiency in Autoimmune Diseases

Many factors have been hypothesized to influence vitamin D status in autoimmune diseases. It is unclear whether the hypothesized alteration of vitamin D3 metabolism is related to the immunopathology of autoimmune diseases or if this is merely an epiphenomenon.

In SLE patients, avoiding sun exposure is usually advised, which is a risk factor for developing vitamin D deficiency. Additional risk factors may be race, ethnicity, and geographic location. Age is another known factor affecting conversion of vitamin D in the skin; those over 70 make about one-quarter the levels of 20 year olds (Holick, 2004a,b).

Antimalarials seem to be a predictor of lower 25(OH)D levels, as hydroxychloroquine in antimalarials is known to inhibit the 1-α hydroxylation of 25(OH)D, thus decreasing the levels of $1,25(OH)_2D_3$. An early observation was calcium malabsorption in corticosteroid-treated patients, which is due to a dose-related abnormality of vitamin D metabolism and not a direct effect of corticosteroids on depressing transmucosal intestinal absorption of calcium (Klein *et al.*, 1977). Administration of a physiologic or near-physiologic dose of synthetic $1,25(OH)_2D_3$ to patients receiving high-dose corticosteroids led to an increase in calcium absorption in all patients.

Other studies measured vitamin D in the context of either bone mineral density and/or fractures. Bone density and muscle strength are often compromised by the frequent use of corticosteroids for disease suppression and by disease itself (Lee *et al.*, 2007). Vitamin D deficiency also causes secondary hyperparathyroidism, which can precipitate osteoporosis and fracture. Cutillas-Marco *et al.* observed that mean serum 25(OH)D levels are significantly lower in cutaneous lupus erythematosus than controls and are associated with higher levels of parathyroid hormone (Cutillas-Marco *et al.*, 2010). Several studies demonstrated that vitamin D supplementation may improve muscle strength and reduce falls (Broe *et al.*, 2007). Vitamin D can also be important in preventing several complications of lupus, such as cognitive dysfunction, metabolic syndrome, and infection (Hypponen *et al.*, 2008; Przybelski and Binkley, 2007).

Interestingly, Wright *et al.* suggest that being overweight is an important risk factor for vitamin D deficiency in SLE patients (Wright *et al.*, 2009), which may be because vitamin D is fat-soluble and thus less bioavailable in overweight individuals.

Otherwise, inflammation, a hallmark of autoimmune diseases, may cause relative hypoparathyroidism by increasing calcium-sensing receptor synthesis. Wright *et al.* observed that the intact PTH is significantly lower in subjects with SLE, even accounting for lower 25(OH)D concentrations (Wright *et al.*, 2009).

Carvalho *et al.* provided an ingenious explanation of the mechanism of vitamin D insufficiency in autoimmune diseases (Carvalho *et al.*, 2007): the potential presence of an inhibitor circulating anti-vitamin D antibodies in these diseases. However, in SLE patients, the low frequency of anti-vitamin D (7 of 171 patients) detected in this study, and demographic features, organ involvement, SLE-DAI score, and the presence of these antibodies did not relate to serum levels of 25(OH)D, expect for anti-dsDNA antibodies, in which anti-vitamin D antibodies were strongly associated with these antibodies.

VIII. Vitamin D and Undifferentiated Connective Tissue Disease

The evolution of disease with an immune pathogenetic background is usually slow and progressive. The term undifferentiated connective tissue disease (UCTD) has been used since 1980 to describe a group of connective tissue disorders (CTDs) that were recognized as being in the early stages of a CTD but did not yet meet the standard criteria for a well-defined CTDs. A great deal of information is available regarding the clinical and serological profile of UCTD and the rate of evolution into well-defined CTD (Bodolay *et al.*, 2003; Mosca *et al.*, 1998, 2007). About 30–40% of patients with UCTD will evolve to defined CTD during years of follow-up. The higher rate of disease evolution can be seen mostly between the first and second year. Of UCTD patients, 50–60% remain undifferentiated, while in 10–20% of patients the symptoms subside and never evolve into a well-defined CTD. Less data are available concerning predictive factors for this transition.

The most frequent clinical manifestations of UCTD are polyarthralgy/polyarthritis, Raynaud's phenomenon, serositis (pleuritis, pericarditis), photosensitive rash; xerostomia, and xerophthalmia, as well as central nervous system involvement, similar to patients with well-established CTDs. During a patient's follow-up period, new organ manifestations can appear, and existing clinical and immunological abnormalities can increase in intensity or become permanent. Evolving to SLE and other systemic autoimmune diseases, including Mixed Connective Tissue Disease (MCTD); Systemic Sclerosis (SSc); Sjögren's syndrome (SS); polymyositis/dermatomyositis; RA; and systemic vasculitis has also been described. The clinical observations demonstrate that the presence of some autoantibody is predictive for progression to certain CTDs. For example, the presence of anti-dsDNA antibodies, anti-phospholipid antibodies, and clinical manifestations such as serositis and photosensitivity rash are predictive for progression to SLE, while xerostomia or xerophtalmia and anti-SSA or anti-SSB antibodies are strongly associated with progression to SS.

The pathogenesis of UCTD, like many rheumatic diseases, is not well understood. However, the clinical symptoms and the presence of the auto-antibodies in UCTD patients suggest that many of the same immunological mechanisms that play a role in different well-established CTDs may also be involved in UCTD. Szodoray *et al.* observed that in patients with UCTD, changes in the Th1/Th2 rate toward Th1 increased with IFN-γ production (Szodoray *et al.*, 2008). In this same study, the relative and absolute number of Tregs was found to be decreased compared with controls; moreover, in patients who developed definitive CTDs, the number of Tregs was further decreased. A significant increase in the IL-10 producing Tr1 regulatory cells was determined in UCTD patients when compared with healthy controls, and a further increase in patients progressing into definitive CTDs was established. One large cohort study analyzed the circulating levels and seasonal variance in levels of 25(OH)D_3 in patients with UCTD, raising the possibility that vitamin D deficiency may contribute to the progression into well-defined CTDs (Zold *et al.*, 2008). According to this study, circulating levels of vitamin D fluctuate seasonally in UCTD patients, with low levels of 25(OH)D in the winter months and higher levels during the summer months. The 25(OH)D levels of UCTD patients were significantly lower than in the control group during both the summer and winter periods. Nevertheless, 41% of these same UCTD patients (67 of 161) showed vitamin D insufficiency in the summer months and more became vitamin D deficient during the wintertime. Vitamin D insufficiency was positively correlated to the probability of developing dermatological symptoms (photosensitivity, vasculitis, and erythema) as well as pleuritis. The presence of anti-U1-RNP, anti-SSA, and anti-CCP occurred more frequently in patients with vitamin D insufficiency. Interestingly, those patients who developed a well-defined CTD during follow-up had lower levels of vitamin D compared with patients who remained in UCTD stage. In 25 patients with UCTD, the Th1/Treg imbalance improved after 5 weeks of oral 0.5 μg/day alfacalcidol treatment, as it inhibited Th17 cells and increased the number of Tregs (Zold *et al.*, 2010). In parallel, alfacalcidol treatment decreased both Th1- (IL-12 and IFN-γ) and Th17-related (IL-23, IL-17, IL-6) cytokine levels in UCTD patients and increased soluble IL-10 levels.

IX. Vitamin D and Systemic Sclerosis

SSc is a chronic autoimmune disease characterized by vasculopathy, diffuse fibrosis of the skin, and various internal organ and complex immune abnormalities, and is four times more common among women than men but rare among children. Symptoms of SSc may occur as part of MCTD, and some people with MCTD develop severe SSc. SSc can occur in limited forms; for example, it sometimes affects just the skin or only certain parts of the skin or as CREST (*c*alcinosis, *R*aynaud's phenomenon, *e*sophageal dysmotility, *s*clerodactyly, and *t*elangiectasias) syndrome. However, SSc often causes damage that is widespread throughout the body, which is called diffuse SSc.

The cause of SSc is unknown; the pathogenesis is complex, and it appears to involve the endothelium, fibroblasts, and immunological mediators. In SSc, the vascular damage, immunologic activation, and collagen deposition are influenced by four major factors: T-cells, fibroblasts, B cells, and cytokines/chemokines. T-cells are a major component of the infiltrate in skin and lung, and exhibit increased expression of activation markers and show signs of antigen-driven expansion. Reports in the literature conflict in terms of the role of T-cells and Th1/Th2 cytokine balance in SSc. Some studies support Th1 activation in the peripheral blood with production of IFNγ, while others predict preferential involvement of Th2 cells in SSc with increased levels of IL-4 and IL-13. Gourh *et al.* report that SSc patients have high levels of TNFα, IL-6, and IFNγ and low levels of IL-17 and IL-23, but the disease duration and the presence of SSc autoantibodies influence these cytokine profiles (Gourh *et al.*, 2009). Otherwise, levels of a number of cellular mediators are elevated in patients with SSc, including chemokines (e.g., CC chemokine ligand 2) (Abraham and Distler, 2007), endothelin (ET)-1 (Abraham and Dashwood, 2008), CTGF (Matucci-Cerinic and Seibold, 2008), and the natural tissue inhibitor of metalloproteinases. Aberrant TGF-β and matrix-modulating protein expression is also implicated in the pathogenesis of fibrosis in SSc. As with the regulation of extracellular matrix deposition, these compounds are critical for regulation of cytokines and chemokines, which in turn play significant roles in the progression of CTDs.

In a highly cell-specific manner, Vitamin D compounds have been demonstrated to alter cellular proliferation through multiple mechanisms, most prominently via effects on cell cycle progression, apoptosis, and differentiation (Dusso *et al.*, 2005; Masuda and Jones, 2006; Nagpal *et al.*, 2005). Studies in VDR knockout mice show that vitamin D/VDR signaling plays an important role in controlling the growth of normal tissues (Welsh *et al.*, 2002). Artaza *et al.* showed a direct antifibrotic effect of vitamin D on cells of murine origin. TGF-β is an important cytokine of fibrotic disorders such as SSc (Artaza and Norris, 2009). *In vitro*, incubation of mesencymal multipotens cells with vitamin D reduced the expression of TGF-β and concomitantly decreased the expression of collagen I and collagen III. Nevertheless, vitamin D enhances the expression of some antifibrotic factors such as matrix metalloproteinase-8, a collagen breakdown inducer; bone morphogenic protein-7, an antagonist of renal fibrosis induced by TGF-β; and follistatin, which inhibits the profibrotic mediator myostatin (Artaza and Norris, 2009).

Active vitamin D reduces the TGF-β1-induced upregulation of mesencymal cell markers and abnormal expression of epithelial cell markers *in vitro*. Subsequently, under TGF-β1 stimulation, $1,25(OH)_2D_3$ acts to differentiate lung epithelial cells into myofibroblast (Ramirez *et al.*, 2010).

Low levels of vitamin D are frequent in patients with SSc, and vitamin D status can be a contributing factor of this disease process. Different studies report that vitamin D insufficiency was found in 63–86% of these patients and deficiency in 95–35%, depending on geographical factors and vitamin D supplementation (Calzolari *et al.*, 2009; Caramaschi *et al.*, 2010; Vacca *et al.*, 2009). A significant negative correlation was found between low vitamin D levels and the European Disease Activity Score, and a more significant correlation was found with acute-phase reactants (Vacca *et al.*, 2009). It should be noted that patients with vitamin D deficiency had more severe disease than patients with vitamin D insufficiency. The vitamin D deficiency was more frequently associated with late nailfold videocapillaroscopy pattern and lower DLCO (a pulmonary function test with diffusing lung capacity for carbon monoxide adjusted to hemoglobin) values, which supports the possible connection between vitamin D levels and disease phenotype (Caramaschi *et al.*, 2010). At the same time, data conflict regarding the association between low levels of vitamin D and the systolic pulmonary artery pressure estimated by echocardiography and the presence or absence of lung fibrosis (Vacca *et al.*, 2009). Research findings from previous small studies suggest no association between 25(OH)D levels and other disease features, such as limited or diffuse form, gastrointestinal involvement, cutaneous ulcers, and joint involvement (Calzolari *et al.*, 2009).

The vitamin D status in SSc is potentially related to several factors. Dermal fibrous thickening with capillary damage could lead to a reduced drawing of previtamin D3 synthesized from 7-dehydocholesterol by UVB radiation in the epidermis; gastrointestinal involvement and malabsorption of dietary vitamin D could play an additional role; moreover, many patients with SSc experience a remarkable impairment in physical functioning. Another cause of vitamin D deficiency in patients is that in some countries, food is not enriched with vitamin D and vitamin supplementation is uncommon.

Little data exist regarding vitamin D administration in SSc patients. Vacca *et al.* reported the failure of standard-dose supplementation to correct hypovitaminosis in patients with SSc (Vacca *et al.*, 2009). Five of seven pediatric patients with linear scleroderma showed improvement of their lesions after oral 0.25 μg/daily dose calcitriol treatment.

Dermatologists generally use the topical form of vitamin D3, calcipotriene, to treat local scleroderma. Calcipotriene appears to help block skin cell production and has anti-inflammatory properties and may prove beneficial when combined with low-dose ultraviolet A1 phototherapy.

X. Vitamin D and Sjögren's Syndrome

Sjögren's syndrome (SS) is a chronic autoimmune disorder characterized by dysfunction and destruction of the exocrine glands associated with lymphocytic infiltrates and immunological hyperactivity. Salivary and lacrimal glands are the most affected, leading to mouth and eye dryness, but similar lymphoid infiltrates may involve other organs such as lungs, liver, skeletal muscle, and kidneys. The disorder can occur alone (primary SS) or in association with another autoimmune disease (secondary SS). Polyclonal B cell activation with hypergammaglobulinemia and the presence of a broad range of autoantibodies, including IgM and IgA rheumatoid factors, as well as antinuclear antibodies, are characteristic of the syndrome; the development of the syndrome is due to a complex interplay of various cytokines and immune cells. Polyclonal B cell activation is a pronounced and convenient marker of disturbed immune regulation in this disease. The changed vitamin D metabolism affects immune reactivities and contributes to polyclonal B cell activation. 1,25(OH)$_2$D$_3$ regulates the proliferation and differentiation of activated human B cells. Vitamin D binding protein (DBP) binds the vitamin D metabolites with high affinity and may play a role as a neutral acute-phase reactant (Swamy and Ray, 1996). In primary SS, the serum concentration of DBP is normal and no significant associations are found between DBP and susceptibility to primary SS (Mitchell *et al.*, 1985; Muller *et al.*, 1990). Data in the literature show that serum levels of 25(OH)D are decreased in primary SS; moreover, levels of 25(OH)D correlate inversely with levels of soluble interleukin-2 receptor, status indices for global disease, total exocrine disease, surface exocrine disease, internal organ exocrine disease, and mediator-induced disease (Bang and Asmussen, 1999; Muller *et al.*, 1990). Bang *et al.* reported that this reduced level of 25(OH)D was stable over the observed 2-year period (Bang and Asmussen, 1999). There was a significantly positive correlation between the concentration of circulating 25(OH)D and IgG titers, but a negative correlation between 25(OH)D concentrations and IgM rheumatoid factor in patients with SS (Muller *et al.*, 1990). However, there is no significantly decreased peripheral level of 1,25(OH)D in primary SS, a level that did not correlate with clinical/immunopathological status. There is no data on the effect of vitamin D supplementation in SS patients.

XI. Vitamin D and Systemic Lupus Erythematosus

Systemic lupus erythematosus (SLE) is a prototypic autoimmune disease characterized by the production of antibodies in the components of the cell nucleus in association with a diverse array of clinical manifestations. The primary pathological findings in patients with SLE are inflammation, vasculitis, immune complex deposition, and vasculopathy. The disease is the result of a complex of immunological aberrations that involve B cells, T-cells, and cells of monocytic lineage, characterized by polyclonal B cell activation, increased numbers of antibody-producing cells, hypergammaglobulinemia, autoantibody production, and immune complex formation. It appears that excessive and uncontrolled T-cells help differentiate and shift Th1 to Th2 immune responses and lead to B cell hyperactivity and the production of pathogenic autoantibodies.

Vitamin D has been studied in two different murine (MRL/lpr and NZB/NZW mouse) models of lupus. These mice spontaneously developed SLE-like symptoms and human SLE mimicking syndromes.

Administration of 1,25(OH)D vitamin to MRL/lpr mice resulted in a loss of dermatologic manifestations (i.e., alopecia, necrosis of the ear, and scab formation) of SLE-like disease and decreased proteinuria (Lemire *et al.*, 1992). Moreover, a trend of reduced serum titers for anti-ssDNA antibodies was observed at 18 weeks of vitamin D treatment. In another study of MRL/lpr mice, the effect of 1,25D was similar to that of high-dose corticosteroids with significant prevention of disease (Koizumi *et al.*, 1985). In a third study with MRL/lpr mice, 1,25(OH)D vitamin given daily prevented proteinuria and pathologic renal disease and improved survival (DeLuca and Cantorna, 2001). In a fourth study, the VDR ligand 22-oxa-1,25(OH)D vitamin prolonged the lifespan of MRL/l mice, decreased proteinuria, and slightly reduced the severity of renal arteritis, granuloma formation, and knee joint arthritis (Abe *et al.*, 1990). However, a single study of intraperitoneal treatment with weekly administration of vitamin D in NZB/W mice reported no prolongation of survival or other beneficial effects (Vaisberg *et al.*, 2000). It should be noted that these mice were not vitamin D deficient, as murine vitamin D deficiency is almost impossible to achieve. Limited assessment of disease, inadequate dosing, and small sample sizes may account for the lack of observed efficacy.

The immunomodulatory effects of vitamin D are mediated through its nuclear receptor. Few studies have examined the interesting question of whether there is connection between VDR polymorphism and vitamin D deficiency in patients with SLE. Four studies have reported the VDR gene *BsmI* polymorphisms in SLE patients and the relationship of polymorphisms to the susceptibility and clinical manifestations of SLE with diverse results. Studies of Japanese and Chinese patients found an association of the BB genotype with disease. The study in Japan of 58 patients with SLE established that the BB genotype might trigger the development of SLE and that the BB genotype is associated with lupus nephritis (Ozaki *et al.*, 2000). The other study, in Taiwan with the population of 47 Chinese SLE patients, found an increased distribution of VDR BB genotype and B allelic frequencies, but indicated no association between the frequency of VDR allelic variations and clinical manifestations, laboratory profiles, and lupus nephritis (Huang *et al.*, 2002a,b). A study of Thai patients could not replicate these results; no association was found between VDR gene *BsmI* polymorphism and SLE in 101 Thai patients with lupus (Sakulpipatsin *et al.*, 2006). In a similar study in Iran, no association was found of VDR gene *BsmI* polymorphisms with the presence of SLE, disease activity index (SLEDAI), SLE damage score, and major organ involvement (Abbasi *et al.*, 2010).

In clinical practice, several methods have been used to determine a potential link between vitamin D status and lupus, including case control, cohort, and retrospective observational studies.

The Nurse's Health Study I and II prospective cohorts showed that vitamin D intake is not associated with risk of SLE or RA (Costenbader *et al.*, 2008). The limitations of these studies for lupus include the relatively small number of incident lupus cases (190), lack of data on sunscreen use, and applicability to only Caucasian female populations (97–98% Caucasian). 25(OH)D was not measured. The Nurse's Health Study I demonstrated low levels of vitamin D among SLE patients in Canada (O'Regan *et al.*, 1979). 1,25(OH)D levels were measured in 12 adolescents with SLE and seven had low levels. In a cross-sectional study, Huisman *et al.* demonstrated that the 25(OH)D, 1,25(OH)D and PTH levels in 25 Caucasian SLE and 25 patients with fibromyalgia had no significant difference; half were vitamin D deficient (Huisman *et al.*, 2001).

Several studies have addressed vitamin D deficiency in SLE patients. A case-control study of 25(OH)D and 1,25(OH)D and PTH in 21 SLE, 29 RA, 12 osteoarthritis, and 72 normal controls was performed in Copenhagen (Muller *et al.*, 1995). 25(OH)D levels in these SLE patients were found to be significantly lower than in the osteoarthritis patients and normal controls, but no significant difference in 1,25(OH)D levels was found. Lower 25(OH)D levels in SLE patients were found in additional cross-sectional case control studies (Carvalho *et al.*, 2007; Chen *et al.*, 2007; Kamen *et al.*, 2006). Kamen *et al.* found lower levels of 25(OH)D in 123 recently diagnosed SLE patients, with increased prevalence in Caucasians. In their study, critically low vitamin D levels (<10 ng/ml) were found in 22 SLE cases, with the presence of renal disease and photosensitivity being the predictors of vitamin D deficiency. In terms of disease activity, published results are controversial. Borba *et al.* reported lower levels of 25(OH)D in 12 SLE patients with high disease activity compared to 24 patients with minimal disease activity and 26 controls (Borba *et al.*, 2009). Becker *et al.* confirm these results: in Germany they found that 34 of 57 SLE patients with high disease activity had severe vitamin D depletion (Becker *et al.*, 2001). Cutolo *et al.* also found inverse association between serum levels of 25(OH)D and disease activity in 46 patients with SLE (Cutolo *et al.*, 2009). In contrast, in other studies of SLE patients, no relationship was found between vitamin D deficiency or insufficiency and clinical disease manifestation of SLE (Muller *et al.*, 1995; Orbach *et al.*, 2007; Ruiz-Irastorza *et al.*, 2008).

Data in the literature are limited in terms of the effect of vitamin D supplementation on the disease procession of SLE. Recently, *in vitro* data suggest that vitamin D supplementation effects on the IFN-α axis regarding DC differentiation and maturation are similar to that of normal DC. Although there is no consensus regarding the exact impact of vitamin D supplementation, it may have benefits beyond bone health for these patients.

In the most of the studies, increased disease symptoms in SLE patients with very low levels of vitamin D suggest a role for supplementation with exogenous vitamin D to optimize therapeutic outcomes. However, the possibility that such treatment could lead to increased autoantibody levels requires further study.

XII. Vitamin D and Rheumatoid Arthritis

RA is a chronic, progressive systemic inflammatory disorder that affects the synovial joints and can lead to joint destruction. The etiopathogenic process leading to disease development and progression is not completely understood, although various cells of the immune system and of synovial origin may be involved (Klareskog *et al.*, 2004). Numerous cytokines are expressed and are functionally active in the synovial tissue once the disease has developed (McInnes and Schett, 2007).

In samples of synovial fluid, Raza *et al.* observed increased levels of the Th2 cytokines IL-4 and IL-13, but not IFN-γ, during the first months of development of RA. IL-17, a proinflammatory cytokine produced by Th17 cells, was also detected at higher levels in early compared with late disease (Raza *et al.*, 2005). The extensive analysis of cytokines includes several key factors such as human leukocyte antigen (HLA), intercellular adhesion molecule (ICAM), IFN, IL, vascular cell adhesion molecule (VCAM), and TNF. Interestingly, these factors demonstrate the involvement of Th1, Th2, and Treg cells as well as signs of more general immune activation (Jorgensen *et al.*, 2008).

Active vitamin D may exert major immunomodulatory effects on RA (DeLuca and Zierold, 1998) that are possibly based on the effects on activated synovial macrophages, resulting in positive regulation of the anti-inflammatory cytokines IL-4 and TGF-β (Cantorna *et al.*, 1998). $1{,}25(OH)_2D_3$ decreases the production of IFN-γ, IL-2, and IL-5 in Th1 cells and inhibits Th1 proliferation (Mahon *et al.*, 2003), while increasing the production of IL-4 and proliferation of Th2 cells, which results in an immunosuppressive action. The recognized immunomodulatory properties of $1,25(OH)_2D_3$ could be important in rheumatoid tissues, in which the inflammatory response is a characteristic feature. VDR has been demonstrated in macrophages, chondrocytes, and synoviocytes in rheumatoid synovium and sites of cartilage erosion in patients with RA, but not in tissues from control subjects (Tetlow *et al.*, 1999). Tetlow *et al.* demonstrated that the IL-1β-activated synovial fibroblasts and chondrocytes *in vitro* showed significant and different responses to $1,25(OH)_2D_3$ exposure with regard to MMP and PGE_2 production, and this could be one trigger for cartilage damage in RA.

The presence of certain VDR genotypes has been associated with low BMD in elderly populations and with accelerated bone loss in patients with RA. Four VDR gene polymorphisms, namely *Fok1*, *BsmI*, *ApaI*, and *Taq1*, have been studied in RA. *Fok1* polymorphism is found in a greater frequency in the RA population as compared to controls, and it is speculated that this polymorphism may contribute to disease susceptibility; however, the mechanisms are yet to be elucidated (Maalej *et al.*, 2005). The distributions of VDR allelic frequencies were similar in patients and controls and therefore no influence of VDR polymorphisms on RA susceptibility has been demonstrated (Garcia-Lozano *et al.*, 2001). However, in an analysis of the clinical features of the different VDR-related genetic subgroups, the BB/tt genotype, defined by the *BsmI* and *TaqI* restriction site polymorphisms, was identified to be weakly associated with early onset RA in female patients. The BB polymorphism *BsmI* of the VDR gene in RA results in clinically more severe disease as evidenced by higher erythrocyte sedimentation rate (ESR) values, disease activity counts, number of DMARDs used, and amount of glucocorticoids taken (Gomez-Vaquero *et al.*, 2007), a higher degree of bone loss and osteoclastic activity, a lower bone mineral density score, and higher titre values of rheumatoid factor as compared to patients without this polymorphism (Rass *et al.*, 2006).

The collagen-induced arthritis model is the most commonly used arthritis model for human RA. Cantorna *et al.* tested two different animal models of arthritis: murine Lyme and collagen-induced (Cantorna *et al.*, 1998). Supplementation with $1,25(OH)_2D_3$ vitamin of an adequate diet fed to mice infected with *Borrelia burgdorferi* minimized or prevented the symptoms of Lyme arthritis. Mice immunized with type II collagen also developed arthritis, the symptoms of which were prevented by dietary supplementation with $1,25(OH)_2D_3$ vitamin. $1,25(OH)_2D_3$ vitamin given to mice with early symptoms of collagen-induced arthritis prevented the progression to severe arthritis compared with untreated controls.

Epidemiological data indicate that more than 60% of RA patients have vitamin D insufficiency and that 16% have 25(OH)D levels in the range of vitamin D deficiency (Aguado *et al.*, 2000). The age-old observation that the seasons influence the disease activity of RA may be true: a higher prevalence of RA seems common among North when compared to

South Europe. The variations of 25(OH)D levels between summer and winter were found to be significant in RA (Cutolo *et al.*, 2006).

Results conflict in terms of whether vitamin D is a factor in RA initiation. Low baseline intake of vitamin D in the Iowa Women's Healthy Study was related to subsequent development of RA (Merlino *et al.*, 2004). Other studies found no difference between 25(OH)D levels in patients who later developed RA and controls (Nielen, 2006). Results are contradictory regarding the correlation between disease activity and vitamin D levels. Some studies report correlation between disease activity in RA or ankylosing spondylitis and 1,25$(OH)_2D_3$ levels, but not 25(OH)D metabolites (Kroger *et al.*, 1993; Lange *et al.*, 2005; Oelzner *et al.*, 1998). Patel *et al.* reported that cross-sectionally, the associations with the various markers of disease activity and severity are stronger for 25(OH)D than 1,25$(OH)_2D_3$ in patients with early polyarthritis (Patel *et al.*, 2007). In a 3-month open-label trial on 19 patients with RA, high-dose oral alphacalcidol therapy showed a positive effect on disease activity in 89% of patients (Andjelkovic *et al.*, 1999). However, Braun-Moscovici *et al.* found no correlation between disease activity (DAS28) and 25(OH)D or PTH levels (Braun-Moscovici *et al.*, 2009). Furthermore, plasma 25(OH)D levels are not associated with RA-related autoantibodies in unaffected individuals at increased risk for RA (Feser *et al.*, 2009).

The incidence of generalized osteoporosis is associated with arthritis severity in RA and increased osteoporotic verebral and hip fracture risk (Lodder *et al.*, 2003). Studies examining the effect of vitamin D supplementation on risk for falls yield conflicting result, but it seems vitamin D may be of some benefit (Jackson *et al.*, 2007).

REFERENCES

Abbasi, M., Rezaieyazdi, Z., Afshari, J. T., Hatef, M., Sahebari, M., and Saadati, N. (2010). Lack of association of vitamin D receptor gene *Bsm*I polymorphisms in patients with systemic lupus erythematosus. *Rheumatol. Int.* **30,** 1537–1539.

Abe, J., Nakamura, K., Takita, Y., Nakano, T., Irie, H., and Nishii, Y. (1990). Prevention of immunological disorders in MRL/l mice by a new synthetic analogue of vitamin D3: 22-oxa-1 alpha, 25-dihydroxyvitamin D3. *J. Nutr. Sci. Vitaminol. Tokyo* **36,** 21–31.

Abraham, D., and Dashwood, M. (2008). Endothelin—Role in vascular disease. *Rheumatology (Oxford)* **47**(Suppl. 5), v23–v24.

Abraham, D., and Distler, O. (2007). How does endothelial cell injury start? The role of endothelin in systemic sclerosis. *Arthritis Res. Ther.* **9**(Suppl. 2), S2.

Adams, J. S., Sharma, O. P., Gacad, M. A., and Singer, F. R. (1983). Metabolism of 25-hydroxyvitamin D3 by cultured pulmonary alveolar macrophages in sarcoidosis. *J. Clin. Invest.* **72,** 1856–1860.

Adorini, L. (2003). Tolerogenic dendritic cells induced by vitamin D receptor ligands enhance regulatory T cells inhibiting autoimmune diabetes. *Ann. NY Acad. Sci.* **987,** 258–261.

Aguado, P., del Campo, M. T., Garces, M. V., Gonzalez-Casaus, M. L., Bernad, M., Gijon-Banos, J., *et al.* (2000). Low vitamin D levels in outpatient postmenopausal women from a rheumatology clinic in Madrid, Spain: Their relationship with bone mineral density. *Osteoporos. Int.* **11,** 739–744.

Andjelkovic, Z., Vojinovic, J., Pejnovic, N., Popovic, M., Dujic, A., Mitrovic, D., *et al.* (1999). Disease modifying and immunomodulatory effects of high dose 1 alpha (OH) D3 in rheumatoid arthritis patients. *Clin. Exp. Rheumatol.* **17,** 453–456.

Artaza, J. N., and Norris, K. C. (2009). Vitamin D reduces the expression of collagen and key profibrotic factors by inducing an antifibrotic phenotype in mesenchymal multipotent cells. *J. Endocrinol.* **200,** 207–221.

Baeke, F., Etten, E. V., Overbergh, L., and Mathieu, C. (2007). Vitamin D3 and the immune system: Maintaining the balance in health and disease. *Nutr. Res. Rev.* **20,** 106–118.

Bang, B., Asmussen, K., Sorensen, O. H., and Oxholm, P. (1999). Reduced 25-hydroxyvitamin D levels in primary Sjogren's syndrome. Correlations to disease manifestations. *Scand. J. Rheumatol.* **28,** 180–183.

Becker, A., Fischer, R., and Schneider, M. (2001). Bone density and 25-OH vitamin D serum level in patients with systemic lupus erythematosus. *Z. Rheumatol.* **60,** 352–358.

Berer, A., Stockl, J., Majdic, O., Wagner, T., Kollars, M., Lechner, K., *et al.* (2000). 1,25-Dihydroxyvitamin D(3) inhibits dendritic cell differentiation and maturation in vitro. *Exp. Hematol.* **28,** 575–583.

Bettelli, E., Carrier, Y., Gao, W., Korn, T., Strom, T. B., Oukka, M., *et al.* (2006). Reciprocal developmental pathways for the generation of pathogenic effector TH17 and regulatory T cells. *Nature* **441,** 235–238.

Bettelli, E., Korn, T., and Kuchroo, V. K. (2007). Th17: The third member of the effector T cell trilogy. *Curr. Opin. Immunol.* **19,** 652–657.

Bischoff-Ferrari, H. A., Giovannucci, E., Willett, W. C., Dietrich, T., and Dawson-Hughes, B. (2006). Estimation of optimal serum concentrations of 25-hydroxyvitamin D for multiple health outcomes. *Am. J. Clin. Nutr.* **84,** 18–28.

Bodolay, E., Csiki, Z., Szekanecz, Z., Ben, T., Kiss, E., Zeher, M., *et al.* (2003). Five-year follow-up of 665 Hungarian patients with undifferentiated connective tissue disease (UCTD). *Clin. Exp. Rheumatol.* **21,** 313–320.

Borba, V. Z., Vieira, J. G., Kasamatsu, T., Radominski, S. C., Sato, E. I., and Lazaretti-Castro, M. (2009). Vitamin D deficiency in patients with active systemic lupus erythematosus. *Osteoporos. Int.* **20,** 427–433.

Braun-Moscovici, Y., Toledano, K., Markovits, D., Rozin, A., Nahir, A. M., and Balbir-Gurman, A. (2009). Vitamin D level: Is it related to disease activity in inflammatory joint disease? *Rheumatol. Int.*

Broe, K. E., Chen, T. C., Weinberg, J., Bischoff-Ferrari, H. A., Holick, M. F., and Kiel, D. P. (2007). A higher dose of vitamin d reduces the risk of falls in nursing home residents: A randomized, multiple-dose study. *J. Am. Geriatr. Soc.* **55,** 234–239.

Brown, S. J. (2006). The role of vitamin D in multiple sclerosis. *Ann. Pharmacother.* **40,** 1158–1161.

Calzolari, G., Data, V., Carignola, R., and Angeli, A. (2009). Hypovitaminosis D in systemic sclerosis. *J. Rheumatol.* **2844,** 36.

Cantorna, M. T., Woodward, W. D., Hayes, C. E., and DeLuca, H. F. (1998). 1, 25-dihydroxyvitamin D3 is a positive regulator for the two anti-encephalitogenic cytokines TGF-beta 1 and IL-4. *J. Immunol.* **160,** 5314–5319.

Caramaschi, P., Dalla, G. A., Ruzzenente, O., Volpe, A., Ravagnani, V., Tinazzi, I., *et al.* (2010). Very low levels of vitamin D in systemic sclerosis patients. *Clin. Rheumatol.* **29,** 1419–1425.

Carvalho, J. F., Blank, M., Kiss, E., Tarr, T., Amital, H., and Shoenfeld, Y. (2007). Anti-vitamin D, vitamin D in SLE: Preliminary results. *Ann. NY Acad. Sci.* **1109,** 550–557.

Chapuy, M. C., Preziosi, P., Maamer, M., Arnaud, S., Galan, P., Hercberg, S., *et al.* (1997). Prevalence of vitamin D insufficiency in an adult normal population. *Osteoporos. Int.* **7,** 439–443.

Chen, Z., and O'Shea, J. J. (2008). Th17 cells: A new fate for differentiating helper T cells. *Immunol. Res.* **41,** 87–102.

Chen, S., Sims, G. P., Chen, X. X., Gu, Y. Y., Chen, S., and Lipsky, P. E. (2007). Modulatory effects of 1, 25-dihydroxyvitamin D3 on human B cell differentiation. *J. Immunol.* **179,** 1634–1647.

Costenbader, K. H., Feskanich, D., Holmes, M., Karlson, E. W., and Benito-Garcia, E. (2008). Vitamin D intake and risks of systemic lupus erythematosus and rheumatoid arthritis in women. *Ann. Rheum. Dis.* **67,** 530–535.

Cutillas-Marco, E., Morales-Suarez-Varela, M., Marquina-Vila, A., and Grant, W. (2010). Serum 25-hydroxyvitamin D levels in patients with cutaneous lupus erythematosus in a Mediterranean region. *Lupus* **19,** 810–814.

Cutolo, M., Otsa, K., Laas, K., Yprus, M., Lehtme, R., Secchi, M. E., *et al.* (2006). Circannual vitamin d serum levels and disease activity in rheumatoid arthritis: Northern versus Southern Europe. *Clin. Exp. Rheumatol.* **24,** 702–704.

Cutolo, M., Otsa, K., Paolino, S., Yprus, M., Veldi, T., and Seriolo, B. (2009). Vitamin D involvement in rheumatoid arthritis and systemic lupus erythaematosus. *Ann. Rheum. Dis.* **68,** 446–447.

Daniel, C., Sartory, N. A., Zahn, N., Radeke, H. H., and Stein, J. M. (2008). Immune modulatory treatment of trinitrobenzene sulfonic acid colitis with calcitriol is associated with a change of a T helper (Th) 1/Th17 to a Th2 and regulatory T cell profile. *J. Pharmacol. Exp. Ther.* **324,** 23–33.

DeLuca, H. F. (1988). The vitamin D story: A collaborative effort of basic science and clinical medicine. *FASEB J.* **2,** 224–236.

DeLuca, H. F., and Cantorna, M. T. (2001). Vitamin D: Its role and uses in immunology. *FASEB J.* **15,** 2579–2585.

DeLuca, H. F., and Zierold, C. (1998). Mechanisms and functions of vitamin D. *Nutr. Rev.* **56,** S4–S10.

Dimeloe, S., Nanzer, A., Ryanna, K., and Hawrylowicz, C. (2010). Regulatory T cells, inflammation and the allergic response—The role of glucocorticoids and Vitamin D. *J. Steroid Biochem. Mol. Biol.* **120,** 86–95.

Dusso, A. S., Brown, A. J., and Slatopolsky, E. (2005). Vitamin D. *Am. J. Physiol. Renal. Physiol.* **289,** F8–F28.

Feser, M., Derber, L. A., Deane, K. D., Lezotte, D. C., Weisman, M. H., Buckner, J. H., *et al.* (2009). Plasma 25, OH vitamin D concentrations are not associated with rheumatoid arthritis (RA)-related autoantibodies in individuals at elevated risk for RA. *J. Rheumatol.* **36,** 943–946.

Fritsche, J., Mondal, K., Ehrnsperger, A., Andreesen, R., and Kreutz, M. (2003). Regulation of 25-hydroxyvitamin D3–1 alpha-hydroxylase and production of 1 alpha, 25-dihydroxyvitamin D3 by human dendritic cells. *Blood* **102,** 3314–3316.

Garcia-Lozano, J. R., Gonzalez-Escribano, M. F., Valenzuela, A., Garcia, A., and Nunez-Roldan, A. (2001). Association of vitamin D receptor genotypes with early onset rheumatoid arthritis. *Eur. J. Immunogenet.* **28,** 89–93.

Gauzzi, M. C., Purificato, C., Donato, K., Jin, Y., Wang, L., Daniel, K. C., *et al.* (2005). Suppressive effect of 1alpha, 25-dihydroxyvitamin D3 on type I IFN-mediated monocyte differentiation into dendritic cells: Impairment of functional activities and chemotaxis. *J. Immunol.* **174,** 270–276.

Gomez-Vaquero, C., Fiter, J., Enjuanes, A., Nogues, X., Diez-Perez, A., and Nolla, J. M. (2007). Influence of the BsmI polymorphism of the vitamin D receptor gene on rheumatoid arthritis clinical activity. *J. Rheumatol.* **34,** 1823–1826.

Gourh, P., Arnett, F. C., Assassi, S., Tan, F. K., Huang, M., Diekman, L., *et al.* (2009). Plasma cytokine profiles in systemic sclerosis: Associations with autoantibody subsets and clinical manifestations. *Arthritis Res. Ther.* **11,** R147.

Gregori, S., Casorati, M., Amuchastegui, S., Smiroldo, S., Davalli, A. M., and Adorini, L. (2001). Regulatory T cells induced by 1 alpha, 25-dihydroxyvitamin D3 and mycophenolate mofetil treatment mediate transplantation tolerance. *J. Immunol.* **167,** 1945–1953.

Holick, M. F. (1994). McCollum Award Lecture, 1994: Vitamin D—New horizons for the 21st century. *Am. J. Clin. Nutr.* **60,** 619–630.

Holick, M. F. (2004a). Sunlight and vitamin D for bone health and prevention of autoimmune diseases, cancers, and cardiovascular disease. *Am. J. Clin. Nutr.* **80,** 1678S–1688S.

Holick, M. F. (2004b). Vitamin D: Importance in the prevention of cancers, type 1 diabetes, heart disease, and osteoporosis. *Am. J. Clin. Nutr.* **79,** 362–371.

Holick, M. F. (2005). 25-OH-vitamin D assays. *J. Clin. Endocrinol. Metab.* **90,** 3128–3129.

Holick, M. F. (2006). High prevalence of vitamin D inadequacy and implications for health. *Mayo Clin. Proc.* **81,** 353–373.

Holick, M. F. (2007). Vitamin D deficiency. *N. Engl. J. Med.* **357,** 266–281.

Holick, M. F., and Chen, T. C. (2008). Vitamin D deficiency: A worldwide problem with health consequences. *Am. J. Clin. Nutr.* **87,** 1080S–1086S.

Huang, C. M., Wu, M. C., Wu, J. Y., and Tsai, F. J. (2002a). No association of vitamin D receptor gene start codon fok 1 polymorphisms in Chinese patients with systemic lupus erythematosus. *J. Rheumatol.* **29,** 1211–1213.

Huang, C. M., Wu, M. C., Wu, J. Y., and Tsai, F. J. (2002b). Association of vitamin D receptor gene BsmI polymorphisms in Chinese patients with systemic lupus erythematosus. *Lupus* **11,** 31–34.

Huisman, A. M., White, K. P., Algra, A., Harth, M., Vieth, R., Jacobs, J. W., *et al.* (2001). Vitamin D levels in women with systemic lupus erythematosus and fibromyalgia. *J. Rheumatol.* **28,** 2535–2539.

Hypponen, E., Boucher, B. J., Berry, D. J., and Power, C. (2008). 25-hydroxyvitamin D, IGF-1, and metabolic syndrome at 45 years of age: A cross-sectional study in the 1958 British Birth Cohort. *Diabetes* **57,** 298–305.

Iannuzzi, M. C., Rybicki, B. A., and Teirstein, A. S. (2007). Sarcoidosis. *N. Engl. J. Med.* **357,** 2153–2165.

Jackson, C., Gaugris, S., Sen, S. S., and Hosking, D. (2007). The effect of cholecalciferol (vitamin D3) on the risk of fall and fracture: A meta-analysis. *QJM* **100,** 185–192.

Jorgensen, K. T., Wiik, A., Pedersen, M., Hedegaard, C. J., Vestergaard, B. F., Gislefoss, R. E., *et al.* (2008). Cytokines, autoantibodies and viral antibodies in premorbid and postdiagnostic sera from patients with rheumatoid arthritis: Case-control study nested in a cohort of Norwegian blood donors. *Ann. Rheum. Dis.* **67,** 860–866.

Kamen, D. L., Cooper, G. S., Bouali, H., Shaftman, S. R., Hollis, B. W., and Gilkeson, G. S. (2006). Vitamin D deficiency in systemic lupus erythematosus. *Autoimmun. Rev.* **5,** 114–117.

Klareskog, L., Alfredsson, L., Rantapaa-Dahlqvist, S., Berglin, E., Stolt, P., and Padyukov, L. (2004). What precedes development of rheumatoid arthritis? *Ann. Rheum. Dis.* **63**(Suppl. 2), ii28–ii31.

Klein, R. G., Arnaud, S. B., Gallagher, J. C., DeLuca, H. F., and Riggs, B. L. (1977). Intestinal calcium absorption in exogenous hypercortisonism. Role of 25-hydroxyvitamin D and corticosteroid dose. *J. Clin. Invest.* **60,** 253–259.

Koizumi, T., Nakao, Y., Matsui, T., Nakagawa, T., Matsuda, S., Komoriya, K., *et al.* (1985). Effects of corticosteroid and 1, 24R-dihydroxy-vitamin D3 administration on lymphoproliferation and autoimmune disease in MRL/MP-lpr/lpr mice. *Int. Arch. Allergy Appl. Immunol.* **77,** 396–404.

Koren, R., Ravid, A., Rotem, C., Shohami, E., Liberman, U. A., and Novogrodsky, A. (1986). 1, 25-Dihydroxyvitamin D3 enhances prostaglandin E2 production by monocytes. A mechanism which partially accounts for the antiproliferative effect of 1, 25(OH) 2D3 on lymphocytes. *FEBS Lett.* **205,** 113–116.

Kroger, H., Penttila, I. M., and Alhava, E. M. (1993). Low serum vitamin D metabolites in women with rheumatoid arthritis. *Scand. J. Rheumatol.* **22,** 172–177.

Kuruto-Niwa, R., Nakamura, M., Takeishi, K., and Nozawa, R. (1998). Transcriptional regulation by C/EBP alpha and -beta in the expression of the gene for the MRP14 myeloid calcium binding protein. *Cell Struct. Funct.* **23,** 109–118.

Lange, U., Teichmann, J., Strunk, J., Muller-Ladner, U., and Schmidt, K. L. (2005). Association of 1.25 vitamin D3 deficiency, disease activity and low bone mass in ankylosing spondylitis. *Osteoporos. Int.* **16,** 1999–2004.

Lee, C., Almagor, O., Dunlop, D. D., Chadha, A. B., Manzi, S., Spies, S., *et al.* (2007). Association between African American race/ethnicity and low bone mineral density in women with systemic lupus erythematosus. *Arthritis Rheum.* **57,** 585–592.

Lemire, J. M. (1995). Immunomodulatory actions of 1, 25-dihydroxyvitamin D3. *J. Steroid Biochem. Mol. Biol.* **53,** 599–602.

Lemire, J. M., Adams, J. S., Sakai, R., and Jordan, S. C. (1984). 1 alpha, 25-dihydroxyvitamin D3 suppresses proliferation and immunoglobulin production by normal human peripheral blood mononuclear cells. *J. Clin. Invest.* **74,** 657–661.

Lemire, J. M., Ince, A., and Takashima, M. (1992). 1, 25-Dihydroxyvitamin D3 attenuates the expression of experimental murine lupus of MRL/l mice. *Autoimmunity* **12,** 143–148.

Lim, W. C., Hanauer, S. B., and Li, Y. C. (2005). Mechanisms of disease: Vitamin D and inflammatory bowel disease. *Nat. Clin. Pract. Gastroenterol. Hepatol.* **2,** 308–315.

Linker-Israeli, M., Elstner, E., Klinenberg, J. R., Wallace, D. J., and Koeffler, H. P. (2001). Vitamin D(3) and its synthetic analogs inhibit the spontaneous in vitro immunoglobulin production by SLE-derived PBMC. *Clin. Immunol.* **99,** 82–93.

Liu, P. T., Stenger, S., Li, H., Wenzel, L., Tan, B. H., Krutzik, S. R., *et al.* (2006). Toll-like receptor triggering of a vitamin D-mediated human antimicrobial response. *Science* **311,** 1770–1773.

Lodder, M. C., Haugeberg, G., Lems, W. F., Uhlig, T., Orstavik, R. E., Kostense, P. J., *et al.* (2003). Radiographic damage associated with low bone mineral density and vertebral deformities in rheumatoid arthritis: The Oslo-Truro-Amsterdam (OSTRA) collaborative study. *Arthritis Rheum.* **49,** 209–215.

Maalej, A., Petit-Teixeira, E., Michou, L., Rebai, A., Cornelis, F., and Ayadi, H. (2005). Association study of VDR gene with rheumatoid arthritis in the French population. *Genes Immun.* **6,** 707–711.

Mahon, B. D., Wittke, A., Weaver, V., and Cantorna, M. T. (2003). The targets of vitamin D depend on the differentiation and activation status of CD4 positive T cells. *J. Cell. Biochem.* **89,** 922–932.

Malabanan, A., Veronikis, I. E., and Holick, M. F. (1998). Redefining vitamin D insufficiency. *Lancet* **351,** 805–806.

Martineau, A. R., Wilkinson, K. A., Newton, S. M., Floto, R. A., Norman, A. W., Skolimowska, K., *et al.* (2007). IFN-gamma- and TNF-independent vitamin D-inducible human suppression of mycobacteria: The role of cathelicidin LL-37. *J. Immunol.* **178,** 7190–7198.

Masuda, S., and Jones, G. (2006). Promise of vitamin D analogues in the treatment of hyperproliferative conditions. *Mol. Cancer Ther.* **5,** 797–808.

Matsuoka, L. Y., Wortsman, J., Dannenberg, M. J., Hollis, B. W., Lu, Z., and Holick, M. F. (1992). Clothing prevents ultraviolet-B radiation-dependent photosynthesis of vitamin D3. *J. Clin. Endocrinol. Metab.* **75,** 1099–1103.

Matucci-Cerinic, M., and Seibold, J. R. (2008). Digital ulcers and outcomes assessment in scleroderma. *Rheumatology (Oxford)* **47**(Suppl. 5), v46–v47.
McInnes, I. B., and Schett, G. (2007). Cytokines in the pathogenesis of rheumatoid arthritis. *Nat. Rev. Immunol.* **7,** 429–442.
Merlino, L. A., Curtis, J., Mikuls, T. R., Cerhan, J. R., Criswell, L. A., and Saag, K. G. (2004). Vitamin D intake is inversely associated with rheumatoid arthritis: Results from the Iowa Women's Health Study. *Arthritis Rheum.* **50,** 72–77.
Mitchell, R. J., Fabb, S. A., and Whittingham, S. (1985). Serum protein polymorphisms in patients with primary Sjogren's syndrome. *Hum. Hered.* **35,** 302–305.
Mosca, M., Tavoni, A., Neri, R., Bencivelli, W., and Bombardieri, S. (1998). Undifferentiated connective tissue diseases: The clinical and serological profiles of 91 patients followed for at least 1 year. *Lupus* **7,** 95–100.
Mosca, M., Tani, C., and Bombardieri, S. (2007). Undifferentiated connective tissue diseases (UCTD): A new frontier for rheumatology. *Best Pract. Res. Clin. Rheumatol.* **21,** 1011–1023.
Mosser, D. M., and Zhang, X. (2008). Interleukin-10: New perspectives on an old cytokine. *Immunol. Rev.* **226,** 205–218.
Muller, K., Oxholm, P., Sorensen, O. H., Thymann, M., Hoier-Madsen, M., and Bendtzen, K. (1990). Abnormal vitamin D3 metabolism in patients with primary Sjogren's syndrome. *Ann. Rheum. Dis.* **49,** 682–684.
Muller, K., Kriegbaum, N. J., Baslund, B., Sorensen, O. H., Thymann, M., and Bentzen, K. (1995). Vitamin D3 metabolism in patients with rheumatic diseases: Low serum levels of 25-hydroxyvitamin D3 in patients with systemic lupus erythematosus. *Clin. Rheumatol.* **14,** 397–400.
Nagpal, S., Na, S., and Rathnachalam, R. (2005). Noncalcemic actions of vitamin D receptor ligands. *Endocr. Rev.* **26,** 662–687.
Nakae, S., Nambu, A., Sudo, K., and Iwakura, Y. (2003). Suppression of immune induction of collagen-induced arthritis in IL-17-deficient mice. *J. Immunol.* **171,** 6173–6177.
Nielen, M. M., Van, S. D., Lems, W. F., van de Stadt, R. J., de Koning, M. H., Reesink, H. W., *et al.* (2006). Vitamin D deficiency does not increase the risk of rheumatoid arthritis: Comment on the article by Merlino et al. *Arthritis Rheum* **54,** 3719–3720.
O'Regan, S., Chesney, R. W., Hamstra, A., Eisman, J. A., O'Gorman, A. M., and DeLuca, H. F. (1979). Reduced serum 1, 25-(OH)2 vitamin D3 levels in prednisone-treated adolescents with systemic lupus erythematosus. *Acta Paediatr. Scand.* **68,** 109–111.
Oberg, F., Botling, J., and Nilsson, K. (1993). Functional antagonism between vitamin D3 and retinoic acid in the regulation of CD14 and CD23 expression during monocytic differentiation of U-937 cells. *J. Immunol.* **150,** 3487–3495.
Oelzner, P., Muller, A., Deschner, F., Huller, M., Abendroth, K., Hein, G., *et al.* (1998). Relationship between disease activity and serum levels of vitamin D metabolites and PTH in rheumatoid arthritis. *Calcif. Tissue Int.* **62,** 193–198.
Orbach, H., Zandman-Goddard, G., Amital, H., Barak, V., Szekanecz, Z., Szucs, G., *et al.* (2007). Novel biomarkers in autoimmune diseases: Prolactin, ferritin, vitamin D, and TPA levels in autoimmune diseases. *Ann. NY Acad. Sci.* **1109,** 385–400.
Ozaki, Y., Nomura, S., Nagahama, M., Yoshimura, C., Kagawa, H., and Fukuhara, S. (2000). Vitamin-D receptor genotype and renal disorder in Japanese patients with systemic lupus erythematosus. *Nephron* **85,** 86–91.
Patel, S., Farragher, T., Berry, J., Bunn, D., Silman, A., and Symmons, D. (2007). Association between serum vitamin D metabolite levels and disease activity in patients with early inflammatory polyarthritis. *Arthritis Rheum.* **56,** 2143–2149.

Pedersen, A. W., Holmstrom, K., Jensen, S. S., Fuchs, D., Rasmussen, S., Kvistborg, P., *et al.* (2009). Phenotypic and functional markers for 1alpha, 25-dihydroxyvitamin D(3)-modified regulatory dendritic cells. *Clin. Exp. Immunol.* **157,** 48–59.
Penna, G., and Adorini, L. (2000). 1 Alpha, 25-dihydroxyvitamin D3 inhibits differentiation, maturation, activation, and survival of dendritic cells leading to impaired alloreactive T cell activation. *J. Immunol.* **164,** 2405–2411.
Penna, G., Roncari, A., Amuchastegui, S., Daniel, K. C., Berti, E., Colonna, M., *et al.* (2005). Expression of the inhibitory receptor ILT3 on dendritic cells is dispensable for induction of CD4+Foxp3+ regulatory T cells by 1, 25-dihydroxyvitamin D3. *Blood* **106,** 3490–3497.
Przybelski, R. J., and Binkley, N. C. (2007). Is vitamin D important for preserving cognition? A positive correlation of serum 25-hydroxyvitamin D concentration with cognitive function. *Arch. Biochem. Biophys.* **460,** 202–205.
Ramirez, A. M., Wongtrakool, C., Welch, T., Steinmeyer, A., Zugel, U., and Roman, J. (2010). Vitamin D inhibition of pro-fibrotic effects of transforming growth factor beta1 in lung fibroblasts and epithelial cells. *J. Steroid Biochem. Mol. Biol.* **118,** 142–150.
Rass, P., Pakozdi, A., Lakatos, P., Zilahi, E., Sipka, S., Szegedi, G., *et al.* (2006). Vitamin D receptor gene polymorphism in rheumatoid arthritis and associated osteoporosis. *Rheumatol. Int.* **26,** 964–971.
Raza, K., Falciani, F., Curnow, S. J., Ross, E. J., Lee, C. Y., Akbar, A. N., *et al.* (2005). Early rheumatoid arthritis is characterized by a distinct and transient synovial fluid cytokine profile of T cell and stromal cell origin. *Arthritis Res. Ther.* **7,** R784–R795.
Ross, T. K., Darwish, H. M., and DeLuca, H. F. (1994). Molecular biology of vitamin D action. *Vitam. Horm.* **49,** 281–326.
Rucker, D., Allan, J. A., Fick, G. H., and Hanley, D. A. (2002). Vitamin D insufficiency in a population of healthy western Canadians. *CMAJ* **166,** 1517–1524.
Ruiz-Irastorza, G., Egurbide, M. V., Olivares, N., Martinez-Berriotxoa, A., and Aguirre, C. (2008). Vitamin D deficiency in systemic lupus erythematosus: Prevalence, predictors and clinical consequences. *Rheumatol (Oxford)* **47,** 920–923.
Sadeghi, K., Wessner, B., Laggner, U., Ploder, M., Tamandl, D., Friedl, J., *et al.* (2006). Vitamin D3 down-regulates monocyte TLR expression and triggers hyporesponsiveness to pathogen-associated molecular patterns. *Eur. J. Immunol.* **36,** 361–370.
Sakulpipatsin, W., Verasertniyom, O., Nantiruj, K., Totemchokchyakarn, K., Lertsrisatit, P., and Janwityanujit, S. (2006). Vitamin D receptor gene BsmI polymorphisms in Thai patients with systemic lupus erythematosus. *Arthritis Res. Ther.* **8,** R48.
Scherberich, J. E., Kellermeyer, M., Ried, C., and Hartinger, A. (2005). 1-alpha-calcidol modulates major human monocyte antigens and toll-like receptors TLR 2 and TLR4 in vitro. *Eur. J. Med. Res.* **10,** 179–182.
Schwalfenberg, G. (2007). Not enough vitamin D: Health consequences for Canadians. *Can. Fam. Physician* **53,** 841–854.
Staeva-Vieira, T. P., and Freedman, L. P. (2002). 1, 25-dihydroxyvitamin D3 inhibits IFN-gamma and IL-4 levels during in vitro polarization of primary murine CD4+ T cells. *J. Immunol.* **168,** 1181–1189.
Steingrimsdottir, L., Gunnarsson, O., Indridason, O. S., Franzson, L., and Sigurdsson, G. (2005). Relationship between serum parathyroid hormone levels, vitamin D sufficiency, and calcium intake. *JAMA* **294,** 2336–2341.
Swamy, N., and Ray, R. (1996). Affinity labeling of rat serum vitamin D binding protein. *Arch. Biochem. Biophys.* **333,** 139–144.
Szodoray, P., Nakken, B., Barath, S., Gaal, J., Aleksza, M., Zeher, M., *et al.* (2008). Progressive divergent shifts in natural and induced T-regulatory cells signify the transition from undifferentiated to definitive connective tissue disease. *Int. Immunol.* **20,** 971–979.

Tetlow, L. C., Smith, S. J., Mawer, E. B., and Woolley, D. E. (1999). Vitamin D receptors in the rheumatoid lesion: Expression by chondrocytes, macrophages, and synoviocytes. *Ann. Rheum. Dis.* **58,** 118–121.

Thomas, M. K., Lloyd-Jones, D. M., Thadhani, R. I., Shaw, A. C., Deraska, D. J., Kitch, B. T., *et al.* (1998). Hypovitaminosis D in medical inpatients. *N. Engl. J. Med.* **338,** 777–783.

Uitterlinden, A. G., Fang, Y., van Meurs, J. B., Pols, H. A., and Van Leeuwen, J. P. (2004). Genetics and biology of vitamin D receptor polymorphisms. *Gene* **338,** 143–156.

Vacca, A., Cormier, C., Piras, M., Mathieu, A., Kahan, A., and Allanore, Y. (2009). Vitamin D deficiency and insufficiency in 2 independent cohorts of patients with systemic sclerosis. *J. Rheumatol.* **36,** 1924–1929.

Vaisberg, M. W., Kaneno, R., Franco, M. F., and Mendes, N. F. (2000). Influence of cholecalciferol (vitamin D3) on the course of experimental systemic lupus erythematosus in F1 (NZBxW) mice. *J. Clin. Lab. Anal.* **14,** 91–96.

van Halteren, A. G., van, E. E., de Jong, E. C., Bouillon, R., Roep, B. O., and Mathieu, C. (2002). Redirection of human autoreactive T-cells Upon interaction with dendritic cells modulated by TX527, an analog of 1,25 dihydroxyvitamin D(3). *Diabetes* **51,** 2119–2125.

Vieth, R., Cole, D. E., Hawker, G. A., Trang, H. M., and Rubin, L. A. (2001). Wintertime vitamin D insufficiency is common in young Canadian women, and their vitamin D intake does not prevent it. *Eur. J. Clin. Nutr.* **55,** 1091–1097.

Wang, T. T., Nestel, F. P., Bourdeau, V., Nagai, Y., Wang, Q., Liao, J., *et al.* (2004). Cutting edge: 1, 25-Dihydroxyvitamin D3 is a direct inducer of antimicrobial peptide gene expression. *J. Immunol.* **173,** 2909–2912.

Welsh, J., Wietzke, J. A., Zinser, G. M., Smyczek, S., Romu, S., Tribble, E., *et al.* (2002). Impact of the Vitamin D3 receptor on growth-regulatory pathways in mammary gland and breast cancer. *J. Steroid Biochem. Mol. Biol.* **83,** 85–92.

Wright, T. B., Shults, J., Leonard, M. B., Zemel, B. S., and Burnham, J. M. (2009). Hypovitaminosis D is associated with greater body mass index and disease activity in pediatric systemic lupus erythematosus. *J. Pediatr.* **155,** 260–265.

Yim, S., Dhawan, P., Ragunath, C., Christakos, S., and Diamond, G. (2007). Induction of cathelicidin in normal and CF bronchial epithelial cells by 1, 25-dihydroxyvitamin D(3). *J. Cyst. Fibros.* **6,** 403–410.

Zhu, J., and Paul, W. E. (2008). CD4 T cells: Fates, functions, and faults. *Blood* **112,** 1557–1569.

Zold, E., Szodoray, P., Gaal, J., Kappelmayer, J., Csathy, L., Gyimesi, E., *et al.* (2008). Vitamin D deficiency in undifferentiated connective tissue disease. *Arthritis Res. Ther.* **10,** R123.

Zold, E., Szodoray, P., Kappelmayer, J., Gaal, J., Csathy, L., Barath, S., *et al.* (2010). Impaired regulatory T-cell homeostasis due to vitamin D deficiency in undifferentiated connective tissue disease. *Scand. J. Rheumatol.* **39,** 490–497.

CHAPTER TWELVE

Key Roles of Vitamins A, C, and E in Aflatoxin B_1-Induced Oxidative Stress

Lokman Alpsoy* *and* Mehmet Emir Yalvac†

Contents

Abstract

Aflatoxins (*Aspergillus flavus* toxins) are one of the natural toxic molecules which are produced by a group of fungi called Aspergillus. Foods and drinks contaminated with aflatoxins cause global health and environmental problems. Today in many developing countries, these toxins are leading cause of some liver cancers and serious gastrointestinal problems. Aflatoxins, which are well known to be mutagenic, carcinogenic, hepatotoxic, and immunosuppressive, exert inhibitory effects on biological processes including DNA synthesis, DNA-dependent RNA synthesis, DNA repair, and protein synthesis. Aflatoxins B_1 (AFB_1) is the most widespread oxidative agent of the aflatoxins. Numerous diverse compounds and extracts have been reported to reduce the aflatoxins induced oxidative stress in the body. Most of these inhibitors including phenylpropanoids, terpenoids, alkaloids, and vitamins are originally derived from plants. Among these, being essential biomolecules, vitamins are used as coenzymes in very significant biological reactions. They also function as nonenzymatic antioxidative agents protecting the cells from oxidative stress-induced toxicity and transformation. This chapter reviews the mechanism of

* Fatih University, Science and Art Faculty, Department of Biology, Buyukcekmece, Istanbul, Turkey
† Yeditepe University, Faculty of Engineering and Architecture, Department of Genetics and Bioengineering, Istanbul, Turkey

Vitamins and Hormones, Volume 86
ISSN 0083-6729, DOI: 10.1016/B978-0-12-386960-9.00012-5

AFB_1-induced oxidative stress and focuses on the protective effects of vitamins A, C, and E on reducing this stress.

I. Aflatoxins and AFB_1

Aflatoxins (*Aspergillus flavus* toxins) are biologically active secondary metabolites mostly produced by certain species of Aspergillus molds including *Aspergillus parasiticus*, *Aspergillus nominus*, and *Aspergillus flavus* (Bedard and Massey, 2006). The aflatoxin-producing fungi are widely found in nature and can grow over a wide range of environmental conditions where organic sources and moisture are present (Holmquist *et al.*, 1983). Many of daily consumed products such as cereal grains, oil seeds, and fermented beverages made from grains, milk, cheese, meat, nuts, and fruit juices might be contaminated with aflatoxins (Bullerman, 1986). Aflatoxins were initially reported to be the cause of "Turkey-X-disease" in 1960 (Asao *et al.*, 1965). So far, many different types of aflatoxins such as aflatoxin B_1 (AFB_1), aflatoxin G_1 (AFG_1), aflatoxin G_2 (AFG_2), aflatoxin M_1 (AFM_1), aflatoxin M_2 (AFM_2), aflatoxin P_1 (AFP_1), and aflatoxin Q_1 (AFQ_1) were determined and characterized (Verma, 2004). AFB_1 (fluoresces blue under UV light) and to a lesser extent AFG_1 (fluoresces greenish yellow under UV light) are detected in aflatoxin-contaminated foods and drinks. When metabolically oxidized, *in vivo* inactive AFB_2 and AFG_2 turn into AFB_1 and AFG_1, respectively. AFM_1 and M_2 are formed *in vivo* upon hydroxylation of AFB_1 and AFG_1 which might be consumed by aflatoxin-contaminated milk, milk products, or meat (Verma, 2004).

Analogous to fatty acid biosynthesis, aflatoxins' polyketide backbones are formed by polymerization of acetate and nine malonate monomers by a polyketide synthetase (Bhatnagar *et al.*, 1992; Dutton, 1988). Being almost insoluble in water, aflatoxins are soluble in moderately polar organic solvents. They are also unstable in highly acidic (pH below 3) and basic (pH above 10) conditions having melting points between 237 °C (AFG_1) and 299 °C (AFM_1). Aflatoxins on contaminated food are not affected from normal cooking conditions but they can be completely demolished by autoclaving in the presence of ammonia or by treatment with bleach (IARC, 1976, 1993).

Contamination of food and feed by aflatoxins is a global problem, as aflatoxin-producing fungi are able to infect a wide variety of crops. Consumption of food or feed highly contaminated with aflatoxins was reported to cause many severe health problems including hepatotoxicity, teratogenicity, immunotoxicity, and cancers (Trail *et al.*, 1995). IARC accepts AFB_1 as a group I carcinogen, as it is very commonly found carcinogenic and oxidative agent (Cotty and Bhatnagar, 1994). Avoid of aflatoxins is not an only health problem but it has also economic impacts such as causing loss of billions of dollars in farming which turns to be a big burden on a country's economy. Occurrence of aflatoxins contaminated crops varies depending on the country's geographical location in the world. It was shown that the highest levels of aflatoxins exist in the countries which are in tropical and subtropical regions (Verma, 2004). In order to restrict the ingestion of aflatoxins from foods and feeds, there are regulations all over the world. In Africa, there is still lack of regulation in about 40% of the countries which reports the existence of common aflatoxin-related health problems. European Union is much stricter than United States and rest of the world having elaborate regulations regarding aflatoxins (Fig. 12.1).

Aflatoxins are considered to be one of the major risk factors of human hepatocellular carcinoma (Mcglynn *et al.*, 1995). It was also reported that dietary and inhalation exposure to AFB_1 increases the risk of lung cancer (Dvorackova, 1984, Massey, 2000). Aflatoxins are also considered to be biological weapons which can ensure direct exposure to aflatoxins or poison the foodstuff (Massey *et al.*, 1995). It has been shown that aflatoxins exist in food chain and can be transmitted from mother to the fetus or infants via cord blood or breast milk (Denning *et al.*, 1990; Srivastava *et al.*, 2001) Even inhalation of AFB_1-contaminated grain dust was reported to be carcinogenic for some individuals (Hayes *et al.*, 1984). Both *in vitro* and *in vivo* studies indicate that AFB_1 causes modifications in expression of p53 gene, an important tumor suppressor gene, by inducing a transversion mutation in the coding sequence of the gene (Hainaut and Vahakangas, 1997;

Country	Aflatoxin Limit (μg/kg)	Total Aflatoxin (μg/kg)	AFB1 (μg/kg)	Reference	Food
Germany	5	44 μg/kg	13 μg/kg	EFSA, 2009	Chocochip almond, hazelnut, cookies
France	10	7.9 μg/kg	7.3 μg/kg	EFSA, 2008	Ponni rice
UK	10	52 μg/kg	47 μg/kg	EFSA, 2009	Corn meal and retail packs
China	20	27.44 μg/kg	29.05 μg/kg	Wang et al., 2007	Corn, peeled peanut, rice, etc.
USA	10	57–244 μg/kg	44–214 μg/kg	Trucksess, 2002	Raw almonds, Brazil nuts, walnuts, etc.
Kenya	20	0–2687 μg/kg	5–50 μg/kg	Mutegi et al., 2009; Kenji et al., 2000	Peanut; Malted maize, finger millet
Brazil	20	1.4–557 μg/kg	21.3 μg/kg	Marklinder et al., 2005; Sekiyama et al., 2005	Brazil nuts; Corn grits
Turkey	10	0.2–32.3 μg/kg	0.1–44.7 μg/kg	Colak et al., 2006	Red scaled, red and black pepper.

Figure 12.1 Country-based aflatoxin limits and detected total aflatoxin and AFB_1 levels in foods.

Mace *et al.*, 1997). It is suggested that AFB_1 induced p53 mutation might be closely linked to cancer formation in liver and pulmonary tissues (Ball *et al.*, 1995; Klein *et al.*, 2002; Lasky and Magder, 1997).

II. Molecular Mechanisms of AFB_1 Toxicity

The reasons of AFB_1-induced cellular transformation and cytotoxicity, forming adducts with DNA, RNA, and proteins; inhibition of RNA and protein synthesis; formation of lipid peroxides; loss of membrane integrity; cell lysis; degranulation of endoplasmic reticulum; abnormal calcium accumulation in the cell; and disrupted sodium pump were reviewed in detail by Verma (2004). AFB_1 is metabolized by the cytochrome P-450 enzymes and converted to metabolites including AFM_1, aflatoxicol (AFL), $AFLH_1$, AFP_1, AFB_2, and AFB_1-2, 2-dihydrodiol (Fig. 12.2).

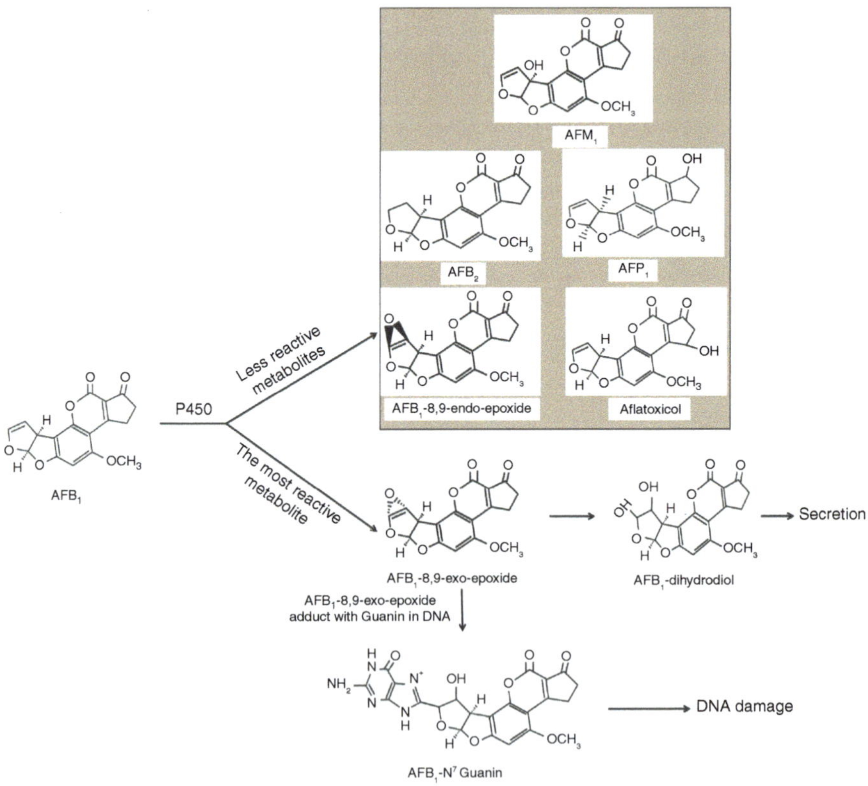

Figure 12.2 Metabolism of AFB_1.

One of the AFB_1, exo-8,9 epoxide, appeared to be most reactive epoxide combining DNA bases and altering its structure (Hendrickse, 1991). It was shown that 8,9-epoxide forms DNA adduct primarily at N7 position of guanine giving rise to mutagenicity and increased cancer risk (Denissenko *et al.*, 1999; Wang and Groopman, 1999). AFB_1 was also reported to increase formation of reactive oxygen species (ROS) such as superoxide radical anion, hydrogen peroxide, and lipid hydro peroxides (Halliwell and Gutteridge, 1999), probably by altering electron transport system attacking and changing the structure of the mitochondria (Hoehler *et al.*, 1996). Altered calcium permeability in mitochondria membrane leads to reduction in activity of the antioxidant enzyme glutathione peroxidase and glutathione reductase (Turrens, 1991). It was shown that 8,9-epoxide increases lipid peroxidation followed by loss of membrane stability and hindering of membrane bound enzyme activity (Toskulkao and Glinsukon, 1988). Decline in activity of antioxidant enzymes or abnormally increased oxidant levels induce oxidative stress in the cells. AFB_1 was linked with increase in ROS which results in reduction of antioxidant enzyme activities or the essential substrates of these enzymes leaving cells vulnerable to oxidation-induced DNA, RNA, protein, and lipid damage (Bedard and Massey, 2006; Clayson *et al.*, 1994; Shen *et al.*, 1995).

III. Inhibition of AFB_1-Induced Oxidative Stress and Toxicity

Various foods, food additives, drugs, and xenobiotics were investigated for their effect on AFB_1-macromolecule adduct formation or their relation with antioxidant defense mechanism. As antioxidant nutrients, some vitamins (A, C, and E) and their precursors act as superoxide anion scavengers. The data obtained from *in vitro* and *in vivo* studies suggest that vitamins and some food additives such as butylated hydroxyanisole (BHA) and butylated hydroxytoluene (BHT) are very efficacious in preventing mycotoxin-induced damages in the cells (Atroshi *et al.*, 2000). For example, different forms of vitamin A (retinol, retinal, retinoic acid, and retinal esters) inhibited AFB_1–DNA adduct (8-hydroxydeoxy-guanosine (8-OHdG)) formation by regulating the metabolism of AFB_1 conducted by cytochrome P450 (CYP450) enzyme system (Aboobaker *et al.*, 1997; Bhattacharya *et al.*, 1984). Vitamin A was also reported to induce the activity of glutathione S-transferase (GST) which is responsible for detoxification of AFB_1-epoxide.

Unlike vitamin A, water-soluble vitamins exerted less significant inhibitory effect on AFB_1–DNA adduct formations (Bhattacharya *et al.*, 1984). Riboflavin was reported to induce DNA repair machinery enzymes very efficiently avoiding DNA adducts (Webster *et al.*, 1996c). It was shown that vitamin C, vitamin B6, and folic acid inhibit mutagenesis in bacterial systems, suggesting that different vitamins subdue the oxidative stress differently (Bhattacharya *et al.*, 1984, 1987). Several studies indicated that diet including BHA or BHT might protect AFB_1-caused mutagenicity by both lowering AFB_1–DNA binding and inducing activity of glutathione S-transferase (Chang and Bjeldanes, 1987).

GST, uridine diphosphate glucuronyl transferase (UDPGT), and CYP450 enzymes are stimulated by many drugs such as phenobarbital, Aroclor 1254 (Dragan and Pitot, 1994), oltipraz (Primiano *et al.*, 1995), and ethoxyquin (Kensler *et al.*, 1986) which enable regulation of AFB_1 metabolism and inhibition of AFB_1-induced carcinogenesis. Plant-derived molecules dimethyl diphenyl bicarboxylate (DDB) (Liu *et al.*, 1995), crocetin (a natural carotenoid), and geniposide (Wang *et al.*, 1991) are well-known herbal drugs which increase glutathione (GSH) levels inhibiting AFB_1-induced DNA binding. However, a unique hormone, cortisol, elevates the toxicity of AFB_1 as it increases the metabolism of the AFB_1. forming its toxic derivatives (Chentanez *et al.*, 1988). Alcohol consumption prior to AFB_1 exposure was demonstrated to increase the damage in the liver by triggering AFB_1 metabolism (Sahaphong *et al.*, 1992). In addition to a diet rich in vitamin and other antioxidant molecules, the evidences represented that food restriction decreases the rate of chemical-induced cancers including AFB_1-induced liver tumors in animal models (Allaben *et al.*, 1991; Pariza and Boutwell, 1987; Tannenbaum, 1942). This might be due to the modified metabolism of chemicals during food restriction resulting in less amount of reactive mutagens (Pollard and Luckert, 1985).

IV. Interaction Between Dietary Factors and AFB_1 Toxicity

Our food seems to contain both our medicine and molecules which make us sick. Food mutagens causing oxidative damage are actually very well tolerated by our body's enzymatic defense system and by the antioxidative nutrients we daily consume. Unfortunately, inadequate consumption of essential dietary factors or abnormal dietary behaviors such as overeating blocks this toleration capacity. A well-known food mutagen, AFB_1, was shown to be associated with sporadic forms of severe diseases including cancers by forming highly reactive oxidizing agents after being metabolized. It is obvious that damage caused by chronic exposure to AFB_1 cannot be inhibited by antioxidative enzymes solely, but intake of some nutrients plays key roles in reducing the risks linked to AFB_1 (Goldman and Shields, 2003). The studies showed that formation of AFB_1–DNA adducts can be reduced by intake of some nutrients including vitamin A, vitamin C, riboflavin, carnitine, and plant extracts avoiding the risk of initiation of carcinogenesis (Ayub and Sachan, 1997). The diet rich of carbohydrate but poor of protein and fat was shown to enhance formation of AFB_1–DNA adducts (Mandel *et al.*, 1992; Nyathi *et al.*, 1993). Blocking the synthesis of AFB_1-epoxide, sulfur-rich protein diet was suggested to prevent AFB_1 mutagenicity (Bhattacharya *et al.*, 1987). L-carnitine supplementation was linked to lower triacylglycerol and higher AFB_1 levels in the plasma of rats after AFB_1 exposure, suggesting that carnitine reduces microsomal metabolism of AFB_1, thus reducing the toxicity (Sachan and Ayub, 1992; Sachan and Yatim, 1991). Unsaturated corn oil and olive oil were not found to have a significant inhibitory effect on AFB_1–DNA formation (Brennan-Craddock *et al.*, 1990; Newberne *et al.*, 1979). However, high-fat diet was suggested to decrease uptake of AFB_1 by hepatocytes, thus reducing the AFB_1-epoxide production (Nyathi *et al.*, 1993). It was reported that essential oils from different plants reduce the microsomal enzyme-mediated metabolism of AFB_1 in a dose-dependent manner causing fall in production of AFB_1–DNA adducts (Hashim *et al.*, 1994). Interacting with the microsomal enzymes, copper and selenium elements were shown to reduce AFB_1-induced mutagenicity *in vitro* (Francis *et al.*, 1988), but the effect of selenium in reducing the levels of AFB_1–DNA adducts was significant only in rats (Bhattacharya *et al.*, 1984). High consumption of cruciferous vegetables was demonstrated to reduce the risk of urinary and colorectal cancers by inhibiting AFB_1–DNA adduct formation and increasing GST activity and excretion of AFB_1 in rats (Chang and Bjeldanes, 1987).

Like vitamin E, the carotenoids (naturally found in some foods, such as carrots, red tomatoes, butter, cheese, paprika, palm oil, and red salmon) are lipid soluble antioxidants which scavenge the ROS and peroxide radicals (Chaudiere and Ferrari-Iliou, 1999; Fukuzawa *et al.*, 1998). Some carotenoids (beta-carotene, alpha-carotene, gamma-carotene, and beta-cryptoxanthin) can be converted to vitamin A (retinol) which has also has antioxidant property (Keys and Zimmerman, 1999). Another lipid soluble antioxidant is Ubiquinol-10 (coenzyme Q10, ubiquinone 50), which scavenges free radicals generated in liposomal membranes, thus preventing lipid peroxidation (Frei *et al.*, 1990; Shi *et al.*, 1999). Among the water-soluble antioxidants, vitamin C (ascorbate) is unique, as it is very effective in scavenging superoxide, hydrogen peroxide, hydroxyl radicals, hypochlorous acid, aqueous peroxyl radicals, and singlet oxygen (Levine *et al.*, 1999). Other vitamins, riboflavin (Webster *et al.*, 1996a,b) and vitamin A2, were reported to inhibit formation of AFB_1–DNA adducts (Aboobaker *et al.*, 1997). It is widely accepted that among all vitamins, vitamins A, C, and E have the greatest capacity to prevent AFB_1-induced oxidative stress. Therefore, the antioxidative roles of these vitamins will be summarized separately in this study.

V. Vitamin A

Vitamin A has three active forms such as retinol, retinal, and retinoic acid (retinoids), which are essential for various biological events such as vision, reproduction, growth, and maintenance of epithelial tissues (Champe *et al.*, 2007). Some carotenoids such as beta-carotene produced by plants are considered as precursors of vitamin A, as they are converted to retinal in our body. Foods with animal origin such as liver, kidney, cream, butter, and egg yolk are rich of vitamin A. However, plant foods serve as the source of carotenoids rather than vitamin A. The recommended dietary allowance (RDA) for adults is 1000 retinol equivalents (RE) for males and 800 RE for females (1 RE = 1 mg of retinol, 6 mg of β-carotene, or 12 mg of other carotenoids). There exist two possible theories explaining the mechanism of antimutagenic and antioxidative effects of vitamin A. The first one is inhibitory role of vitamin A on cytochrome P450-mediated metabolism of mutagens or carcinogens such as AFB_1. The second one is preventing mutagenic epoxides from binding to the DNA by forming epoxides and competing with mutagenic epoxides in reacting with DNA (De Flora and Ramel, 1988; Zile *et al.*, 1986) Retinol, retinal, all-trans retinoic acid, and two retinal esters were demonstrated to inhibit the adduct formation in a dose-dependent manner. They interact with microsomal enzyme components resulting in reduced the bioactivation of AFB_1 (Firozi *et al.*, 1986). Retinol (vitamin A) and beta-carotene were shown to reduce the AFB_1-induced genotoxicity mainly by inhibiting sister chromatid exchanges (SCE) (Deng *et al.*, 1988; Huang *et al.*, 1982; Sinha and Dharmshila, 1994), thus suppressing AFB_1-induced hepatocarcinogenicity. It was also shown that vitamin A has roles in maintaining number and normal morphology of sperms after AFB_1-induced toxicity (Sinha and Dharmshila, 1994).

As precursors of vitamin A, many carotenoids such as lycopene and β-carotene work as quenchers inactivating electronically excited molecules such as singlet molecular oxygen and other free radicals. Anticarcinogenic properties of carotenoids might be associated being part of nonenzymatic antioxidant defense systems. For example, lycopene and beta-carotene were shown to reduce the oxidative DNA damage and enhance the immune defense by stimulating increase of lymphocytes in blood (Alexander *et al.*, 1985; Bendich and Shapiro, 1986; Mathews-Roth and Krinsky, 1985). It was shown that, at certain doses, carotenoids increases chemotaxis and phagocytosis of monocytes and peritoneal macrophages which exposed to AFB_1 (Chang and Hamilton, 1979) and turkey (Neldon-Ortiz and Qureshi, 1991). *In vitro* studies showed that lycopene and beta-carotene are effective in inhibiting the AFB_1-induced toxicity on human hepatocytes (Hep3G) by decreasing apoptosis and the level of AFB_1-guanine adducts. These carotenoids also avoided AFB_1-induced mutations in p53 tumor suppressor gene and inhibited the metabolism of AFB_1 (Reddy *et al.*, 2006). Another *in vitro* study presented that carotenoids inhibit the growth of human colon carcinoma cells by inducing apoptosis (Briviba *et al.*, 2001).

VI. Vitamin C

Vitamin C (ascorbic acid: AA) is mainly utilized as an electron donor which is well documented in hydroxylation of prolyle and lysyle residues of collagen, the most abundant protein in our body, strengthening the connective tissue and helping wound healing. Humans cannot produce their own vitamin C but they are dependent on fruits and vegetables which are rich in vitamin C such as citrus fruits, tomato, strawberry, pepper, cabbage, and leafy greens. Vitamin C cannot be stored in the body, and excess vitamin C is excreted in urine. Daily RDA for vitamin C is 90 mg/day for men and 75 mg/day for women. The smokers must take at least 35 mg/day, as their vitamin C level in their plasma is lower than that of nonsmokers (Lykkesfeldt *et al.*, 1997). In combination with vitamin E, long-term AA supplementation was demonstrated to lower oxidative stress-induced DNA damage in mononuclear blood cells of smokers (Moller *et al.*, 2004). Consuming less than 5 mg of vitamin C per day gives rise to scurvy disease characterized by sore, spongy gums, loose teeth, fragile blood vessels, swollen joints, and anemia (Champe *et al.*, 2007). All these symptoms are related to deficiency in production of collagen and strong connective tissue. The researches have represented that diet rich in vitamin C might be associated with reduced risk of chronic diseases and certain type cancers despite the fact that supplementation of antioxidants including vitamin C did not show persuading therapeutic potential in clinical trials (Champe *et al.*, 2007).

Unlike vitamin E, vitamin C is a significant water-soluble antioxidant in plasma helping to reduce the effect of oxidative stress. As it is water soluble, it can easily react with free radical in extracellular body fluids (Bendich, 1990). Vitamin C exerts its antioxidant effects in both direct and indirect ways. In the direct way, AA scavenges the free radicals formed as a byproduct of metabolic reactions (Dawson *et al.*, 1990). During this process, AA is first reduced to semidehydroascorbyl radical and then to dehydroascorbate (Pietri *et al.*, 1994). Dehydroascorbate can be converted back to AA by the selenoenzyme thioredoxin reductase (May *et al.*, 1998) or interacting with reduced glutathione (May *et al.*, 1996). In indirect way, AA helps recycling of oxidized vitamin E thus supplying active vitamin E fighting against lipid peroxidation (Netke *et al.*, 1997). It has been reported that besides lowering AFB_1-related lipid peroxidation, AA inhibits the binding of AFB_1 to DNA (Yu *et al.*, 1994). AA was found to abbreviate the adverse effects of AFB_1 on the semen production and testosterone levels in male rabbits. This might suggest that AA might be essential for reproduction system work properly (Salem *et al.*, 2001). AA functions in hydroxylation of some oxidases which are responsible for detoxification of different pesticides, heavy metals, steroids, and other xenobiotics (Dawson *et al.*, 1990; Flodin, 1990; Tucker and Halver, 1984). A subfamily of cytochrome P450, CYP3A, includes monooxygenases which catalyze many reactions involved in detoxification of drugs and many other xenobiotics (Lamba *et al.*, 2003). It was suggested that AA protects the animals from acute toxicity of AFB_1 by activating AFB_1-epoxide hydroxylase, aldehyde reductase, and CYP3A enzymes located in the enterocytes (Netke *et al.*, 1997).

VII. Vitamin E

Vitamin E is the most notable lipid soluble antioxidant having two main groups: tocopherols and tocotrienols both of which have four types designated as α-, β-, γ-, and δ-tocopherols and tocotrienols (Esterbauer *et al.*, 1991). Although all these forms of vitamin E have antioxidative properties to some extent, the body mainly utilizes α-tocopherol (Arita *et al.*, 1995). Tocopherols are transported either by lipoproteins or by some specific lipid-binding proteins. These proteins belong to the Sec14 superfamily consisting around 500 distinct proteins (Saito *et al.*, 2007). One of these proteins, α-tocopherol transfer protein (α-TTP), preferentially transports α-tocopherol having less affinity for non-α-tocopherol forms of vitamin E which might explain why body mainly utilizes α-tocopherol (Hosomi *et al.*, 1997). α-TTP−/− mice develop neurological defects and infertility (Noguchi *et al.*, 2003). In addition to this, some mutations in α-TTP gene were shown to be associated with neurological disorders in man (Sontag and Parker, 2007). Further, α-tocopherol was shown to have highest scavenging capacity of free radicals among all other forms of vitamin E (Traber and Atkinson, 2007). The RDA for vitamin E varies between 15 and 19 mg in adults, but it is highly related to the intake of polyunsaturated fatty acids (PUFAs) which are targeted by free radicals. Vegetable oils (sunflower, soy bean, and corn oil), whole grain products, nuts, and seeds are rich sources of vitamin E. On the contrary, the animal-derived foods contain low amount of vitamin E. Therapeutic effects of vitamin E on diseases which are closely related to the oxidative stress have not been shown so far, but there are lots of studies demonstrating that vitamin E protects cell membranes by preventing lipid peroxidation. α-Tocopherol reacts with peroxyl radicals—depending on its methylation state of the chromanol ring and the saturation grade of the side chain—forming tocopheroxyl radicals (Brigelius-Flohe, 2009). Tocopheroxyl radicals are converted into tocopherols by reacting with ascorbate (May *et al.*, 1998), reduced glutathione, urate (Kagan and Tyurina, 1998), or ubiquinol (Q10H2) (Bowry and Stocker, 1993). Vitamin E has been shown to play role in various enzymes' activities by enabling their translocation to the membrane (Kempna *et al.*, 2004) or affecting their transcriptional activation process (Khor and Ng, 2000). It is reported that a tocopherol affects the expression of many genes which involves in apoptosis, cell growth, inflammation, transmitter release, and metabolism (Zingg and Azzi, 2004). Despite this fact, it is still being questioned if vitamin E is a tremendous regulator of various biochemical activities or its role is only limited to prevention of lipid peroxidation of long-chain PUFAs, which are functional units of cell membranes. PUFAs are important for membrane integrity and function as signaling molecules of cells in response to environmental stimuli.

The role of vitamin E in reducing the oxidative stress caused by AFB_1 was shown by many reports. Chlopkiewicz (1991) showed that vitamin E can reduce the mutagenicity of both aflatoxin and adriamycin in liver (Chlopkiewicz *et al.*, 1991). Vitamin E dietary intake was shown to decrease AFB_1-induced genotoxicity by modifying the hepatic microsomal cytochrome P-450 activities (Cassand *et al.*, 1993). Metabolism of AFB_1 is reduced by α-tocopherol reducing the radical formation, which might be one of the protective roles of vitamin E (Ibeh and Saxena, 1998). However, it has been shown that vitamin E increases the abundance or activity of biomarkers associated with oxidative stress in a dose-dependent manner (Alpsoy *et al.*, 2009) (Fig. 12.3).

It was shown that oral intake of vitamin E (2 mg/day) improves steroidogenesis, biochemical and histopathological parameters altered by aflatoxin treatment in mice (Verma and Nair, 2001, 2002). α-Tocopherol possesses high affinity for aflatoxin reducing its bioactive roles in forming lipid peroxides (Odin, 1997). It also enables regular transportation of phosphate ions in the membranes of mitochondria by inhibiting peroxidative changes in the membranes caused by hydroxyl radicals (Shen *et al.*, 1994). After being metabolized by CYP450, AFB_1 is converted to its bioactive forms such as AFM1 which was shown to be suppressed in animal feed with vitamin E supplements (Emerole *et al.*, 1984). Undoubtedly, initiation of cancer is a result of changes in DNA which results in upregulation of oncogenes and downregulation of tumor suppressor genes. There are evidences that AFB_1 induces mutagenic changes in DNA by forming AFB_1–DNA adducts. It was reported that vitamin E is not able to reduce AFB_1–DNA adducts like vitamins C and A (Yu *et al.*, 1994) suggesting that vitamins might have complex roles in prevention of AFB_1-induced carcinogenesis which is closely related to antioxidative fighters (enzymatic and nonenzymatic) of the body. Vitamins A, C, and E were reported to reduce the cancer initiation caused by AFB_1 treatment in the liver

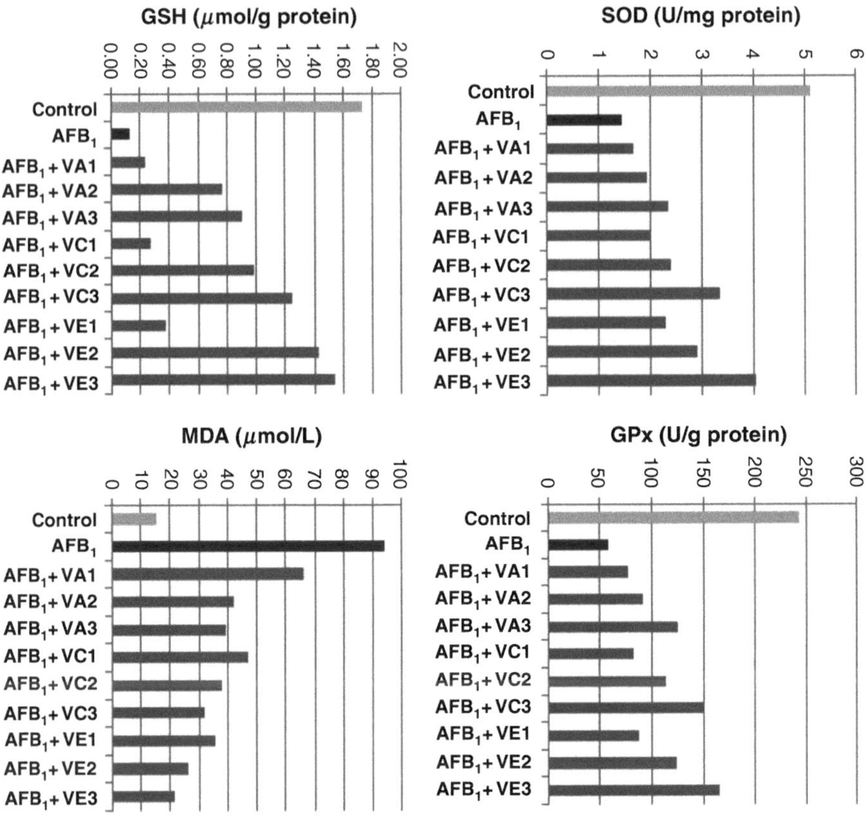

Figure 12.3 Effect of vitamins A, C, and D on the levels of oxidative stress markers in human lymphocytes exposed to AFB_1. SOD: superoxide dimutase, MDA: malondialdehyde, GPx: glutathion peroxidase, GSH: glutathion. AFB1: 5 μM AFB_1, AFB_1 + VA1: 5 μM AFB_1 + 0.5 μM vitamin A, AFB_1 + VA2: 5 μM AFB_1 + 1 μM vitamin A, AFB_1 + VA3: 5 μM AFB_1 + 1.5 μM vitamin A, AFB_1 + VC1: 5 μM AFB_1 + 25 μM vitamin C, AFB_1 + VC2: 5 μM AFB_1 + 50 μM vitamin C, AFB_1 + VC3: 5 μM AFB_1 + 100 μM vitamin C, AFB_1 + VE1: 5 μM AFB_1 + 50 μM vitamin E, AFB_1 + VE2: 5 μM AFB_1 + 100 μM vitamin E, AFB_1 + VE3: 5 μM AFB_1 + 200 μM vitamin E.

(Nyandieka *et al.*, 1990) which might be because of their inhibition of microsomal enzymes carrying out *in vitro* metabolism of AFB_1 (Wheeler *et al.*, 2006). Studies represent that vitamins A, C, and E exert antioxidative and antimutagenic activity against AFB_1 at premetabolic, metabolic, or postmetabolic levels. It is also certain that they have a very complex way of action together against AFB_1 and the other mutagens depending on the many factors related to the physiological state of the body, character of the diet, eating habits, or type of the mutagens. Based on the literature, in Fig. 12.4, we tried to illustrate the roles of vitamins A, C, and E in reducing the AFB_1-induced oxidative stress and mutagenicity.

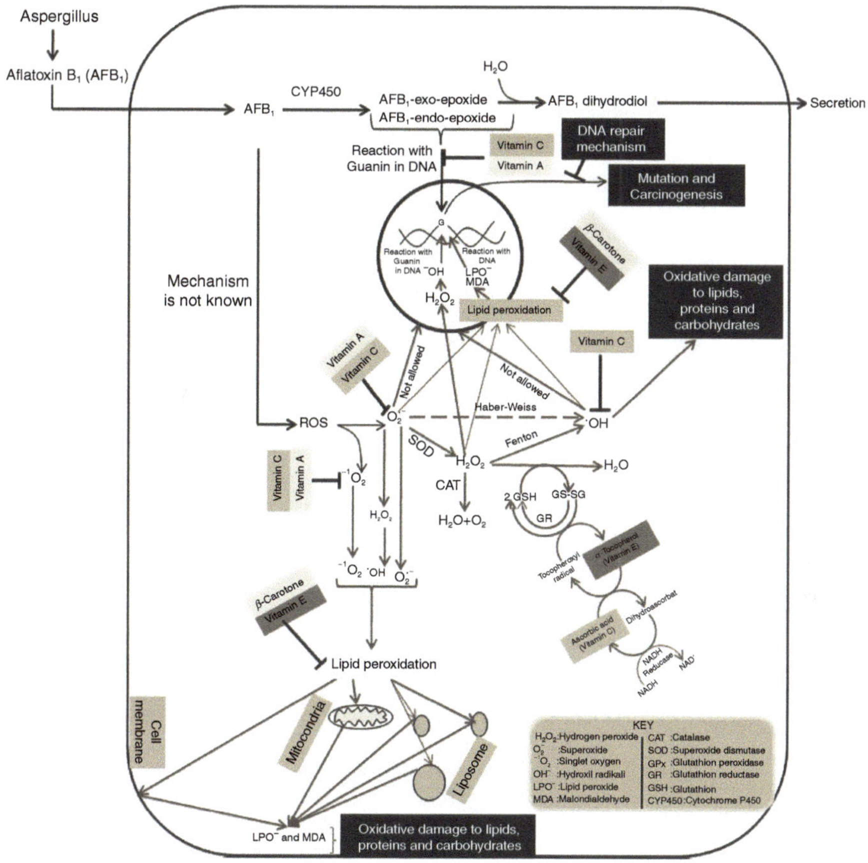

Figure 12.4 Complex roles of vitamins A, C, and E in reducing the AFB_1-induced oxidative stress and mutagenicity.

VIII. Conclusion and Future Remarks

There are two major obligations to be performed in fighting against aflatoxin-associated health problems in all over the world. The first obligation is to take measures including strict control of aflatoxin-contaminated food and feed in a professional way. The second obligation is to conduct high-quality scientific research on reducing the hazardous effects of aflatoxins in our body. Vitamins A, C, and E were shown to play a great role in reducing the oxidative stress induced by aflatoxins including AFB_1. However, the studies performed so far seem to be insufficient in explaining how these vitamins exactly achieve this protective role. The reasons of this problem might be differences between the cell culture conditions and *in vivo* conditions, as well as biochemical, physiological, and genetic variations between the model animals and human beings. Based on the literature, it might be suggested that vitamins A, C, and E have a very complex network of relations in reducing the stress caused by AFB_1. The capacity of vitamins to scavenge the radicals formed by AFB_1 exposure appears to increase when they are consumed together instead of taking them as separate supplements. Further, the effective doses of the vitamins against oxidative stress and relationship of vitamins with nonvitamin nutrients must be investigated to recommend precise public health measures.

ACKNOWLEDGMENT

We thank Dr. Fikrettin Sahin from Yeditepe University for constructive discussions.

REFERENCES

Aboobaker, V. S., *et al.* (1997). Inhibition of microsomal activation of aflatoxin B1 by 3-dehydroretinol and 3-dehydroretinyl palmitate. *Indian J. Exp. Biol.* **35,** 1125–1127.

Alexander, M., *et al.* (1985). Oral beta-carotene can increase the number of OKT4+ cells in human blood. *Immunol. Lett.* **9,** 221–224.

Allaben, W. T., *et al.* (1991). Dietary Restriction and Toxicological Endpoints: A Historical Perspective. Springer-Verlag, Berlin, Germany.

Alpsoy, L., *et al.* (2009). The antioxidant effects of vitamin A, C, and E on aflatoxin B1-induced oxidative stress in human lymphocytes. *Toxicol. Ind. Health* **25,** 121–127.

Arita, M., *et al.* (1995). Human alpha-tocopherol transfer protein: cDNA cloning, expression and chromosomal localization. *Biochem. J.* **306**(Pt. 2), 437–443.

Asao, T., *et al.* (1965). The structures of aflatoxins B and G. *J. Am. Chem. Soc.* **87,** 882–886.

Atroshi, F., *et al.* (2000). Liver enzyme activities of rats exposed to ochratoxin A and T-2 toxin with antioxidants. *Bull. Environ. Contam. Toxicol.* **64,** 586–592.

Ayub, M., and Sachan, D. (1997). Dietary factors affecting aflatoxin Bi carcinogenicity. *Mal. J. Nutr.* **3,** 161–179.

Ball, R. W., *et al.* (1995). Comparative activation of aflatoxin B-1 by mammalian pulmonary tissues. *Toxicol. Lett.* **75,** 119–125.

Bedard, L. L., and Massey, T. E. (2006). Aflatoxin B1-induced DNA damage and its repair. *Cancer Lett.* **241,** 174–183.

Bendich, A. (1990). Antioxidant Micro Nutrients and Immune Responses. New York Academy of Science, New York.

Bendich, A., and Shapiro, S. S. (1986). Effect of beta-carotene and canthaxanthin on the immune responses of the rat. *J. Nutr.* **116,** 2254–2262.

Bhatnagar, D., *et al.* (1992). Oxidation-reduction reactions in biosynthesis of secondary metabolites. *In* "Handbook of Applied Micology: Mycotoxins in Ecological Systems," (D. Bhatnagar, E.B. Lillehoj, and D.L. Arora, Eds.), pp. 255–286. New York.

Bhattacharya, R. K., *et al.* (1984). Factors modulating the formation of DNA adduct by aflatoxin-B1 in vitro. *Carcinogenesis* **5,** 1359–1362.

Bhattacharya, R. K., *et al.* (1987). Modifying role of dietary factors on the mutagenicity of aflatoxin B1: In vitro effect of vitamins. *Mutat. Res.* **188,** 121–128.

Bowry, V. W., and Stocker, R. (1993). Tocopherol-mediated peroxidation. The prooxidant effect of vitamin E on the radical-initiated oxidation of human low-density lipoprotein. *J. Am. Chem. Soc.* **115,** 6029–6044.

Brennan-Craddock, W. E., *et al.* (1990). Dietary fat modifies the in vivo mutagenicity of some food-borne carcinogens. *Mutat. Res.* **230,** 49–54.

Brigelius-Flohe, R. (2009). Vitamin E: The shrew waiting to be tamed. *Free Radic. Biol. Med.* **46,** 543–554.

Briviba, K., *et al.* (2001). Beta-carotene inhibits growth of human colon carcinoma cells in vitro by induction of apoptosis. *Biol. Chem.* **382,** 1663–1668.

Bullerman, L. B. (1986). Mycotoxins and food safety. *Food Technol.* **40,** 59–66.

Cassand, P., *et al.* (1993). Effect of vitamin E dietary intake on in vitro activation of aflatoxin B1. *Mutat. Res.* **319,** 309–316.

Champe, P. C., *et al.* (2007). Lippincott's Illustrated Reviews: Biochemistry. North American Edition Wolters Kluwer/Lippincott Williams and Wilkins, New York.

Chang, Y., and Bjeldanes, L. F. (1987). R-goitrin- and BHA-induced modulation of aflatoxin B1 binding to DNA and biliary excretion of thiol conjugates in rats. *Carcinogenesis* **8,** 585–590.

Chang, C. F., and Hamilton, P. B. (1979). Impairment of phagocytosis in chicken monocytes during aflatoxicosis. *Poult. Sci.* **58,** 562–566.

Chaudiere, J., and Ferrari-Iliou, R. (1999). Intracellular antioxidants: From chemical to biochemical mechanisms. *Food Chem. Toxicol.* **37,** 949–962.

Chentanez, T., *et al.* (1988). Effects of cortisol pretreatment on the acute hepatotoxicity of aflatoxin B1. *Toxicol. Lett.* **42,** 237–248.

Chlopkiewicz, B., *et al.* (1991). An evaluation of antimutagenic properties of vitamin E. *Acta Pol. Pharm.* **48,** 33–34.

Clayson, D. B., *et al.* (1994). Oxidative DNA-damage—The effects of certain genotoxic and operationally nongenotoxic carcinogens. *Mutat. Res.* **317,** 25–42.

Colak, H., *et al.* (2006). Determination of aflatoxin contamination in red-scaled, red and black pepper by ELISA and HPLC. *J. Food Drug Anal.* **14,** 292–296.

Cotty, P. J., and Bhatnagar, D. (1994). Variability among atoxigenic *Aspergillus flavus* strains in ability to prevent aflatoxin contamination and production of aflatoxin biosynthetic pathway enzymes. *Appl. Environ. Microbiol.* **60,** 2248–2251.

Dawson, E. B., *et al.* (1990). Relationship between ascorbic acid and male fertility. *World Rev. Nutr. Diet.* **62,** 1–26.

De Flora, S., and Ramel, C. (1988). Mechanisms of inhibitors of mutagenesis and carcinogenesis. Classification and overview. *Mutat. Res.* **202,** 285–306.

Deng, D. J., *et al.* (1988). Effect of beta-carotene on sister chromatid exchanges induced by MNNG and aflatoxin B1 in V79 cells. *Zhonghua Zhong Liu Za Zhi* **10,** 89–91.

Denissenko, M. F., *et al.* (1999). Quantitation and mapping of aflatoxin B1-induced DNA damage in genomic DNA using aflatoxin B1-8, 9-epoxide and microsomal activation systems. *Mutat. Res., Fundam. Mol. Mech. Mutagen.* **425,** 205–211.

Denning, D. W., *et al.* (1990). Transplacental transfer of aflatoxin in humans. *Carcinogenesis* **11,** 1033–1035.

Dragan, Y. P., and Pitot, H. C. (1994). Aflatoxin Carcinogenesis in the Context of the Multistage Nature of Cancer. Academic Press, New York.

Dvorackova, I., and Polster, M. (1984). Relation between aflatoxin producing aspergilloma and lung carcinoma. Microbiologie-Aliments-Nutrition. **2,** 187–192.

Dutton, M. F. (1988). Enzymes and aflatoxin biosynthesis. *Microbiol. Rev.* **52,** 274–295.

EFSA, Rapid Alert System for Food and Feed (RASFF) (2008). https://webgate.ec.europa.eu/rasff-window/portal/index.cfm?event=notificationsList.

EFSA, Rapid Alert System for Food and Feed (RASFF) (2009). https://webgate.ec.europa.eu/rasff-window/portal/index.cfm?event=notificationsList.

Emerole, G. O., *et al.* (1984). Effect of dietary vitamin E (alpha-tocopherol) on aflatoxin B metabolism. *Eur. J. Drug Metab. Pharmacokinet.* **9,** 295–300.
Esterbauer, H., *et al.* (1991). Role of vitamin-E in preventing the oxidation of low-density-lipoprotein. *Am. J. Clin. Nutr.* **53,** S314–S321.
Firozi, P. F., *et al.* (1986). Modulation by certain factors of metabolic activation of aflatoxin B1 as detected in vitro in a simple fluorimetric assay. *Chem. Biol. Interact.* **58,** 173–184.
Flodin, N. W. (1990). Micronutrient supplements: Toxicity and drug interactions. *Prog. Food Nutr. Sci.* **14,** 277–331.
Francis, A. R., *et al.* (1988). Modifying role of dietary factors on the mutagenicity of aflatoxin B1: In vitro effect of trace elements. *Mutat. Res.* **199,** 85–93.
Frei, B., *et al.* (1990). Ubiquinol-10 is an effective lipid-soluble antioxidant at physiological concentrations. *Proc. Natl. Acad. Sci. USA* **87,** 4879–4883.
Fukuzawa, K., *et al.* (1998). Rate constants for quenching singlet oxygen and activities for inhibiting lipid peroxidation of carotenoids and alpha-tocopherol in liposomes. *Lipids* **33,** 751–756.
Goldman, R., and Shields, P. G. (2003). Food mutagens. *J. Nutr.* **133**(Suppl. 3), 965S–973S.
Hainaut, P., and Vahakangas, K. (1997). p53 as a sensor of carcinogenic exposures: Mechanisms of p53 protein induction and lessons from p53 gene mutations. *Pathol. Biol. (Paris)* **45,** 833–844.
Halliwell, B., and Gutteridge, J. M. C. (1999). Oxidative Stress: Adaptation Damage, Repair and Death. Oxford University Press, New York.
Hashim, S., *et al.* (1994). Modulatory effects of essential oils from spices on the formation of DNA adduct by aflatoxin B1 in vitro. *Nutr. Cancer* **21,** 169–175.
Hayes, R. B., *et al.* (1984). Aflatoxin exposures in the industrial-setting—An epidemiological-study of mortality. *Food Chem. Toxicol.* **22,** 39–43.
Hendrickse, R. G. (1991). Clinical implications of food contaminated by aflatoxins. *Ann. Acad. Med. Singapore* **20,** 84–90.
Hoehler, D., *et al.* (1996). Model studies on free radical generation induced by different mycotoxins in yeast and bacteria. *FASEB J.* **10,** 790–796.
Holmquist, G. U., *et al.* (1983). Influence of temperature, Ph, water activity and anti-fungal agents on growth of *Aspergillus-flavus* and Aspergillus-parasiticus. *J. Food Sci.* **48,** 778–782.
Hosomi, A., *et al.* (1997). Affinity for alpha-tocopherol transfer protein as a determinant of the biological activities of vitamin E analogs. *FEBS Lett.* **409,** 105–108.
Huang, C. C., *et al.* (1982). Retinol (vitamin A) inhibits sister chromatid exchanges and cell cycle delay induced by cyclophosphamide and aflatoxin B1 in Chinese hamster V79 cells. *Carcinogenesis* **3,** 1–5.
IARC (1976). Some Naturally Occurring Substances. IARC Monographs on the Evaluation of Carcinogenic Risk of Chemicals to Humans, Vol. 10 International Agency for Research on Cancer, Lyon, France 353.
IARC (1993). Some Naturally Occurring Substances: Food Items and Constituents, Heterocyclic Aromatic Amines, and Mycotoxins. IARC Monographs on the Evaluation of Carcinogenic Risk of Chemicals to Humans, Vol. 56. International Agency for Research on Cancer, Lyon, France, 571.
Ibeh, I. N., and Saxena, D. K. (1998). Effect of alpha-tocopherol supplementation on the impact of aflatoxin B1 on the testes of rats. *Exp. Toxicol. Pathol.* **50,** 221–224.
Kagan, V. E., and Tyurina, Y. Y. (1998). Recycling and redox cycling of phenolic antioxidants. *Ann. NY Acad. Sci.* **854,** 425–434.
Kempna, P., *et al.* (2004). Inhibition of HMC-1 mast cell proliferation by vitamin E: Involvement of the protein kinase B pathway. *J. Biol. Chem.* **279,** 50700–50709.

Kenji, G. M., *et al.* (2000). Aflatoxin Contamination of Kenyan Maize Flour and Malted Kenyan and Malawian Grains. Scientific Reports of the Faculty of Agriculture, Vol. 89. Okayama University, pp. 5–7.

Kensler, T. W., *et al.* (1986). Modulation of aflatoxin metabolism, aflatoxin-N7-guanine formation, and hepatic tumorigenesis in rats fed ethoxyquin: Role of induction of glutathione S-transferases. *Cancer Res.* **46,** 3924–3931.

Keys, S. A., and Zimmerman, W. F. (1999). Antioxidant activity of retinol, glutathione, and taurine in bovine photoreceptor cell membranes. *Exp. Eye Res.* **68,** 693–702.

Khor, H. T., and Ng, T. T. (2000). Effects of administration of alpha-tocopherol and tocotrienols on serum lipids and liver HMG CoA reductase activity. *Int. J. Food Sci. Nutr.* **51**(Suppl.), S3–S11.

Klein, P. J., *et al.* (2002). Biochemical factors underlying the age-related sensitivity of turkeys to aflatoxin B-1. *Comp. Biochem. Physiol. C Toxicol. Pharmacol.* **132,** 193–201.

Lamba, V., *et al.* (2003). Hepatic CYP2B6 expression: Gender and ethnic differences and relationship to CYP2B6 genotype and CAR (constitutive androstane receptor) expression. *J. Pharmacol. Exp. Ther.* **307,** 906–922.

Lasky, T., and Magder, L. (1997). Hepatocellular carcinoma p53 G>T transversions at codon 249: The fingerprint of aflatoxin exposure? *Environ. Health Perspect.* **105,** 392–397.

Levine, M., *et al.* (1999). Criteria and recommendations for vitamin C intake. *JAMA* **281,** 1415–1423.

Liu, T. Y., *et al.* (1995). Mechanistic study of the inhibition of aflatoxin b1-induced hepatotoxicity by dimethyl 4, 4'-dimethoxy-5, 6, 5', 6'-dimethylenedioxy biphenyl-2, 2'-dicarboxylate. *Cancer Lett.* **89,** 201–205.

Lykkesfeldt, J., *et al.* (1997). Ascorbic acid and dehydroascorbic acid as biomarkers of oxidative stress caused by smoking. *Am. J. Clin. Nutr.* **65,** 959–963.

Mace, K., *et al.* (1997). Aflatoxin B1-induced DNA adduct formation and p53 mutations in CYP450-expressing human liver cell lines. *Carcinogenesis* **18,** 1291–1297.

Mandel, H. G., *et al.* (1992). Effect of dietary-protein level on aflatoxin-B1 actions in the liver of weanling rats. *Carcinogenesis* **13,** 1853–1857.

Marklinder, I., *et al.* (2005). Consumers' ability to discriminate aflatoxin-contaminated Brazil nuts. *Food Addit. Contam.* **22,** 56–64.

Massey, T. E., *et al.* (1995). Biochemical and molecular aspects of mammalian susceptibility to aflatoxin B-1 carcinogenicity. *Proc. Soc. Exp. Biol. Med.* **208,** 213–227.

Massey T. E., *et al.* (2000). Mechanisms of aflatoxin B1 lung tumorigenesis. *Exp. Lung Res.* **26,** 673–683.

Mathews-Roth, M. M., and Krinsky, N. I. (1985). Carotenoid dose level and protection against UV-B induced skin tumors. *Photochem. Photobiol.* **42,** 35–38.

May, J. M., *et al.* (1996). Ascorbate recycling in human erythrocytes: Role of GSH in reducing dehydroascorbate. *Free Radic. Biol. Med.* **20,** 543–551.

May, J. M., *et al.* (1998). Protection and recycling of alpha-tocopherol in human erythrocytes by intracellular ascorbic acid. *Arch. Biochem. Biophys.* **349,** 281–289.

Mcglynn, K. A., *et al.* (1995). Susceptibility to hepatocellular-carcinoma is associated with genetic-variation in the enzymatic detoxification of aflatoxin B-1. *Proc. Natl. Acad. Sci. USA* **92,** 2384–2387.

Moller, P., *et al.* (2004). Vitamin C supplementation decreases oxidative DNA damage in mononuclear blood cells of smokers. *Eur. J. Nutr.* **43,** 267–274.

Mutegi, C. K., *et al.* (2009). Prevalence and factors associated with aflatoxin contamination of peanuts from Western Kenya. *Int. J. Food Microbiol.* **130,** 27–34.

Neldon-Ortiz, D. L., and Qureshi, M. A. (1991). Direct and microsomal activated aflatoxin B1 exposure and its effects on turkey peritoneal macrophage functions in vitro. *Toxicol. Appl. Pharmacol.* **109,** 432–442.

Netke, S. P., *et al.* (1997). Ascorbic acid protects guinea pigs from acute aflatoxin toxicity. *Toxicol. Appl. Pharmacol.* **143,** 429–435.
Newberne, P. M., *et al.* (1979). Effects of dietary-fat on hepatic mixed-function oxidases and hepatocellular carcinoma induced by aflatoxin-B1 in rats. *Cancer Res.* **39,** 3986–3991.
Noguchi, N., *et al.* (2003). Inhibition of THP-1 cell adhesion to endothelial cells by alpha-tocopherol and alpha-tocotrienol is dependent on intracellular concentration of the antioxidants. *Free Radic. Biol. Med.* **34,** 1614–1620.
Nyandieka, H. S., *et al.* (1990). Association of reduction of Afb1-induced liver-tumors by antioxidants with increased activity of microsomal-enzymes. *Indian J. Med. Res. B* **92,** 332–336.
Nyathi, C. B., *et al.* (1993). The effect of diet on aflatoxin-B(1) binding to hepatic macromolecules in rats. *Res. Commun. Chem. Pathol. Pharmacol.* **82,** 199–207.
Odin, A. P. (1997). Vitamins as antimutagens: Advantages and some possible mechanisms of antimutagenic action. *Mutat. Res.* **386,** 39–67.
Pariza, M. W., and Boutwell, R. K. (1987). Historical perspective: Calories and energy expenditure in carcinogenesis. *Am. J. Clin. Nutr.* **45,** 151–156.
Pietri, S., *et al.* (1994). Ascorbyl free radical: A noninvasive marker of oxidative stress in human open-heart surgery. *Free Radic. Biol. Med.* **16,** 523–528.
Pollard, M., and Luckert, P. H. (1985). Tumorigenic effects of direct- and indirect-acting chemical carcinogens in rats on a restricted diet. *J. Natl. Cancer Inst.* **74,** 1347–1349.
Primiano, T., *et al.* (1995). Intermittent dosing with oltipraz: Relationship between chemoprevention of aflatoxin-induced tumorigenesis and induction of glutathione S-transferases. *Cancer Res.* **55,** 4319–4324.
Reddy, L., *et al.* (2006). Aflatoxin B1-induced toxicity in HepG2 cells inhibited by carotenoids: Morphology, apoptosis and DNA damage. *Biol. Chem.* **387,** 87–93.
Sachan, D., and Ayub, M. (1992). Suppression of aflatoxin B1-induced lipid abnormalities and macromolecule-adduct formation by L-carnitine. *J. Environ. Pathol. Toxicol. Oncol.* **11,** 205–210.
Sachan, D. S., and Yatim, A. M. (1991). Modulation of aflatoxin-B1 (Afb1) toxicity by L-carnitine. *FASEB J.* **5,** A712.
Sahaphong, S., *et al.* (1992). Enhanced hepatotoxicity of aflatoxin B1 in the rat by ethanol: Ultrastructural changes. *Toxicol. Lett.* **61,** 89–98.
Saito, K., *et al.* (2007). The lipid-binding SEC14 domain. *Biochim. Biophys. Acta* **1771,** 719–726.
Salem, M. H., *et al.* (2001). Protective role of ascorbic acid to enhance semen quality of rabbits treated with sublethal doses of aflatoxin B(1). *Toxicology* **162,** 209–218.
Sekiyama, B. L., *et al.* (2005). Aflatoxins, ochratoxin a and zearalenone in maize-based food products. *Braz. J. Microbiol.* **36,** 289–294.
Shen, H. M., *et al.* (1994). Aflatoxin B1-induced lipid peroxidation in rat liver. *Toxicol. Appl. Pharmacol.* **127,** 145–150.
Shen, H. M., *et al.* (1995). Aflatoxin B1-induced 8-hydroxydeoxyguanosine formation in rat hepatic DNA. *Carcinogenesis* **16,** 419–422.
Shi, H. L., *et al.* (1999). Comparative study on dynamics of antioxidative action of alpha-tocopheryl hydroquinone, ubiquinol, and alpha-tocopherol, against lipid peroxidation. *Free Radic. Biol. Med.* **27,** 334–346.
Sinha, S. P., and Dharmshila, K. (1994). Vitamin A ameliorates the genotoxicity in mice of aflatoxin B1-containing *Aspergillus flavus* infested food. *Cytobios* **79,** 85–95.
Sontag, T. J., and Parker, R. S. (2007). Comparative influence of major structural features of tocopherols and tocotrienols on kinetics of their omega-oxidation by cellular and microsomal tocopherol-omega -hydroxylase. *J. Lipid Res.* **48,** 1090–1098.
Srivastava, V. P., *et al.* (2001). Aflatoxin M-1 contamination in commercial samples of milk and dairy products in Kuwait. *Food Addit. Contam.* **18,** 993–997.

Tannenbaum, A. (1942). The genesis and growth of tumors. II. Effects of caloric restriction per se. *Cancer Res.* **2,** 460–467.

Toskulkao, C., and Glinsukon, T. (1988). Hepatic lipid-peroxidation and intracellular calcium accumulation in ethanol potentiated aflatoxin-B1 toxicity. *J. Pharmacobio-Dynam.* **11,** 191–197.

Traber, M. G., and Atkinson, J. (2007). Vitamin E, antioxidant and nothing more. *Free Radic. Biol. Med.* **43,** 4–15.

Trail, F., *et al.* (1995). Molecular biology of aflatoxin biosynthesis. *Microbiology* **141**(Pt. 4), 755–765.

Trucksess, M. W., *et al.* (2002). Occurrence of aflatoxins and fumonisins in Incaparina from Guatemala. *Food Addit. Contam.* **19,** 671–675.

Tucker, B. W., and Halver, J. E. (1984). Ascorbate-2-sulfate metabolism in fish. *Nutr. Rev.* **42,** 173–179.

Turrens, J. F. (1991). The potential of antioxidant enzymes as pharmacological agents in vivo. *Xenobiotica* **21,** 1033–1040.

Verma, R. J. (2004). Aflatoxin cause DNA damage. *Int. J. Hum. Genet.* **4,** 231–236.

Verma, R. J., and Nair, A. (2001). Vitamin E ameliorates aflatoxin-induced biochemical changes in the testis of mice. *Asian J. Androl.* **3,** 305–309.

Verma, R. J., and Nair, A. (2002). Effect of aflatoxins on testicular steroidogenesis and amelioration by vitamin E. *Food Chem. Toxicol.* **40,** 669–672.

Wang, J. S., and Groopman, J. D. (1999). DNA damage by mycotoxins. *Mutat. Res., Fundam. Mol. Mech. Mutagen.* **424,** 167–181.

Wang, J., *et al.* (2007). Contamination of aflatoxins in different kinds of foods in China. *Biomed. Environ. Sci.* **20,** 483–487.

Wang, C. J., *et al.* (1991). Modulatory effect of crocetin on aflatoxin B1 cytotoxicity and DNA adduct formation in C3H10T1/2 fibroblast cell. *Cancer Lett.* **56,** 1–10.

Webster, R. P., *et al.* (1996a). Effect of different vitamin a status on carcinogen-induced DNA damage and repair enzymes in rats. *In Vivo* **10,** 113–118.

Webster, R. P., *et al.* (1996b). Modulation of carcinogen-induced DNA damage and repair enzyme activity by dietary riboflavin. *Cancer Lett.* **98,** 129–135.

Wheeler, J. L., *et al.* (2006). In vitro metabolism of aflatoxin B1 with microsomal enzymes in the presence of selected nutrients. *J. Food Sci.* **52,** 1432–1433.

Yu, M. W., *et al.* (1994). Influence of vitamins A, C, and E and beta-carotene on aflatoxin B1 binding to DNA in woodchuck hepatocytes. *Cancer* **73,** 596–604.

Zile, M. H., *et al.* (1986). Effect of moderate vitamin A supplementation and lack of dietary vitamin A on the development of mammary tumors in female rats treated with low carcinogenic dose levels of 7, 12-dimethylbenz(a)anthracene. *Cancer Res.* **46,** 3495–3503.

Zingg, J. M., and Azzi, A. (2004). Non-antioxidant activities of vitamin E. *Curr. Med. Chem.* **11,** 1113–1133.

CHAPTER THIRTEEN

Vitamin D, Vitamin D Receptor, and Cathelicidin in the Treatment of Tuberculosis

P. Selvaraj

Contents

Abstract

Vitamin D plays a major role in bone mineral density and calcium homeostasis. Apart from its classical action, the active form of vitamin D [1,25-dihydroxyvitamin D_3 (1,25$(OH)_2D_3$)] influences the innate and adaptive immune functions through

Department of Immunology, Tuberculosis Research Centre, Indian Council of Medical Research, Chennai, India

Vitamins and Hormones, Volume 86
ISSN 0083-6729, DOI: 10.1016/B978-0-12-386960-9.00013-7

vitamin D receptor (VDR) that are present in various cells of the immune system. Vitamin D deficiencies have been associated with development of tuberculosis (TB) disease, caused by *Mycobacterium tuberculosis*. Vitamin D_3 is shown to enhance macrophage phagocytosis of *M. tuberculosis* and increases the production of antimicrobial peptide cathelicidin and killing of *M. tuberculosis*. During the preantibiotic era, exposure to sunlight and supplementation of vitamin D were the methods of choice for treatment of TB. Vitamin D supplementation showed sputum clearance and radiological improvement and reduction in mortality among human immunodeficiency virus (HIV)-infected patients with TB. VDR gene polymorphisms regulate the immunomodulatory effect of vitamin D_3 and are associated with faster sputum conversion during anti-TB treatment. The emerging evidences regarding immunomodulatory properties of vitamin D_3 have rekindled interest in vitamin D as an adjunct to anti-TB therapy. The current review explains the important potential application of vitamin D in enhancing the innate immunity to TB and the role of VDR gene variants on anti-TB treatment.

I. Introduction

Vitamins (vital amines) are organic compounds that are required in trace amounts in the diet because they cannot be synthesized in sufficient quantities by an organism (Rosenberg, 2007). Vitamins and their metabolites are essential for a large number of physiological processes, fulfilling diverse functions as hormones and antioxidants, as regulators of tissue growth and differentiation, in embryonic development, and in calcium metabolism (Rosenberg, 2007). Vitamin D has received particular attention owing to recent discoveries of its multifaceted interactions with the immune system (Liu *et al.*, 2006, 2007).

Tuberculosis (TB), caused by *Mycobacterium tuberculosis*, remains a major cause of morbidity and mortality around the world (Dye, 2006). The current treatment of TB involves the use of multiple drugs and interruption of the treatment leads to multidrug-resistant TB (WHO report, 2008).

Pharmacologic doses of vitamin D were used to treat TB during the preantibiotic era, but this practice fell out of widespread use with the introduction of effective antituberculous chemotherapy. Interest in this area has recently been rekindled due to emerging evidences regarding the immunomodulatory properties of 1,25-dihydroxyvitamin D_3 (vitamin D_3), an active form of vitamin D, *in vitro*. In this chapter, vitamin D metabolism and the mechanism of action, vitamin D and immunity to TB, vitamin D in TB treatment, and the role of vitamin D receptor (VDR) polymorphisms in treatment response to TB are discussed.

II. Vitamin D Metabolism

Vitamin D_3 (1,25$(OH)_2D_3$), the most physiologically relevant form of vitamin D, is synthesized in the skin from 7-dehydrocholesterol (Holick, 2007), a process which depends on sunlight, specifically ultraviolet B radiation (wavelengths of 270–300 nm). Alternatively, it can be acquired in the diet or in vitamin supplements (Holick, 2007). Vitamin D_3 or cholecalciferol is hydroxylated in the liver into 25-hydroxyvitamin D_3 (25$(OH)D_3$) by 25-hydroxylase. Finally, 25$(OH)D_3$ is hydroxylated by 1α-hydroxylase in the kidney into 1,25-dihydroxyvitamin D_3 (1,25$(OH)_2D_3$),the most physiologically active vitamin D_3 metabolite (Holick, 2007). In addition, vitamin D_3 can also be metabolized by immune cells such as activated T cells, macrophages, and dendritic cells (DCs) (Holick, 2007; Sigmundsdottir *et al.*, 2007). In this manner, the active form of 1,25$(OH)_2D_3$ is concentrated locally in the lymphoid microenvironments that contain physiologically high concentrations of vitamin D_3, thereby increasing its specific action and also limiting potentially undesirable systemic effects, such as hypercalcemia and increased bone resorption (van Etten and Mathieu, 2005). Finally, the enzyme 24-hydroxylase, which is most abundant in the kidney and intestine (Akeno *et al.*, 1997), catabolizes 1,25$(OH)_2D_3$ to its inactive metabolite, calcitroic acid, which is then excreted in the bile.

III. Immunomodulatory Role of Vitamin D

The influence of Vitamin D_3 metabolites on the immune system, particularly of 1,25$(OH)_2D_3$, has been known for more than 20 years (Lemire *et al.*, 1984; Rigby *et al.*, 1984). Under *in vitro* conditions, 1,25 $(OH)_2D_3$ exerts a marked decrease in T-cell proliferation (Rigby *et al.*, 1984), the expression of interleukin-2 (IL-2) (Bhalla *et al.*, 1986) and interferon-γ (IFN-γ) mRNA and protein in T cells (Reichel *et al.*, 1987) and $CD8^+$ T-cell-mediated cytotoxicity (Meehan *et al.*, 1992). The antiproliferative effect has been suggested to be due to the decrease in IL-2 production, and exogenous IL-2 addition partially restores the proliferation (Matsui *et al.*, 1985). These inhibitory effects of 1,25$(OH)_2D_3$ are more pronounced in the memory T-cell compartment (Muller and Bendtzen, 1992), which is concomitant with higher expression of VDR in effector and memory T cells compared with naïve T cells (Veldman *et al.*, 2000). Moreover, 1,25$(OH)_2D_3$ enhances nonspecific T-cell suppressor activity, as measured by the ability of 1,25$(OH)_2D_3$-treated T cells to suppress primary mixed-lymphocyte reactions and cytotoxic T-cell responses (Meehan *et al.*, 1992). The overall effect of 1,25$(OH)_2D_3$ on T cells is to block the induction of T-helper-1 (Th1)-cell cytokines, particularly IFN-γ, while promoting Th2-cell responses by enhancing IL-4 production (van Etten and Mathieu, 2005).

The activity of 1,25$(OH)_2D_3$ on effector T-cell differentiation is further enhanced by its effect on antigen-presenting DCs, in which it suppresses the synthesis of IL-12, a cytokine that promotes Th1-cell responses (Penna and Adorini, 2000). In addition to its inhibitory effects on T cells, 1,25$(OH)_2D_3$ decreases B-cell proliferation, plasma-cell differentiation, and IgG secretion (Chen *et al.*, 2007; Lemire *et al.*, 1984).This suggests that vitamin D_3 influences both cellular and humoral immune functions.

Although 1,25$(OH)_2D_3$ primarily has inhibitory effects on the adaptive immune response, some of its effects on innate immunity are stimulatory. For example, 1,25$(OH)_2D_3$ can stimulate circulating human monocyte proliferation *in vitro* (Ohta *et al.*, 1985) and has been shown to increase the production of both IL-1 and the bactericidal peptide cathelicidin by monocytes and macrophages (Bhalla *et al.*, 1986).

IV. Cathelicidin and Vitamin D

Among the various components of the innate immune system, antimicrobial peptides have a role as effectors and are involved in killing of a broad spectrum of microbes (Bals *et al.*, 1998). One of the best characterized families of antimicrobial peptides is defensins which are small cationic cystine-rich peptides of broad antimicrobial activity (Ganz and Lehrer, 1994). A human homolog of these β-defensins called human β-defensin-1 (hBD-1) has been described (Bensch *et al.*, 1995). Another family of peptide antibiotics that is receiving increased attention is the cathelicidins (Agerberth *et al.*, 1995). The only cathelicidin present in human is hCAP-18, which contains a 30-residue signal region, a 103-residue polypeptide corresponding to the conserved cathelin-like proregion, and the 37-residue peptide LL-37 at the C terminus. LL-37 becomes antimicrobially active on release from the proregion by the action of proteinase 3 (Sorensen *et al.*, 2001).

LL-37 is produced by various cell types including neutrophils, lung epithelial cells, keratinocytes, monocytes, mast cells, and γδ T cells (Agerberth *et al.*, 2000; Di Nardo *et al.*, 2003; Frohm *et al.*, 1997). The synthetic peptide LL-37 is known to have antibiotic activity against a number of gram-negative and gram-positive organisms including *Pseudomonas aeruginosa*, *Salmonella typhimurium*, *Escherichia coli*, *Listeria monocytogenes*, *Staphylococcus epidermidis*, *Staphylococcus aureus* (Bals *et al.*, 1998; Turner *et al.*, 1998).

Apart from antimicrobial activities, host defense peptides have pleiotrophic immunomodulatory activities. LL-37 has been demonstrated to be a chemoattractant for neutrophils, monocytes, and subsets of T cells (De *et al.*, 2000). LL-37 is also shown to induce IL-8, a potent chemokine for neutrophils and monocytes. Moreover, LL-37 also upregulated the chemokine receptors CXCR4, CCR2, and IL-8RB, suggesting that LL-37 is a multifunctional modulator of innate immune response (Scott *et al.*, 2002).

The promoter region of the *hCAP18* gene contains multiple VDR-response elements, and stimulation with 1,25-VitD_3 *ex vivo* enhances hCAP18 expression in keratinocytes, monocytes, and neutrophils (Wang *et al.*, 2004). Further, the 1,25-VitD_3-dependent induction of LL-37 contributes to the microbicidal activity of macrophages against *M. tuberculosis* (Segaert, 2008). The role of 1,25-VitD_3 in the induction of hCAP18 and LL-37 in keratinocytes is brought out during wound healing process, with cytokine TGFβ1 upregulating the expression of the VitD_3-activating enzyme CYP27B1, which subsequently leads to VitD_3 activation and increased levels of hCAP18 and LL-37 in the wounded tissue (Schauber *et al.*, 2007). Oral intake of vitamin D_3 in rickets patients for 4 weeks significantly increased the hCAP18 expression in neutrophils compared to age-matched healthy controls without vitamin D_3, indicating the potential role of vitamin D_3 as a regulator of the innate immune response (Misawa *et al.*, 2009). The hormonal form of vitamin D_3 induced the expression of pro-LL-37 in isolated neutrophil progenitors and in Epstein–Barr virus-transformed B cells from patients with severe congenital neutropenia (Karlsson *et al.*, 2008). 1,25$(OH)_2D_3$ induces expression of the human cathelicidin antimicrobial peptide (*CAMP*) gene in acute myeloid leukemia (AML), immortalized keratinocyte, and colon cancer cell lines as well as normal human bone marrow (BM)-derived macrophages and fresh BM cells from two normal individuals and one AML patient (Gombart *et al.*, 2005). Moreover, 1,25$(OH)_2D_3$ enhances the induction of antimicrobial proteins and secretion of antimicrobial activity against pathogens including *P. aeruginosa*, revealing the potential role of its analogues in the treatment of opportunistic infections (Wang *et al.*, 2004).

V. Vitamin D Receptor

Vitamin D_3 exerts its action through VDR which is a ligand-dependent transcription factor belonging to the superfamily of steroid/thyroid hormone receptors (Pinette *et al.*, 2003). The gene encoding the VDR is located on chromosome 12cen-ql2, contains 11 exons, and spans approximately 75 kilo base (kb) of genomic DNA (Miyamoto *et al.*, 1997; Taymans *et al.*, 1999). Macrophages and DCs constitutively express VDR, whereas its expression in T cells is upregulated following activation (Veldman *et al.*, 2000). In monocytes and macrophages, 1,25$(OH)_2D_3$ enhances the expression of VDR and the cytochrome P450 protein CYP27B1 through several toll-like receptors (TLRs) which are associated with innate immunity (Liu *et al.*, 2006).

In the absence of its ligand vitamin D, VDR is present in the cytoplasm and upon ligand binding it translocates to the nucleus and exerts its actions. Retinoid X receptor (RXR), a nuclear receptor for 9-*cis* retinoic acid, is an obligate partner of VDR in mediating $1{,}25(OH)_2D_3$ action (Kim *et al.*, 2005; Kliewer *et al.*, 1992). The VDR protein is modular in nature, and it can be functionally divided into three regions with well-characterized functions. The NH_2-terminal region contains a ligand-independent transactivation function-1 (AF-1). The central region contains the DNA-binding domain consisting of two C2–C2 type zinc fingers, which target the receptor to vitamin D response elements (VDREs), and the C-terminal region contains a multifunctional domain harboring the ligand-binding domain, the RXR heterodimerization motif, and a ligand-dependent transactivation function (AF-2). Upon ligand binding, conformational change occurs leading to an enhancement of VDR–RXR heterodimer formation (Cheskis and Freedman, 1994).

A. VDR and transcription

The VDR–RXR heterodimer binds to VDREs located in the promoter regions of target genes. This binding leads to the recruitment of additional coregulatory proteins necessary for chromatin modification and transcriptional activation (Mckenna *et al.*, 1999). The successful formation of these multiprotein complexes containing VDR and RXR, histone-modifying enzymes, and regulatory components of the basal transcriptional apparatus is instrumental to changes in $1{,}25(OH)_2D_3$-mediated gene transcription (Kim *et al.*, 2005). VDR can either positively or negatively regulate the expression of certain genes by binding to the VDREs present in their promoter regions (Dong *et al.*, 2003; Griffin *et al.*, 2007; Pinette *et al.*, 2003) or inhibit the expression of some genes by antagonizing the action of certain transcription factors, such as nuclear factor (NF)-AT and NF-κB (Alroy *et al.*, 1995; Harant *et al.*, 1997).

B. VDR gene polymorphisms

The *VDR* gene contains more than 25 known polymorphisms, although more than 100 are expected based on the observed genome-wide analysis. Single nucleotide changes producing amino acid substitutions in the DNA and ligand-binding domains are the predominant type of mutations found in the *VDR* gene (Malloy *et al.*, 1997).

Three adjacent 3′-untranslated region (UTR) polymorphisms for *Bsm*I, *Apa*I, and *Taq*I are the most frequently studied VDR gene polymorphisms.

*Bsm*I (A/G) and *Apa*I (G/T) restriction site polymorphisms occur in the intron separating exons VIII and IX and do not affect any splicing site or transcription factor binding site (Faraco *et al.*, 1989; Morrison *et al.*, 1992). A T/C nucleotide substitution (ATT to ATC) leading to a synonymous change at codon 352 (isoleucine) in exon IX has also been described (Hustmyer *et al.*, 1993) and is detected by the restriction enzyme *Taq*I. Although the *Taq*I site is present in the coding region of *VDR* gene, it does not alter the amino acid sequence of the encoded protein. The less frequent allele of *Taq*I site designated as t has been associated with higher levels of VDR mRNA expression (Morrison *et al.*, 1994).

The presence of a T/C transition polymorphism (ATG to ACG) at the first of two potential translation initiation sites in exon II (Baker *et al.*, 1988) has been defined using the *Fok*I restriction endonuclease (Gross *et al.*, 1996). The Cdx-2 polymorphism (1e-G-1739A) is a G to A variation in a Cdx (caudal-related homeodomain protein) binding site in the 1e promoter region, and this site is suggested to play an important role in intestinal-specific transcription of the *VDR* gene, thereby influencing vitamin D-regulated calcium absorption (Arai *et al.*, 2001). A1012G polymorphism is located upstream of transcription start site in 1A promoter region of the *VDR* gene. The A allele of A1012G polymorphism allows expression of a putative binding site in the VDR promoter for GATA-3, a transcription factor which directs polarization of naïve T cells to Th2 cells (Halsall *et al.*, 2004). Several studies have associated VDR gene polymorphisms with susceptibility or resistance to various infectious and noninfectious diseases (Hill, 1998, 2001).

VI. Tuberculosis

M. tuberculosis, the causative organism for the development of TB disease, is a facultative intracellular bacterial parasite that can spread by inhalation of a minimal dose (one to five bacilli). The first immune defense response to *M. tuberculosis* infection begins with the innate immune system, involving the epithelial cells and alveolar macrophages (AM) in the airways. This initial response is strengthened by recruitment of neutrophils, which are among the first cells to arrive at the site of infection (Cosma *et al.*, 2003; Rivas-Santiago *et al.*, 2008). Macrophages phagocytize the bacilli, but the normal destruction of bacilli by macrophages can be interrupted by the defense mechanisms of the mycobacteria. One of the potential pathways through which the mycobacteria prevent their own destruction involves glycosylated phosphatidylinositol lipoarabinomannan, a compound of the mycobacterial cell membrane. Lipoarabinomannan is translocated to the phagosome wall, interrupting the normal maturation of the phagosome and its further fusion with the lysosome (Cosma *et al.*, 2003; Hmama *et al.*, 2004).

Thus protected from host defenses, the viable mycobacteria reproduce inside the macrophages and can also migrate to other tissues. However, a localized inflammatory response promotes the recruitment of T lymphocytes, which leads to the formation of a granuloma (Houben *et al.*, 2006) to wall off the spread of the infection. The TB infection is usually contained inside the granuloma, and the infection may remain dormant, or latent, for many years. However, immunodeficiency secondary to an event such as coinfection with human immunodeficiency virus (HIV) or malnutrition can lead to activation of the disease (Martineau *et al.*, 2007a; Russell, 2001).

Although TB is a highly infective disease, only 1 in 10 infected persons may become sick with active TB (WHO report, 2008). The susceptibility to active disease can be influenced by environmental and host genetic factors or by gene–environment interactions. Host genetic factors may influence not only the host susceptibility to active TB but also host response to treatment (Hill, 2006).

A. Vitamin D and immunity to TB

$1,25(OH)_2D_3$ induces antimycobacterial activity *in vitro* in both monocytes/macrophages (Crowle *et al.*, 1987; Rook *et al.*, 1986) and the expression of cathelicidin in macrophages (Selvaraj *et al.*, 2009). The biological mechanisms through which vitamin D modulates the immune system to fight against *M. tuberculosis* infection are still under study (Kaufmann, 2006; Zasloff, 2006). $1,25(OH)_2D_3$ increases the phagocytic potential of macrophages (Selvaraj *et al.*, 2004), promotes phagolysosome fusion via phosphoinositide 3-kinase signaling pathway, and rescues from inhibition of phagolysosome fusion in *Mycobacterium*-infected macrophages (Hmama *et al.*, 2004). $1,25(OH)_2D_3$ also modulates immune responses by binding nuclear VDR, where it upregulates protective innate host responses (including induction of nitric oxide synthase (Rockett *et al.*, 1998) and cathelicidin (Liu *et al.*, 2006)) and downregulates IFN-γ gene expression by downregulating activity of the IFN-γ promoter (Cippitelli and Santoni, 1998). Vitamin D_3 differentially modulates production of cytokines in response to *M. tuberculosis* antigens by predominantly suppressing IL-12p40 and IFN-γ production in a dose-dependent manner and restricting acquired immune response against TB by regulating cytokine production (Vidyarani *et al.*, 2007). Moreover, $1,25(OH)_2D_3$ suppresses the intracellular expression of IFN-γ and TNF-α by $CD3^+CD4^+$ and $CD3^+CD8^+$ T cells (Prabhu Anand *et al.*, 2009).

B. Vitamin D deficiency and TB

Several recent studies in different populations have associated a deficiency in vitamin D with increased risk of TB (Gibney *et al.*, 2008; Sasidharan *et al.*, 2002; Ustianowski *et al.*, 2005). A meta-analysis study revealed that vitamin D levels were lower in persons with TB than in controls (Nnoaham and Clarke, 2008). An association study determined that the Gc2/Gc2 genotype of vitamin D-binding protein with low vitamin D serum concentration was a susceptibility factor for active TB in Gujarati Asian patients from London (Martineau *et al.*, 2009a). However, no association was detected in patients from Brazil or South Africa, who were less likely to be vitamin D deficient (Martineau *et al.*, 2009a). Moreover, a study carried out in south Indian population also revealed an increased plasma level of $1,25(OH)_2D_3$ in PTB patients, suggesting no association with vitamin D deficiency in population living in a tropical country where exposure to sunlight is very frequent than in Western countries (Selvaraj *et al.*, 2009).

C. Vitamin D and cathelicidin in TB

Information on the role of antimicrobial peptides in the immunity against TB is scanty. A study has shown that mycobacterial infection induced the production of cathelicidin in A549 epithelial cells, AM, neutrophils, and monocyte-derived macrophages (MDM) with AM being the most efficient producer. However, peptide expression was not detectable in tuberculous granulomas suggesting that LL-37 participates only during early infection (Rivas-Santiago *et al.*, 2008). It has been shown that LL-37 can be induced in MDM by stimulation of TLRs TLR-2, TLR-4, and TLR-9 by *M. tuberculosis* components (Rivas-Santiago *et al.*, 2008).

Although the antimicrobial effects of vitamin D have been previously documented and reduced vitamin D status is known to be associated with susceptibility to *M. tuberculosis* infection, only recently it was demonstrated that TLR stimulation in human macrophages induces the enzyme that catalyzes conversion of $25(OH)D_3$ to active $1,25(OH)_2D_3$ and the expression of VDR and relevant downstream targets of VDR including cathelicidin and play a role as a key link between TLR activation and antibacterial responses in innate immunity (Liu *et al.*, 2006). Though $1,25(OH)_2D_3$ downregulates Th1 cytokine response, it strongly upregulated the cathelicidin gene, *hCAP18*. Intracellular hCAP18 protein was also increased by $1,25(OH)_2D_3$ and synthetic LL-37, the antimicrobial peptide derived from hCAP18, reduced the growth of *M. tuberculosis* directly up to 75% under *in vitro* condition. These findings indicate that vitamin D mediates protection against TB by "nonclassical" mechanisms, including the induction of antimicrobial peptide such as cathelicidin (Martineau *et al.*, 2007b).

Autophagy plays an important role in maintaining cellular homeostasis by degrading the damaged cytosolic components in the cell. Autophagy and vitamin D_3-mediated innate immunity have been shown to confer protection against infection with *M. tuberculosis*. Vitamin D induces autophagy-related genes *Beclin-1* and *Atg5* via cathelicidin in human monocytes. Vitamin D_3 also induced the colocalization of mycobacterial phagosomes with autophagosomes in human macrophages in a cathelicidin-dependent manner. This indicates that human cathelicidin, a protein that has direct antimicrobial activity, also serves as a mediator of vitamin D_3-induced autophagy (Yuk *et al.*, 2009).

VII. Vitamin D and Treatment of TB

A. Heliotherapy (sunlight treatment)

In 1855, Rikli, a Swiss doctor, opened a thermal treatment station in Slovenia. In 1903, Finsen was awarded the Nobel Prize for Medicine for successful treatment of cutaneous TB (lupus vulgaris) with ultraviolet (UV) radiation, and this marked the start of modern phototherapy. Rollier from Switzerland opened a hospital to treat TB by using graded sun exposure in 1903. In 1922, popularity of sunlight treatment was increased and "Committee on Sunlight" and Light Department was established in the UK at London Hospital to widespread adoption of sun exposure practices (Roelandts, 2002).

B. Cod liver oil

Cod liver oil, rich in vitamin D, was first advocated for the treatment of TB in 1770, and it was widely used for this purpose in the nineteenth century. In 1833, Henkel, a German doctor, reported on the successful use of cod liver oil in the treatment of TB. In 1841, Bennett, a Scottish physician, published medical uses of cod liver oil, including TB. Five cases report of improvement in TB symptoms, but two relapsed after stopping cod liver oil. In 1849, Williams reported that "the pure fresh oil from the liver of the cod is more beneficial in the treatment of TB." The hospital for consumption and diseases of the chest in London published outcomes of cod liver oil in TB treatment. The outcome was 18% disease arrested, 63% improved, and 19% unchanged. In 1855, Woods from Philadelphia, USA, attributed the 19% fall in deaths due to the use of cod liver oil for TB between 1847 and 1852 (Grad, 2004).

C. Vitamin D trials in TB

Charpy pioneered the use of pharmacological doses of vitamin D_2 to treat cutaneous TB. The regime consisted of oral doses of 600,000 international units (IU) vitamin D_2 administered weekly for the first 3 months, fortnightly for the next 3 months; he subsequently adopted a more intensive regime: 600,000 IU vitamin D_2 three times per week for the first week, twice a week for the next 3 weeks, then weekly for the next 4 months

(Charpy, 1950). No toxic symptoms were reported with either regime (Dowling and Prosser Thomas, 1946). Two phases of clinical response were described: in the initial 2–3 weeks cutaneous lesions became inflamed; patients with coexisting tuberculous cervical adenitis sometimes developed exacerbation of lymphadenopathy during this period. In the second phase, beginning at 5–6 weeks, cutaneous lesions began to fibrose (Fielding and Maloney, 1951). In 1952, one case series study administered 200,000 IU of D_2 three times per week to 35 patients with pulmonary TB and cutaneous TB. They observed good response in 19 patients out of 35. Four individuals developed hypercalcemia (Trautwein and Stein, 1952). In 1967, another study reported rapid liquefaction of caseating necrosis and decreased fibrotic sequelae in pulmonary TB patients who had undergone 600,000 IU D_2 every 10 days for up to 4 months (Brincourt, 1967). The repeated oral supplementation with 15 mg (600,000 IU) of vitamin D_2 as supplementary treatment to antibiotics in 150 patients with no control group resulted effect on dissolving cavities (Brincourt, 1969). In an Egyptian study, 24 children received vitamin D at 1000 and 10,000 IU/day and showed more evident clinical and radiographic improvement (Morcos *et al.*, 1998). In Tanzanian study, multivitamin supplement including vitamin D in a randomized clinical trial reported 50% reduction in mortality among HIV-infected patients with TB (Range *et al.*, 2006). Another trial of vitamin D supplementation in Indonesian pulmonary TB patients suggested more rapid sputum clearance and radiological improvement, but the trial was small, the process of randomization was not described, and the safety profile including calcium levels was not assessed (Nursyam *et al.*, 2006).

Martineau *et al.* (2007a) reviewed three randomized controlled trials (RCTs) and 10 prospective case series studies in which vitamin D was administered to patients with pulmonary TB. The impact of vitamin D supplementation on TB outcome could not be assessed in the included studies, most studies were conducted in the 1950s. The trials were identified as being of poor quality and used ergocalciferol (vitamin D_2), which is less efficacious than cholecalciferol (vitamin D_3) (Armas *et al.*, 2004). In another study, patients received 100,000 IU of cholecalciferol or placebo during inclusion, and this was repeated 5–8 months after inclusion but no improvement was observed due to insufficient dose (Wejse *et al.*, 2009). A study conducted in multiethnic cohort of TB patients, a single oral dose of 2.5 mg vitamin D_2, corrected hypovitaminosis D at 1 week postdose and induced a 109.5 nmol/l mean increase in their serum 25(OH)D concentration. No patient receiving vitamin D_2 experienced hypercalcemia. The results revealed that a single oral dose of 2.5 mg vitamin D_2 corrects hypovitaminosis D at 1 week but not at 8 weeks postdose in TB patients (Martineau *et al.*, 2009b).

Some of the epidemiological studies (Nnoaham and Clarke, 2008), but not all (Gibney *et al.*, 2008), suggest that a fall in serum vitamin D leads to activation of latent TB. If this is the case, then an important potential application for vitamin D is as an adjunctive therapy in latently infected individuals to prevent TB reactivation. Vitamin D supplementation in latently infected TB patients demonstrated immunological improvement, compared to vitamin D-supplemented healthy people and controls, in functional whole blood assay (BCG-lux assay), which measures the ability of whole blood to restrict luminescence, and thus growth, of recombinant reporter mycobacteria *in vitro* (Martineau *et al.*, 2007c).

D. Vitamin D and hypercalcemia

Hypercalcemia has been observed in patients with active TB during the early phases of treatment (Sharma, 2000). Vitamin D toxicity was observed that there can be an abnormal hypercalcemic response to vitamin D administered with antitubercular therapy, which led to a decline in vitamin D therapy (Narang *et al.*, 1984). The possibility of hypercalcemia would necessitate careful vitamin D dose selection and monitoring and indeed could limit the potential of vitamin D as an adjunctive therapy. The use of vitamin D_3 analogues or combination therapy with bisphosphonates has been proposed to exploit the immunomodulatory properties of vitamin D while avoiding possible hypercalcemia and increased bone turnover (van Etten and Mathieu, 2005).

E. VDR gene polymorphisms and susceptibility to TB

Several association studies on VDR gene polymorphisms with TB in various populations (Yim and Selvaraj, 2010) revealed a differential susceptibility or resistance to TB. This may be due to different ethnicity, gene–environment interaction, and variation in environmental factors between geographically separated areas. However, a meta-analysis study revealed that *FokI* ff and *BsmI* bb genotypes are associated with susceptibility to TB in Asians but not in Africans and South Americans (Gao *et al.*, 2010).

F. VDR gene polymorphisms and treatment response

The *FokI* and *TaqI* VDR gene polymorphisms are shown to be associated with susceptibility to TB and faster sputum conversion time following anti-TB treatment among inhabitants of an area in the outskirts of Lima, Peru, where the incidence of TB is very high (Roth *et al.,* 2004). Sputum mycobacterial culture and auramine stain conversions were significantly faster among participants with the *FokI* FF genotype compared to participants with the non-FF genotypes and *Taq*I Tt genotype compared to patients with TT genotype (Roth *et al.,* 2004).

A cohort of pulmonary TB patients in a South African admixed population was investigated to determine whether VDR gene polymorphisms *FokI*, *ApaI*, and *TaqI* are associated with TB susceptibility or time to sputum conversion, and to investigate other clinical and demographic factors affecting the rate of response to treatment (Babb *et al.*, 2007). During treatment, a faster smear conversion was observed with VDR genotypes *ApaI* AA and *TaqI* TT and Tt as compared to the *ApaI* aa and *TaqI* tt VDR genotypes, respectively. For the categorization between "fast respondents" and "slow respondents," there was a significant trend to a faster smear conversion in those with a VDR *FokI* f allele and for a faster culture conversion in patients with the *ApaI* A allele. The results suggested that the time taken for an individual to convert to sputum negativity while on anti-TB therapy can be independently predicted by the VDR genotype (Babb *et al.*, 2007). Further studies on the association between VDR polymorphisms and response to TB treatment will enlighten the role of VDR gene polymorphisms and response to anti-TB treatment.

VIII. Conclusion

The importance of vitamin D in the treatment of TB was emphasized during the preantibiotic era, and exposure to sunlight and supplementation of vitamin D were useful. Various clinical trials with vitamin D were attempted to find out the suitability of vitamin D as an adjunctive therapy for TB or latent TB, and the impact was sputum clearance of *M. tuberculosis,* clinical and radiological improvement in patients with TB. Vitamin D exerts good treatment response in some studies, while no response was observed in some other studies. Further, though vitamin D deficiency is associated with TB susceptibility and a fall in serum vitamin D leads to activation of latent TB, few studies reveal that some patients are less likely to be vitamin D deficient. Moreover, the active metabolites of vitamin D enhance the innate immunity by upregulating the production of the antimicrobial peptide cathelicidin in normal subjects and in patients with vitamin D deficiency. However, in patients with higher vitamin D level and hypercalcemic conditions, supplementation of vitamin D may not have any significant effect on the induction of cathelicidin. Further, VDR gene polymorphisms while associated with faster sputum conversion during anti-TB treatment in patients with TB, the effect of vitamin D on the sputum conversion may be altered by differential expression of VDR. Though vitamin D could be a potential immunomodulatory agent for clinical use, the above issues as well as vitamin D-induced hypercalcemia should be kept in mind while designing prospective clinical trials with optimal vitamin D supplementation which may adjuvant the TB treatment.

ACKNOWLEDGMENTS

The author thanks Mr. M. Harishankar and Mr. Brijendra Singh (doctoral students of Dr. P. Selvaraj), Tuberculosis Research Centre, Chennai, India, for their help in preparing this chapter.

REFERENCES

Agerberth, B., Gunne, H., Odeberg, J., Kogner, P., Boman, H. G., and Gudmundsson, G. H. (1995). FALL-39, a putative human peptide antibiotic, is cysteine-free and expressed in bone marrow and testis. *Proc. Natl. Acad. Sci. USA* **92,** 195–199.

Agerberth, B., Charo, J., Werr, J., Olsson, B., Idali, F., Lindbom, L., Kiessling, R., Jornvall, H., Wigzell, H., and Gudmundsson, G. H. (2000). The human antimicrobial and chemotactic peptides LL-37 and alpha-defensins are expressed by specific lymphocyte and monocyte populations. *Blood* **96,** 3086–3093.

Akeno, N., Saikatsu, S., Kawane, T., and Horiuchi, N. (1997). Mouse vitamin D-24-hydroxylase: Molecular cloning, tissue distribution, and transcriptional regulation by 1alpha,25-dihydroxyvitamin D3. *Endocrinology* **138,** 2233–2240.

Alroy, I., Towers, T. L., and Freedman, L. P. (1995). Transcriptional repression of the interleukin-2 gene by vitamin D3: Direct inhibition of NFATp/AP-1 complex formation by a nuclear hormone receptor. *Mol. Cell. Biol.* **15,** 5789–5799.

Arai, H., Miyamoto, K. I., Yoshida, M., Yamamoto, H., Taketani, Y., Morita, K., Kubota, M., Yoshida, S., Ikeda, M., Watabe, F., Kanemasa, Y., and Takeda, E. (2001). The polymorphism in the caudal-related homeodomain protein Cdx-2 binding element in the human vitamin D receptor gene. *J. Bone Miner. Res.* **16,** 1256–1264.

Armas, L. A., Hollis, B. W., and Heaney, R. P. (2004). Vitamin D2 is much less effective than vitamin D3 in humans. *J. Clin. Endocrinol. Metab.* **89,** 5387–5391.

Babb, C., van der Merwe, L., Beyers, N., Pheiffer, C., Walzl, G., Duncan, K., van Helden, P., and Hoal, E. G. (2007). Vitamin D receptor gene polymorphisms and sputum conversion time in pulmonary tuberculosis patients. *Tuberculosis (Edinb)* **87,** 295–302.

Baker, A. R., McDonnell, D. P., Hughes, M., Crisp, T. M., Mangelsdorf, D. J., Haussler, M. R., Pike, J. W., Shine, J., and O'Malley, B. W. (1988). Cloning and expression of full-length cDNA encoding human vitamin D receptor. *Proc. Natl. Acad. Sci. USA* **85,** 3294–3298.

Bals, R., Wang, X., Zasloff, M., and Wilson, J. M. (1998). The peptide antibiotic LL-37/hCAP-18 is expressed in epithelia of the human lung where it has broad antimicrobial activity at the airway surface. *Proc. Natl. Acad. Sci. USA* **95,** 9541–9546.

Bensch, K. W., Raida, M., Magert, H. J., Schulz-Knappe, P., and Forssmann, W. G. (1995). hBD-1: A novel beta-defensin from human plasma. *FEBS Lett.* **368,** 331–335.

Bhalla, A. K., Amento, E. P., and Krane, S. M. (1986). Differential effects of 1,25-dihydroxyvitamin D3 on human lymphocytes and monocyte/macrophages: Inhibition of interleukin-2 and augmentation of interleukin-1 production. *Cell. Immunol.* **98,** 311–322.

Brincourt, J. (1967). Does calciferol have a liquifying action on caseum? *Poumon Coeur* **23,** 841–851.

Brincourt, J. (1969). Liquefying effect on suppurations of an oral dose of calciferol. *Presse Méd.* **77,** 467–470.

Charpy, J. (1950). Aspects of vitamin and functional substance therapy in dermatology. *Bull. Méd.* **64,** 555–559.

Chen, S., Sims, G. P., Chen, X. X., Gu, Y. Y., Chen, S., and Lipsky, P. E. (2007). Modulatory effects of 1,25-dihydroxyvitamin D3 on human B cell differentiation. *J. Immunol.* **179,** 1634–1647.

Cheskis, B., and Freedman, L. P. (1994). Ligand modulates the conversion of DNA-bound vitamin D3 receptor (VDR) homodimers into VDR-retinoid X receptor heterodimers. *Mol. Cell. Biol.* **14,** 3329–3338.

Cippitelli, M., and Santoni, A. (1998). Vitamin D3: A transcriptional modulator of the interferon-gamma gene. *Eur. J. Immunol.* **28,** 3017–3030.

Cosma, C. L., Sherman, D. R., and Ramakrishnan, L. (2003). The secret lives of the pathogenic mycobacteria. *Annu. Rev. Microbiol.* **57,** 641–676.

Crowle, A. J., Ross, E. J., and May, M. H. (1987). Inhibition by 1,25(OH)2-vitamin D3 of the multiplication of virulent tubercle bacilli in cultured human macrophages. *Infect. Immun.* **55,** 2945–2950.

De, Y., Chen, Q., Schmidt, A. P., Anderson, G. M., Wang, J. M., Wooters, J., Oppenheim, J. J., and Chertov, O. (2000). LL-37, the neutrophil granule- and epithelial cell-derived cathelicidin, utilizes formyl peptide receptor-like 1 (FPRL1) as a receptor to chemoattract human peripheral blood neutrophils, monocytes, and T cells. *J. Exp. Med.* **192,** 1069–1074.

Di Nardo, A., Vitiello, A., and Gallo, R. L. (2003). Cutting edge: Mast cell antimicrobial activity is mediated by expression of cathelicidin antimicrobial peptide. *J. Immunol.* **170,** 2274–2278.

Dong, X., Craig, T., Xing, N., Bachman, L. A., Paya, C. V., Weih, F., McKean, D. J., Kumar, R., and Griffin, M. D. (2003). Direct transcriptional regulation of RelB by 1alpha,25-dihydroxyvitamin D3 and its analogs: Physiologic and therapeutic implications for dendritic cell function. *J. Biol. Chem.* **278,** 49378–49385.

Dowling, G. B., and Prosser Thomas, E. W. (1946). Treatment of lupus vulgaris with calciferol. *Lancet* **1,** 919–922.

Dye, C. (2006). Global epidemiology of tuberculosis. *Lancet* **367,** 938–940.

Faraco, J. H., Morrison, N. A., Baker, A., Shine, J., and Frossard, P. M. (1989). ApaI dimorphism at the human vitamin D receptor gene locus. *Nucleic Acids Res.* **17,** 2150.

Fielding, J., and Maloney, J. J. (1951). Calciferol, streptomycin, and para-aminosalicylic acid in pulmonary tuberculosis. *Lancet* **2,** 614–617.

Frohm, M., Agerberth, B., Ahangari, G., Stahle-Backdahl, M., Liden, S., Wigzell, H., and Gudmundsson, G. H. (1997). The expression of the gene coding for the antibacterial peptide LL-37 is induced in human keratinocytes during inflammatory disorders. *J. Biol. Chem.* **272,** 15258–15263.

Ganz, T., and Lehrer, R. I. (1994). Defensins. *Curr. Opin. Immunol.* **6,** 584–589.

Gao, L., Tao, Y., Zhang, L., and Jin, Q. (2010). Vitamin D receptor genetic polymorphisms and tuberculosis: Updated systematic review and meta-analysis. *Int. J. Tuberc. Lung Dis.* **14,** 15–23.

Gibney, K. B., MacGregor, L., Leder, K., Torresi, J., Marshall, C., Ebeling, P. R., and Biggs, B. A. (2008). Vitamin D deficiency is associated with tuberculosis and latent tuberculosis infection in immigrants from sub-Saharan Africa. *Clin. Infect. Dis.* **46,** 443–446.

Gombart, A. F., Borregaard, N., and Koeffler, H. P. (2005). Human cathelicidin antimicrobial peptide (CAMP) gene is a direct target of the vitamin D receptor and is strongly up-regulated in myeloid cells by 1,25-dihydroxyvitamin D3. *FASEB J.* **19,** 1067–1077.

Grad, R. (2004). Cod and the consumptive: A brief history of cod-liver oil in the treatment of pulmonary tuberculosis. *Pharm. Hist.* **46,** 106–120.

Griffin, M. D., Dong, X., and Kumar, R. (2007). Vitamin D receptor-mediated suppression of RelB in antigen presenting cells: A paradigm for ligand-augmented negative transcriptional regulation. *Arch. Biochem. Biophys.* **460,** 218–226.

Gross, C., Eccleshall, T. R., Malloy, P. J., Villa, M. L., Marcus, R., and Feldman, D. (1996). The presence of a polymorphism at the translation initiation site of the vitamin D receptor gene is associated with low bone mineral density in postmenopausal Mexican-American women. *J. Bone Miner. Res.* **11,** 1850–1855.

Halsall, J. A., Osborne, J. E., Potter, L., Pringle, J. H., and Hutchinson, P. E. (2004). A novel polymorphism in the 1A promoter region of the vitamin D receptor is associated with altered susceptibility and prognosis in malignant melanoma. *Br. J. Cancer* **91,** 765–770.

Harant, H., Andrew, P. J., Reddy, G. S., Foglar, E., and Lindley, I. J. (1997). 1alpha,25-Dihydroxyvitamin D3 and a variety of its natural metabolites transcriptionally repress nuclear-factor-kappaB-mediated interleukin-8 gene expression. *Eur. J. Biochem.* **250,** 63–71.

Hill, A. V. (1998). The immunogenetics of human infectious diseases. *Annu. Rev. Immunol.* **16,** 593–617.

Hill, A. V. (2001). Immunogenetics and genomics. *Lancet* **357,** 2037–2041.

Hill, A. V. (2006). Aspects of genetic susceptibility to human infectious diseases. *Annu. Rev. Genet.* **40,** 469–486.

Hmama, Z., Sendide, K., Talal, A., Garcia, R., Dobos, K., and Reiner, N. E. (2004). Quantitative analysis of phagolysosome fusion in intact cells: Inhibition by mycobacterial lipoarabinomannan and rescue by an 1alpha,25-dihydroxyvitamin D3-phosphoinositide 3-kinase pathway. *J. Cell Sci.* **117,** 2131–2140.

Holick, M. F. (2007). Vitamin D deficiency. *N. Engl. J. Med.* **357,** 266–281.

Houben, E. N., Nguyen, L., and Pieters, J. (2006). Interaction of pathogenic mycobacteria with the host immune system. *Curr. Opin. Microbiol.* **9,** 76–85.

Hustmyer, F. G., DeLuca, H. F., and Peacock, M. (1993). ApaI, BsmI, EcoRV and TaqI polymorphisms at the human vitamin D receptor gene locus in Caucasians, blacks and Asians. *Hum. Mol. Genet.* **2,** 487.

Karlsson, J., Carlsson, G., Larne, O., Andersson, M., and Putsep, K. (2008). Vitamin D3 induces pro-LL-37 expression in myeloid precursors from patients with severe congenital neutropenia. *J. Leukoc. Biol.* **84,** 1279–1286.

Kaufmann, S. H. (2006). Tuberculosis: Back on the immunologists' agenda. *Immunity* **24,** 351–357.

Kim, S., Shevde, N. K., and Pike, J. W. (2005). 1,25-Dihydroxyvitamin D3 stimulates cyclic vitamin D receptor/retinoid X receptor DNA-binding, co-activator recruitment, and histone acetylation in intact osteoblasts. *J. Bone Miner. Res.* **20,** 305–317.

Kliewer, S. A., Umesono, K., Mangelsdorf, D. J., and Evans, R. M. (1992). Retinoid X receptor interacts with nuclear receptors in retinoic acid, thyroid hormone and vitamin D3 signalling. *Nature* **355,** 446–449.

Lemire, J. M., Adams, J. S., Sakai, R., and Jordan, S. C. (1984). 1 alpha,25-Dihydroxyvitamin D3 suppresses proliferation and immunoglobulin production by normal human peripheral blood mononuclear cells. *J. Clin. Invest.* **74,** 657–661.

Liu, P. T., Stenger, S., Li, H., Wenzel, L., Tan, B. H., Krutzik, S. R., Ochoa, M. T., Schauber, J., Wu, K., Meinken, C., Kamen, D. L., Wagner, M., *et al.* (2006). Toll-like receptor triggering of a vitamin D-mediated human antimicrobial response. *Science* **311,** 1770–1773.

Liu, P. T., Stenger, S., Tang, D. H., and Modlin, R. L. (2007). Cutting edge: Vitamin D-mediated human antimicrobial activity against *Mycobacterium tuberculosis* is dependent on the induction of cathelicidin. *J. Immunol.* **179,** 2060–2063.

Malloy, P. J., Eccleshall, T. R., Gross, C., Van Maldergem, L., Bouillon, R., and Feldman, D. (1997). Hereditary vitamin D resistant rickets caused by a novel mutation in the vitamin D receptor that results in decreased affinity for hormone and cellular hyporesponsiveness. *J. Clin. Invest.* **99,** 297–304.

Martineau, A. R., Honecker, F. U., Wilkinson, R. J., and Griffiths, C. J. (2007a). Vitamin D in the treatment of pulmonary tuberculosis. *J. Steroid Biochem. Mol. Biol.* **103,** 793–798.

Martineau, A. R., Wilkinson, K. A., Newton, S. M., Floto, R. A., Norman, A. W., Skolimowska, K., Davidson, R. N., Sorensen, O. E., Kampmann, B., Griffiths, C. J., and Wilkinson, R. J. (2007b). IFN-gamma- and TNF-independent vitamin D-inducible human suppression of mycobacteria: The role of cathelicidin LL-37. *J. Immunol.* **178,** 7190–7198.

Martineau, A. R., Wilkinson, R. J., Wilkinson, K. A., Newton, S. M., Kampmann, B., Hall, B. M., Packe, G. E., Davidson, R. N., Eldridge, S. M., Maunsell, Z. J., Rainbow, S. J., Berry, J. L., *et al.* (2007c). A single dose of vitamin D enhances immunity to mycobacteria. *Am. J. Respir. Crit. Care Med.* **176,** 208–213.

Martineau, A. R., Leandro, A. C., Anderson, S. T., Newton, S. M., Wilkinson, K. A., Nicol, M. P., Pienaar, S. M., Skolimowska, K. H., Rocha, M. A., Rolla, V. C., Levin, M., Davidson, R. N., *et al.* (2009a). Association between Gc genotype and susceptibility to TB is dependent on vitamin D status. *Eur. Respir. J.* **35,** 1106–1112.

Martineau, A. R., Nanzer, A. M., Satkunam, K. R., Packe, G. E., Rainbow, S. J., Maunsell, Z. J., Timms, P. M., Venton, T. R., Eldridge, S. M., Davidson, R. N., Wilkinson, R. J., and Griffiths, C. J. (2009b). Influence of a single oral dose of vitamin D(2) on serum 25-hydroxyvitamin D concentrations in tuberculosis patients. *Int. J. Tuberc. Lung Dis.* **13,** 119–125.

Matsui, T., Nakao, Y., Koizumi, T., Nakagawa, T., and Fujita, T. (1985). 1,25-Dihydroxyvitamin D3 regulates proliferation of activated T-lymphocyte subsets. *Life Sci.* **37,** 95–101.

McKenna, N. J., Lanz, R. B., and O'Malley, B. W. (1999). Nuclear receptor coregulators: Cellular and molecular biology. *Endocr. Rev.* **20,** 321–344.

Meehan, M. A., Kerman, R. H., and Lemire, J. M. (1992). 1,25-Dihydroxyvitamin D3 enhances the generation of nonspecific suppressor cells while inhibiting the induction of cytotoxic cells in a human MLR. *Cell. Immunol.* **140,** 400–409.

Misawa, Y., Baba, A., Ito, S., Tanaka, M., and Shiohara, M. (2009). Vitamin D(3) induces expression of human cathelicidin antimicrobial peptide 18 in newborns. *Int. J. Hematol.* **90,** 561–570.

Miyamoto, K., Kesterson, R. A., Yamamoto, H., Taketani, Y., Nishiwaki, E., Tatsumi, S., Inoue, Y., Morita, K., Takeda, E., and Pike, J. W. (1997). Structural organization of the human vitamin D receptor chromosomal gene and its promoter. *Mol. Endocrinol.* **11,** 1165–1179.

Morcos, M. M., Gabr, A. A., Samuel, S., Kamel, M., el Baz, M., el Beshry, M., and Michail, R. R. (1998). Vitamin D administration to tuberculous children and its value. *Boll. Chim. Farm.* **137,** 157–164.

Morrison, N. A., Yeoman, R., Kelly, P. J., and Eisman, J. A. (1992). Contribution of trans-acting factor alleles to normal physiological variability: Vitamin D receptor gene polymorphism and circulating osteocalcin. *Proc. Natl. Acad. Sci. USA* **89,** 6665–6669.

Morrison, N. A., Qi, J. C., Tokita, A., Kelly, P. J., Crofts, L., Nguyen, T. V., Sambrook, P. N., and Eisman, J. A. (1994). Prediction of bone density from vitamin D receptor alleles. *Nature* **367,** 284–287.

Muller, K., and Bendtzen, K. (1992). Inhibition of human T lymphocyte proliferation and cytokine production by 1,25-dihydroxyvitamin D3. Differential effects on CD45RA+ and CD45R0+ cells. *Autoimmunity* **14,** 37–43.

Narang, N. K., Gupta, R. C., and Jain, M. K. (1984). Role of vitamin D in pulmonary tuberculosis. *J. Assoc. Physicians India* **32,** 185–188.

Nnoaham, K. E., and Clarke, A. (2008). Low serum vitamin D levels and tuberculosis: A systematic review and meta-analysis. *Int. J. Epidemiol.* **37,** 113–119.

Nursyam, E. W., Amin, Z., and Rumende, C. M. (2006). The effect of vitamin D as supplementary treatment in patients with moderately advanced pulmonary tuberculous lesion. *Acta Med. Indones.* **38,** 3–5.

Ohta, M., Okabe, T., Ozawa, K., Urabe, A., and Takaku, F. (1985). 1 alpha,25-Dihydroxyvitamin D3 (calcitriol) stimulates proliferation of human circulating monocytes in vitro. *FEBS Lett.* **185,** 9–13.

Penna, G., and Adorini, L. (2000). 1 alpha,25-Dihydroxyvitamin D3 inhibits differentiation, maturation, activation, and survival of dendritic cells leading to impaired alloreactive T cell activation. *J. Immunol.* **164,** 2405–2411.

Pinette, K. V., Yee, Y. K., Amegadzie, B. Y., and Nagpal, S. (2003). Vitamin D receptor as a drug discovery target. *Mini Rev. Med. Chem.* **3,** 193–204.

Prabhu Anand, S., Selvaraj, P., and Narayanan, P. R. (2009). Effect of 1,25 dihydroxyvitamin D3 on intracellular IFN-gamma and TNF-alpha positive T cell subsets in pulmonary tuberculosis. *Cytokine* **45,** 105–110.

Range, N., Changalucha, J., Krarup, H., Magnussen, P., Andersen, A. B., and Friis, H. (2006). The effect of multi-vitamin/mineral supplementation on mortality during treatment of pulmonary tuberculosis: A randomised two-by-two factorial trial in Mwanza, Tanzania. *Br. J. Nutr.* **95,** 762–770.

Reichel, H., Koeffler, H. P., Tobler, A., and Norman, A. W. (1987). 1 alpha,25-Dihydroxyvitamin D3 inhibits gamma-interferon synthesis by normal human peripheral blood lymphocytes. *Proc. Natl. Acad. Sci. USA* **84,** 3385–3389.

Rigby, W. F., Stacy, T., and Fanger, M. W. (1984). Inhibition of T lymphocyte mitogenesis by 1,25-dihydroxyvitamin D3 (calcitriol). *J. Clin. Invest.* **74,** 1451–1455.

Rivas-Santiago, B., Hernandez-Pando, R., Carranza, C., Juarez, E., Contreras, J. L., Aguilar-Leon, D., Torres, M., and Sada, E. (2008). Expression of cathelicidin LL-37 during *Mycobacterium tuberculosis* infection in human alveolar macrophages, monocytes, neutrophils, and epithelial cells. *Infect. Immun.* **76,** 935–941.

Rockett, K. A., Brookes, R., Udalova, I., Vidal, V., Hill, A. V., and Kwiatkowski, D. (1998). 1,25-Dihydroxyvitamin D3 induces nitric oxide synthase and suppresses growth of *Mycobacterium tuberculosis* in a human macrophage-like cell line. *Infect. Immun.* **66,** 5314–5321.

Roelandts, R. (2002). The history of phototherapy: Something new under the sun? *J. Am. Acad. Dermatol.* **46,** 926–930.

Rook, G. A., Steele, J., Fraher, L., Barker, S., Karmali, R., O'Riordan, J., and Stanford, J. (1986). Vitamin D3, gamma interferon, and control of proliferation of *Mycobacterium tuberculosis* by human monocytes. *Immunology* **57,** 159–163.

Rosenberg, I. H. (2007). Challenges and opportunities in the translation of the science of vitamins. *Am. J. Clin. Nutr.* **85,** 325S–327S.

Roth, D. E., Soto, G., Arenas, F., Bautista, C. T., Ortiz, J., Rodriguez, R., Cabrera, L., and Gilman, R. H. (2004). Association between vitamin D receptor gene polymorphisms and response to treatment of pulmonary tuberculosis. *J. Infect. Dis.* **190,** 920–927.

Russell, D. G. (2001). *Mycobacterium tuberculosis*: Here today, and here tomorrow. *Nat. Rev. Mol. Cell Biol.* **2,** 569–577.

Sasidharan, P. K., Rajeev, E., and Vijayakumari, V. (2002). Tuberculosis and vitamin D deficiency. *J. Assoc. Physicians India* **50,** 554–558.

Schauber, J., Dorschner, R. A., Coda, A. B., Buchau, A. S., Liu, P. T., Kiken, D., Helfrich, Y. R., Kang, S., Elalieh, H. Z., Steinmeyer, A., Zugel, U., Bikle, D. D., *et al.* (2007). Injury enhances TLR2 function and antimicrobial peptide expression through a vitamin D-dependent mechanism. *J. Clin. Invest.* **117,** 803–811.

Scott, M. G., Davidson, D. J., Gold, M. R., Bowdish, D., and Hancock, R. E. (2002). The human antimicrobial peptide LL-37 is a multifunctional modulator of innate immune responses. *J. Immunol.* **169,** 3883–3891.

Segaert, S. (2008). Vitamin D regulation of cathelicidin in the skin: Toward a renaissance of vitamin D in dermatology? *J. Invest. Dermatol.* **128,** 773–775.

Selvaraj, P., Chandra, G., Jawahar, M. S., Rani, M. V., Rajeshwari, D. N., and Narayanan, P. R. (2004). Regulatory role of vitamin D receptor gene variants of Bsm I, Apa I, Taq I, and Fok I polymorphisms on macrophage phagocytosis and lymphoproliferative response to mycobacterium tuberculosis antigen in pulmonary tuberculosis. *J. Clin. Immunol.* **24,** 523–532.

Selvaraj, P., Prabhu Anand, S., Harishankar, M., and Alagarasu, K. (2009). Plasma 1,25 dihydroxy vitamin D3 level and expression of vitamin d receptor and cathelicidin in pulmonary tuberculosis. *J. Clin. Immunol.* **29,** 470–478.

Sharma, O. P. (2000). Hypercalcemia in granulomatous disorders: A clinical review. *Curr. Opin. Pulm. Med.* **6,** 442–447.

Sigmundsdottir, H., Pan, J., Debes, G. F., Alt, C., Habtezion, A., Soler, D., and Butcher, E. C. (2007). DCs metabolize sunlight-induced vitamin D3 to 'program' T cell attraction to the epidermal chemokine CCL27. *Nat. Immunol.* **8,** 285–293.

Sorensen, O. E., Follin, P., Johnsen, A. H., Calafat, J., Tjabringa, G. S., Hiemstra, P. S., and Borregaard, N. (2001). Human cathelicidin, hCAP-18, is processed to the antimicrobial peptide LL-37 by extracellular cleavage with proteinase 3. *Blood* **97,** 3951–3959.

Taymans, S. E., Pack, S., Pak, E., Orban, Z., Barsony, J., Zhuang, Z., and Stratakis, C. A. (1999). The human vitamin D receptor gene (VDR) is localized to region 12cen-q12 by fluorescent in situ hybridization and radiation hybrid mapping: Genetic and physical VDR map. *J. Bone Miner. Res.* **14,** 1163–1166.

Trautwein, H., and Stein, E. (1952). Vitamin D2 and pulmonary tuberculosis; effects and therapeutic results. *Beitr. Klin. Tuberk. Spezif. Tuberkuloseforsch.* **107,** 295–313.

Turner, J., Cho, Y., Dinh, N. N., Waring, A. J., and Lehrer, R. I. (1998). Activities of LL-37, a cathelin-associated antimicrobial peptide of human neutrophils. *Antimicrob. Agents Chemother.* **42,** 2206–2214.

Ustianowski, A., Shaffer, R., Collin, S., Wilkinson, R. J., and Davidson, R. N. (2005). Prevalence and associations of vitamin D deficiency in foreign-born persons with tuberculosis in London. *J. Infect.* **50,** 432–437.

van Etten, E., and Mathieu, C. (2005). Immunoregulation by 1,25-dihydroxyvitamin D3: Basic concepts. *J. Steroid Biochem. Mol. Biol.* **97,** 93–101.

Veldman, C. M., Cantorna, M. T., and DeLuca, H. F. (2000). Expression of 1,25-dihydroxyvitamin D(3) receptor in the immune system. *Arch. Biochem. Biophys.* **374,** 334–338.

Vidyarani, M., Selvaraj, P., Jawahar, M. S., and Narayanan, P. R. (2007). 1,25 Dihydroxyvitamin D3 modulated cytokine response in pulmonary tuberculosis. *Cytokine* **40,** 128–134.

Wang, T. T., Nestel, F. P., Bourdeau, V., Nagai, Y., Wang, Q., Liao, J., Tavera-Mendoza, L., Lin, R., Hanrahan, J. W., Mader, S., and White, J. H. (2004). Cutting edge: 1,25-dihydroxyvitamin D3 is a direct inducer of antimicrobial peptide gene expression. *J. Immunol.* **173,** 2909–2912.

Wejse, C., Gomes, V. F., Rabna, P., Gustafson, P., Aaby, P., Lisse, I. M., Andersen, P. L., Glerup, H., and Sodemann, M. (2009). Vitamin D as supplementary treatment for tuberculosis: A double-blind, randomized, placebo-controlled trial. *Am. J. Respir. Crit. Care Med.* **179,** 843–850.

World Health Organization (2008). Global Tuberculosis Control—Surveillance, Planning, Financing. WHO Report 2008 World Health Organization, Geneva.

Yim, J. J., and Selvaraj, P. (2010). Genetic susceptibility in tuberculosis. *Respirology* **15,** 241–256.

Yuk, J. M., Shin, D. M., Lee, H. M., Yang, C. S., Jin, H. S., Kim, K. K., Lee, Z. W., Lee, S. H., Kim, J. M., and Jo, E. K. (2009). Vitamin D3 induces autophagy in human monocytes/macrophages via cathelicidin. *Cell Host Microbe* **6,** 231–243.

Zasloff, M. (2006). Fighting infections with vitamin D. *Nat. Med.* **12,** 388–390.

CHAPTER FOURTEEN

Vitamin D Endocrine System and the Immune Response in Rheumatic Diseases

Maurizio Cutolo,* M. Plebani,† Yehuda Shoenfeld,‡,§ Luciano Adorini,¶ *and* Angela Tincani‖

Contents

Abstract

Epidemiological evidence indicates a significant association between vitamin D deficiency and an increased incidence of autoimmune diseases. The presence of vitamin D receptors (VDRs) in the cells of the immune system and the fact that several of these cells produce the vitamin D hormone suggested that vitamin D could have immunoregulatory properties, and now potent immunomodulatory activities on dendritic cells, Th1 and Th17 cells, as well as B cells have been confirmed. Serum levels of vitamin D have been found to be significantly lower in patients with systemic lupus erythematosus, undifferentiated connective tissue

* Rheumatology, Research Laboratories and Academic Unit of Clinical Rheumatology, Postgraduate Academic School of Rheumatology, University of Genova, Genova, Italy
† Department of Laboratory Medicine, University Hospital of Padova, Padova, Italy
‡ Department of Medicine 'B', Zabludowicz Center for Autoimmune Diseases, Sheba Medical Center (Affiliated to Tel-Aviv University), Tel-Hashomer, Israel
§ Incumbent of the Laura Schwarz-Kipp Chair for Research of Autoimmune Diseases, Tel-Aviv University, Tel-Aviv, Israel
¶ Intercept Pharmaceuticals, Corciano (Perugia), Italy
‖ Rheumatology and Clinical Immunology, Spedali Civili and University of Brescia, Brescia, Italy

Vitamins and Hormones, Volume 86
ISSN 0083-6729, DOI: 10.1016/B978-0-12-386960-9.00014-9

disease, and type-1 diabetes mellitus than in the healthy population. In addition, it was also found that lower levels of vitamin D were associated with higher disease activity in rheumatoid arthritis. Promising clinical results together with evidence for the regulation of multiple immunomodulatory mechanisms by VDR agonists represent a sound basis for further exploration of their potential in the treatment of rheumatic autoimmune disorders.

Abbreviations

APS	antiphospholipid syndrome
ECLAM	European Consensus Lupus Activity Measurement
HCQ	hydroxychloroquine
MS	multiple sclerosis
NHD	normal healthy donors
OR	odds ratio
PM/DM	polymyositis/dermatomyositis
RA	rheumatoid arthritis
SLE	systemic lupus erythematosus
SLEDAI	systemic lupus erythematosus disease activity index
SLICC	systemic lupus international collaborating clinics
SSc	systemic sclerosis
USA	United States of America
VAS	visual analogue scale

I. Introduction

Several observations suggest that nonclassical metabolism and response to vitamin D might have a significant role in human physiology beyond skeletal and calcium homeostasis (Adams and Hewison, 2008). Epidemiological evidence indicates a significant association between vitamin D deficiency and an increased incidence of autoimmune diseases (Cutolo, 2009). Serum levels of vitamin D have been found to be significantly lower in patients with systemic lupus erythematosus (SLE), undifferentiated connective tissue disease (UCTD), and type-1 diabetes mellitus than in the healthy population (Cutolo and Otsa, 2008).

In addition, it was also found that lower levels of vitamin D were associated with higher disease activity in rheumatoid arthritis (RA) (Cutolo *et al.*, 2006a). An inverse correlation has been described between the supplementation of vitamin D and the development of type-1 diabetes mellitus and multiple sclerosis (Littorin *et al.*, 2006).

A detailed analysis on the role of vitamin D endocrine system and the immune response in rheumatic diseases is reported here.

II. Function and Biochemical Measures of Vitamin D

Vitamin D is essential for a vast number of physiologic processes, and as such, appropriate levels are necessary or advantageous for optimal health (Stechschulte *et al.*, 2009). Current dogma holds that vitamin D, through its hormonal form 1,25$(OH)_2$D (calcitriol), is a central regulation of calcium homeostasis. Calcitriol achieves this role mainly through a vitamin D receptor (VDR)-mediated mechanism in which the hormone directly regulates gene expression at the transcriptional level.

The majority of the body's 1,25$(OH)_2$D is synthesized in the primary renal tubules of the kidney, but synthesis also occurs in numerous extrarenal sites in cells that express CYP27B1 (1α-hydroxylase enzyme) (Jones *et al.*, 2007). Renal production of 1,25$(OH)_2$D occurs in response to decreased levels of circulating Ca^{2+}, which stimulates the production of parathyroid hormone (PTH). PTH, in turn, induces the production of CYP27B1 by primary renal tubules.

As circulating levels of 1,25$(OH)_2$D rise, it suppresses its own production via a negative feedback loop in which the VDR binds to the CYP27B1 promoter to repress its expression. 1,25$(OH)_2$D increases the uptake of Ca^{2+} by the intestine, which leads to a decrease in PTH levels. In addition, 1,25$(OH)_2$D induces FGF-23 in osteocytes that represses PTH production. Further, vitamin D induces the production of CYP24, a mitochondrial cytochrome P450 enzyme that catabolizes both 1,25$(OH)_2$D and 25(OH) D, thus limiting its own production.

Extrarenal production of vitamin D occurs in bone, epithelial cells of the skin, lung and colon, parathyroid glands, and immune cells. The wide distribution of 1α-hydroxylase enzyme (CYP27B1) is believed to augment the kidney-produced 1,25$(OH)_2$D with locally produced 1,25$(OH)_2$D within its target cells to promote further roles for vitamin D in addition to the classical functions in calcium homeostasis.

The conformationally flexible 1,25$(OH)_2$D can interact with the VDR localized in the cell nucleus to generate genomic responses and in caveolae with the plasma membrane VDR to generate rapid responses. Therefore, the spectrum of vitamin D-dependent genes is not limited to a handful of specific Ca-related genes but is broad and probably encompasses hundreds or even thousands. Most dividing cell types, normal and malignant, can express VDR and respond to 1,25$(OH)_2$D, and the VDR is expressed in at least 30 different target tissues. Functions of vitamin D in the immune system, skin, muscle, pancreas, kidney, and brain have led to claims that 1,25$(OH)_2$D, the biologically active hormone, is involved in the pathogenesis of psoriasis, certain types of cancer, multiple sclerosis, type 1 diabetes, blood pressure regulation, muscle weakness, cardiovascular disease, and microbial infections.

There is growing evidence, in fact, that vitamin D may regulate different cellular processes associated with carcinogenesis (differentiation, proliferation, and apoptosis) and play a role in protecting against heart disease, diabetes, asthma, and reduced muscle tone (Giovannucci, 2009). Although extensive research has been done on vitamin D, the molecular and cellular mechanisms responsible for its many benefits have not been fully elucidated and the list of nontraditional vitamin deficiency-associated diseases and conditions continues to grow.

The increasing recognition of the contribution of 25-hydroxyvitamin D deficiency to many clinical problems promotes a significant debate regarding diagnosis of vitamin D deficiency and circulating concentration defining vitamin D deficiency.

Currently, we do not know all the roles of vitamin D, but we know that a large body of data (Jesudason *et al.*, 2002; Lips, 2001; Malabanan *et al.*, 1998; Vieth *et al.*, 2003) suggest multiple potential benefits, with risk of adverse consequences minimized at least to levels around 75 nmol/l (30 ng/ml) (Cavalier *et al.*, 2008).

The growing interest in vitamin D promoted a recent upsurge in requests for 25 vitamin D evaluation, increasing the need for reliable measurement. Although several available assays can measure serum 25 $(OH)_2$D concentrations, they have methodological limitations.

The major difficulty in measuring 25(OH)D is attributable to the molecule itself. 25(OH)D is probably the most hydrophobic compound measured by protein binding assay (PBA), which constitutes either competitive PBA or radioimmunoassay (RIA). 25(OH)D's lipophilic nature renders it especially vulnerable to the matrix effects of any PBA. Anything present in the sample assay vessel that is not present in the calibrator assay vessel can cause matrix effects. These matrix effect substances are usually lipid, but in the newer direct assays, they could be anything contained in the serum or plasma sample. These matrix factors change the ability of the binding agent, antibody, or binding protein to associate with 25(OH)D in the sample or standard in an equal fashion. When this occurs, it markedly diminishes the assay's validity.

The fact that the molecule exists in two forms, 25(OH)D_2 and 25(OH) D_3, compounds the difficulties with its measurement by PBA. Another problem for the quantification of 25(OH)D_3 could be the strong binding of the molecule to its specific binding protein (vitamin D-binding protein,

VDBP) with variable affinities. The hydrophobic nature of 25(OH)D, its binding to a specific binding protein (VDBP) with high affinity and with lower affinities to lipoproteins and albumin, and the impact of sample matrix on assay performance make determination of 25(OH)D represent no easy task. An additional aspect of vitamin D measurement that has received only limited investigation is within-individual biological variability that not only reflects seasonal variability but also requires a stable intake or a trough concentration time of measuring (Holick, 2009a).

High variability in 25(OH)D measurements due to utilized test and assay technologies, the lack of equity of 25(OH)D_2 and 25(OH)D_3 metabolite recognition (the problems of the immunoassays inability to measure 25-hydroxyvitamin D_2) (Binkley *et al.*, 2008), and the lack of a reference method often confound proper assessment of vitamin D status. The methods available for the assessment of 25(OH)D concentrations represent a variety of different methodologies to release 25(OH)D from its protein bond with consecutive quantification of the molecule.

The generation of specific antibodies has facilitated development of RIA and chemiluminescence assays that, together with competitive PBAs, are compatible with various clinical chemistry platforms. These assays employ a chemical release of the analyte from the VDBP followed by a classical immunoassay. This procedure may lead to interference with VDBP if entire chemical release of 25(OH)D from its binding protein and irreversible denaturation of VDBP are not achieved or if there is interference of serum matrix factors (e.g., lipids) in the final immunological reaction.

Another new arrival on the methodologies scene has been the liquid chromatography–tandem mass spectroscopy (LC–MS/MS) vitamin D assays that utilize a comparable chemical sample purification and combine the excellent resolving power of high-performance liquid chromatography (HPLC) with the molecular fragmentation and mass/charge-based detection of mass spectrometry. Sample prepurification guarantees assessment of 25(OH)D concentration without any interfering sample compounds. The suitability for routine measurement of the 25-hydroxyvitamin D metabolites makes LC–MS/MS, interference-free method, an ideal tool for measuring 25-hydroxyvitamin D_2 and D_3 (Glendenning *et al.*, 2006).

At first glance, LC–MS/MS appeared to offer several advantages over immunoassay including improved accuracy and better measurement of 25-hydroxyvitamin D_2, but the performance of these assays in the DEQAS (vitamin D external quality assessment schemes) has not reflected this optimistic belief showing poor interlaboratory agreement (Carter *et al.*, 2004; Roth *et al.*, 2008).

Obvious problems, in fact, exist with assay standardization like errors in the preparation of standards in different matrices, use of different internal standard material, alternative approaches to calibration, and the lack of an international standard material. Therefore, it is of prime importance that an internationally agreed standard material for both 25-hydroxyvitamin D_2 and D_3 needs to be produced that can be utilized worldwide to improve not only LC–MS/MS consistency but also immunoassay comparability.

Such an improvement in assay performance would hopefully lead to a more consistent definition of vitamin D deficiency with better comparability between clinical trials using different outcomes to measure vitamin D deficiency. In addition, an improved outcome for patients receiving vitamin D supplementation should be seen, as the target total 25-hydroxyvitamin D concentration achieved in such trials would have greater comparability between the studies (Carter and Jones, 2009; Fraser, 2009).

Currently, a general consensus exists on some key points of vitamin D measurement that should be summarized as follows: (a) choose an assay that measures both 25(OH)D_2 and 25(OH)D_3; (b) when using an assay that separates 25(OH)D_2 and 25(OH)D_3 (i.e., HPLC or LC/MS–MS), indicate the sum of the two compounds (25OHD_2 + 25OHD_3) as the main results in your laboratory report; (c) participate to an external quality assessment scheme that provides materials commutable to patient specimens; and (d) report appropriate levels for vitamin D deficiency and toxicity in addition to reference levels obtained in well-selected reference subjects.

III. Vitamin D and Autoimmunity

In recent years, vitamin D attracted a significant amount of attention due to its wide range of classical and nonclassical biological activities. The latter include the role of vitamin D, an immune modulator which possesses immune-regulatory and anti-inflammatory properties (Arnson *et al.*, 2007; Shoenfeld *et al.*, 2009).

A large body of evidence confirm that vitamin D interferes with multiple intracellular pathways thereby orchestrating the differentiation, maturation, and activation of both the innate and adaptive components of the immune systems. These modulator effects are mediated mostly through binding of vitamin D to VDR which is constitutively expressed on various cells such as lymphocytes and monocytes (Penna and Adorini, 2000; van Etten and Mathieu, 2005).

Several components of the innate immune system such as monocytes, macrophages, dendritic cells (DCs), and toll-like receptors (TLR) are directly subjected to vitamin D impact (Penna and Adorini, 2000; Sdeghi *et al.*, 2006; van Etten and Mathieu, 2005). *In vitro* studies have showed that the active form of vitamin D significantly reduces the expression of MHC class II molecules, TLR 2, and TLR 4 on monocytes and suppresses their differentiation into DCs.

Vitamin D also inhibits DCs' surface expression of costimulatory molecules such as CD40, CD80, and CD86, thereby decreasing DCs' ability to provide a secondary signal to T cell and inhibiting T cell activation and secretion of the Th1-polarizing cytokine interleukin (IL)-12 (Lyakh *et al.*, 2005; Xu *et al.*, 1993). The inhibition of IL-12 secretion is achieved through the direct interaction of active vitamin D bound to VDR with nuclear factor (NF)-κB thus suppressing NF-κB-induced transcription of IL-12 (Lyakh *et al.*, 2005; Xu *et al.*, 1993).

Further, treatment of DCs with vitamin D leads to upregulation of immunoglobulin-like transcripts-3 (ILT3), and ILT3 expressed by DCs is involved in induction of CD4+Foxp3+ regulatory T cells (Adorini *et al.*, 2003). Therefore, vitamin D reduces the antigen presenting capabilities of DCs and enhances the production of DCs with tolerogenic phenotypes which in parallel inhibit DC-dependent T cell activation and favor the induction of regulatory, rather than effector, T cell response.

Direct effects of vitamin D on both arms of the adaptive immune system have also been documented via inhibition of antibody secretion and autoantibody production by B cells as well as a direct effect on T cells (Linker-Israeli *et al.*, 2001a).

Vitamin D inhibits T cell proliferation, cytokine secretion, and cell cycle progression. Moreover, the activation of T cells expressing VDR by vitamin D promotes a Th-2 phenotype with IL-4 and IL-5 production while suppressing Th1 activity and cytokines production such as interferon-gamma (IFN-γ) and IL-2 (Linker-Israeli *et al.*, 2001a; van Etten and Mathieu, 2005).

The development of a highly skewed T lymphocyte population is largely mediated by upregulation of IL-4 (Linker-Israeli *et al.*, 2001a). Additionally, vitamin D promotes IL-5 and IL-10 production, which further tilts the T cell response toward Th2 dominance (Arnson *et al.*, 2007).

The transcription and production of Th1 cytokines, namely IFN-γ and IL-2, are also directly inhibited by vitamin D, and thereby further decreases the recruitment activation and proliferation of Th1 lymphocytes (van Etten and Mathieu, 2005). These Th1-related cytokines are considered to be key mediators of autoimmune diseases, while Th2-related cytokines such as IL-4, IL-5, and IL-13 have more regulatory functions. Thus via directly and indirectly inhibiting the synthesis of Th1 cytokines and by polarization toward a Th2 phenotype, vitamin D may eventually attenuate autoimmunity.

Another T cell subset, the Th17 cells has recently emerged as a third independent subset which of critical importance in the pathogenesis of several autoimmune diseases (Bettelli *et al.*, 2007). The cytokines TGFβ and IL-6 are essential for the initial differentiation of Th17 cells. Vitamin D inhibits the expression of IL-6 protein, thus negatively affecting the differentiation of Th17 cells (Stockinger, 2007).

These multifacet associations between vitamin D and different arms of the immune system define the close alliance between its deficiency and malfunctions of the immune system, such as increased autoimmunity and reduced response to certain infectious agents (van Etten and Mathieu, 2005).

Low levels of vitamin D were documented in animal models as well as in human autoimmune diseases. In the experimental model of autoimmune encephalomyelitis (EAE), the combination of vitamin D and dexamethasone could prevent autoimmune demyelination in an antigen-specific manner (van Etten and Mathieu, 2005). In MRL/lpr mice that spontaneously develops SLE-like disease, administration of active vitamin D starting at 1 month of age resulted in reduction of circulating autoantibodies, proteinuria, SLE-like skin lesions, and significantly improved longevity (Shoenfeld *et al.*, 2009).

Another study of NOD mice that are genetically prone to develop type 1 diabetes demonstrated vitamin D deficiency in early life to be a cause of a more aggressive presentation of the disease (Carvalho *et al.*, 2007; van Etten and Mathieu, 2005).

Human epidemiological studies have indicated a significant association between VDR polymorphisms or low levels of vitamin D and increased prevalence of a variety of autoimmune diseases. Additionally, for several systemic and organ-specific autoimmune diseases, such as multiple sclerosis, diabetes mellitus, SLE, and autoimmune thyroid diseases, latitudinal gradients of increasing disease rates were inversely associated with sunlight–ultraviolet radiation exposure and thus vitamin D synthesis (Shapira *et al.*, 2010).

Among SLE patients, lower levels of vitamin D were documented compared to healthy subjects, and vitamin D deficiency was documented in 65–75% of patients in different studies (Cutolo *et al.*, 2009; Sdeghi *et al.*, 2006). Moreover, we have recently demonstrated an association between low levels of vitamin D and higher SLE disease activity (Amital *et al.*, 2010). Similarly, increased prevalence of vitamin D deficiency was reported in patients with RA (Cutolo *et al.*, 2009), type I diabetes mellitus (Hypponen *et al.*, 2001), multiple sclerosis (Hypponen *et al.*, 2001), autoimmune thyroid diseases (Shapira *et al.*, 2010; Shoenfeld *et al.*, 2009), and others.

Last but not the least, the supplementation of vitamin D has shown effectiveness in reducing and treating autoimmune diseases. Treatment with high dose of vitamin D (2000 IU/day) was found to be beneficial in preventing the development of type 1 diabetes when given prophylactic. This was documented by Hypponen *et al.* (2001) in a birth cohort study of more than 10,000 subjects that received high doses of vitamin D resulting in a 78% reduction of type 1 diabetes development.

Others reported vitamin D supplementation to be associated with diminishing exacerbations of multiple sclerosis and reducing pain and C-reactive protein levels in patients with rheumatoid and psoriatic arthritis (PA) (Amital *et al.*, 2010; Andjelkovic *et al.*, 1999a; Huckins *et al.*, 1990).

Taking it all together, it seems that vitamin D effects on the immune system may be utilized to diminish autoimmunity and support supplementation as a preventive as well as a therapeutic measurement.

IV. SLE and Other Systemic Autoimmune Diseases

There are growing epidemiological data for 25-OH vitamin D inadequacy in patients with SLE. This is actually not surprising, as SLE patients are at greater risk for suboptimal vitamin D levels due to strongly recommended sun avoidance and use of sunscreens. Current efforts aim to establish whether low levels of serum vitamin D are associated SLE activity and severity.

Supplementation with 25-OH vitamin D in SLE patients has been traditionally used for the prevention of corticosteroid-induced osteoporosis (Bertsias *et al.*, 2008). For this reason, initial hints at vitamin D inadequacy in SLE came from studies of bone health. The very first report was on a small cohort of 12 SLE teenagers who were receiving corticosteroids (O'Regan *et al.*, 1979). Low levels of 1,25-OH vitamin D were described in seven of them. Further studies evaluated the levels of 25-OH vitamin D in relation to bone mineral density (BMD) or fractures. A study took into consideration newly diagnosed SLE patients, long-standing SLE on corticosteroids, and age-matched controls (Teichmann *et al.*, 1999). The lowest mean value of 25-OH vitamin D was found in the group of treated SLE (19.6 ng/ml vs. 40.45 of healthy controls), suggesting a possible iatrogenic origin of the problem. A more recent study on 107 SLE from the Netherlands found 25-OH vitamin D deficiency (<25 nmol/l) in 8% of the patients, with a significant association with a low BMD (Bultink *et al.*, 2005).

Prompted by the growing evidence in animal models for a regulatory *in vivo* role for vitamin D in ameliorating autoimmune diseases, subsequent clinical studies in SLE were mainly designed for assessing the prevalence of vitamin D deficiency and its relationships with disease activity and severity.

Most of the studies were cross-sectional and assessed vitamin D inadequacy as both insufficiency and deficiency, being <30 and <10 ng/ml the most common cutoff values, respectively. To note that cutoff values and units of measurement (ng/ml vs. nmol/ml) may be different from study to study. A vitamin D inadequacy in SLE patients was detected in every study, with a variable prevalence (see Table 14.1).

A control group was present in most of the studies, usually including healthy individuals. In a few studies, patients with RA, fibromyalgia (FM), or other autoimmune diseases (myositis, thyroiditis, multiple sclerosis) were included as disease controls (Chen *et al.*, 2007; Huisman *et al.*, 2001; Müller *et al.*, 1995; Orbach *et al.*, 2007).

Table 14.1 Studies assessing the prevalence of 25-OH vitamin D inadequacy in SLE patients and its association with disease activity/severity

Reference	SLE patients (number, ethnicity)	Controls (number, diagnosis)	25-OH vitamin D status	Clinical associations/ correlations with serum levels of 25-OH vitamin D
Müller *et al.* (1995)	21 patients from Denmark	29 RA, 12 osteoarthritis, NHD	Significantly lower levels in SLE in comparison to osteoarthritis and NHD	No associations with clinical disease manifestations
Huisman *et al.* (2001)	25 females, Caucasian	25 females with primary fibromyalgia	<50 nmol/l: 56% SLE; 48% controls	Not done. Subanalysis of 1,25 $(OH)_2$ vitamin D: lower in SLE patients taking HCQ than in SLE not taking HCQ
Kamen *et al.* (2006)	123 recently diagnosed males and females (South Carolina, USA: Caucasian and African American)	240 age- and sex-matched NHD	Mean (ng/ml): 21.6 in SLE; 27.4 in NHD <30 ng/ml: 67% of SLE African Americans $<$ Caucasians	Critically low levels (<10 ng/ml) in 18% SLE had renal disease and photosensitivity as predictors (OR 13.3 and 12.9, respectively)
Chen *et al.* (2007)	57 males and females (China)	29 RA, 28 NHD	Mean (ng/ml): 11.5 in SLE; 54.6 in RA; 59.2 in NHD SLE significantly lower than RA and NHD	No correlations with disease activity (SLEDAI) and disease manifestations
Orbach *et al.* (2007)	138 males and females (several European countries and Israeli)	229 SSc, 196 PM/DM, 56 RA, 160 APS, 150 MS, 100 thyroid autoimmune diseases, European NHD	Mean (ng/ml): 11.9 in SLE; 11.0 in SSc; 13.8 PM/DM; 9.3 in RA; 11.9 in APS; 13.7 in MS; 11.0 in thyroid autoimmune diseases; 21.6 in NHD	Not done

Cutolo and Otsa (2008)	Patients from northern Europe (Estonia) and southern Europe (Italy)	NHD from the same geographical areas	25-OH vitamin D levels significantly lower in SLE patients compared with their controls No difference between SLE patients from Estonia and those from Italy	Negative correlation between 25-OH vitamin levels and SLE activity (ECLAM; SLEDAI)
Kamen and Aranow (2008)	200 males and females (African American, Hispanic, Caucasian, Asian)	Not reported	Levels in African American and Hispanics were statistically lower than in Caucasian or Asians. A significant number of African Americans and Hispanics had severe deficiency (<10 ng/ml)	Not reported
Ruiz-Irastorza *et al.* (2008)	92 males and females (Spain: 98% white)	Not present	<30 mg/ml: 75% <10 ng/ml: 15%	Female sex, treatment with HCQ, and treatment with calcium and vitamin D were associated with higher levels of 25-OH vitamin D
			Mean: 22 ng/ml	Photosensitivity and photoprotection were predictors of vitamin D inadequacy (OR = 3.5 and OR = 5.7, respectively)
Thudi *et al.* (2008)	37 females (Texas: Caucasian, African American, Hispanic)	Not present	<80 nmol/l: 65% <47.7 nmol/l: 20% No difference between ethnicities	Patients <47.7 nmol/l had higher disease activity measures (VAS global, VAS fatigue, combined score)

(*continued*)

Table 14.1 (*continued*)

Reference	SLE patients (number, ethnicity)	Controls (number, diagnosis)	25-OH vitamin D status	Clinical associations/ correlations with serum levels of 25-OH vitamin D
Borba *et al.* (2009)	36 females (Brazil: White, Black, Asian)	26 age- and sex-matched NHD	Mean (ng/ml): 17.4 in active SLE; 44.6 in quiescent SLE; 37.8 in NHD (statistically significant) No difference between ethnicities	Disease activity (SLEDAI) was inversely correlated with 25-OH vitamin D levels
Damanhouri (2009)	165 males and females (Saudi Arabia)	214 SLE-free volunteers	<30 ng/ml: 98.8% of SLE, 55% of controls <20 ng/ml: 89.7% of SLE, 20% of controls	No differences between males and females
Wright *et al.* (2009)	38 pediatric patients (North America: 47% black)	207 pediatric NHD	Mean (ng/ml): 18.0 in SLE; 22.3 in NHD <30 ng/ml: 76% of SLE, 79% of NHD <10 ng/ml: 37% of SLE, 9% of NHD Black SLE patients more deficient than white SLE patients	Vitamin D inadequacy (<30 ng/ml) was associated with overweight (greater body mass index). Greater SLE disease activity index scores were observed in patients with <20 ng/ml
Wu *et al.* (2009)	181 females (North America: White, African American, Hispanic, Asian)	Not present	Mean (ng/ml): 27.1 <30 ng/ml: 62.2% <15 ng/ml: 20%	Lower 25-OH vitamin D levels were associated with higher SLE disease activity (SLEDAI) and damage scores (SLICC)

Amital *et al.* (2010)	378 males and females from several European countries and Israeli	Not present	Mean (ng/ml): 23.9 in patients assessed with SLEDAI; 27.6 in patients assessed with ECLAM	Patients with active disease had lower mean vitamin D concentrations than patients with quiescent disease (17.8 vs. 24.3 ng/ml)
Kim *et al.* (2010)	104 females (Korea)	49 female NHD	Mean (ng/ml): 42.5 in SLE; 52.7 in NHD <30 ng/ml: 16.3% of SLE, 4.1% of NHD	No association with disease manifestations/activity (SLEDAI) nor with steroid or HCQ intake
Ruiz-Irastorza *et al.* (2010)	80 males and females (Spain: 98% white)	Not present	<30 mg/ml: 71% <5 ng/ml: 6% Mean: 24.8 ng/ml	Significant inverse correlation between 25-OH vitamin D levels and the VAS fatigue. No correlation with disease activity (SLEDAI) and damage (SLICC)
Toloza *et al.* (2010)	124 females (Caucasians, African American, Asian, other)	Not present	<80 nmol/l: 66.7% <40 nmol/l: 17.9% No difference between ethnicities	Season, glucocorticoid exposure, and serum creatinine were correlated to 25-OH vitamin D levels. No association with disease activity

Some studies also addressed the ethnicity issue (Borba *et al.*, 2009; Kamen and Aranow, 2008; Kamen *et al.*, 2006; Thudi *et al.*, 2008; Toloza *et al.*, 2010; Wright *et al.*, 2009; Wu *et al.*, 2009). Vitamin D deficiency is indeed more prevalent in patients with darker skin due to the reduced conversion of 7-dehydrocholesterol to vitamin D.

Still controversial is the association between vitamin D inadequacy and SLE manifestations/activity/severity. The outcomes of different studies are summarized in Table 14.1.

Only one prospective study is currently available on the effect of oral supplementation on serum 25-OH vitamin D levels and lupus activity (Ruiz-Irastorza *et al.*, 2008). Although the mean 25-OH vitamin D level of the whole cohort was significantly higher after supplementation, 71% of the patients had still values less than 30 ng/ml. A beneficial effect was reported on fatigue, while no correlations were seen between variations of SLE activity and severity and changes in 25-OH vitamin D levels. This study underlines for the first time that the usual oral regimen of vitamin D3 (median dose 800 UI/day) seems not sufficient for correcting vitamin D inadequacy and to have benefit on disease activity.

Vitamin D inadequacy has been investigated in other systemic autoimmune diseases, although not as extensively as in SLE. Zold *et al.* analyzed a cohort of 161 patients with UCTD and found lower levels of 25-OH vitamin D in comparison to healthy controls, during both summer and winter (Zold *et al.*, 2008). Interestingly, those patients with lower levels were more likely to progress into a definite connective tissue disease (CTD) over time. The large study by Orbach *et al.* included 229 systemic sclerosis, 196 dermatomyositis/polymyositis, and 160 antiphospholipid syndrome; mean values of 25-OH vitamin D were 11.0, 13.8, and 11.9 ng/ml, respectively, being 21.6 ng/ml the mean of normal controls (Orbach *et al.*, 2007).

In conclusion, vitamin D inadequacy appears to be widespread in several systemic autoimmune diseases. SLE has been widely investigated, but no definitive conclusions have been drawn on the relationship between 25-OH vitamin D status and disease activity/severity.

Such discordant results may be mainly related to methodological issues. First, studies may not be directly compared due to the use of different assays for 25-OH vitamin D detection; even if a similar assay is used, the actual poor interlaboratory agreement may affect the results, as described in the previous chapters. Second, SLE cohorts may differ for several variables which may alter the interpretation of 25-OH vitamin D levels (e.g., ethnicity, season, geographical area, dietary intake and/or supplementation, SLE treatments—particularly corticosteroids).

Clarification of the relationship between SLE activity and 25-OH vitamin D is certainly of major interest, as vitamin D appears to be a novel, cheap, and safe immunomodulant therapy in SLE.

V. Vitamin D and Rheumatoid Arthritis

It is evident that both genetic and environmental factors affect prevalence of autoimmune diseases. Therefore, the fact that vitamin D as a true steroid hormone (common structure with glucocorticoids, as both synthesized from cholesterol) has been implicated as a factor in different autoimmune diseases suggests that vitamin D might be one of the environmental factors that normally participate in the control of self-tolerance. Several rheumatic diseases such as RA, PA, or overlap syndromes like UCTD are characterized by low-serum levels of vitamin D often correlated to the severity of the diseases.

RA is an autoimmune disorder of multifactorial etiology in which both genetic and nongenetic factors (i.e., infectious, hormonal, genetic) contribute to disease susceptibility. Vitamin D may exert immunomodulatory effects, and hypovitaminosis D together with higher prevalence of RA seems common among North when compared to South Europe (Sokka, 2010). Recently, greater intake of vitamin D was associated with a lower risk of RA, as well as lower vitamin D was found associated with higher disease activity (Merlino *et al.*, 2004a; Oelzner *et al.*, 1998).

However, other authors argue that these results found an inverse association between vitamin D and lower risk of RA, by means of questionnaires to measure dietary vitamin D intake (Nielen *et al.*, 2006a). These authors found no differences on 25(OH)D_3 serum levels between patients who later developed RA and healthy donors.

To explain these contrasting conclusions, it must be considered that direct measurement of vitamin D in serum is a more accurate estimate of vitamin D levels than is a dietary questionnaire, especially without taking sun exposure into account (Merlino *et al.*, 2004a).

As lower vitamin D serum levels have been also associated with higher RA disease activity, in a recent study were evaluated serum 25(OH)D_3 levels in 64 female RA patients from north Europe (Estonia/EP) and 54 RA patients from south Europe (Italy/IP) during winter and summer and were correlated with the disease activity score (DAS28) (Cutolo *et al.*, 2006b). Normal female controls were Italians and Estonians age-matched subjects, respectively. 25(OH)D_3 levels were found significantly higher in IP versus EP ($p = 0.0116$) both in winter and in summer (58.9 ± 5.4 vs. 35.1 ± 1.9 and 65.2 ± 5.4 vs. 46.4 ± 2.3 nmol/l, respectively). However, the variations (increase) of 25(OH)D_3 levels between summer and winter time were found significant in both IP and EP ($p = 0.0005$). Differences were observed also between controls and between summer and winter, confirming a circannual rhythm (Cutolo *et al.*, 2007).

Interestingly, a significant inverse correlation between 25(OH)D_3 and DAS28 was found in summer in IP ($r = -0.57, p < 0.0001$) and in winter in EP ($r = -0.40$, $p < 0.05$). In addition, mean DAS28 scores were found generally higher in EP versus IP, and the difference was more evident in winter (4.19 ± 1.24 vs. 3.73 ± 1.69, respectively).

Another recent study showed that clinical improvement in RA patient treated with $1{,}25(OH)_2D_3$ strongly correlated with the immunomodulating potential of vitamin D administration. Dual effects on lymphocyte proliferation and apoptosis were observed (Andjelkovic *et al.*, 1999b). More recently, in unadjusted analyses, vitamin D concentrations were inversely associated with baseline pain ($p = 0.04$), swollen joints ($p = 0.04$), and DAS28 ($p = 0.05$) in African American early RA patients (Craig *et al.*, 2010).

VI. Vitamin D and Psoriasis/Psoriatic Arthritis

Interestingly, psoriasis and associated arthritis (PA) are characterized by hyperproliferation and abnormal differentiation of keratinocytes, and inflammation involving skin and joints.

1,25-Dihydroxyvitamin D_3, which is used for the treatment of psoriasis, binds to VDR and modulates gene transcription.

In a recent study, among 19 PA patients investigated, 10 were treated with 0.25 μg oral alphacalcidol twice daily for 6 months, while 9 other patients served as controls (Gaál *et al.*, 2009). In the peripheral blood of the treated group but not in the controls, a statistically significant decrease was observed in the percentage of CD3/CD69-positive-activated and CD8-positive IFN-γ-producing T cells and in the serum level of IFN-γ during the first 3 months and also in the clinical activity of the disease during the whole 6-month follow-up period. The results of the study indicate that systemic alphacalcidol treatment exert an immunomodulatory effect on PA patients.

However, a possible VDR gene FokI, ApaI, and TaqI polymorphisms and related resistance to vitamin D effects were evaluated in Turkish familial psoriasis patients (psoriasis vulgaris and PA) and healthy subjects (Dayangac-Erden *et al.*, 2007).

T allele frequency was found significantly increased (91.7%: $p \leq 0.05$). In addition, with regard to response to calcipotriol treatment, in non-responsive patients, TT genotype and T allele frequencies were higher than they were in the controls (63.6% vs. 35%: $p \leq 0.025$, 81.8% vs. 59.5%: $p \leq 0.01$, respectively).

The study demonstrated that VDR gene polymorphisms may play a role in partial resistance to calcipotriol therapy and therefore to higher expression of PA in these populations.

VII. Vitamin D and Overlap Syndromes

It has been estimated that 25–50% of patients referred to tertiary rheumatology centers do not have a clearly defined autoimmune rheumatic disease or present with features of two or more rheumatic diseases. Several of these patients are classified as having an UCTD.

Generally, 60% of UCTD patients remains in an undifferentiated stage. About 30–40% develops and reaches the stage of a well-defined systemic autoimmune disease during 5 years follow-up with SLE being most common (5–32%).

In a recent study, serum levels of vitamin D were found significantly lower in UCTD patients compared with controls in both summer and winter periods (UCTD summer: 33 ± 13.4 ng/ml vs. control: 39.9 ± 11.7 ng/ml, $p = 0.01$; UCTD winter: 27.8 ± 12.48 ng/ml vs. control: 37.8 ± 12.3 ng/ml, $p = 0.0001$) (Zold *et al.*, 2008).

Interestingly, the presence of dermatological symptoms (photosensitivity, erythema, and chronic discoid rash) and pleuritis was associated with low levels of vitamin D.

During the average follow-up period of 2.3 years, 35 of 161 patients (21.7%) with UCTD further developed into well-established CTD.

Patients who progressed into CTDs had lower vitamin D levels than those who remained in the UCTD stage (vitamin D levels: CTD: 14.7 ± 6.45 ng/ml vs. UCTD: 33.0 ± 13.4 ng/ml, $p = 0.0001$).

In conclusion, patients with UCTD show a seasonal variance in levels of vitamin D and these levels were significantly lower than in controls during the corresponding seasons. In addition, the study suggests that vitamin D deficiency in UCTD patients may play a role in the subsequent progression into well-defined CTDs, confirming that all CTDs might be influenced by low vitamin D levels.

VIII. Vitamin D Supplementation and VDR Agonists in the Treatment of Rheumatic Diseases

Although there is no consensus on optimal serum levels of $25(OH)D_3$, a reliable indicator of vitamin D status, vitamin D deficiency is usually defined by $25(OH)D_3$ levels below 20 ng/ml (Holick, 2009b). Mounting evidence indicates a high prevalence of vitamin D deficiency in the general population, and this has been linked to increased frequency of autoimmune diseases, in addition to bone diseases and cancer (Holick, 2007).

Even in sunny Mediterranean countries, a surprisingly high incidence of vitamin D deficiency has been found in patients with inflammatory joint diseases, including RA, PA, and ankylosing spondylitis (Braun-Moscovici *et al.*, 2009).

Estimated baseline dietary vitamin D intake has been found to be inversely correlated with the risk of developing RA in an inception cohort study (Merlino *et al.*, 2004b). In contrast, a small study of blood donors who subsequently developed RA did not show any difference in baseline pre-RA vitamin D levels compared with controls (Nielen *et al.*, 2006b). In addition, plasma $25(OH)D_3$ levels are not associated with RA-related autoantibodies, anticyclic citrullinated peptide antibodies, or rheumatoid factors, in individuals at elevated risk for RA (Feser *et al.*, 2009), although an association between serum vitamin D metabolite levels and disease activity was observed in patients with early inflammatory polyarthritis (Patel *et al.*, 2007). These discrepancies are reflected by epidemiologic analysis showing strong ecologic and case–control evidence that vitamin D reduces the risk of several autoimmune diseases, such as multiple sclerosis and type 1 diabetes, with evidence also for RA (Grant, 2006). Similarly, case–control studies have shown significantly lower $25(OH)D_3$ levels in SLE patients (Kamen *et al.*, 2006). However, in large prospective cohorts of women, increasing levels of vitamin D intake were not associated with the relative risk of developing either SLE or RA (Costenbader *et al.*, 2008).

Collectively, these data suggest low vitamin D status as an environmental factor affecting rheumatic disease prevalence, indicating the need for vitamin D supplementation. In RA patients with vitamin D insufficiency, correction of vitamin D deficiency is important for the management of osteoporosis and for modifying falls and fracture risks.

Vitamin D supplementation in this patient group may also reduce RA disease activity, based on the well-established anti-inflammatory and immunomodulatory properties of the vitamin D system (Adorini and Penna, 2008). A prevailing view indicates that optimal vitamin D status is achieved with a 25(OH)D3 serum concentration above 75 nmol/l, suggesting a dose of 95 μg/day (3800 IU) for individuals above 55 nmol/l and a dose of 125 μg/day (5000 IU) for those below that threshold (Aloia *et al.*, 2008).

Compared to vitamin D supplementation, treatment with VDR agonists, like $1,25(OH)_2D_3$ and its analogs, is expected to result in higher efficacy and more rapid onset of action, both in RA and in SLE patients. VDR agonists have been tested preclinically in two RA models, Lyme arthritis and collagen-induced arthritis (Cantorna *et al.*, 1998). Infection of mice with *Borrelia burgdorferi*, the causative agent of human Lyme arthritis, produces acute arthritic lesions with footpad and ankle swelling. Supplementation with $1,25(OH)_2D_3$ to mice infected with *B. burgdorferi* minimized or prevented these symptoms, and the same treatment could also inhibit collagen-induced arthritis, preventing the progression to severe arthritis when given to mice with early symptoms (Cantorna *et al.*, 1998). VDR agonists displayed a similar capacity to prevent and suppress already established collagen-induced arthritis without inducing hypercalcemia (Larsson *et al.*, 1998). 1,25$(OH)_2D_3$ contributes to the regulation of MMPs and PGE2 production by human articular chondrocytes in osteoarthritic cartilage, suggesting immunomodulatory effects also in human RA (Tetlow and Woolley, 1999).

Efficacy of VDR agonists has also been shown in SLE models. Administration of the 22-oxa derivative of 1,25$(OH)_2D_3$ significantly prolongs the average life span of MRLlpr/lpr mice, a mouse strain spontaneously developing a SLE-like syndrome with immunological features similar to human SLE, and induces a significant reduction in proteinuria, renal arteritis, granuloma formation, and knee joint arthritis (Abe *et al.*, 1990). In the same mouse strain, treatment with 1,25$(OH)_2D_3$ could reduce proteinuria and anti-ssDNA antibody levels. In addition, dermatological lesions, like alopecia, necrosis of the ear, and scab formation, were also completely inhibited by 1,25$(OH)_2D_3$ therapy (Lemire *et al.*, 1992). These data suggest a beneficial role of VDR agonists in the treatment of human SLE, also considering that reduced levels of 1,25$(OH)_2D_3$ in SLE patients may contribute to B cell hyperactivity (Chen *et al.*, 2007). Indeed, *in vitro* treatment with VDR agonists can significantly reduce cell proliferation and IgG production, both polyclonal and anti-dsDNA, while enhancing B cell apoptosis in lymphocytes from SLE patients (Linker-Israeli *et al.*, 2001b).

VDR agonists have widespread clinical application, but hypercalcemia is a dose-limiting side effect that prevents sustained systemic administration. Thus, the exquisite anti-inflammatory, protolerogenic, and immunoregulatory properties exerted by VDR agonists have been clinically exploited so far only partially in the treatment of autoimmune conditions due to their calcemic liability, the major side effect of this class of agents potentially leading to hypercalciuria and hypercalcemia, and in severe cases eventually to tissue calcification. To overcome this limitation, several thousands of 1,25$(OH)_2D_3$ analogs, with a wider therapeutic window than 1,25 $(OH)_2D_3$ itself, have been synthetized. VDR agonists with lower calcemic liability compared to 1,25$(OH)_2D_3$ have been identified and shown effective in experimental models of autoimmune diseases and allograft rejection (Mathieu and Adorini, 2002).

Importantly, tissue-selective VDR agonists, with a wider therapeutic index compared to the natural hormone 1,25$(OH)_2D_3$, have been identified (Ma *et al.*, 2006). Unfortunately, the clinical translation of VDR agonists has been disappointingly slow.

Only one small open-label intervention study with the VDR agonist 1,25$(OH)D_3$ (alphacalcidiol) in patients with established RA has been published (Andjelkovic *et al.*, 1999c). This was a 3-month open-label trial in 19 patients being treated with standard DMARD therapy for acute RA.

Their regular drug regimen was maintained during the trial, and oral alphacalcidiol 2 μg/day was added. After 3 months, oral alphacalcidiol therapy showed a positive effect on disease activity in 89% of the patients. No side effects were observed.

Nevertheless, these promising clinical results together with the accumulating evidence for the regulation of multiple immunomodulatory mechanisms by VDR agonists represent a sound basis for further exploration of their potential in the treatment of rheumatic autoimmune disorders (Adorini and Penna, 2008).

IX. Conclusions

Serum levels of vitamin D have been confirmed to be significantly lower in patients with autoimmune diseases such as RA, SLE, PA, UCTD as well as type-1 diabetes mellitus and multiple sclerosis than in the healthy population. In addition, it was also found that lower levels of vitamin D were associated with higher disease activity at least in RA and SLE.

The reason is that vitamin D exerts potent immunomodulatory activities on DCs, Th1 and Th17 cells, as well as B cells.

Therefore, promising clinical results together with evidence for the regulation of multiple immunomodulatory mechanisms by VDR agonists represent the basis for further testing of their efficacy in the treatment of rheumatic autoimmune disorders.

REFERENCES

Abe, J., *et al.* (1990). Prevention of immunological disorders in MRL/l mice by a new synthetic analogue of vitamin D3: 22-oxa-1 alpha, 25-dihydroxyvitamin D3. *J. Nutr. Sci. Vitaminol. (Tokyo)* **36,** 21–31.

Adams, J. S., and Hewison, M. (2008). Unexpected actions of vitamin D: New perspectives on the regulation of innate and adaptive immunity. *Nat. Clin. Pract. Endocrinol. Metab.* **4,** 80–90.

Adorini, L., and Penna, G. (2008). Control of autoimmune diseases by the vitamin D endocrine system. *Nat. Clin. Pract. Rheumatol.* **4,** 404–412.

Adorini, L., Penna, G., Giarratana, N., and Uskokovic, M. (2003). Tolerogenic dendritic cells induced by vitamin D receptor ligands enhance regulatory T cells inhibiting allograft rejection and autoimmune diseases. *J. Cell. Biochem.* **88,** 227–233.

Aloia, J. F., *et al.* (2008). Vitamin D intake to attain a desired serum 25-hydroxyvitamin D concentration. *Am. J. Clin. Nutr.* **87,** 1952–1958.

Amital, H., Szekanecz, Z., Szücs, G., Dankó, K., Nagy, E., Csépány, T., Corocher, N., Agmon-Levin, N., Orbach, H., Zandman-Goddard, G., and Shoenfeld, Y. (2010). Serum concentrations of 25-OH Vitamin D in SLE patients are inversely related to disease activity—Is it time to routinely supplement SLE patients with vitamin D? *Ann. Rheum. Dis.* **69,** 1155–1157.

Andjelkovic, Z., Vojinovic, J., Pejnovic, N., Popovic, M., Dujic, A., Mitrovic, D., *et al.* (1999a). Disease modifying and immunomodulatory effects of high dose 1 alpha (OH) D3 in rheumatoid arthritis patients. *Clin. Exp. Rheumatol.* **17,** 453–456.

Andjelkovic, Z., Vojinovic, J., Pejnovic, N., *et al.* (1999b). Disease modifying and immunomodulatory effects of high dose 1 alpha (OH) D3 in rheumatoid arthritis patients. *Clin. Exp. Rheumatol.* **17,** 453–456.

Andjelkovic, Z., *et al.* (1999c). Disease modifying and immunomodulatory effects of high dose 1 alpha (OH) D3 in rheumatoid arthritis patients. *Clin. Exp. Rheumatol.* **17,** 453–456.

Arnson, Y., Amital, H., and Shoenfeld, Y. (2007). Vitamin D and autoimmunity: New aetiological and therapeutic considerations. *Ann. Rheum. Dis.* **66,** 1137–1142.

Bertsias, G., Ioannidis, J. P., Boletis, J., Bombardieri, S., Cervera, R., Dostal, C., Font, J., Gilboe, I. M., Houssiau, F., Huizinga, T., Isenberg, D., Kallenberg, C. G., *et al.* (2008). EULAR recommendations for the management of systemic lupus erythematosus. Report of a Task Force of the EULAR Standing Committee for International Clinical Studies Including Theurapeutics. *Ann. Rheum. Dis.* **67,** 195–205.

Bettelli, E., Korn, T., and Kuchroo, V. K. (2007). Th17: The third member of the effector T cell trilogy. *Curr. Opin. Immunol.* **19,** 652–657.

Binkley, N., Krueger, D., Gemar, D., and Drezner, M. K. (2008). Correlation among 25-hydroxy-vitamin D assays. *J. Clin. Endocrinol. Metab.* **93,** 1804–1808.

Borba, V. Z. C., Vieira, J. G. H., Kasamatsu, T., Radominski, S. C., Sato, E. I., and Lazaretti-Castro, M. (2009). Vitamin D deficiency in patients with active systemic lupus erythematosus. *Osteoporos. Int.* **20,** 427–433.

Braun-Moscovici, Y., *et al.* (2009). Vitamin D level: Is it related to disease activity in inflammatory joint disease? *Ann Rheum Dis.* 2010 Jun; **69**(6), 1155–1157.

Bultink, I. E., Lems, W. F., Kostense, P. J., Dijkmans, B. A., and Voskuyl, A. E. (2005). Prevalence of and risk factors for low bone mineral density and vertebral fractures in patients with systemic lupus erythematosus. *Arthritis Rheum.* **52**(7), 2044–2050.

Cantorna, M. T., *et al.* (1998). 1,25-Dihydroxycholecalciferol inhibits the progression of arthritis in murine models of human arthritis. *J. Nutr.* **128,** 68–72.

Carter, G. D., and Jones, J. C. (2009). Use of a common standard improves the performance of liquid chromatography-tandem mass spectrometry methods for serum 25-hydroxyvitamin D. *Ann. Clin. Biochem.* **46,** 79–81.

Carter, G. D., Carter, R., Jones, J., and Berry, J. (2004). How accurate are assays for 25-hydroxyvitamin D? Data from the international vitamin D external quality assessment scheme. *Clin. Chem.* **50,** 2195–2197.

Carvalho, J. F., Blank, M., Kiss, E., Tarr, T., Amital, H., and Shoenfeld, Y. (2007). Anti-vitamin D, vitamin D in SLE: Preliminary results. *Ann. N. Y. Acad. Sci.* **1109,** 550–557.

Cavalier, E., Wallace, M., Knox, S., Mistretta, V. I., Cormier, C., and Souberbielle, J. C. (2008). Serum vitamin D measurement may not reflect what you give to your patients. *J. Bone Miner. Res.* **23,** 1864–1865.

Chen, S., Sims, G. P., Chen, X. X., Gu, Y. Y., Chen, S., and Lipsky, P. E. (2007). Modulatory effects of 1,25-dihydroxyvitamin D3 on human B cell differentiation. *J. Immunol.* **179,** 1634–1647.

Costenbader, K. H., *et al.* (2008). Vitamin D intake and risks of systemic lupus erythematosus and rheumatoid arthritis in women. *Ann. Rheum. Dis.* **67,** 530–535.

Craig, S. M., Yu, F., Curtis, J. R., Alarcón, G. S., Conn, D. L., Jonas, B., Callahan, L. F., Smith, E. A., Moreland, L. W., Bridges, S. L., Jr., and Mikuls, T. R. (2010). Vitamin D status and its associations with disease activity and severity in African Americans with recent-onset rheumatoid arthritis. *J. Rheumatol.* **37,** 275–281.

Cutolo, M. (2009). Vitamin D and autoimmune rheumatic diseases. *Rheumatology (Oxford)* **48,** 210–212.

Cutolo, M., and Otsa, K. (2008). Review: Vitamin D, immunity and lupus. *Lupus* **17,** 6–10.

Cutolo, M., Otsa, K., Laas, K., Yprus, M., Lehtme, R., Secchi, M. E., Sulli, A., Paolino, S., and Seriolo, B. (2006a). Circannual vitamin D serum levels and disease activity in rheumatoid arthritis: Northern versus Southern Europe. *Clin. Exp. Rheumatol.* **24,** 702–704.

Cutolo, M., Otsa, K., Laas, K., *et al.* (2006b). Circannual vitamin D serum levels and disease activity in rheumatoid arthritis: Northern versus Southern Europe. *Clin. Exp. Rheumatol.* **24,** 702–704.

Cutolo, M., Otsa, K., Yprus, M., *et al.* (2007). Vitamin D and rheumatoid arthritis: Comment on the letter by Nielen et al.. *Arthritis Rheum.* **56,** 1719–1720.

Cutolo, M., Otsa, K., Paolino, S., Yprus, M., Veldi, T., and Seriolo, B. (2009). Vitamin D involvement in rheumatoid arthritis and systemic lupus erythaematosus. *Ann. Rheum. Dis.* **68,** 446–447.

Damanhouri, L. H. (2009). Vitamin D deficiency in Saudi patients with systemic lupus erythematosus. *Saudi Med J.* **30**(10), 1291–1295. PubMed PMID: 19838436.

Dayangac-Erden, D., Karaduman, A., and Erdem-Yurter, H. (2007). Polymorphisms of vitamin D receptor gene in Turkish familial psoriasis patients. *Arch. Dermatol. Res.* **99,** 487–491.

Feser, M., *et al.* (2009). Plasma 25,OH vitamin D concentrations are not associated with rheumatoid arthritis (RA)-related autoantibodies in individuals at elevated risk for RA. *J. Rheumatol.* **36,** 943–946.

Fraser, W. D. (2009). Standardization of vitamin D assays: Art or science? *Ann. Clin. Biochem.* **46,** 3–4.

Gaál, J., Lakos, G., Szodoray, P., Kiss, J., Horváth, I., Horkay, E., Nagy, G., and Szegedi, A. (2009). Immunological and clinical effects of alphacalcidol in patients with psoriatic arthropathy: Results of an open, follow-up pilot study. *Acta Derm. Venereol.* **89,** 140–144.

Giovannucci, E. (2009). Expanding roles of vitamin D. *J. Clin. Endocrinol. Metab.* **94,** 418–420.

Glendenning, P., Taranto, M., Noble, J. M., *et al.* (2006). Current assays overestimate 25-hydroxyvitamin D3 and underestimate 25-hydroxyvitamin D2 compared with HPLC: Need for assay-specific decision limits and metabolite-specific assays. *Ann. Clin. Biochem.* **43,** 23–30.

Grant, W. B. (2006). Epidemiology of disease risks in relation to vitamin D insufficiency. *Prog. Biophys. Mol. Biol.* **92,** 65–79.

Holick, M. F. (2007). Vitamin D deficiency. *N. Engl. J. Med.* **357,** 266–281.

Holick, M. F. (2009a). Vitamin D status: Measurement, interpretation, and clinical application. *Ann. Epidemiol.* **19,** 73–78.

Holick, M. F. (2009b). Vitamin D status: Measurement, interpretation, and clinical application. *Ann. Epidemiol.* **19,** 73–78.

Huckins, D., Felson, D. T., and Holick, M. (1990). Treatment of psoriatic arthritis with oral 1,25-dihydroxyvitamin D3: A pilot study. *Arthritis Rheum.* **33,** 1723–1727.

Huisman, A. M., White, K. P., Algra, A., Harth, M., Vieth, R., Jacobs, J. W. G., Bijlsma, J. W. J., and Bell, D. A. (2001). Vitamin D levels in women with systemic lupus erythematosus and fibromyalgia. *J. Rheumatol.* **28,** 2535–2539.

Hypponen, E., Laara, E., Reunanen, A., Jarvelin, M. R., and Virtanen, S. M. (2001). Intake of vitamin D and risk of type 1 diabetes: A birth-cohort study. *Lancet* **358,** 1500–1503.

Jesudason, D., Need, A. G., Horowitz, M., O'Loughlin, P. D., Morris, H. A., and Nordin, B. E. (2002). Relationship between serum 25-hydroxyvitamin D and bone resorption markers in vitamin D insufficiency. *Bone* **31,** 626–630.

Jones, G., Horst, R., Carter, G., and Makin, H. L. J. (2007). Contemporary diagnosis and treatment of vitamin D-related disorders. *J. Bone Miner. Res.* **22**(S2), V11–V15.

Kamen, D., and Aranow, C. (2008). Vitamin D in systemic lupus erythematosus. *Curr. Opin. Rheumatol.* **20,** 532–537.

Kamen, D. L., Cooper, G. S., Bouali, H., Shaftman, S. R., Hollis, B. W., and Gilkeson, G. S. (2006). Vitamin D deficiency in systemic lupus erythematosus. *Autoimmun. Rev.* **5,** 114–117.

Kim, H. A., Sung, J. M., Jeon, J. Y., Yoon, J. M., and Suh, C. H. (2010). Vitamin D may not be a good marker of disease activity in Korean patients with systemic lupus erythematosus. *Rheumatol Int.* [Epub ahead of print] PubMed PMID: 20352222.

Larsson, P., *et al.* (1998). A vitamin D analogue (MC 1288) has immunomodulatory properties and suppresses collagen-induced arthritis (CIA) without causing hypercalcaemia. *Clin. Exp. Immunol.* **114,** 277–283.

Lemire, J. M., *et al.* (1992). 1,25-Dihydroxyvitamin D3 attenuates the expression of experimental murine lupus of MRL/l mice. *Autoimmunity* **12,** 143–148.

Linker-Israeli, M., Elstner, E., Klinenberg, J. R., Wallace, D. J., and Koeffler, H. P. (2001a). Vitamin D(3) and its synthetic analogs inhibit the spontaneous in vitro immunoglobulin production by SLE-derived PBMC. *Clin. Immunol.* **99,** 82–93.

Linker-Israeli, M., *et al.* (2001b). Vitamin D(3) and its synthetic analogs inhibit the spontaneous in vitro immunoglobulin production by SLE-derived PBMC. *Clin. Immunol.* **99,** 82–93.

Lips, P. (2001). Vitamin D deficiency and secondary hyperparathyroidism in the elderly: Consequences for bone loss and fractures and therapeutic implications. *Endocr. Rev.* **22,** 477–501.

Littorin, B., Blom, P., Scholin, A., Arnqvist, H. J., Blohme, G., Bolinder, J., Ekbom-Schnell, A., Eriksson, J. W., Gudbjornsdottir, S., Nystrom, L., Ostman, J., and Sundkvist, G. (2006). Lower levels of plasma 25-hydroxyvitamin D among young adults at diagnosis of autoimmune type 1 diabetes compared with control subjects: Results from the nationwide Diabetes Incidence Study in Sweden (DISS). *Diabetologia* **49,** 2847–2852.

Lyakh, L. A., Sanford, M., Chekol, S., Young, H. A., and Roberts, A. B. (2005). TGF-beta and vitamin D3 utilize distinct pathways to suppress IL-12 production and modulate rapid differentiation of human monocytes into CD83+ dendritic cells. *J. Immunol.* **15,** 2061–2070.

Ma, Y., *et al.* (2006). Identification and characterization of noncalcemic, tissue-selective, nonsecosteroidal vitamin D receptor modulators. *J. Clin. Invest.* **116,** 892–904.

Malabanan, A., Veronikis, I. E., and Holick, M. F. (1998). Redefining vitamin D insufficiency. *Lancet* **351,** 805–806.

Mathieu, C., and Adorini, L. (2002). The coming of age of 1,25-dihydroxyvitamin D(3) analogs as immunomodulatory agents. *Trends Mol. Med.* **8,** 174–179.

Merlino, L. A., Curtis, J., Mikuls, T. R., *et al.* (2004a). Vitamin D intake is inversely associated with rheumatoid arthritis: Results from the Iowa Women's Health Study. *Arthritis Rheum.* **50,** 72–77.

Merlino, L. A., *et al.* (2004b). Vitamin D intake is inversely associated with rheumatoid arthritis: Results from the Iowa Women's Health Study. *Arthritis Rheum.* **50,** 72–77.

Müller, K., Kriegbaum, N. J., Baslund, B., Sorensen, O. H., Thymann, M., and Bentzen, K. (1995). Vitamin D3 metabolism in patients with rheumatic diseases: Low serum levels of 25-hydroxyvitamin D3 in patients with systemic lupus erythematosus. *Clin. Rheumatol.* **14,** 397–400.

Nielen, M. M., van Schaardenburg, D., Lems, W., *et al.* (2006a). Vitamin D deficiency does not increase the risk of rheumatoid arthritis: Comment on the article by Merlino et al.. *Arthritis Rheum.* **54,** 3719–3720.

Nielen, M. M., *et al.* (2006b). Vitamin D deficiency does not increase the risk of rheumatoid arthritis: Comment on the article by Merlino et al.. *Arthritis Rheum.* **54,** 3719–3720.

O'Regan, S., Chesney, R. W., Hamstra, A., Eisman, J. A., O'Gorman, A. M., and Deluca, H. F. (1979). Reduced serum 1,25-(OH)2 vitamin D3 levels in prednisone-treated adolescents with systemic lupus erythematosus. *Acta Paediatr. Scand.* **68,** 109–111.

Oelzner, P., Muller, A., Deschner, F., *et al.* (1998). Relationship between disease activity and serum levels of vitamin D metabolites and PTH in rheumatoid arthritis. *Calcif. Tissue Int.* **62,** 193–198.

Orbach, H., Zandman-Goddard, G., Amital, H., Barak, V., Szekanecz, Z., Szucs, G., Danko, K., Nagy, E., Csepany, T., Carvalho, J. F., Doria, A., and Shoenfeld, Y. (2007). Novel biomarkers in autoimmune diseases. Prolactin, ferritin, vitamin D, and TPA levels in autoimmune diseases. *Ann. N. Y. Acad. Sci.* **1109,** 385–400.

Patel, S., *et al.* (2007). Association between serum vitamin D metabolite levels and disease activity in patients with early inflammatory polyarthritis. *Arthritis Rheum.* **56,** 2143–2149.

Penna, G., and Adorini, L. (2000). 1Alpha,25-dihydroxyvitamin D3 inhibits differentiation, maturation, activation, and survival of dendritic cells leading to impaired alloreactive T cell activation. *J. Immunol.* **164,** 2405–2411.

Roth, H. J., Schmidt-Gayk, H., Weber, H., and Niederau, C. (2008). Accuracy and clinical implications of seven 25-hydroxyvitamin D methods compared with liquid chromatography-tandem mass spectrometry as a reference. *Ann. Clin. Biochem.* **45,** 153–159.

Ruiz-Irastorza, G., Egurbide, M. V., Olivares, N., Martinez-Berriotxoa, A., and Aguirre, C. (2008). Vitamin D deficiency in systemic lupus erythematosus: Prevalence, predictors and clinical consequences. *Rheumatology* **47,** 920–923.

Ruiz-Irastorza, G., Gordo, S., Olivares, N., Egurbide, M. V., and Aguirre, C. (2010). Changes in vitamin D levels in patients with systemic lupus erythematosus: Effects on fatigue, disease activity, and damage. *Arthritis Care Res. (Hoboken).* **62**(8), 1160–1165. PubMed PMID: 20235208.

Sdeghi, K., Wessner, B., Laggner, U., *et al.* (2006). Vitamin D3 down-regulates monocyte TLR expression and triggers hyporesponsiveness to pathogen-associated molecular patterns. *Eur. J. Immunol.* **36,** 361–370.

Shapira, Y., Agmon-Levin, N., and Shoenfeld, Y. (2010). Defining and analyzing geoepidemiology and human autoimmunity. *J. Autoimmun.* **34,** J168–J177.

Shoenfeld, N., Amital, H., and Shoenfeld, Y. (2009). The effect of melanism and vitamin D synthesis on the incidence of autoimmune disease. *Nat. Clin. Pract. Rheumatol.* **5,** 99–105.

Sokka, T. (2010). Rheumatoid arthritis data bases in Finland. *Clin. Exp. Rheumatol.* **23** (Suppl. 39), S201–S204.

Stechschulte, S. A., Kirsner, R. S., and Federman, F. G. (2009). Vitamin D: Bone and beyond, rationale and recommendations for supplementation. *Am. J. Med.* **122,** 793–802.

Stockinger, B. (2007). Th17 cells: An orphan with influence. *Immunol. Cell Biol.* **85,** 83–84.

Teichmann, J., Lange, U., Stracke, H., Federlin, K., and Bretzel, R. G. (1999). Bone metabolism and bone mineral density of systemic lupus erythematosus at the time of diagnosis. *Rheumatol. Int.* **18,** 137–140.

Tetlow, L. C., and Woolley, D. E. (1999). The effects of 1 alpha,25-dihydroxyvitamin D(3) on matrix metalloproteinase and prostaglandin E(2) production by cells of the rheumatoid lesion. *Arthritis Res.* **1,** 63–70.

Thudi, A., Yin, S., Wandstrat, A. E., Quan-Zhen, L., and Olsen, N. J. (2008). Vitamin D levels and disease status in Texas patients with systemic lupus erythematosus. *Am. J. Med. Sci.* **335,** 99–104.

Toloza, S. M. A., Cole, D. E. C., Gladman, D. D., Ibanez, D., and Urowitz, M. B. (2010). Vitamin D insufficiency in a large female SLE cohort. *Lupus* **19,** 13–19.

van Etten, E., and Mathieu, C. (2005). Immunoregulation by 1,25-dihydroxyvitamin D3: Basic concepts. *J. Steroid Biochem. Mol. Biol.* **97,** 93–101.

Vieth, R., Ladak, Y., and Walfish, P. G. (2003). Age-related changes in the 25-hydroxyvitamin D versus parathyroid hormone relationship suggest a different reason why older adults require more vitamin D. *J. Clin. Endocrinol. Metab.* **88,** 185–191.

Wright, T. B., Shults, J., Leonard, M. B., Zemel, B. S., and Burnham, J. M. (2009). Hypovitaminosis D is associated with greater body mass index and disease activity in pediatric systemic lupus erythematosus. *J. Pediatr.* **155,** 260–265.

Wu, P. W., Rhew, E. Y., Dyer, A. R., Dunlop, D. D., Langman, C. B., Price, H., Sutton-Tyrrel, K., McPherson, D. D., Edmundowicz, D., Kondos, G. T., and Ramsey-Goldman, R. (2009). 25-Hydroxyvitamin D and cardiovascular risk factors in women with systemic lupus erythematosus. *Arthritis Rheum.* **61,** 1387–1395.

Xu, H., Soruri, A., Gieseler, R. K., and Peters, J. H. (1993). 1,25-Dihydroxyvitamin D3 exerts opposing effects to IL-4 on MHC class-II antigen. *Scand. J. Immunol.* **38,** 535–540.

Zold, E., Szodoray, P., Gaal, J., Kappelmayer, J., Csathy, L., Gyimesi, E., Zeher, M., Szegedi, G., and Bodolay, E. (2008). Vitamin D deficiency in undifferentiated connective tissue disease. *Arthritis Res. Ther.* **10,** R123.

CHAPTER FIFTEEN

L-Carnitine and Intestinal Inflammation

Geneviève Fortin

Contents

Abstract

The intestinal barrier is one of the most dynamic surfaces of the body. It is here where a single layer of epithelial cells mediates the intricate encounters that occur between the host's immune system and a multitude of potential threats present in the intestinal lumen. Several key factors play an important role in the final outcome of this interaction, including the state of oxidative stress, the level of activation of the immune cells, and the integrity of the epithelial barrier. This chapter describes the main evidence demonstrating the impact that L-carnitine has on each of these factors. These findings, combined with the demonstrated safety profile of L-carnitine, underscore the potential therapeutic value of L-carnitine supplementation in humans suffering from intestinal inflammation and highlight the functional data supporting an association between Crohn's disease and mutations in the L-carnitine transporter genes.

Department of Experimental Medicine, McGill University, Montreal, Quebec, Canada

Vitamins and Hormones, Volume 86
ISSN 0083-6729, DOI: 10.1016/B978-0-12-386960-9.00015-0

I. L-CARNITINE

A. Function

L-carnitine (γ-trimethylamino-β-hydroxybutyric acid) (Fig. 15.1) is a derivative of the amino acid lysine and is found in nearly all cells of the body. Although it was once thought to be a vitamin and was originally called "vitamin B_T," this turned out to be a misnomer when it was discovered that it could be biosynthesized in humans, mainly in the liver and kidneys. Nevertheless, under certain conditions, the physiological demand for L-carnitine may exceed an individual's capacity to synthesize it, thereby classifying it as a conditionally essential nutrient. Carnitine exists as two stereoisomers. While L-carnitine is biologically active, its enantiomer, D-carnitine, is believed to be biologically inactive (Liedtke *et al.*, 1982).

Dietary sources of L-carnitine include mainly meat and dairy products, with only very small amounts found in plants. L-Carnitine is transported across the cell membrane by two main organic cation transporters (OCTNs), OCTN1 and OCTN2. OCTNs are widely expressed in human tissues, including the heart, skeletal muscle, kidney, placenta, brain, and intestine. While OCTN1 is a multispecific and pH-dependent OCTN with lower affinity for L-carnitine, OCTN2, which has 75.8% sequence homology with OCTN1, functions as an Na^+-dependent transporter with greater affinity for L-carnitine (Tamai *et al.*, 1998).

Once inside the cell, the main physiological function of L-carnitine is to shuttle long-chain fatty acids (LCFA) across the mitochondrial membranes, where they are processed by β-oxidation to produce biological energy in the form of adenosine triphosphate (ATP). Thus, L-carnitine is most concentrated in tissues that use fatty acids as their primary fuel, such as skeletal and cardiac muscle. As depicted in Fig. 15.2, this transport requires three enzymes, which are located on the mitochondrial outer (CPTI) and inner (CPTII and translocase) membranes. Therefore, L-carnitine is primarily responsible for chaperoning activated fatty acids (acyl-CoA) into the mitochondrial matrix for energy production.

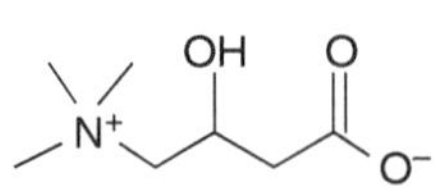

Figure 15.1 Chemical structure of L-carnitine.

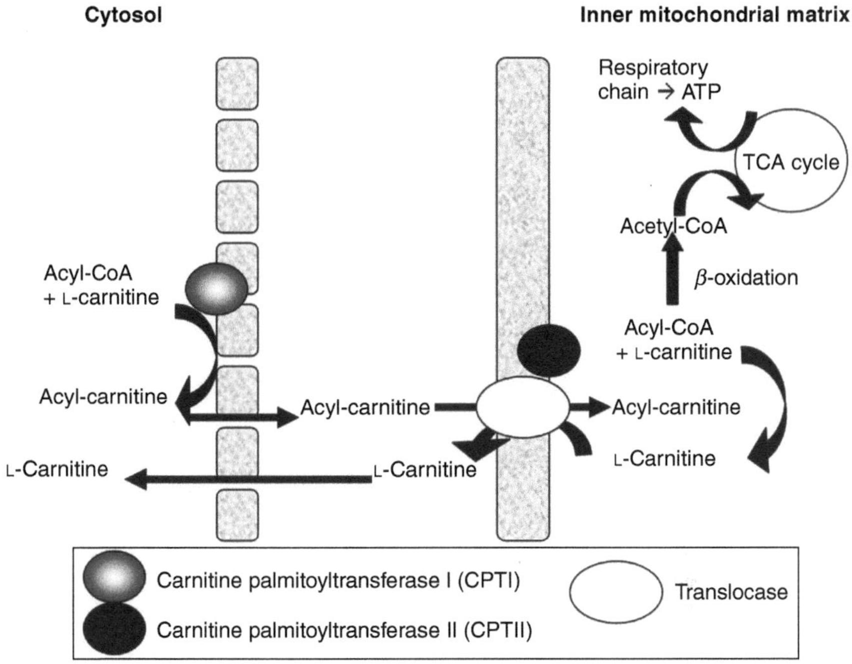

Figure 15.2 L-Carnitine in mitochondrial long-chain fatty acid transportation.

B. Carnitine deficiency

Primary carnitine deficiency is an autosomal recessive metabolic disorder caused by a deficiency in the carnitine transporters. The initial signs and symptoms of this disorder occur during infancy or early childhood and often include brain function abnormalities, cardiomyopathy, confusion, vomiting, muscle weakness, and hypoglycemia. Some patients may also experience serious complications, such as heart failure, liver disease, coma, and sudden unexpected death. Secondary carnitine deficiency occurs more commonly than primary carnitine deficiency and is most often associated with dialysis in chronic renal failure, although it can also be induced by intestinal resection, severe infection, and liver disease.

BALB/cByJ mice are an inbred substrain of BALB/c mice and are a useful tool for studying carnitine deficiency using an animal model. These mice were discovered to be short-chain acyl-CoA dehydrogenase (SCAD)-deficient by screening naturally occurring, "spontaneous" mutant mice for the excretion of urinary organic acids (Wood *et al.*, 1989). These mice display a defect in the conversion of short-chain fatty acids (SCFA) such as butyrate into acetyl-CoA, which is important for the generation of ATP by in the Krebs cycle. Butyrate therefore accumulates inside the mitochondria and is converted to butyryl-L-carnitine by carnitine acetyltransferase. During this conversion, carnitine stores are used up, resulting in carnitine deficiency (Wood *et al.*, 1989). This carnitine deficiency then impairs the uptake of LCFA, because carnitine is necessary for their mitochondrial transport. Therefore, BALB/cByJ mice display several biochemical abnormalities, including a form of secondary carnitine deficiency (Turnbull *et al.*, 1984).

C. Therapeutic applications of L-carnitine

The most frequent therapeutic application of L-carnitine therapy is in the treatment of primary and secondary L-carnitine deficiencies. However, it has also been successfully used as an adjunct therapy in treating conditions related to myocardial ischemia, such as myocardial infarctions (Lopaschuk, 2000), heart failure (Rizos, 2000), and angina pectoris (Cacciatore *et al.*, 1991), as well as in the treatment of intermittent claudication in peripheral arterial disease (Hiatt, 2004), in HIV/AIDS (Moretti *et al.*, 1998), and male infertility (Lenzi *et al.*, 2004). The therapeutic benefits of L-carnitine in these diseases were mainly attributed to its role in energy metabolism and as an antioxidant, as discussed in further detail later in this chapter.

Presently, intravenous and oral L-carnitine are available by prescription for the treatment of primary and secondary L-carnitine deficiencies. Doses for L-carnitine therapy are determined on a patient-by-patient basis, but are generally in the range of 500–6000 mg/day. This would translate into ~10–100 mg/kg based on an average weight of 70 kg. A number of clinical trials in the fields of heart disease, atherosclerosis, chronic renal failure/dialysis, Alzheimer's disease, HIV/AIDS, and male infertility have also addressed the therapeutic efficacy of similar doses of L-carnitine.

L-carnitine is also available without a prescription as a nutritional supplement and has been used at a dose of 40–80 mg/kg to improve athletic performance (Marconi *et al.*, 1985; Vecchiet *et al.*, 1990). In all these settings, L-carnitine therapy was well tolerated and no toxic effects of L-carnitine overdose have been reported. Nevertheless, L-carnitine supplementation was said to be associated with some mild side effects, including nausea, vomiting, diarrhea, and a "fishy" body odor at doses above 3000 mg/day.

II. Intestinal Inflammation

A. Pathological processes leading to intestinal inflammation

There are many potential causes for intestinal inflammation. As shown in Table 15.1, these can generally be categorized as either intestinal diseases or intestinal disorders.

Table 15.1 Pathologies of the gastrointestinal tract resulting in inflammation

Intestinal diseases	
Gastroenteritis	Inflammation of the stomach and the intestines, with vomiting and diarrhea, usually as a result of a bacterial or viral infection (Encarta® World English Dictionary, 2009)
Appendicitis	Inflammation of the appendix, causing severe pain (Encarta® World English Dictionary, 2009)
Celiac disease	A disease characterized by sensitivity to gluten, with chronic inflammation and atrophy of the mucosa of the upper small intestine (Lippincott Williams & Wilkins, 2008)
Crohn's disease	A chronic inflammatory disease of unknown cause, involving the terminal ileum and less frequently other parts of the gastrointestinal tract; characterized by patchy deep ulcers that may cause fistulas, and narrowing and thickening of the bowel by fibrosis and lymphocytic infiltration (Lippincott Williams & Wilkins, 2008)
Ulcerative colitis	A chronic disease of unknown cause characterized by ulceration of the colon and rectum, with rectal bleeding, mucosal crypt abscesses, inflammatory pseudopolyps, abdominal pain, and diarrhea (Lippincott Williams & Wilkins, 2008)
Intestinal disorders	
Irritable bowel syndrome (IBS)	A condition characterized by gastrointestinal signs and symptoms including constipation, diarrhea, gas, and bloating, all in the absence of organic pathology. Associated with uncoordinated contractions of the large intestine. Some patients with IBS have an increased number of inflammatory cells in the colonic and ileal mucosa. Previous episodes of infectious enteritis, genetic factors, undiagnosed food allergies, and changes in bacterial microflora may all play a role in promoting and perpetuating this low-grade inflammatory process (Lippincott Williams & Wilkins, 2008; Barbara *et al.*, 2002)
Diverticulosis	Presence of a number of diverticula of the intestine, common in middle age (Lippincott Williams & Wilkins, 2008)

Although currently there is a paucity of data describing the role of L-carnitine in most of the pathologies described in Table 15.1, there have been a number of publications describing the links between L-carnitine and the development and treatment of Crohn's disease, a member of the inflammatory bowel disease (IBD) family, of which ulcerative colitis is the other member. This chapter will therefore focus mainly on the role of L-carnitine in Crohn's disease.

Crohn's disease is caused by the aberrant activation of cells of both the innate and the adaptive immune systems, resulting in a "vicious cycle" of inflammation within the digestive tract. In the intestinal tissues, activated $CD4^+$ T cells induce the release of proinflammatory mediators such as cytokines, chemokines, and reactive oxygen species (ROS) from innate and epithelial cells. The swelling that results from this ongoing inflammatory process can cause pain and can make the intestines empty frequently, resulting in diarrhea.

Crohn's disease can be distinguished from ulcerative colitis, in that the inflammation associated with Crohn's disease is transmural, while the inflammatory changes in ulcerative colitis typically involve only the superficial mucosal and submucosal layers of the intestinal wall. Additionally, in Crohn's disease, the inflammation is often discontinuous, patchy, and segmental and results in the formation of granulomas (aggregation of macrophages). It can affect the patient anywhere in the gastrointestinal tract from the mouth to the anus, but most commonly involves the ileum and the colon. In contrast, the inflammatory changes in ulcerative colitis typically extend proximally from the rectum up to varying degrees in the colon, but do not affect any other portion of the digestive tract. Moreover, the extraintestinal manifestations characteristic of Crohn's disease are not observed in UC patients.

B. Common treatments for intestinal inflammation

The treatment for Crohn's disease has changed dramatically over the past decade with the introduction of biological therapy and the increased use of immunomodulators. Biological therapies, such as anti-TNFα agents, allow a more profound control of intestinal inflammation compared with conventional therapies and often result in improved clinical parameters, including mucosal healing. Although many of these therapies can induce rapid mucosal healing, improve the quality of life, and help to avoid hospitalization and surgery in many Crohn's disease patients, some do not respond at all or eventually develop infusion reactions and delayed serum-sickness and secondary loss of effectiveness of therapy.

However, probiotics, prebiotics, and nutritional supplements have also attracted a great deal of interest for the treatment of intestinal inflammation, including Crohn's disease, and usually display a low efficacy but high safety profile. There certainly still is a need to develop new therapeutic regimens to treat Crohn's disease.

III. L-Carnitine and Intestinal Inflammation

A. OCTNs and their association with Crohn's disease

The IBD5 locus on chromosome 5q31 was originally described in a Canadian population (Rioux *et al.*, 2000). Subsequent studies identified a 250-kb risk haplotype within this locus that was significantly associated with Crohn's disease (Armuzzi *et al.*, 2003; Giallourakis *et al.*, 2003; Mirza *et al.*, 2003; Rioux *et al.*, 2001). However, due to strong linkage disequilibrium in this area, there remains a degree of uncertainty as to the identity of the causal variant within this region. This is further compounded by the fact that this region contains several genes implicated in the maintenance of epithelial integrity and/or immunoregulation, including *interferon regulatory factor-1* (*IRF1*), *IL-4*, *IL-5*, *IL-13*, *PDZ and LIM domain protein 4* (*PDLIM4*), and *prolyl 4-hydroxylase α-2 subunit precursor* (*P4HA2*), in addition to *OCTN1* and *OCTN2* (Van Limbergen *et al.*, 2007).

Nevertheless, polymorphisms in *OCTN1* (*SLC22A4*, missense substitution 1672C → T) and the *OCTN2* promoter (*SLC22A5*, transversion −207 G → C) were originally proposed as the causal variants in patients of European decent, since these two SNPs constituted a two-point risk haplotype for Crohn's disease, demonstrating strong association independently of genotype at other SNPs in the IBD5 locus (Peltekova *et al.*, 2004). Furthermore, these SNPs translated into reduced function and expression of OCTN1 and OCTN2, respectively, and in functional impairments in L-carnitine uptake (Peltekova *et al.*, 2004; Vermeire *et al.*, 2005). A subsequent study noted an association between pediatric-onset Crohn's disease and *OCTN1/2* mutations (Cucchiara *et al.*, 2007). Similar to *NOD2* mutations, the association of *OCTN1/2* mutations to Crohn's disease susceptibility has only been observed in Western populations, with no documented association in a Chinese population (Li *et al.*, 2008). Several reports in Western populations have also questioned the causative role for *OCTN1/2* mutations in the IBD5 locus (Noble *et al.*, 2005). One such study found that several other genes, including *IRF1*, *PDLIM*, and *P4HA2*, may be equally as likely to contain the IBD5 causal variant as the *OCTN* genes (Silverberg *et al.*, 2007). Another study reported that no definitive conclusions could be drawn about *OCTN* variants as causative genes in pediatric Crohn's disease (Babusukumar *et al.*, 2006). Interestingly, one study found that while mutations in *OCTN1/2* did not play a role in the susceptibility to Crohn's disease in the Flemish population, they did alter the phenotypic expression of the disease since *OCTN1/2* variants were associated with the development of perianal and penetrating Crohn's disease (Vermeire *et al.*, 2005).

Although *OCTN1* and *OCTN2* are thought to be widely expressed, *in situ* hybridization data suggested that the expression of both genes was limited to the intestinal epithelium, macrophages, and T cells, but not B cells (Peltekova *et al.*, 2004). This is of particular interest, since a recent study demonstrated that L-carnitine does not exert any immunosuppressive effect on B cells, but does suppress the activation and cytokine production of macrophages, and dendritic cells (DCs) and T cells, the cells that are prominently implicated in Crohn's disease pathogenesis (Fortin *et al.*, 2009). Interestingly, *OCTN* mutations were also shown to increase susceptibility to rheumatoid arthritis (RA; Tokuhiro *et al.*, 2003), further underscoring the implication of these genes in chronic inflammatory diseases.

B. Antioxidant activities of L-carnitine

Oxidative stress is caused by an imbalance in the production of ROS, such as oxygen ions, free radicals, and peroxides, and a biological system's ability to quench them or repair damaged tissues. ROS have the potential to damage various cellular components, including the lipids of the various membranes of the cell and the DNA and RNA. To dampen the destructive effects of ROS, tissues are equipped with an intricate antioxidant system, which includes the production of enzymes such as superoxide dismutases, catalases, glutathione peroxidases, and peroxiredoxins. Small-molecule antioxidants such as Vitamin C, Vitamin E, uric acid, and glutathione also play an important role in the defense against ROS.

Oxidative stress is known to play a pathogenic role in several diseases such as atherosclerosis, Parkinson's disease, heart disease, myocardial infarction, Alzheimer's disease, and chronic fatigue syndrome. While an enhanced production of ROS has been demonstrated in the inflamed tissues of Crohn's disease patients, their role in disease pathogenesis has not been fully understood. It is believed that T cell-derived IL-2 and IFN-γ activate tissue macrophages to release a variety of proinflammatory cytokines and mediators, including TNF-α, IL-1β, IL-12, nitric oxide (NO), and ROS. While this mechanism is critical for the protection from pathogens, uncontrolled mucosal immune responses may result in tissue damage and the perpetuation of chronic intestinal inflammation.

Many diet components or natural compounds act as antioxidants to suppress the production of ROS and play a critical role in preventing inflammation and cancer (Frenkel, 1992; Halliwell and Gutteridge, 1984). Recent studies have demonstrated that L-carnitine can act as an antioxidant and protect from ROS-induced tissue damage (Rauchova *et al.*, 2002; Wang *et al.*, 2007). In fact, L-carnitine was more effective at inhibiting lipid peroxidation than both trolox and Vitamin E, two widely recognized antioxidants (Gulcin, 2006). Moreover, by promoting the mitochondrial transport of LCFAs and the generation of ATP by β-oxidation, L-carnitine acts to reduce the cellular oxygen concentration and the generation of ROS (Fritz and Marquis, 1965; Rebouche, 1992; Rebouche and Engel, 1980). By acting as an antioxidant in the gastrointestinal tract, L-carnitine may promote an anti-inflammatory local tissue environment.

C. Immunosuppressive properties of L-carnitine

Apart from its antioxidant properties, L-carnitine has also been shown to be directly immunosuppressive by inducing the activation and nuclear translocation of the glucocorticoid receptor alpha (GRα) in mice (Alesci *et al.*, 2003). In the absence of glucocorticoids, GRα is normally found in the cytoplasm, bound to receptor-associated proteins (RAP) that maintain a level of inactivity. However, upon ligand binding, the RAP dissociate from GRα, leading to its activation, translocation into the nucleus, homodimerization, and the transcription of many genes (Bamberger *et al.*, 1996). L-Carnitine is thought to function as an allosteric regulator of GRα, binding to an area outside the glucocorticoid-binding pocket, but ultimately resulting in conformational changes similar to those induced by glucocorticoids. The evidence to support this hypothesis comes mainly from competitive binding assays, where L-carnitine administration reduced the affinity of GRα for dexamethasone while, at the same time, inducing GRα translocation to the nucleus and the transcription of glucocorticoid-responsive genes (Manoli *et al.*, 2004). In support of this, pharmacological doses of L-carnitine markedly suppressed lipopolysaccharide (LPS)-induced cytokine production and improved survival rates during cachexia and septic shock (Winter *et al.*, 1995). Although L-carnitine has been shown to activate GRα and mimic some of the effects of glucocorticoids on immune function, it was also proved to protect osteoblasts from apoptosis (Colucci *et al.*, 2005) and may therefore exert the beneficial anti-inflammatory effects of glucocorticoids without the serious side effects on bone.

The immunosuppressive properties of L-carnitine were further supported both *in vitro* and *in vivo* in a recent study. *In vitro*, LCAR dose-dependently suppressed DC and macrophage costimulatory molecule expression and inhibited purified $CD4^+$ T cell activation and cytokine production (Fortin *et al.*, 2009). T cells isolated from Balb/cByJ mice were hyperactivated, suggesting that an endogenous reduction in L-carnitine levels may predispose an individual to enhanced immune responses. The supplementation of the cell cultures with exogenous L-carnitine had an immunosuppressive effect in cells isolated from both Balb/c and Balb/cByJ mice (Fortin *et al.*, 2009).

These findings have a significant clinical importance since, as discussed earlier, mutations in the *OCTN1* and *OCTN2* genes have been shown to result in poor L-carnitine transport and have been linked to increased susceptibility to Crohn's disease (Peltekova *et al.*, 2004). Although the molecular events involved in the immunosuppressive characteristics of

L-carnitine *in vitro* were not investigated in the study by Fortin *et al.*, the previously described antioxidant and GRα-activating properties of L-carnitine are likely to play an important role.

In vivo, treatment with L-carnitine successfully reduced body weight loss, cytokine production, and intestinal inflammation in TNBS colitis, a murine model of Crohn's disease (Fortin *et al.*, 2009). TNBS colitis mimics human Crohn's disease in that it generates mucosal inflammation which is dependent upon the presence of bacteria in the gut lumen and results in the transmural infiltration of mononuclear cells (Neurath *et al.*, 1995). Although once thought to be primarily driven by adaptive immune responses, innate cells are now recognized as playing a key role in the initiation phase of TNBS colitis (Santucci *et al.*, 2007). T cells, however, are likely implicated in the amplification and perpetuation of inflammation (Sheibanie *et al.*, 2007). In support of their *in vitro* data, Fortin *et al.* also demonstrated that systemic administration of free L-carnitine was effective in treating TNBS colitis. This protection was characterized by an improvement in all clinical and histological criteria in mice treated with daily injections of L-carnitine and was associated with a suppressive effect on the colonic mRNA expression and serum levels of IL-1β and IL-6. Importantly, LCAR was also effective in dampening antigen-specific T cell responses in the colon-draining lymph nodes of mice with chronic TNBS colitis (Fortin *et al.*, 2009).

In humans, evidence of an immunosuppressive role for L-carnitine lies in the observation that TNFα levels were reduced after *ex vivo* stimulation of human neutrophils with *Staphylococcus aureus* (Fattorossi *et al.*, 1993) and after L-carnitine supplementation in surgical and AIDS patients (De Simone *et al.*, 1993; Delogu *et al.*, 1993).

D. Protection of the intestinal epithelial barrier

The primary evidence to support a role for L-carnitine in the protection of the intestinal epithelial barrier comes from the observation that mice deficient in OCTN2, one of the carnitine transporters, develop spontaneous atrophy of intestinal epithelial cells and colonic inflammation (Shekhawat *et al.*, 2007). The pathology observed in these mice was mainly attributed to alterations in the intestinal and colonic structure and morphology, as a result of enhanced apoptosis of gut epithelial cells and a subsequent breakdown in barrier function (Shekhawat *et al.*, 2007).

A study investigating the role of carnitine transporters in butyrate metabolism in colonocytes demonstrated a protective role of the local administration of carnitine-loaded liposomes in TNBS colitis (D'Argenio *et al.*, 2006). Since carnitine is required for beta-oxidation, it was suggested that a reduction in carnitine uptake could lead to impaired fatty acid oxidation in intestinal epithelial cells and to cell injury. This hypothesis was investigated by examining the expression of the carnitine transporters and butyrate metabolism in colonocytes in TNBS colitis. The expression of the carnitine transporters was decreased in inflammatory samples at both the translational and the functional levels (D'Argenio *et al.*, 2006). Butyrate oxidation was also affected in colonocytes isolated from TNBS-treated rats, which could be corrected by treatment with carnitine-loaded liposomes *in vitro* (D'Argenio *et al.*, 2006). The administration of these carnitine-loaded liposomes *in vivo* reduced the severity of colitis, suggesting that carnitine depletion in colonocytes is associated with the inability to maintain normal butyrate metabolism and protect from inflammation (D'Argenio *et al.*, 2006).

IV. Conclusions and Future Directions

The intestinal barrier is one of the most dynamic surfaces of the body. It is here where a single layer of epithelial cells mediates the intricate encounters that occur between the underlying cells of the host's immune system and a multitude of potential threats, including food antigens, bacteria, viruses, parasites, and more. Several key factors play an important role in the final outcome of this interaction, including the state of oxidative stress, the level of activation of the immune cells, and the integrity of the epithelial barrier. This chapter described how L-carnitine plays a role in each of these key factors.

First, L-carnitine can act as an antioxidant and protect from ROS-induced tissue damage. Second, L-carnitine can suppress the activation and cytokine production of both innate and adaptive immune cells. Third, L-carnitine promotes the integrity of the intestinal epithelial barrier. These functions of L-carnitine were further supported by data from two independent investigators who both demonstrated a beneficial therapeutic effect of L-carnitine using an animal model of intestinal inflammation.

While the association between mutations in the *OCTN* genes and Crohn's disease susceptibility has not been replicated worldwide, the extensive functional data demonstrating an important role for L-carnitine in intestinal homeostasis support the aforementioned candidate gene in predisposing individuals to Crohn's disease. These findings, combined with the demonstrated safety profile of L-carnitine, highlight the potential therapeutic value of L-carnitine supplementation in humans suffering from intestinal inflammation.

REFERENCES

Alesci, S., *et al.* (2003). L-carnitine: A nutritional modulator of glucocorticoid receptor functions. *FASEB J.* **17,** 1553–1555.

Armuzzi, A., *et al.* (2003). Genotype–phenotype analysis of the Crohn's disease susceptibility haplotype on chromosome 5q31. *Gut* **52,** 1133–1139.

Babusukumar, U., *et al.* (2006). Contribution of OCTN variants within the IBD5 locus to pediatric onset Crohn's disease. *Am. J. Gastroenterol.* **101,** 1354–1361.
Bamberger, C. M., *et al.* (1996). Molecular determinants of glucocorticoid receptor function and tissue sensitivity to glucocorticoids. *Endocr. Rev.* **17,** 245–261.
Barbara, G., *et al.* (2002). A role for inflammation in irritable bowel syndrome? *Gut* **51,** i41–i44.
Cacciatore, L., *et al.* (1991). The therapeutic effect of L-carnitine in patients with exercise-induced stable angina: A controlled study. *Drugs Exp. Clin. Res.* **17,** 225–235.
Colucci, S., *et al.* (2005). L-carnitine and isovaleryl L-carnitine fumarate positively affect human osteoblast proliferation and differentiation in vitro. *Calcif. Tissue Int.* **76,** 458–465.
Cucchiara, S., *et al.* (2007). Role of CARD15, DLG5 and OCTN genes polymorphisms in children with inflammatory bowel diseases. *World J. Gastroenterol.* **13,** 1221–1229.
D'Argenio, G., *et al.* (2006). Experimental colitis: Decreased Octn2 and Atb0+ expression in rat colonocytes induces carnitine depletion that is reversible by carnitine-loaded liposomes. *FASEB J.* **20,** 2544–2546.
De Simone, C., *et al.* (1993). High dose L-carnitine improves immunologic and metabolic parameters in AIDS patients. *Immunopharmacol. Immunotoxicol.* **15,** 1–12.
Delogu, G., *et al.* (1993). Anaesthetics modulate tumour necrosis factor alpha: Effects of L-carnitine supplementation in surgical patients. Preliminary results. *Mediators Inflamm.* **2,** S33–S36.
Encarta® World English Dictionary [North American Edition] (2009). Developed for Microsoft by Bloomsbury Publishing Plc.
Fattorossi, A., *et al.* (1993). Regulation of normal human polyrnorphonuclear leucocytes by carnitine. *Mediators Inflamm.* **2,** S37–S41.
Fortin, G., *et al.* (2009). L-carnitine, a diet component and organic cation transporter OCTN ligand, displays immunosuppressive properties and abrogates intestinal inflammation. *Clin. Exp. Immunol.* **156,** 161–171.
Frenkel, K. (1992). Carcinogen-mediated oxidant formation and oxidative DNA damage. *Pharmacol. Ther.* **53,** 127–166.
Fritz, I. B., and Marquis, N. R. (1965). The role of acylcarnitine esters and carnitine palmityltransferase in the transport of fatty acyl groups across mitochondrial membranes. *Proc. Natl. Acad. Sci. USA* **54,** 1226–1233.
Giallourakis, C., *et al.* (2003). IBD5 is a general risk factor for inflammatory bowel disease: Replication of association with Crohn disease and identification of a novel association with ulcerative colitis. *Am. J. Hum. Genet.* **73,** 205–211.
Gulcin, I. (2006). Antioxidant and antiradical activities of L-carnitine. *Life Sci.* **78,** 803–811.
Halliwell, B., and Gutteridge, J. M. (1984). Lipid peroxidation, oxygen radicals, cell damage, and antioxidant therapy. *Lancet* **1,** 1396–1397.
Hiatt, W. R. (2004). Carnitine and peripheral arterial disease. *Ann. NY Acad. Sci.* **1033,** 92–98.
Lenzi, A., *et al.* (2004). A placebo-controlled double-blind randomized trial of the use of combined l-carnitine and l-acetyl-carnitine treatment in men with asthenozoospermia. *Fertil. Steril.* **81,** 1578–1584.
Li, M., *et al.* (2008). OCTN and CARD15 gene polymorphism in Chinese patients with inflammatory bowel disease. *World J. Gastroenterol.* **14,** 4923–4927.
Liedtke, A. J., *et al.* (1982). Metabolic and mechanical effects using L- and D-carnitine in working swine hearts. *Am. J. Physiol.* **243,** H691–H697.
Lippincott Williams & Wilkins (2008). Stedman's Medical Dictionary for the Health Professions and Nursing. Lippincott Williams & Wilkins, Philadelphia, PA.
Lopaschuk, G. (2000). Regulation of carbohydrate metabolism in ischemia and reperfusion. *Am. Heart J.* **139,** S115–S119.

Manoli, I., *et al.* (2004). Modulatory effects of L-carnitine on glucocorticoid receptor activity. *Ann. NY Acad. Sci.* **1033,** 147–157.
Marconi, C., *et al.* (1985). Effects of L-carnitine loading on the aerobic and anaerobic performance of endurance athletes. *Eur. J. Appl. Physiol. Occup. Physiol.* **54,** 131–135.
Mirza, M. M., *et al.* (2003). Genetic evidence for interaction of the 5q31 cytokine locus and the CARD15 gene in Crohn disease. *Am. J. Hum. Genet.* **72,** 1018–1022.
Moretti, S., *et al.* (1998). Effect of L-carnitine on human immunodeficiency virus-1 infection-associated apoptosis: A pilot study. *Blood* **91,** 3817–3824.
Neurath, M. F., *et al.* (1995). Antibodies to interleukin 12 abrogate established experimental colitis in mice. *J. Exp. Med.* **182,** 1281–1290.
Noble, C. L., *et al.* (2005). The contribution of OCTN1/2 variants within the IBD5 locus to disease susceptibility and severity in Crohn's disease. *Gastroenterology* **129,** 1854–1864.
Peltekova, V. D., *et al.* (2004). Functional variants of OCTN cation transporter genes are associated with Crohn disease. *Nat. Genet.* **36,** 471–475.
Rauchova, H., *et al.* (2002). Hypoxia-induced lipid peroxidation in rat brain and protective effect of carnitine and phosphocreatine. *Neurochem. Res.* **27,** 899–904.
Rebouche, C. J. (1992). Carnitine function and requirements during the life cycle. *FASEB J.* **6,** 3379–3386.
Rebouche, C. J., and Engel, A. G. (1980). Tissue distribution of carnitine biosynthetic enzymes in man. *Biochim. Biophys. Acta* **630,** 22–29.
Rioux, J. D., *et al.* (2000). Genomewide search in Canadian families with inflammatory bowel disease reveals two novel susceptibility loci. *Am. J. Hum. Genet.* **66,** 1863–1870.
Rioux, J. D., *et al.* (2001). Genetic variation in the 5q31 cytokine gene cluster confers susceptibility to Crohn disease. *Nat. Genet.* **29,** 223–228.
Rizos, I. (2000). Three-year survival of patients with heart failure caused by dilated cardiomyopathy and L-carnitine administration. *Am. Heart J.* **139,** S120–S123.
Santucci, L., *et al.* (2007). GITR modulates innate and adaptive mucosal immunity during the development of experimental colitis in mice. *Gut* **56,** 52–60.
Sheibanie, A. F., *et al.* (2007). The proinflammatory effect of prostaglandin E2 in experimental inflammatory bowel disease is mediated through the IL-23–>IL-17 axis. *J. Immunol.* **178,** 8138–8147.
Shekhawat, P. S., *et al.* (2007). Spontaneous development of intestinal and colonic atrophy and inflammation in the carnitine-deficient jvs (OCTN2(−/−)) mice. *Mol. Genet. Metab.* **92,** 315–324.
Silverberg, M. S., *et al.* (2007). Refined genomic localization and ethnic differences observed for the IBD5 association with Crohn's disease. *Eur. J. Hum. Genet.* **15,** 328–335.
Tamai, I., *et al.* (1998). Molecular and functional identification of sodium ion-dependent, high affinity human carnitine transporter OCTN2. *J. Biol. Chem.* **273,** 20378–20382.
Tokuhiro, S., *et al.* (2003). An intronic SNP in a RUNX1 binding site of SLC22A4, encoding an organic cation transporter, is associated with rheumatoid arthritis. *Nat. Genet.* **35,** 341–348.
Turnbull, D. M., *et al.* (1984). Short-chain acyl-CoA dehydrogenase deficiency associated with a lipid-storage myopathy and secondary carnitine deficiency. *N. Engl. J. Med.* **311,** 1232–1236.
Van Limbergen, J., *et al.* (2007). Genetics of the innate immune response in inflammatory bowel disease. *Inflamm. Bowel Dis.* **13,** 338–355.
Vecchiet, L., *et al.* (1990). Influence of L-carnitine administration on maximal physical exercise. *Eur. J. Appl. Physiol. Occup. Physiol.* **61,** 486–490.
Vermeire, S., *et al.* (2005). Association of organic cation transporter risk haplotype with perianal penetrating Crohn's disease but not with susceptibility to IBD. *Gastroenterology* **129,** 1845–1853.

Wang, C., *et al.* (2007). L-carnitine protects neurons from 1-methyl-4-phenylpyridinium-induced neuronal apoptosis in rat forebrain culture. *Neuroscience* **144,** 46–55.
Winter, B. K., *et al.* (1995). Effects of L-carnitine on serum triglyceride and cytokine levels in rat models of cachexia and septic shock. *Br. J. Cancer* **72,** 1173–1179.
Wood, P. A., *et al.* (1989). Short-chain acyl-coenzyme A dehydrogenase deficiency in mice. *Pediatr. Res.* **25,** 38–43.

CHAPTER SIXTEEN

Vitamin D and Inflammatory Bowel Disease

Sandro Ardizzone,* Andrea Cassinotti,* Maurizio Bevilacqua,[†] Mario Clerici,[‡,§] *and* Gabriele Bianchi Porro*

Contents

Abstract

Crohn's disease (CD) and ulcerative colitis (UC) are the main forms of inflammatory bowel disease (IBD), chronic relapsing-remitting inflammatory conditions of uncertain origin affecting the gastrointestinal tract.

Much effort has recently been made both in defining the mechanisms underlying the development of IBD, and in broadening the spectrum of effective treatment. Substantial progress has been made in characterising immune-cell populations and inflammatory mediators in IBD.

1,25-Dihydroxyvitamin D_3 [1,25$(OH)_2D_3$], the bioactive form of Vitamin D_3, besides having well-known control findings of calcium and phosphorus metabolism, bone formation and mineralization, also has a role in the maintenance of immune- omeostasis. The immune-regulatory role of vitamin D affects both the innate and adaptive immune system contributing to the immune-tolerance of self-structures. Impaired vitamin D supply/regulation, amongst other factors, leads to the development of autoimmune processes in animal models of various autoimmune diseases, including IBD. The administration of vitamin D in these animals leads to improvement of immune-mediated symptoms. Future studies now need to focus on the potential of vitamin D and its derivatives as therapeutic adjuncts in the treatment of IBD. © 2011 Elsevier Inc.

* Department of Gastroenterology, "L. Sacco" University Hospital, Milan, Italy
† Endocrinology Unit, Department of Clinical Science, "L. Sacco" University Hospital, Milan, Italy
‡ Chair of Immunology, DISP LITA Vialba, University of Milan, Milan, Italy
§ DISTeB LITA Segrate, University of Milan, Milan, Italy

Vitamins and Hormones, Volume 86
ISSN 0083-6729, DOI: 10.1016/B978-0-12-386960-9.00016-2

I. Introduction

Crohn's disease (CD) and ulcerative colitis (UC) are the main forms of inflammatory bowel disease (IBD), chronic relapsing–remitting inflammatory conditions of uncertain origin affecting the gastrointestinal tract (Podolsky, 1991).

Much effort has recently been made both in defining the mechanisms underlying the development of IBD and in broadening the spectrum of effective treatment (Baumgart and Carding, 2007). It is now widely accepted that IBD results from an inappropriate response of a defective mucosal immune system to unknown luminal antigens (probably environmental or infective, including indigenous microflora) in a genetically predisposed subject (Ardizzone and Bianchi Porro, 2002). Substantial progress has been made in characterizing immune cell populations and inflammatory mediators in IBD. In particular, IBD develops due to an immune-mediated attack by pathogenic T cells that overproduce interleukin-17 (IL-17) and interferon-gamma (IFN)-γ and a few regulatory cells (Fiocchi, 2008; Scaldaferri and Fiocchi, 2007).

1,25-Dihydroxyvitamin D_3 [1,25$(OH)_2D_3$], the bioactive form of vitamin D_3, besides having well-known control findings of calcium and phosphorus metabolism, bone formation, and mineralization, also has a role in the maintenance of immune homeostasis. The immune regulatory role of vitamin D affects both the innate and adaptive immune system contributing to the immune-tolerance of self-structures. Impaired vitamin D supply/regulation, among other factors, leads to the development of autoimmune processes in animal models of various autoimmune diseases. The administration of vitamin D in these animals leads to improvement of immune-mediated symptoms. Moreover, in human autoimmune diseases, such as multiple sclerosis, rheumatoid arthritis, systemic lupus erythematosus, and possibly also type I diabetes, IBD, and autoimmune prostatitis, the pathogenic role of vitamin D has been described (Adorini and Penna, 2008; Szodoray *et al.*, 2008).

With this background, we aimed to review the regulation of immune responses, highlighting its potentially beneficial effects in the treatment of IBD.

A. Vitamin D and the immune system

Vitamin D_3 is hydroxylated in the liver to produce 25$(OH)D_3$, a reliable indicator of vitamin D status, and is further hydroxylated in the kidney to form the active hormone 1,25$(OH)_2D_3$ (Holick, 2007).

A major source of vitamin D results from its manufacture via a photolysis reaction in the skin, and vitamin D available from sunlight exposure is significantly less in northern climates and especially low during the winter (Fiocchi, 2008; Szodoray *et al.*, 2008). In addition, dietary intake of vitamin D is problematic as there are few foods that are naturally rich in vitamin D. There is mounting evidence for a link between vitamin D availability either from sunshine or from diet and the prevalence of autoimmune diseases (Lai and Gallo, 2009).

The biological effects of vitamin D_3 are mediated by the vitamin D receptor (VDR), which belongs to the superfamily of nuclear hormone receptors and is expressed in most cell types. Ligand binding induces conformational changes in the VDR, which promote heterodimerization with the retinoid X receptor and the recruitment of corepressor and coactivator proteins. Thus, the VDR functions as a ligand-activated transcription factor that binds to vitamin D-responsive elements in the promoter region of vitamin D-responsive genes, and ultimately influences the rate of RNA-polymerase-II-mediated transcription of these genes (Wang *et al.*, 2004).

Vitamin D and the VDR have been shown to be important regulators of the immune system. In particular, vitamin D and VDR deficiency exacerbates experimental autoimmune diseases such as IBD. IBD develops due to an immune-mediated attack by pathogenic T cells that overproduce IL-17 and IFN-γ and a few regulatory cells. VDR knockout mice have twice as many T cells making IL-17 and IFN-γ than wild-type mice. In addition, vitamin D and the VDR are required for normal numbers of regulatory T cells (iNKT and CD8aa) that have been shown to suppress experimental IBD. In the absence of vitamin D and the VDR, autoimmunity occurs in the gastrointestinal tract due to increased numbers of IL-17 and IFN-γ secreting T cells and a concomitant reduction in regulatory T cells (Adorini and Penna, 2008; Holick, 2007; Szodoray *et al.*, 2008; Weber *et al.*, 2005).

Recent research has begun to unravel important roles of vitamin D in the regulation of innate immunity (Gombart *et al.*, 2005; Lai and Gallo, 2009; Liu *et al.*, 2006; Wang *et al.*, 2004; Weber *et al.*, 2005). Unlike the adaptive immune system, the innate immune system is responsible for nonspecific defense against pathogens. Stimulation of this system triggers the release of cytokines and chemokines, which are important for the culmination of the innate immune response, as well as recruitment and activation of cells of the adaptive immune system to the site of infection. In response to bacterial pathogens, the innate immune response includes the production and release of antimicrobial peptides (AMPs). Treatment of several cell lines or primary cell cultures with 1,25D induced the expression of two AMPs, human b-defensin 2 *(DEFB2/DEFB4/HBD2)* and cathelicidin AMP (CAMP). Moreover, conditioned media from 1,25D-treated cells acquired the capacity to kill bacteria, including the pathogen *Pseudomonas aeruginosa*. While the effect of 1,25D alone on *DEFB2/HBD2* was only modest, recent work detailed later has shown that 1,25D in combination with other signaling pathways leads to robust stimulation of DEF2/HBD2 expression. By contrast, induction of CAMP was particularly strong and subsequent follow-up studies have shown that CAMP expression is widely regulated by 1,25D both *in vitro* and *in vivo*. The innate immune system uses pattern recognition receptors to detect the presence of conserved molecular motifs characteristic of certain families of pathogens. Toll-like receptors (TLRs) are transmembrane proteins that induce an innate immune response after detecting components of extracellular microbes, such as bacterial lipopolysaccharide by TLR4, or lipoprotein in the case of TLR2. Importantly, TLR2/1 stimulation by *Mycobacterium tuberculosis* lipoprotein induces the expression of both the VDR and CYP27B1; stimulated macrophages thus acquire the capacity to respond to circulating levels of 25D, underlying the central role of vitamin D signaling in human innate immune responses. The 1,25D produced stimulates the expression of CAMP, which colocalizes with mycobacteria in infected macrophages.

While etiology of IBD is unknown, a rich list of genetic susceptibility markers has been identified, and it is likely that a combination of these and environmental cues or infections triggers the full manifestation of these inflammatory conditions. Variants in the *NOD2/CARD15/IBD1* locus are associated with the strongest risk of development of CD (Hugot *et al.*, 2001). *NOD2* encodes a protein that is a member of a family of intracellular pattern recognition receptors (Inohara *et al.*, 2003). *NOD2* recognizes modified forms of muramyl dipeptide (MDP), a lysosomal breakdown product of bacterial peptidoglycan. A recent work has shown that *NOD2* is particularly sensitive to the *N*-glycolyl form of MDP produced by mycobacteria (Coulombe *et al.*, 2009). Remarkably, major *NOD2* variants associated with CD contain frameshift or point mutations that encode proteins incapable of recognizing MDP, and are thus inactive signaling molecules. *ATG16L1* and *IRGM*, both of which encode proteins required for autophagy, are also CD susceptibility loci (Hampe *et al.*, 2007; Parkes *et al.*, 2007; Rioux *et al.*, 2007). Autophagy is a process that employs autophagosomes to target other damaged organelles, proteins and a number of intracellular pathogens for degradation in lysosomes.

Recent studies have linked *NOD2* function to autophagy (Cooney *et al.*, 2010; Travassos *et al.*, 2010). Activated *NOD2* recruits *ATG16L1* to the cell membrane at the site of bacterial entry (Travassos *et al.*, 2010). *ATG16L1* is an essential component of protein complexes that control autophagy (Mizushima *et al.*, 2003). Stimulation of *NOD2* induced autophagy and clearance of pathogen. However, the introduction of mutations common to CD for either *NOD2 or ATG16L1* abrogated this effect, strongly suggesting a functional role for these mutations in the pathogenesis of CD (Travassos *et al.*, 2010). Taken together, these data suggest that at least a subset of the genetic predisposition to CD results from defects in the detection and/or processing of intracellular pathogens by the innate immune system.

Recently, it has been found that transcription of the *NOD2* gene was stimulated directly by the 1,25D-bound VDR. Regulation of *NOD2* expression by 1,25D is noteworthy for several reasons. Signaling through *NOD2* induces the function of the nuclear factor (NF)-κB transcription factor, which in turn induces expression of *DEFB2/HBD2* (Verway *et al.*, 2010; Wang *et al.*, 2010). We found that pretreatment with 1,25D to induce *NOD2*, followed by incubation with MDP, led to stimulation of NF-κB function and synergistic induction of *DEFB2/HBD2* expression (Wang *et al.*, 2010). Significantly, this synergism, along with induction of NF-κB function, was absent in macrophages from patients homozygous for inactivating *NOD2* mutations. Taken together with previous work, these data demonstrated that 1,25D is both a direct and an indirect inducer of the *NOD2–DEFB2/HBD2* innate immune pathway.

The observation that *NOD2* is a 1,25D target gene also links vitamin D signaling to autophagy. Stimulation of *NOD2* expression by 1,25D implies that it would boost autophagy at least in part by enhancing *NOD2* function. In addition, recent work has shown that 1,25D-stimulated CAMP production enhanced autophagy in mycobacteria-infected macrophages (Yuk *et al.*, 2009). Previous studies revealed that CAMP expressed in 1,25D-treated cells colocalized with mycobacteria in phagolysosomal structures (Holick, 2007). Ablation of CAMP expression decreased the number of autophagosomes in 1,25D-treated cells (Yuk *et al.*, 2009). While this study is intriguing, it is not clear whether CAMP functioned to enhance autophagy directly or indirectly by reducing bacterial viability due to its AMP activity.

The effect of 1,25D alone on CAMP expression is strong (Gombart *et al.*, 2005; Liu *et al.*, 2006; Wang *et al.*, 2004; Weber *et al.*, 2005). Thus, the effects of 1,25D-induced CAMP on autophagy may be at least partially independent of *NOD2* function. This raises the possibility that enhanced CAMP expression may be sufficient to induce clearance of intracellular pathogens despite mutations in the *NOD2* pathway common in CD. Notably, in this regard, adherent-invasive *Escherichia coli* has been detected in ileal lesions in CD. Normal autophagy is sufficient in the clearance of this pathogen, but in the absence of functional *ATG16L1* and *IRGM*, adherent-invasive *Escherichia coli* is able to proliferate (Lapaquette *et al.*, 2010). In addition, there has been a positive correlation between the detection of *Mycobacterium avium* substrain *paratuberculosis* in biopsies from CD patients compared with control samples taken from patients with UC (Feller *et al.*, 2007). While neither has yet to be directly implicated in the etiology of CD, their persistent presence might explain some of the inflammatory complications that manifest in CD.

B. Vitamin D and inflammatory bowel disease

For many years, vitamin D status was defined simply by whether the patient had symptoms of the bone rickets (osteomalacia in adults). However, an entirely new perspective on vitamin D status has arisen from the observation that serum levels of the main circulating form of vitamin D ($25OHD_3$) as high as 75 nM correlate inversely with parathyroid hormone (Chapuy *et al.*, 1997). This has prompted the introduction of a new term, *vitamin D insufficiency*, defined by serum levels of $25OHD_3$ that are suboptimal (<75 nM) but not necessarily rachitic (<20 nM) (Holick, 2007). Unlike serum concentrations of $1,25(OH_2)D_3$, which are primarily defined by the endocrine regulators of the vitamin D-activating enzyme, 1α-hydroxylase, circulating levels of $25OHD_3$ are a direct reflection of vitamin D status, which for any given individual depends on access to vitamin D either through exposure to sunlight or through dietary intake. The net effect of this is that vitamin D status can vary significantly in populations depending on geographic, social, or economic factors. As a result of these new parameters for vitamin D status, vitamin insufficiency is a worldwide epidemic (Hewison, 2010). Moreover, recent studies have shown that in the past 10 years alone, serum vitamin D levels have on average fallen by 20% (Ginde *et al.*, 2009). The key question now being considered is what is the physiologic and clinical effect of global vitamin D insufficiency beyond the classic bone disease such rickets?

Epidemiologic studies have highlighted possible links between vitamin D insufficiency and a wide range of human diseases (Cantorna and Mahon, 2004; Holick, 2007). The incidence of immune-mediated diseases such as multiple sclerosis and IBD has increased in developed countries over the past 50 years. To explain the increased incidence of immune-mediated diseases as well as the geographical restriction of these diseases to the developed world, the hygiene hypothesis has been put forward. The hygiene hypothesis states that reduced exposure to microbial components results in immune dysregulation and T-cell responses that drive immune-mediated disease. In a recent review, Cantorna proposed that other factors in the environment in addition to the hygiene hypothesis are important in the development of the immune response leading to multiple sclerosis and IBD (Cantorna, 2010). In particular, the decreased outdoor activity, increased pollution, and diets that lack adequate vitamin D have combined to create large fluctuations in vitamin D status in developed countries and especially in populations that experience winter (Namgung *et al.*, 1992, 1994). The vitamin D hypothesis proposes that vitamin D regulates the development and function of the immune system and that early childhood and prenatal changes in vitamin D status affect the resultant immune response and the development of autoimmune diseases such as IBD (Cantorna, 2000, 2006).

1. Vitamin D and animal models of IBD

Few studies have correlated vitamin D and IBD. Up to now, the relationship between vitamin D and IBD has been studied mainly with regard to malabsorption and osteoporosis. So far, no attempt has been made to analyze the possible effect that vitamin D therapy may exert upon the course of intestinal disease in man, although it is worthwhile pointing out that current anti-osteoporosis treatment is based upon colecalciferol and not calcitriol, conditioning different pharmacokinetics and pharmacodynamics *in vivo*. Moreover, the fear of potential side effects due to hypercalcemia have led to little attention being focused on this hormone as a possible pharmacological agent for active disease, despite the lack of data on the relationship between dosage and clinical effect.

However, recent data appear to support a pathological link between vitamin D deficiency and the risk of these diseases, in which the hormone suppressed the *in vitro* activation of T-lymphocyte proliferation and prevented the onset of the disease in animal models (Cantorna *et al.*, 2000; Froicu *et al.*, 2003, 2006). Moreover, VDR KO mice were extremely sensitive to dextran sodium sulfate (DSS), with a high colonic expression of tumor necrosis factor (TNF)-α, IL-12, IFN-γ, and IL-10 (Froicu and Cantorna, 2007).

Animal models suggest that VDR plays a critical role in mucosal barrier homeostasis not only by preserving the integrity of junction complexes but also by promoting healing of the colonic epithelium (Kong *et al.*, 2008). Very few studies, performed only in animals, have shown a direct effect of vitamin D on cytokines in IBD models. Zhu *et al.* reported that the hormone inhibited TNF-α in an experimental model of IBD (Zhu *et al.*, 2005). More recently, Daniel *et al.* showed that, in mice TNBS colitis, calcitriol and/or dexamethasone downregulated Th1 parameters and upregulated Th2 markers, thus suggesting a rational for a steroid-sparing effect of calcitriol in IBD (Daniel *et al.*, 2008).

In a recent study (Laverny *et al.*, 2010), 1α,25(OH)(2)-16-ene-20-cyclopropyl-vitamin D(3) (BXL-62) was identified as a potent anti-inflammatory VDR agonist with a low calcemic activity. Its marked anti-inflammatory properties and its capacity to induce VDR primary response genes, like CYP24A1 and CAMP, at lower concentrations than conventional vitamin D, in peripheral blood mononuclear cells (PBMCs) from IBD patients were evaluated. Its higher anti-inflammatory potency compared to 1,25D(3) was demonstrated by the significantly more potent inhibition in PBMCs and in lymphocyte-enriched lamina propria mononuclear cells of the proinflammatory cytokines TNF-α, IL-12/23p40, IL-6, and IFN-γ, both at mRNA and at protein level. The therapeutic efficacy of intrarectal administration of BXL-62 in experimental IBD was shown by its beneficial effects, significantly higher than 1,25D(3), to induce recovery of clinical symptoms of colitis at normocalcemic doses in mice undergoing DSS-induced colitis.

2. Vitamin D and human IBD

Vitamin D and VDR may also play a role in human IBD.

The immunomodulatory effects of vitamin D on Th1/Th2 cytokines were evaluated in an *in vitro* study in patients suffering from IBD (Ardizzone *et al.*, 2009). In this study, nine patients with UC, eight patients with CD, and six healthy controls (HC) were enrolled. Peripheral blood was collected after a drug washout of 15 days and peripheral blood mononuclear cells were stimulated with mitogens alone or in the presence of physiological concentrations of calcitriol (100 pg/mL). Type 1 (IL-2, TNF-α, and IFN-γ) and type 2 (IL-10) cytokine production was assayed. Compared to HC, TNF-α production was significantly higher both in UC ($p = 0.0002$) and in CD ($p = 0.0001$) patients, at baseline and after incubation with calcitriol (UC: $p = 0.0003$; CD: $p = 0.0009$). The effects of calcitriol incubation were (1) reduced IFN-γ ($p = 0.024$) and increased IL-10 ($p = 0.06$) production in UC patients; (2) reduced TNF-α production in CD patients ($p = 0.032$); and (3) no significant effects in HC patients. Calcitriol increased, albeit not significantly, IL-10 production in UC compared to CD patients ($p = 0.09$). These results suggest an important modulatory role of vitamin D in the Th1/Th2 immune response. Moreover, the observation that the effect of this modulation was different in CD compared to UC patients provides an interesting area of research into the pathogenesis and treatment of these inflammatory conditions. First, a modulation of TNF-α was observed in CD, leading to a direct reduction of the single baseline cytokine that appeared higher in both diseases. It is interesting to integrate this observation with the reported synergistic effect of the anti-TNF agent infliximab when coadministered with vitamin D derivatives in an *in vitro* study (Stio *et al.*, 2004). Second, the inhibitory effect on IFN-γ and the apparent stimulation of IL-10 following incubation with vitamin D confirm the more complex immunological scenario in UC and the fact that the hormone actually enforces an anti-inflammatory response and counterbalances the baseline proinflammatory (higher baseline TNF-α levels) milieu featuring the disease.

The therapeutic efficacy of vitamin D_3 treatment was evaluated in patients with CD.

A prospective study to compare the effects of active vitamin D [1,25(OH) 2 vitamin D (aVD)] and plain vitamin D [25(OH) vitamin D (pVD)] on bone metabolism and the clinical course of CD was performed (Miheller *et al.*, 2009). Thirty-seven inactive CD patients were involved in the study and divided into two age-, gender-, and *t*-score-matched groups. Group A was treated with aVD, while group B received pVD. Osteocalcin, β-CrossLaps, osteoprotegerin, and receptor activator NF-κB ligand concentrations were estimated at the start of the study and at 6 weeks and 3 and 12 months. The activity of CD was also measured clinically and by laboratory parameters. At week 6, the Crohn's disease activity index (CDAI) scores and concentration of C-reactive protein decreased (69.44 ± 58.6 vs. 57.0 ± 54.89 and 15.8 ± 23.57 mmol/L vs. 7.81 ± 3.91 mmol/L, respectively, $p < 0.05$) parallel with markers of bone turnover (β-CrossLaps: 0.46 ± 0.21 vs. 0.40 ± 0.25 ng/mL; osteocalcin: 32.29 ± 15.3 vs. 29.98 ± 14.14 ng/mL, $p < 0.05$); however, osteoprotegerin concentration (marker of osteoblast activity) increased (3.96 ± 2.1 vs. 4.58 ± 2.19 pg/mL) in group A, but did not change in group B. Osteocalcin and β-CrossLaps concentrations changed more significantly by the third month; however, these changes disappeared by the 12th month.

Very recently, a randomized double-blind placebo-controlled trial to assess the benefits of oral vitamin D_3 treatment in CD was performed

(Jørgensen *et al.*, 2010). One hundred and eight patients with CD in remission, of which 14 were excluded later, were included. Patients were randomized to receive either 1200 IU vitamin D_3 ($n = 46$) or placebo ($n = 48$) once daily during 12 months. The primary endpoint was clinical relapse. Oral vitamin D_3 treatment with 1200 IU daily increased serum 25OHD from mean 69 (standard deviation [SD] 31 nmol/L) to mean 96 nmol/L (SD 27 nmol/L) after 3 months ($p < 0.001$). The relapse rate was lower among patients treated with vitamin D_3 (6/46 or 13%) than among patients treated with placebo (14/48 or 29%; $p = 0.06$). Thus, oral supplementation with 1200 IU vitamin D_3 significantly increased serum vitamin D levels and insignificantly reduced the risk of relapse from 29% to 13% ($p = 0.06$).

Taken together, the last two studies suggest that vitamin D could be useful in the treatment of CD. However, a better patient selection, vitamin D doses, and clinical end point are necessary in the future clinical trials.

II. Conclusions

In these past decades, an important interaction between vitamin D and immune system was demonstrated. Recent studies have shown a potential physiological role for vitamin D in regulating normal innate and adaptive immunity. Future studies now need to focus on the potential of vitamin D and its derivatives as therapeutic adjuncts in the treatment of IBD.

References

Adorini, L., and Penna, G. (2008). Control of autoimmune diseases by the vitamin D endocrine system. *Nat. Clin. Pract. Rheumatol.* **4,** 404–412.

Ardizzone, S., and Bianchi Porro, G. (2002). Inflammatory bowel disease: New insights into pathogenesis and treatment. *J. Intern. Med.* **252,** 4675–4696.

Ardizzone, S., Cassinotti, A., Trabattoni, D., *et al.* (2009). Immunomodulatory effects of 1,25-dihydroxyvitamin d3 on th1/th2 cytokines in inflammatory bowel disease: An in vitro study. *Int. J. Immunopathol. Pharmacol.* **22,** 63–71.

Baumgart, D. C., and Carding, S. R. (2007). Inflammatory bowel disease: Cause and immunobiology. *Lancet* **369,** 1627–1640.

Cantorna, M. T. (2000). Vitamin D and autoimmunity: Is vitamin D status an environmental factor affecting autoimmune disease prevalence? *Proc. Soc. Exp. Biol. Med.* **223,** 230–233.

Cantorna, M. T. (2006). Vitamin D and its role in immunology: Multiple sclerosis, and inflammatory bowel disease. *Prog. Biophys. Mol. Biol.* **92,** 60–64.

Cantorna, M. T. (2010). Micronutrients and the immune system. Mechanisms underlying the effect of vitamin D on the immune system. *Proc. Nutr. Soc.* **69,** 286–289.

Cantorna, M. T., and Mahon, B. D. (2004). Mounting evidence for vitamin D as an environmental factor affecting autoimmune disease prevalence. *Exp. Biol. Med.* **229,** 1136–1142.

Cantorna, M. T., Munsick, C., Bemiss, C., *et al.* (2000). 1,25-Dihydroxycholecalciferol prevents and ameliorates symptoms of experimental murine inflammatory bowel disease. *J. Nutr.* **130,** 2648–2652.
Chapuy, M. C., Preziosi, P., Maarner, M., *et al.* (1997). Prevalence of vitamin D insufficiency in an adult normal population. *Osteoporos. Int.* **7,** 439–443.
Cooney, R., Baker, J., Brain, O., *et al.* (2010). *NOD2* stimulation induces autophagy in dendritic cells influencing bacterial handling and antigen presentation. *Nat. Med.* **16,** 90–97.
Coulombe, F., Divangahi, M., Veyrier, F., *et al.* (2009). Increased *NOD2*-mediated recognition of *N*-glycolyl muramyl dipeptide. *J. Exp. Med.* **206,** 1709–1716.
Daniel, C., Sartory, N. A., Zahn, N., *et al.* (2008). Immune modulatory treatment of TNBS colitis with calcitriol is associated with a change of a Th1/Th17 to a Th2 and regulatory T cell profile. *J. Pharmacol. Exp. Ther.* **324,** 23–33.
Feller, M., Huwiler, K., Stephan, R., *et al.* (2007). *Mycobacterium avium* subspecies *paratuberculosis* and Crohn's disease: A systematic review and meta-analysis. *Lancet Infect. Dis.* **7,** 607–613.
Fiocchi, C. (2008). What is "physiological" intestinal inflammation and how does it differ from "pathological" inflammation? *Inflamm. Bowel Dis.* **14**(Suppl. 2), S77–S78.
Froicu, M., and Cantorna, M. T. (2007). Vitamin D and the vitamin D receptor are critical for control of the innate immune response to colonic injury. *BMC Immunol.* **8,** 5.
Froicu, M., Weaver, V., Wynn, T. A., *et al.* (2003). A crucial role for the vitamin D receptor in experimental inflammatory bowel diseases. *Mol. Endocrinol.* **17,** 2386–2392.
Froicu, M., Zhu, Y., and Cantorna, M. T. (2006). Vitamin D receptor is required to control gastrointestinal immunity in IL-10 knockout mice. *Immunology* **117,** 310–318.
Ginde, A. A., Liu, M. C., Camargo, C. A., *et al.* (2009). Demographic differences and trends of vitamin D insufficiency in the US population, 2988-2004. *Arch. Intern. Med.* **169,** 626–632.
Gombart, A. F., Borregaard, N., and Koeffler, H. P. (2005). Human cathelicidin antimicrobial peptide (CAMP) gene is a direct target of the vitamin D receptor and is strongly upregulated in myeloid cells by 1,25-dihydroxyvitamin D3. *FASEB J.* **19,** 1067–1077.
Hampe, J., Franke, A., Rosenstiel, P., *et al.* (2007). A genome-wide association scan of nonsynonymous SNPs identifies a susceptibility variant for Crohn disease in *ATG16L1*. *Nat. Genet.* **39,** 207–211.
Hewison, M. (2010). Vitamin D and the immune system: New perspectives on an old theme. *Endocrinol. Metab. Clin. N. Am.* **39,** 365–379.
Holick, M. F. (2007). Vitamin D deficiency. *N. Engl. J. Med.* **357,** 26–81.
Hugot, J.-P., Chamaillard, M., Zouali, H., *et al.* (2001). Association of *NOD2* leucine-rich repeat variants with susceptibility to Crohn's disease. *Nature* **411,** 599–603.
Inohara, N., Ogura, Y., Fontalba, A., *et al.* (2003). Host recognition of bacterial muramyl dipeptide mediated through *NOD2*. *J. Biol. Chem.* **2278,** 5509–5512.
Jørgensen, S. P., Agnholt, J., Glerup, H., *et al.* (2010). Clinical trial: Vitamin D3 treatment in Crohn's disease—A randomized double-blind placebo-controlled study. *Aliment Pharmacol. Ther.* **32,** 377–383.
Kong, J., Zhang, Z., Mush, M. W., *et al.* (2008). Novel role of the vitamin D receptor in maintaining the integrity of the intestinal mucosal barrier. *Am. J. Physiol. Gastrointest. Liver Physiol.* **294**(1), G208–G216.
Lai, Y., and Gallo, R. L. (2009). AMPed up immunity: How antimicrobial peptides have multiple roles in immune defense. *Trends Immunol.* **30,** 131–141.
Lapaquette, P., Glasser, A.-L., Huett, A., Xavier, R. J., and Darfeuille-Michaud, A. (2010). Crohn's disease-associated adherent-invasive *E. coli* are selectively favoured by impaired autophagy to replicate intracellularly. *Cell. Microbiol.* **12,** 99–113.

Laverny, G., Penna, G., Vetrano, S., *et al.* (2010). Efficacy of a potent and safe vitamin D receptor agonist for the treatment of inflammatory bowel disease. *Immunol. Lett.* **131,** 49–58.
Liu, P. T., Stenger, S., Li, H., *et al.* (2006). Toll-like receptor triggering of a vitamin D-mediated human antimicrobial response. *Science* **311,** 1770–1773.
Miheller, P., Muzes, G., Hritz, I., *et al.* (2009). Comparison of the effects of 1,25 dihydroxy-vitamin D and 25 hydroxyvitamin D on bone pathology and disease activity in Crohn's disease patients. *Inflamm. Bowel Dis.* **15,** 1656–1662.
Mizushima, N., Kuma, A., Kobayashi, Y., *et al.* (2003). Mouse Apg16L, a novel WD-repeat protein, targets to the autophagic isolation membrane with the Apg12–Apg5 conjugate. *J. Cell Sci.* **116,** 1679–1688.
Namgung, R., Mimouni, F., Campaigne, B. N., *et al.* (1992). Low bone mineral content in summer-born compared with winterborn infants. *J. Pediatr. Gastroenterol. Nutr.* **15,** 285–288.
Namgung, R., Tsang, R. C., Specker, B. L., *et al.* (1994). Low bone mineral content and high serum osteocalcin and 1,25-dihydroxyvitamin D in summer- versus winter-born newborn infants: An early fetal effect? *J. Pediatr. Gastroenterol. Nutr.* **19,** 220–227.
Parkes, M., Barrett, J. C., Prescott, N. J., *et al.* (2007). Sequence variants in the autophagy gene *IRGM* and multiple other replicating loci contribute to Crohn's disease susceptibility. *Nat. Genet.* **39,** 830–832.
Podolsky, D. K. (1991). Inflammatory bowel disease. *N. Engl. J. Med.* **325,** 928–937.
Rioux, J. D., Xavier, R. J., Taylor, K. D., *et al.* (2007). Genome-wide association study identifies new susceptibility loci for Crohn disease and implicates autophagy in disease pathogenesis. *Nat. Genet.* **39,** 596–604.
Scaldaferri, F., and Fiocchi, C. (2007). Inflammatory bowel disease: Progress and current concepts of etiopathogenesis. *J. Dig. Dis.* **8,** 171–178.
Stio, M., Treves, C., Martinesi, M., *et al.* (2004). Effect of anti-TNF therapy and vitamin D derivatives on the proliferation of peripheral blood mononuclear cells in Crohn's disease. *Dig. Dis. Sci.* **49**(2), 328–335.
Szodoray, P., Nakken, B., and Gaal, J. (2008). The complex role of vitamin D in autoimmune diseases. *Scand. J. Immunol.* **68,** 261–269.
Travassos, L. H., Carneiro, L. A. M., Ramjeet, M., *et al.* (2010). Nod1 and Nod2 direct autophagy by recruiting *ATG16L1* to the plasma membrane at the site of bacterial entry. *Nat. Immunol.* **11,** 55–62.
Verway, M., Behr, M. A., and White, J. H. (2010). Vitamin D, *NOD2*, autophgy and Crohn's disease. *Expert Rev. Clin. Immunol.* **6,** 505–508.
Wang, T.-T., Nestel, F. P., Bourdeau, V., *et al.* (2004). Cutting edge: 1,25-dihydroxyvitamin D3 is a direct inducer of antimicrobial peptide gene expression. *J. Immunol.* **173,** 2909–2912.
Wang, T.-T., Dabbas, B., Laperriere, D., *et al.* (2010). Direct and indirect induction by 1,25-dihydroxyvitamin D3 of the *NOD2*/CARD15-defensin b2 innate immune pathway defective in Crohn disease. *J. Biol. Chem.* **285,** 2227–2231.
Weber, G., Heilborn, J. D., Chamorro Jimenez, C. I., *et al.* (2005). Vitamin D induces the antimicrobial protein hCAP18 in human skin. *J. Invest. Dermatol.* **124,** 1080–1082.
Yuk, J.-M., Shin, D.-M., Lee, H.-M., *et al.* (2009). Vitamin D3 induces autophagy in human monocytes/macrophages via cathelicidin. *Cell Host Microbe* **6,** 231–243.
Zhu, Y., Mahon, B. D., Froicu, M., *et al.* (2005). Calcium and 1alpha,25-dihydroxyvitamin D3 target the TNF-alpha pathway to suppress experimental inflammatory bowel disease. *Eur. J. Immunol.* **35,** 217–224.

CHAPTER SEVENTEEN

Vitamin D Deficiency and Chronic Obstructive Pulmonary Disease: A Vicious Circle

Wim Janssens,* Chantal Mathieu,† Steven Boonen,‡ *and* Marc Decramer*

Contents

Abstract

Vitamin D and vitamin D deficiency strongly interact with different pathogenic mechanisms in COPD. Prevalence of vitamin D deficiency is particularly high in COPD patients, increases with the severity of COPD, and is closely associated with osteoporosis prevalence. Adequate calcium and vitamin D supplementation

* Respiratory Division, University of Leuven, Herestraat 49, Leuven, Belgium
† Division of Endocrinology, University of Leuven, Belgium
‡ Division for Geriatric Medicine and Center of Metabolic Bone Diseases, University of Leuven, Belgium

Vitamins and Hormones, Volume 86
ISSN 0083-6729, DOI: 10.1016/B978-0-12-386960-9.00017-4

in COPD patients with documented deficiencies reduces the risk for falling and osteoporotic fractures, may indirectly reduce morbidity, and may potentially prevent the further deterioration of pulmonary function. Apart from the proven beneficial effects of vitamin D supplements on bone and muscle tissue, many epidemiological studies have putatively linked vitamin D deficiency with a higher risk for cardiovascular, inflammatory and infectious diseases, and cancer, diseases known to be associated with and to contribute significantly to the phenotypic presentation of COPD patients. Different animal and human studies have provided considerable evidence on how vitamin D may affect these processes. The burning question in COPD is whether prevention of vitamin D deficiency or adequate supplementation may reverse the natural course of the disease.

I. Introduction

Chronic obstructive pulmonary disease (COPD) is defined as a chronic disease characterized by airflow limitation that is progressive, not fully reversible, and associated with an abnormal inflammatory response of the lungs to noxious particles or gasses. In Western countries, tobacco smoke is the major cause for COPD, accounting for approximately 90–95% of cases. Despite the deleterious effects of tobacco smoke in these patients, only 20% of smokers develop severe COPD indicating that other factors (biological, hereditary, environmental, etc.) must be involved (Molfino and Coyle, 2008). COPD is a growing public health problem. Currently, it is estimated that 210 million people suffer from COPD worldwide, a number which is still increasing. By 2020, the World Health Organization predicts that COPD will rise from the sixth to the third leading cause of death, next only to cardiovascular disease and cancer (Mathers and Loncar, 2006).

Abnormal inflammation in the smaller airway compartment is believed to be the driving force in the pathogenesis of COPD. Narrowing of the airways by inflammation, mucus production, and irreversible remodeling, together with a progressive loss of aveoli and peripheral airways (emphysema), is resulting in expiratory airflow limitation and disturbed gas exchange (Barnes, 2000). Clinically, COPD might be recognized by a persistent cough, sputum production, and exertional dyspnea but, according to the global obstructive lung disease (GOLD) definition, a correct diagnosis of COPD should be based on spirometry with a postbronchodilator forced expiratory volume in 1 second over forced vital capacity ratio (FEV1/FVC) below 0.7. Subsequently, COPD can be categorized in different stages of severity going from mild, moderate, severe to very severe disease according to FEV1 (Rabe *et al.*, 2007). It should be noted, however, that the majority of COPD patients, especially in the early stages of the disease, report no complaints, do not perform spirometry, and thus are unaware of their smoldering asymptomatic disease. In addition, it has been widely recognized that, apart from FEV1, many other factors critically contribute to severity of the disease presentation.

COPD is typically associated with systemic inflammation and increased comorbidities. Whether these comorbidities are caused by the underlying COPD or just coexist because of common risk factors such as smoking, aging, and inactivity is far from being understood. Their presence, however, unequivocally contributes to clinical deterioration and poor outcome in COPD. Notwithstanding the need for optimal respiratory treatment, comorbidities are now conceived as important targets in the therapeutic approach of the COPD patient (Agusti, 2005; Decramer *et al.*, 2005).

With the progressive loss of pulmonary function, patients become more prone to acute exacerbations of their disease which frequently necessitate hospitalization and may lead to respiratory failure and death (Niewoehner, 2006). Recent studies have indicated that quality of life and health status of patients are mainly determined by the presence and frequency of such exacerbations which, in turn, may lead to a faster decline in FEV1 (Donaldson *et al.*, 2002). Because of chronic inflammation, a disrupted epithelial barrier and an impaired innate immune defense, airways in COPD become more easily infected or chronically colonized by different rods which are believed to be key players in the origin of exacerbations (Sethi *et al.*, 2009). Preventing and treating these infections/exacerbations are therefore of utmost importance in the general approach of COPD.

Over the past years, increasing interest has been attributed to role of vitamin D and vitamin D deficiency in different diseases. Vitamin D deficiency is well known to accelerate bone loss in adults but accumulating evidence also links a low vitamin D nutritional status to highly prevalent chronic illnesses, including common cancers, autoimmune diseases, infectious, and cardiovascular diseases (Bouillon *et al.*, 2008a,b; Holick, 2007). In particular, the relationship between vitamin D deficiency and COPD is intriguing. COPD often integrates an uncontrolled inflammatory and infectious disease process of the airways with different comorbidities such as osteoporosis, cancer, skeletal muscle dysfunction, and cardiovascular disease, all domains which may be affected by vitamin D deficiency (Janssens *et al.*, 2009b). Moreover, vitamin D deficiency worsens with age which on its turn is a risk factor for developing COPD (Chapuy *et al.*, 1997; Dawson-Hughes *et al.*, 2005; Norman *et al.*, 2007).

This chapter aims to discuss the prevalence and determinants of vitamin D deficiency in COPD, the well-known effect of vitamin D in the development and treatment of COPD-associated osteoporosis and its potential role in the uncontrolled inflammatory cascade and systemic consequences of the disease.

II. Prevalence and Determinants of Vitamin D Deficiency in COPD

A. Vitamin D pathway

Vitamin D is obtained by photosynthesis in the skin but can also be derived from nutrition (fatty fish, fish liver oils, and dairy products). Ultraviolet light catalyzes the first step in vitamin D biosynthesis, which is the conversion of *de novo* synthesized 7-dehydrocholesterol into pre-vitamin D that undergoes an isomerization into vitamin D. The next step is a hydroxylation in the liver into 25-OHD, which then circulates in serum. Next, 25-OHD is hydroxylated into the active vitamin D metabolite 1,25-$(OH)_2D$ by 1α-hydroxylase (CYP27B1) in the kidney which is under strict control of serum levels of calcium and phosphate and their regulating hormones such as parathyroid hormone (PTH), calcitonin, and phosphatonins. 1,25-$(OH)_2D$ also induces the expression of a 24-hydroxylase (CYP24A1) which catabolizes both 25-OHD and 1,25-$(OH)_2D$ into biologically inactive, water-soluble metabolites, thereby serving as its own negative feedback regulator. Up to 99% of 25-OHD and 1,25-$(OH)_2D$ are bound to plasma proteins, of which more than 90% are bound to the specific vitamin D-binding protein (DBP) (Speeckaert *et al.*, 2006). These carrier proteins are important for the delivery of substrate (25-OHD) or active hormone (1,25-$(OH)_2D$) to their respective targets organs. 1,25-$(OH)_2D$ produced in the kidney may thus bind to the nuclear vitamin D receptor (VDR) in the intestine, bone, kidney, and parathyroid gland cells, directly or indirectly resulting in the maintenance of calcium and phosphorus levels (DeLuca, 2004; Lips, 2006).

Alternatively, 1α-hydroxylase is also found in several extrarenal tissues with an expression regulated by immune signals instead of mediators of bone and calcium (Overbergh *et al.*, 2000; van Etten and Mathieu, 2005). Upon intracellular activation of systemically delivered 25-OHD, local 1,25-$(OH)_2D$ concentrations may, independently from serum concentrations, exert an autocrine and paracrine function by binding to the nuclear receptor VDR. The vitamin–VDR complex may then activate vitamin D response elements (VDRE) on genes involved in different cellular processes.

B. Vitamin D deficiency in COPD

Because of its long half life, vitamin D status is best measured by total circulating 25-OHD. It reflects the dynamic equilibrium between vitamin D synthesis in the skin by sun exposure, vitamin D intake by food or dietary supplements, and vitamin D degradation by catabolizing enzymes. There is a broad consensus that in view of the calcemic effects, vitamin D insufficiency is best defined as a 25-OHD level below 20 ng/ml (50 nmol/l) (Holick, 2007; Norman *et al.*, 2007). Solely considering its effects on bone, a sensitive parameter to determine vitamin D deficiency is the serum level of PTH. Older data have clearly demonstrated that levels of 25-OHD below 20 ng/ml are sensed by the parathyroids as being insufficient (Lips, 2001). Based on indirect evidence, several experts have suggested that, for non-calcemic effects, serum levels of at least 30 ng/ml (75 nmol/l) are required, but so far, intervention studies to support this are lacking.

Few studies have assessed the prevalence of vitamin D deficiency in COPD by measuring serum levels of 25-OHD. Forli and colleagues reported that in a small sample of advanced COPD patients awaiting lung transplantation, the majority suffered from vitamin D deficiency (25-OHD $<$ 20 ng/ml) (Forli *et al.*, 2004). Similarly, $>$50% of a community-dwelling COPD cohort of 250 patients exhibited insufficient 25-OHD levels (Graat-Verboom *et al.*, 2010). Unfortunately, both studies failed to compare vitamin D status in COPD patients with those in age-, gender-, and smoking-matched control populations. Such matched control population is of crucial importance, as insufficient or deficient vitamin D levels may occur in up to 40–70% of the elderly in the USA and Europe (Chapuy *et al.*, 1997; Dawson-Hughes *et al.*, 2005; Norman *et al.*, 2007). However, very recent data from a Belgian patient cohort of 414 smoking individuals not taking vitamin D supplements demonstrate that COPD patients are more likely to suffer from vitamin D deficiency than matched healthy smokers (Janssens *et al.*, 2009a). A nonsignificant trend toward reduced 25-OHD levels was already apparent in GOLD 1 and 25-OHD levels continued to decrease significantly from GOLD 2 onward. Unsubstituted patients in GOLD 3 and GOLD 4 were vitamin D insufficient in more than 60–77% of cases (Fig. 17.1). Comparable findings were found in the population-based Third National Health and Nutrition Examination Survey (NHANES; cross-sectional survey on 14091 healthy US civilians over 20 years of age) (Black and Scragg, 2005). After adjustment for potential confounders, a strong relationship between serum levels of 25-OHD and pulmonary function, as assessed by FEV1 and FVC, was found. Although the authors did not report a significant correlation with COPD, the association between FEV1 and 25-OHD levels tended to be slightly stronger in the smoking subgroup. Overall, consistent evidence shows that FEV1 and 25-OHD are associated and establishes that a major subgroup of COPD patients is deficient for vitamin D.

C. Determinants of vitamin D deficiency

Many factors may cause vitamin D deficiency in a general population. Reduced synthesis in the skin, disturbed uptake from the gastrointestinal tract, impaired activation in liver or kidneys, sequestration in body fat, and

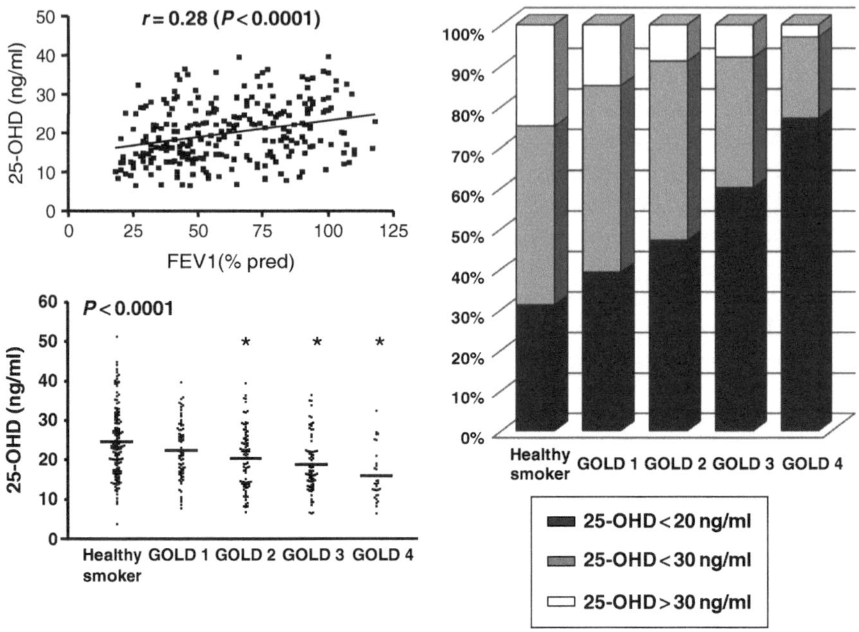

Figure 17.1 Cross-sectional assessment of 25-OHD levels in COPD patients and smoking controls ($n = 414$). (Adapted from Janssens *et al.*, 2009a.)

increased catabolism are all factors known to reduce 25-OHD serum levels (Holick, 2007). For COPD, in particular, the impaired capacity of the skin for vitamin D synthesis by aging and toxic smoke effects, the absence of sun exposure because of disability and reduced outdoor activity, the increased catabolism of vitamin D by glucocorticoids, together with a potentially impaired activation in liver, reduced gastrointestinal uptake, and sequestration in body mass fat, may explain the defective vitamin D status in the majority of COPD patients. In addition, total vitamin D action, by its active form $1,25(OH)_2D$, is impaired in renal failure by decreased 1alpha-hydroxylation. When correcting for FEV1 and diffusing capacity, parameters reflecting the severity and duration of COPD, we found that 25-OHD levels were also determined by genetic variants in the vitamin D-binding gene *GC*, rs7041 and rs4588 (Janssens *et al.*, 2009a). Similar associations have recently been shown in pre- and postmenopausal women (Lauridsen *et al.*, 2005; Sinotte *et al.*, 2009), confirming that these genetic variants of vitamin D-binding protein are independent determinants of 25-OHD levels. It is not entirely clear how a single amino acid change in the vitamin D-binding protein may affect 25-OHD levels, but a change in the glycosylation pattern, with lower affinity and more rapid metabolization of the "mutant" DBP protein, has been suggested as the underlying cause

(Chishimba *et al.*, 2010; Lauridsen *et al.*, 2005; Sinotte *et al.*, 2009). Another important question is whether oral vitamin D supplementation will work for patients with such a genetic defect in *GC*. At present, one small study indicates that risk variants associated with reduced 25-OHD levels are indeed sensitive to vitamin D supplementation (Fu *et al.*, 2009).

III. COPD and Osteoporosis: Role for Vitamin D

A. Osteoporosis

Osteoporosis is a systemic skeletal disorder which is characterized by compromised bone strength resulting in a higher susceptibility to fractures. Bone strength reflects the integration of structural determinants and bone density (BMD). The latter is accurately measured by dual X-ray absorbtiometry (DXA) and used to define osteoporosis. According to the World Health Organization (WHO), T-scores between -1 and -2.5 (i.e., BMD values between -1 and -2.5 standard deviations below the young–adult average) are considered as osteopenia, whereas T-scores of less than -2.5 are defined as osteoporosis, at least in postmenopausal women (Kanis, 1994). Bone tissue is continuously renewed throughout life, and it is estimated that in adults, approximately 25% of trabecular bone and 3% of cortical bone are replaced every year. After reaching peak bone mass at the age of 25–30 years, bone resorption exceeds bone formation, and each remodeling cycle will be associated with some degree of net bone loss, resulting in a mean annual bone loss of 0.5–1% which differs by sex, skeletal site, and age. Key determinants of the rate of bone remodeling and, hence, bone loss are PTH, vitamin D, and sex hormones (Manolagas and Jilka, 1995; Raisz, 2005; Sambrook and Cooper, 2006). At the cellular level, bone remodeling is a complex interplay in which osteoblasts, osteoclasts, and osteocytes work together. Basically, osteoclasts resorb bone, osteoblasts replace bone by the formation of a collagen matrix that subsequently mineralizes, whereas osteocytes and their canicular network serve as sensors to adjust bone responses to mechanical stimuli. The processes of bone formation and bone resorption are coupled by a close interaction between osteoblasts and osteoclasts (Matsuo, 2009). On their surface, osteoblasts constitutively express on their surface the receptor activator of nuclear factor-kB ligand (RANKL). When binding to its receptor RANK on the surface of pre-osteoclast cells, the latter differentiate into mature and activated osteoclasts (Leibbrandt and Penninger, 2008). Additionally, not only osteoblasts but also stromal cell secrete a soluble decoy receptor osteoprotegerin (OPG), which blocks the RANK/RANKL interaction, thereby acting as a physiological regulator of bone turnover (Lacey *et al.*, 1998). Imbalance between RANKL and OPG will result in excessive osteoclast activity and is considered to be one of the main mechanistic pathways involved in osteoporosis. Another less well-understood pathway is the Wnt/β-catenin signaling cascade downstream of a number of osteoblast-activating proteins and receptors. Wnt signaling activates osteoblasts and bone formation, whereas reduced Wnt signaling may contribute to osteoporosis (Patel and Karsenty, 2002). In COPD systemic inflammation, use of corticosteroids and vitamin D deficiency may enhance bone resorption through these signaling pathways.

B. Vitamin D and calcemic effects

Vitamin D plays a key role in the regulation of calcium and bone homeostasis (Lips, 2001). Low levels of vitamin D result in low bioavailability of calcium which stimulates parathyroid glands to increase secretion of PTH, the so-called secondary hyperparathyroidism. In the kidneys, PTH reduces reabsorption of phosphate from the proximal tubule while increasing calcium reabsorption in the distal tubule, resulting in a net increase in calcium/phosphate ratio. More importantly, PTH induces renal 1α-hydroxylase expression, hydroxylation of 25-OHD, and production of active $1,25(OH)_2D$. $1,25(OH)_2D$ enhances intestinal calcium absorption. It also acts on the immature osteoblastic cells to stimulate osteoclastogenesis through the RANKL/RANK regulatory system, with enhanced bone resorption and mobilization of calcium from the bone compartment (Suda *et al.*, 1999). Resulting higher levels of calcium and $1,25(OH)_2D$ have a negative feedback on PTH and will limit resorption of bone. In addition, $1,25(OH)_2D$ enhances OPG expression in mature osteoblasts, further reducing osteoclastogenesis (Baldock *et al.*, 2006).

C. Osteoporosis in COPD

The prevalence of osteoporosis in COPD varies between 9% and 59% depending on the diagnostic methods used, the population studied, and the severity of the underlying respiratory disease (Graat-Verboom *et al.*, 2009). The majority of studies have reported an increased risk for osteoporosis with lower FEV1 (Kjensli *et al.*, 2007; Sin *et al.*, 2003; Vrieze *et al.*, 2007). Osteoporosis is a major health problem because osteoporotic fractures frequently cause significant and long-lasting morbidity in older individuals. At this stage in life, hip fractures and other types of nonvertebral fractures account for most of the burden of osteoporosis, with increased mortality, functional decline, loss of quality of life, and need for institutionalization (Haentjens *et al.*, 2010; Schurch *et al.*, 1996). Mortality in hip fracture patients is close to 20% within 1 year and, of those who do survive the fracture, again some 20% will have to be institutionalized because of the fracture and because of its functional consequences (Schurch *et al.*, 1996).

The exact prevalence of hip fractures in COPD patients has not been studied in detail, but it is to be expected that the impact of such events in disabled COPD patients will be even worse. Spinal fractures should not be underestimated either, particularly not in the context of COPD. Vertebral compression fractures may lead to back pain, significant functional impairments, increased kyphosis with reduced rib cage mobility, and decline of pulmonary function (Leech *et al.*, 1990; Lyles *et al.*, 1993; Nevitt *et al.*, 1998). The overall prevalence of vertebral fractures in an ambulatory COPD population has been investigated by the EOLO study. In a large cohort of close to 3000 participants, more than 40% had one or more vertebral fractures and the prevalence significantly correlated with severity of disease (Nuti *et al.*, 2009). Finally, rib fractures are also associated with osteoporosis. They most frequently occur by falling (Barrett-Connor *et al.*, 2010) but may also be induced by heavy coughing (Hanak *et al.*, 2005). Because they induce thoracic pain, rib fractures may cause hypoventilation and reduce sputum evacuation which may lead to or aggravate exacerbations. However, no study has specifically addressed the prevalence and impact of rib fractures in COPD (Fig. 17.2).

In a general population, female gender, advancing age, a history of fragility fractures, current or former smoking, low body weight or weight loss, and functional limitations are well-established risk factors for osteoporosis and osteoporotic fracture occurrence (Kanis, 2002; Papaioannou *et al.*, 2009), along with the use of systemic glucocorticoids (Kanis *et al.*, 2004; van Staa *et al.*, 2002). As many of these risk factors coincide with COPD especially at the more severe stages, it should be no surprise that osteoporosis and COPD are strongly linked. A recent literature survey of Graat-verboom and colleagues in COPD confirmed low body mass, disease

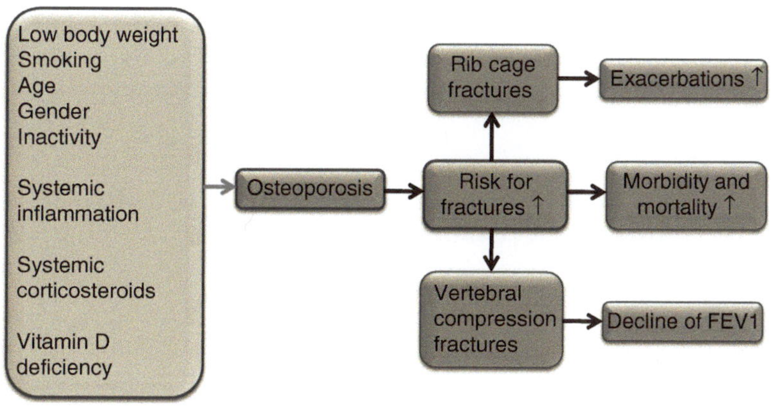

Figure 17.2 Risk factors for osteoporosis in COPD and functional consequences.

severity, use of corticosteroids, age, and female gender to be independent risk factors for osteoporosis (Graat-Verboom *et al.*, 2009). Low levels of vitamin D are highly prevalent in COPD as well and, in these patients, associated with the presence of osteoporosis (Franco *et al.*, 2009; Janssens *et al.*, 2009a).

D. Vitamin D substitution in COPD

Supplementation of calcium and vitamin D enhances bone density, suppresses bone remodeling, and reduces fracture risk in older individuals. However, compliance with supplements is essential, with no long-lasting benefits once calcium and vitamin D have been discontinued (Dawson-Hughes *et al.*, 2000). In a comparative meta-analysis, we found that fracture risk is only reduced when calcium is added to vitamin D (Boonen *et al.*, 2007). In line with these findings, a recent Cochrane review of 45 trials concluded that vitamin D alone was unlikely to be effective in preventing fractures, whereas vitamin D with calcium supplementation did reduce fracture risk (Avenell *et al.*, 2009). Although specific data for COPD patients are currently lacking, the fact that the majority of COPD patients are of older age, have many additional risk factors for osteoporosis, and are more likely to be deficient in vitamin D supports standard supplementation, especially at the more severe stages of disease. It is now accepted that a daily dose of 700–800 IU of vitamin D together with an adequate daily calcium intake (1000 mg) is probably the best strategy to prevent fractures in older subjects (Boonen *et al.*, 2007). Such supplementation regimens restore low serum 25-OHD levels in a general adult population to concentrations above the 20-ng/ml (50 nmol/l) threshold (Bischoff-Ferrari *et al.*, 2006; Vieth, 2007). Patients with COPD—particularly those on systemic corticosteroids—should be considered for a DEXA scan and osteoporosis medication. By integrating BMD measures with clinical risk factor tools such as FRAX, fracture risk may be estimated even more accurately (Kanis, 2002; Kanis *et al.*, 2008). However, for the time being, BMD continues to be the main tool to identify patients who will benefit from therapy.

IV. Airway and Systemic Inflammation in COPD: Link with Vitamin D Pathway

A. Noncalcemic effects of vitamin D

Because the nuclear receptor VDR and the key activating enzyme of 25-OHD (CYP27B1) are widely present in many different cells and tissues, high local 1,25-$(OH)_2D$ concentrations can exert different autocrine and paracrine functions. It is estimated that about 3% of the mouse/human genome is regulated by 1,25-$(OH)_2D$ (Uitterlinden *et al.*, 2004). Directly or indirectly, 1,25-$(OH)_2D$ may control genes that are involved in the regulation of cellular proliferation, differentiation, and apoptosis of healthy and malignant cells. From this perspective, many clinical studies have associated prevalence and incidence of cancer and poor prognosis in cancer patients to low 25-OHD levels (Giovannucci *et al.*, 2006; Lappe *et al.*, 2007). 1,25-$(OH)_2D$ is also a potent immune modulator of the adaptive immune system and different studies clearly associate vitamin D deficiency with autoimmune diseases like type I diabetes, multiple sclerosis, and rheumatoid arthritis (Merlino *et al.*, 2004; Munger *et al.*, 2006; Scragg *et al.*, 2004). Further, vitamin D is boosting the innate immune response upon infection (Baeke *et al.*, 2008) and deficient vitamin D levels have been linked to chronic infections such as tuberculosis and acute viral infections such as influenza (Cannell *et al.*, 2006; Ginde *et al.*, 2009a; Nnoaham and Clarke, 2008). As vitamin D is also involved in skeletal muscle function (Hamilton, 2009) and the cardiovascular system (Ginde *et al.*, 2009b; Wang *et al.*, 2008), it is clear that these noncalcemic effects may extend the potential therapeutic target of vitamin D beyond bone maintenance.

However, most of these noncalcemic effects are based on epidemiological associations or on boosting evidence from animal models, whereas adequately powered placebo-controlled intervention studies to demonstrate causal relationships are often lacking. In contrast to the better defined effects of different doses of vitamin D supplements for osteoporosis, therapeutic benefits, 25-OHD levels to target, and corresponding supplementation doses for noncalcemic effects are still largely based on speculation. Nevertheless, the potential role of the vitamin D pathway in airway inflammation and infection, muscle dysfunction, and systemic consequences of COPD is such an attractive hypothesis, that it definitely merits more attention (Fig. 17.3).

B. Airway inflammation

COPD is characterized by an uncontrolled inflammatory cascade in the distal airways and lung parenchyma. Different inflammatory cells interact with epithelial cells, smooth muscle cells, and endothelial cells leading to a complex interplay of inflammation, tissue destruction, and remodeling. As the pattern of inflammatory cells changes with increasing severity of the disease, it is obvious that different immune mechanisms are involved (Barnes, 2008; Cosio *et al.*, 2002; Hogg *et al.*, 2004). One attractive hypothesis proposes that COPD is initiated by an innate immune response to cigarette smoke which relies on the recognition of tissue damage by toll-like receptors (TLRs) and is driven by epithelial cells, macrophages, and neutrophils. The second step involves the adaptive immune system which is triggered by the maturation of dendritic cells leading to T cell activation and proliferation and resulting in CD8+ cytotoxic T cells, Th1 CD4+ cells, and oligoclonal B cells, all of

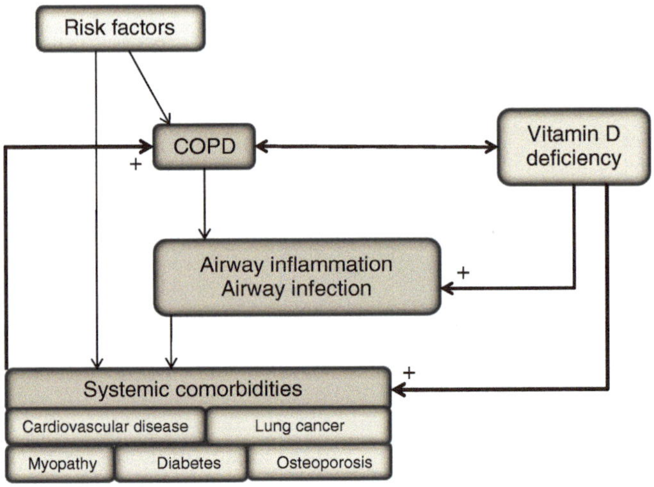

Figure 17.3 Schematic representation of vicious interaction between COPD and vitamin D deficiency.

which are found in organized lymphoid follicles along the airways of patients with severe COPD (Cosio and Agusti, 2010; Cosio *et al.*, 2009). Chronic infection and bacterial colonization, which unequivocally contribute to the further deterioration of the disease, are persistent triggers for this adaptive immune system (Sethi *et al.*, 2009). An alternative explanation is that deliberation of self-antigens upon tissue destruction may initiate an autoimmune reaction (Lee *et al.*, 2007). In the absence of sufficient downregulatory mechanisms (Treg/Th17 disbalance), both foreign and self-antigen-specific immune responses may explain the persistent inflammatory process years after smoking cessation (Brusselle *et al.*, 2009).

Interestingly, vitamin D may control many of these pathways by different mechanisms (Dimeloe *et al.*, 2010; Janssens *et al.*, 2009b). First, 1,25-$(OH)_2D$ appears to act on innate immune cells. It reduces the expression of TLRs which are critical in the induction of the early immune response and the priming of the adaptive immune system (Sadeghi *et al.*, 2006). Via VDRE containing regions on selective genes, 1,25-$(OH)_2D$ also controls the synthesis of antimicrobial peptides like human cathelicidin (hCAP18) and β-defensins (DEFB2 and DEFB4) which are highly expressed in human monocytes, neutrophils, and airway epithelial cells (Bals *et al.*, 1998; Liu *et al.*, 2006; Wang *et al.*, 2004). Second, all cells of the adaptive immune system express VDR, either constitutively or after appropriate immune stimulation. High levels of 1,25-$(OH)_2D$ are potent inhibitors of dendritic cell maturation with lower expression of MHC class II molecules, downregulation of costimulatory molecules, and lower production of proinflammatory cytokines such as IL-2, IL-12, IFN-y, and IL-23 (Baeke *et al.*, 2008;

van Etten and Mathieu, 2005). In several mouse models, 1,25-$(OH)_2D$ also tapers down the adaptive immune system from a Th1/Th17 responses toward a Th2 and regulatory T cell answer (Bouillon *et al.*, 2008a; Daniel *et al.*, 2008; Mathieu and Adorini, 2002; Mathieu *et al.*, 1994). In human, 1,25-$(OH)_2D$ appears to induce IL-10 secreting CD4+ Treg cells both directly or in concert with glucocorticoids (Barrat *et al.*, 2002; Xystrakis *et al.*, 2006).

In chronic smokers or COPD patients, reduced vitamin D levels may thus enhance proinflammatory pathways which, together with reduced downregulatory T cells and impaired innate defense again bacteria and viruses, may lead to clinical disease onset and/or further deterioration. Conversely, restoring 25-OHD levels to optimal values may likely be beneficial. However, only indirect evidence from cross-sectional analyses and intervention studies is currently supporting such hypothesis. For instance, Black and colleagues examined spirometric data from the Third National Health and Nutrition Examination Survey (cross-sectional survey on 14091 US civilians over 20 years of age) (Black and Scragg, 2005). After adjustment for potential confounders, a strong dose–response relationship between serum levels of 25-OHD and pulmonary function was found which may suggest a causal link (Wright, 2005). We recently extended the population-based association between FEV1 and 25-OHD levels from NHANES to a large cohort of COPD patients and suggested that genetic determinants for low vitamin D levels were associated with an increased risk for COPD (Janssens *et al.*, 2009a). Moreover, vitamin D deficiency has been linked with incidence of upper respiratory tract infections in healthy individuals (Ginde *et al.*, 2009a), and associations with asthma severity in childhood (Brehm *et al.*, 2009) and therapeutic benefits in asthma treatment have recently been published (Sutherland *et al.*, 2010). At present, a randomized control trial in COPD patients is ongoing to study potential benefits of vitamin D supplementation on exacerbations.

C. Skeletal muscle dysfunction

Skeletal muscle weakness is a very common observation in moderate to severe COPD and is an independent predictor of respiratory failure and death (Decramer *et al.*, 1997, 1998; Gosselink *et al.*, 1996). Although the underlying mechanism of skeletal muscle dysfunction in COPD is not entirely understood, it is generally accepted that the combination of disuse because of respiratory limitation, with elevated oxidative stress systemic inflammation, hypoxia, and frequent steroid intake are the main causes of deterioration (Decramer *et al.*, 1996, 2008). Different lines of evidence also support a role of vitamin D in skeletal muscle health. Muscle weakness is a prominent feature in rickets and chronic renal failure, and epidemiological studies found a positive association between 25-OHD levels and lower extremity function in older persons (Bischoff-Ferrari *et al.*, 2004a). In elderly individuals, vitamin D status predicts physical performance and its subsequent decline during long-term follow-up (Wicherts *et al.*, 2007). A cross-sectional analysis from NHANES indicated that muscle strength continued to increase throughout the reference range of 9–37 ng/ml of 25-OHD (Bischoff-Ferrari *et al.*, 2004a). Moreover, several double-blind randomized control trials demonstrated that vitamin D supplementation increased muscle strength and balance and reduces the risk of falling in elderly (Bischoff-Ferrari *et al.*, 2004b), at least when used at doses of 800 IU or more.

How vitamin D affects skeletal muscle function is not completely understood. Direct effects through VDR signaling with upregulation of gene expression (for instance, IGF-I), more rapid nongenomic effects on cellular Ca^{2+} influx through VDR like plasma membrane receptors, as well as indirect effects through plasma calcium levels have been implicated (Hamilton, 2009). Further, it is tempting to extrapolate these general observations on vitamin D involvement in skeletal muscle health to the more specific population of COPD patients. A recent publication on VDR genotype polymorphism and quadriceps strength in COPD is in line with this assumption (Hopkinson *et al.*, 2008). Given the impact of muscle weakness on outcome and health status of COPD patients, there is an urgent need for intervention trials with vitamin D to specifically address these questions.

D. Other systemic consequences

Although still defined on pulmonary criteria, COPD is now considered as a chronic disease state which is not confined to the lungs but is typically associated with systemic inflammation and underlying comorbidities (Agusti, 2005; Decramer *et al.*, 2008; Fabbri and Rabe, 2007). The clinical importance of this broader context has been indirectly confirmed by the TORCH study demonstrating that, in a prospective 3-year follow-up of a large cohort of COPD patients, only one-third of deaths could be attributed to respiratory failure, whereas the majority deceased from lung cancer or cardiovascular events (Calverley *et al.*, 2007). In many of these comorbidities, vitamin D deficiency is thought to play an important role. Different epidemiological and cohort studies have linked vitamin D deficiency with an increased risk of type II diabetes, arterial hypertension, and cardiovascular diseases including cardiovascular mortality, congestive heart failure, and peripheral vascular disease (Chiu *et al.*, 2004; Forman *et al.*, 2007; Ginde *et al.*, 2009b; Wang *et al.*, 2008). Besides its downregulatory effect on the renin-angiotensin-aldosteron system and its positive effects on insulin resistance, vitamin D may also reduce inflammatory cytokines and metallo-proteinases with consequent benefits on atherosclerosis, cardiac hypertrophy, and arterial stiffness (Lee *et al.*, 2008). Further, several epidemiologic studies have found a higher risk for different cancers in patients with lower serum 25-OHD levels (Giovannucci *et al.*, 2006), and survival in nonsmall cell lung cancer has been linked to 25-OHD levels and VDR genotypes (Zhou *et al.*, 2006, 2007). Although the underlying mechanisms are still far from being understood, vitamin D-mediated genetic control of proliferation, differentiation, and apoptosis of healthy and cancer cells may potentially be involved.

Whether sufficient vitamin D supplementation will finally reduce cardiovascular or lung cancer mortality in COPD patients is currently not known but, given the abundant indirect evidence for potential benefits, it is certainly worth exploring this.

V. Conclusion

It is increasingly being recognized that the pathogenesis of COPD and its systemic consequences have many putative interactions with the vitamin D pathway. To explore reverse causality and further disentangle these interactions, randomized controlled trials are urgently needed. Only then, the role of vitamin D and the potential effects of vitamin D substitution in COPD on disease progression and on other outcomes than the bone will be revealed.

ACKNOWLEDGMENTS

W. J., S. B., and C. M. are clinical investigators of the Fund for Scientific Research (FWO-Vlaanderen). Steven Boonen is holder of the Leuven University Chair in Gerontology and Geriatrics.

REFERENCES

Agusti, A. G. (2005). Systemic effects of chronic obstructive pulmonary disease. *Proc. Am. Thorac. Soc.* **2,** 367–370.

Avenell, A., Gillespie, W. J., Gillespie, L. D., and O'Connell, D. (2009). Vitamin D and vitamin D analogues for preventing fractures associated with involutional and postmenopausal osteoporosis. *Cochrane Database Syst. Rev.* **2,** CD000227.

Baeke, F., van Etten, E., Gysemans, C., Overbergh, L., and Mathieu, C. (2008). Vitamin D signaling in immune-mediated disorders: Evolving insights and therapeutic opportunities. *Mol. Aspects Med.* **29,** 376–387.

Baldock, P. A., Thomas, G. P., Hodge, J. M., Baker, S. U., Dressel, U., O'Loughlin, P. D., Nicholson, G. C., Briffa, K. H., Eisman, J. A., and Gardiner, E. M. (2006). Vitamin D action and regulation of bone remodeling: Suppression of osteoclastogenesis by the mature osteoblast. *J. Bone Miner. Res.* **21,** 1618–1626.

Bals, R., Wang, X., Zasloff, M., and Wilson, J. M. (1998). The peptide antibiotic LL-37/hCAP-18 is expressed in epithelia of the human lung where it has broad antimicrobial activity at the airway surface. *Proc. Natl. Acad. Sci. USA* **95,** 9541–9546.

Barnes, P. J. (2000). Chronic obstructive pulmonary disease. *N. Engl. J. Med.* **343,** 269–280.

Barnes, P. J. (2008). Immunology of asthma and chronic obstructive pulmonary disease. *Nat. Rev. Immunol.* **8,** 183–192.

Barrat, F. J., Cua, D. J., Boonstra, A., Richards, D. F., Crain, C., Savelkoul, H. F., de Waal-Malefyt, R., Coffman, R. L., Hawrylowicz, C. M., and O'Garra, A. (2002). In vitro generation of interleukin 10-producing regulatory CD4(+) T cells is induced by immunosuppressive drugs and inhibited by T helper type 1 (Th1)- and Th2-inducing cytokines. *J. Exp. Med.* **195,** 603–616.

Barrett-Connor, E., Nielson, C. M., Orwoll, E., Bauer, D. C., and Cauley, J. A. (2010). Epidemiology of rib fractures in older men: Osteoporotic Fractures in Men (MrOS) prospective cohort study. *BMJ* **340,** c1069.

Bischoff-Ferrari, H. A., Dietrich, T., Orav, E. J., Hu, F. B., Zhang, Y., Karlson, E. W., and wson-Hughes, B. (2004a). Higher 25-hydroxyvitamin D concentrations are associated with better lower-extremity function in both active and inactive persons aged > or =60 y. *Am. J. Clin. Nutr.* **80,** 752–758.

Bischoff-Ferrari, H. A., wson-Hughes, B., Willett, W. C., Staehelin, H. B., Bazemore, M. G., Zee, R. Y., and Wong, J. B. (2004b). Effect of vitamin D on falls: A meta-analysis. *JAMA* **291,** 1999–2006.

Bischoff-Ferrari, H. A., Giovannucci, E., Willett, W. C., Dietrich, T., and wson-Hughes, B. (2006). Estimation of optimal serum concentrations of 25-hydroxyvitamin D for multiple health outcomes. *Am. J. Clin. Nutr.* **84,** 18–28.

Black, P. N., and Scragg, R. (2005). Relationship between serum 25-hydroxyvitamin d and pulmonary function in the third national health and nutrition examination survey. *Chest* **128,** 3792–3798.

Boonen, S., Lips, P., Bouillon, R., Bischoff-Ferrari, H. A., Vanderschueren, D., and Haentjens, P. (2007). Need for additional calcium to reduce the risk of hip fracture with vitamin d supplementation: Evidence from a comparative metaanalysis of randomized controlled trials. *J. Clin. Endocrinol. Metab.* **92,** 1415–1423.

Bouillon, R., Bischoff-Ferrari, H., and Willett, W. (2008a). Vitamin D and health: Perspectives from mice and man. *J. Bone Miner. Res.* **23,** 974–979.

Bouillon, R., Carmeliet, G., Verlinden, L., van Etten, E., Verstuyf, A., Luderer, H. F., Lieben, L., Mathieu, C., and Demay, M. (2008b). Vitamin D and human health: Lessons from vitamin D receptor null mice. *Endocr. Rev.* **29,** 726–776.

Brehm, J. M., Celedon, J. C., Soto-Quiros, M. E., Avila, L., Hunninghake, G. M., Forno, E., Laskey, D., Sylvia, J. S., Hollis, B. W., Weiss, S. T., and Litonjua, A. A. (2009). Serum vitamin D levels and markers of severity of childhood asthma in Costa Rica. *Am. J. Respir. Crit. Care Med.* **179,** 765–771.

Brusselle, G. G., Demoor, T., Bracke, K. R., Brandsma, C. A., and Timens, W. (2009). Lymphoid follicles in (very) severe COPD: Beneficial or harmful? *Eur. Respir. J.* **34,** 219–230.

Calverley, P. M., Anderson, J. A., Celli, B., Ferguson, G. T., Jenkins, C., Jones, P. W., Yates, J. C., and Vestbo, J. (2007). Salmeterol and fluticasone propionate and survival in chronic obstructive pulmonary disease. *N. Engl. J. Med.* **356,** 775–789.

Cannell, J. J., Vieth, R., Umhau, J. C., Holick, M. F., Grant, W. B., Madronich, S., Garland, C. F., and Giovannucci, E. (2006). Epidemic influenza and vitamin D. *Epidemiol. Infect.* **134,** 1129–1140.

Chapuy, M. C., Preziosi, P., Maamer, M., Arnaud, S., Galan, P., Hercberg, S., and Meunier, P. J. (1997). Prevalence of vitamin D insufficiency in an adult normal population. *Osteoporos. Int.* **7,** 439–443.

Chishimba, L., Thickett, D. R., Stockley, R. A., and Wood, A. M. (2010). The vitamin D axis in the lung: A key role for vitamin D-binding protein. *Thorax* **65,** 456–462.
Chiu, K. C., Chu, A., Go, V. L., and Saad, M. F. (2004). Hypovitaminosis D is associated with insulin resistance and beta cell dysfunction. *Am. J. Clin. Nutr.* **79,** 820–825.
Cosio, B. G., and Agusti, A. (2010). Update in chronic obstructive pulmonary disease 2009. *Am. J. Respir. Crit. Care Med.* **181,** 655–660.
Cosio, M. G., Majo, J., and Cosio, M. G. (2002). Inflammation of the airways and lung parenchyma in COPD: Role of T cell. *Chest* **121,** 160S–165S.
Cosio, M. G., Saetta, M., and Agusti, A. (2009). Immunologic aspects of chronic obstructive pulmonary disease. *N. Engl. J. Med.* **360,** 2445–2454.
Daniel, C., Sartory, N. A., Zahn, N., Radeke, H. H., and Stein, J. M. (2008). Immune modulatory treatment of trinitrobenzene sulfonic acid colitis with calcitriol is associated with a change of a T helper (Th) 1/Th17 to a Th2 and regulatory T cell profile. *J. Pharmacol. Exp. Ther.* **324,** 23–33.
Dawson-Hughes, B., Harris, S. S., Krall, E. A., and Dallal, G. E. (2000). Effect of withdrawal of calcium and vitamin D supplements on bone mass in elderly men and women. *Am. J. Clin. Nutr.* **72,** 745–750.
Dawson-Hughes, B., Heaney, R. P., Holick, M. F., Lips, P., Meunier, P. J., and Vieth, R. (2005). Estimates of optimal vitamin D status. *Osteoporos. Int.* **16,** 713–716.
Decramer, M., de Bock, V., and Dom, R. (1996). Functional and histologic picture of steroid-induced myopathy in chronic obstructive pulmonary disease. *Am. J. Respir. Crit. Care Med.* **153,** 1958–1964.
Decramer, M., Gosselink, R., Troosters, T., Verschueren, M., and Evers, G. (1997). Muscle weakness is related to utilization of health care resources in COPD patients. *Eur. Respir. J.* **10,** 417–423.
Decramer, M., Gosselink, R., Troosters, T., and Schepers, R. (1998). Peripheral muscle force is a determinant of survival in COPD. *Eur. Respir. J.* **12,** 261S, Abstract.
Decramer, M., De, B. F., Del, P. A., and Marinari, S. (2005). Systemic effects of COPD. *Respir. Med.* **99**(Suppl. B), S3–S10.
Decramer, M., Rennard, S., Troosters, T., Mapel, D. W., Giardino, N., Mannino, D., Wouters, E., Sethi, S., and Cooper, C. B. (2008). COPD as a lung disease with systemic consequences—Clinical impact, mechanisms, and potential for early intervention. *COPD* **5,** 235–256.
DeLuca, H. F. (2004). Overview of general physiologic features and functions of vitamin D. *Am. J. Clin. Nutr.* **80,** 1689S–1696S.
Dimeloe, S., Nanzer, A., Ryanna, K., and Hawrylowicz, C. (2010). Regulatory T cells, inflammation and the allergic response—The role of glucocorticoids and vitamin D. *J. Steroid Biochem. Mol. Biol.* **120,** 86–95.
Donaldson, G. C., Seemungal, T. A., Bhowmik, A., and Wedzicha, J. A. (2002). Relationship between exacerbation frequency and lung function decline in chronic obstructive pulmonary disease. *Thorax* **57,** 847–852.
Fabbri, L. M., and Rabe, K. F. (2007). From COPD to chronic systemic inflammatory syndrome? *Lancet* **370,** 797–799.
Forli, L., Halse, J., Haug, E., Bjortuft, O., Vatn, M., Kofstad, J., and Boe, J. (2004). Vitamin D deficiency, bone mineral density and weight in patients with advanced pulmonary disease. *J. Intern. Med.* **256,** 56–62.
Forman, J. P., Giovannucci, E., Holmes, M. D., Bischoff-Ferrari, H. A., Tworoger, S. S., Willett, W. C., and Curhan, G. C. (2007). Plasma 25-hydroxyvitamin D levels and risk of incident hypertension. *Hypertension* **49,** 1063–1069.
Franco, C. B., Paz-Filho, G., Gomes, P. E., Nascimento, V. B., Kulak, C. A., Boguszewski, C. L., and Borba, V. Z. (2009). Chronic obstructive pulmonary disease

is associated with osteoporosis and low levels of vitamin D. *Osteoporos. Int.* **20,** 1881–1887.

Fu, L., Yun, F., Oczak, M., Wong, B. Y., Vieth, R., and Cole, D. E. (2009). Common genetic variants of the vitamin D binding protein (DBP) predict differences in response of serum 25-hydroxyvitamin D [25(OH)D] to vitamin D supplementation. *Clin. Biochem.* **42,** 1174–1177.

Ginde, A. A., Mansbach, J. M., and Camargo, C. A., Jr. (2009a). Association between serum 25-hydroxyvitamin D level and upper respiratory tract infection in the Third National Health and Nutrition Examination Survey. *Arch. Intern. Med.* **169,** 384–390.

Ginde, A. A., Scragg, R., Schwartz, R. S., and Camargo, C. A., Jr. (2009b). Prospective study of serum 25-hydroxyvitamin D level, cardiovascular disease mortality, and all-cause mortality in older U.S. adults. *J. Am. Geriatr. Soc.* **57,** 1595–1603.

Giovannucci, E., Liu, Y., Rimm, E. B., Hollis, B. W., Fuchs, C. S., Stampfer, M. J., and Willett, W. C. (2006). Prospective study of predictors of vitamin D status and cancer incidence and mortality in men. *J. Natl. Cancer Inst.* **98,** 451–459.

Gosselink, R., Troosters, T., and Decramer, M. (1996). Peripheral muscle weakness contributes to exercise limitation in COPD. *Am. J. Respir. Crit. Care Med.* **153,** 976–980.

Graat-Verboom, L., van den Borne, B. E., Smeenk, F. W., Spruit, M. A., and Wouters, E. F. (2010). Osteoporosis in COPD outpatients based on bone mineral density and vertebral fractures. *J. Bone. Miner. Res.* **27,** Epub.

Graat-Verboom, L., Wouters, E. F., Smeenk, F. W., van den Borne, B. E., Lunde, R., and Spruit, M. A. (2009). Current status of research on osteoporosis in COPD: A systematic review. *Eur. Respir. J.* **34,** 209–218.

Haentjens, P., Magaziner, J., Colon-Emeric, C. S., Vanderschueren, D., Milisen, K., Velkeniers, B., and Boonen, S. (2010). Meta-analysis: Excess mortality after hip fracture among older women and men. *Ann. Intern. Med.* **152,** 380–390.

Hamilton, B. (2010). Vitamin D and human skeletal muscle. *Scand. J. Med. Sci. Sports* **20,** 182–190.

Hanak, V., Hartman, T. E., and Ryu, J. H. (2005). Cough-induced rib fractures. *Mayo Clin. Proc.* **80,** 879–882.

Hogg, J. C., Chu, F., Utokaparch, S., Woods, R., Elliott, W. M., Buzatu, L., Cherniack, R. M., Rogers, R. M., Sciurba, F. C., Coxson, H. O., and Pare, P. D. (2004). The nature of small-airway obstruction in chronic obstructive pulmonary disease. *N. Engl. J. Med.* **350,** 2645–2653.

Holick, M. F. (2007). Vitamin D deficiency. *N. Engl. J. Med.* **357,** 266–281.

Hopkinson, N. S., Li, K. W., Kehoe, A., Humphries, S. E., Roughton, M., Moxham, J., Montgomery, H., and Polkey, M. I. (2008). Vitamin D receptor genotypes influence quadriceps strength in chronic obstructive pulmonary disease. *Am. J. Clin. Nutr.* **87,** 385–390.

Janssens, W., Bouillon, R., Claes, B., Carremans, C., Lehouck, A., Buysschaert, I., Coolen, J., Mathieu, C., Decramer, M., and Lambrechts, D. (2009a). Vitamin D deficiency is highly prevalent in COPD and correlates with variants in the vitamin D binding gene. *Thorax* **65,** 215–220.

Janssens, W., Lehouck, A., Carremans, C., Bouillon, R., Mathieu, C., and Decramer, M. (2009b). Vitamin D beyond bones in chronic obstructive pulmonary disease: Time to act. *Am. J. Respir. Crit. Care Med.* **179,** 630–636.

Kanis, J. A. (1994). Assessment of fracture risk and its application to screening for postmenopausal osteoporosis: Synopsis of a WHO report. WHO Study Group. *Osteoporos. Int.* **4,** 368–381.

Kanis, J. A. (2002). Diagnosis of osteoporosis and assessment of fracture risk. *Lancet* **359,** 1929–1936.

Kanis, J. A., Johansson, H., Oden, A., Johnell, O., de Laet, C., Melton, L. J., III, Tenenhouse, A., Reeve, J., Silman, A. J., Pols, H. A., Eisman, J. A., McCloskey, E. V., *et al.* (2004). A meta-analysis of prior corticosteroid use and fracture risk. *J. Bone Miner. Res.* **19,** 893–899.

Kanis, J. A., Johnell, O., Oden, A., Johansson, H., and McCloskey, E. (2008). FRAX and the assessment of fracture probability in men and women from the UK. *Osteoporos. Int.* **19,** 385–397.

Kjensli, A., Mowinckel, P., Ryg, M. S., and Falch, J. A. (2007). Low bone mineral density is related to severity of chronic obstructive pulmonary disease. *Bone* **40,** 493–497.

Lacey, D. L., Timms, E., Tan, H. L., Kelley, M. J., Dunstan, C. R., Burgess, T., Elliott, R., Colombero, A., Elliott, G., Scully, S., Hsu, H., Sullivan, J., *et al.* (1998). Osteoprotegerin ligand is a cytokine that regulates osteoclast differentiation and activation. *Cell* **93,** 165–176.

Lappe, J. M., Travers-Gustafson, D., Davies, K. M., Recker, R. R., and Heaney, R. P. (2007). Vitamin D and calcium supplementation reduces cancer risk: Results of a randomized trial. *Am. J. Clin. Nutr.* **85,** 1586–1591.

Lauridsen, A. L., Vestergaard, P., Hermann, A. P., Brot, C., Heickendorff, L., Mosekilde, L., and Nexo, E. (2005). Plasma concentrations of 25-hydroxy-vitamin D and 1, 25-dihydroxy-vitamin D are related to the phenotype of Gc (vitamin D-binding protein): A cross-sectional study on 595 early postmenopausal women. *Calcif. Tissue Int.* **77,** 15–22.

Lee, S. H., Goswami, S., Grudo, A., Song, L. Z., Bandi, V., Goodnight-White, S., Green, L., Hacken-Bitar, J., Huh, J., Bakaeen, F., Coxson, H. O., Cogswell, S., *et al.* (2007). Antielastin autoimmunity in tobacco smoking-induced emphysema. *Nat. Med.* **13,** 567–569.

Lee, J. H., O'Keefe, J. H., Bell, D., Hensrud, D. D., and Holick, M. F. (2008). Vitamin D deficiency an important, common, and easily treatable cardiovascular risk factor? *J. Am. Coll. Cardiol.* **52,** 1949–1956.

Leech, J. A., Dulberg, C., Kellie, S., Pattee, L., and Gay, J. (1990). Relationship of lung function to severity of osteoporosis in women. *Am. Rev. Respir. Dis.* **141,** 68–71.

Leibbrandt, A., and Penninger, J. M. (2008). RANK/RANKL: Regulators of immune responses and bone physiology. *Ann. NY Acad. Sci.* **1143,** 123–150.

Lips, P. (2001). Vitamin D deficiency and secondary hyperparathyroidism in the elderly: Consequences for bone loss and fractures and therapeutic implications. *Endocr. Rev.* **22,** 477–501.

Lips, P. (2006). Vitamin D physiology. *Prog. Biophys. Mol. Biol.* **92,** 4–8.

Liu, P. T., Stenger, S., Li, H., Wenzel, L., Tan, B. H., Krutzik, S. R., Ochoa, M. T., Schauber, J., Wu, K., Meinken, C., Kamen, D. L., Wagner, M., *et al.* (2006). Toll-like receptor triggering of a vitamin D-mediated human antimicrobial response. *Science* **311,** 1770–1773.

Lyles, K. W., Gold, D. T., Shipp, K. M., Pieper, C. F., Martinez, S., and Mulhausen, P. L. (1993). Association of osteoporotic vertebral compression fractures with impaired functional status. *Am. J. Med.* **94,** 595–601.

Manolagas, S. C., and Jilka, R. L. (1995). Bone marrow, cytokines, and bone remodeling. Emerging insights into the pathophysiology of osteoporosis. *N. Engl. J. Med.* **332,** 305–311.

Mathers, C. D., and Loncar, D. (2006). Projections of global mortality and burden of disease from 2002 to 2030. *PLoS Med.* **3,** e442.

Mathieu, C., and Adorini, L. (2002). The coming of age of 1, 25-dihydroxyvitamin D(3) analogs as immunomodulatory agents. *Trends Mol. Med.* **8,** 174–179.

Mathieu, C., Waer, M., Laureys, J., Rutgeerts, O., and Bouillon, R. (1994). Prevention of autoimmune diabetes in NOD mice by 1, 25 dihydroxyvitamin D. *Diabetologia* **37,** 552–558.

Matsuo, K. (2009). Cross-talk among bone cells. *Curr. Opin. Nephrol. Hypertens.* **18,** 292–297.

Merlino, L. A., Curtis, J., Mikuls, T. R., Cerhan, J. R., Criswell, L. A., and Saag, K. G. (2004). Vitamin D intake is inversely associated with rheumatoid arthritis: Results from the Iowa Women's Health Study. *Arthritis Rheum.* **50,** 72–77.

Molfino, N. A., and Coyle, A. J. (2008). Gene-environment interactions in chronic obstructive pulmonary disease. *Int. J. Chron. Obstruct. Pulmon. Dis.* **3,** 491–497.

Munger, K. L., Levin, L. I., Hollis, B. W., Howard, N. S., and Ascherio, A. (2006). Serum 25-hydroxyvitamin D levels and risk of multiple sclerosis. *JAMA* **296,** 2832–2838.

Nevitt, M. C., Ettinger, B., Black, D. M., Stone, K., Jamal, S. A., Ensrud, K., Segal, M., Genant, H. K., and Cummings, S. R. (1998). The association of radiographically detected vertebral fractures with back pain and function: A prospective study. *Ann. Intern. Med.* **128,** 793–800.

Niewoehner, D. E. (2006). The impact of severe exacerbations on quality of life and the clinical course of chronic obstructive pulmonary disease. *Am. J. Med.* **119,** 38–45.

Nnoaham, K. E., and Clarke, A. (2008). Low serum vitamin D levels and tuberculosis: A systematic review and meta-analysis. *Int. J. Epidemiol.* **37,** 113–119.

Norman, A. W., Bouillon, R., Whiting, S. J., Vieth, R., and Lips, P. (2007). 13th Workshop consensus for vitamin D nutritional guidelines. *J. Steroid Biochem. Mol. Biol.* **103,** 204–205.

Nuti, R., Siviero, P., Maggi, S., Guglielmi, G., Caffarelli, C., Crepaldi, G., and Gonnelli, S. (2009). Vertebral fractures in patients with chronic obstructive pulmonary disease: The EOLO Study. *Osteoporos. Int.* **20,** 989–998.

Overbergh, L., Decallonne, B., Valckx, D., Verstuyf, A., Depovere, J., Laureys, J., Rutgeerts, O., Saint-Arnaud, R., Bouillon, R., and Mathieu, C. (2000). Identification and immune regulation of 25-hydroxyvitamin D-1-alpha-hydroxylase in murine macrophages73. *Clin. Exp. Immunol.* **120,** 139–146.

Papaioannou, A., Kennedy, C. C., Cranney, A., Hawker, G., Brown, J. P., Kaiser, S. M., Leslie, W. D., O'Brien, C. J., Sawka, A. M., Khan, A., Siminoski, K., Tarulli, G., *et al.* (2009). Risk factors for low BMD in healthy men age 50 years or older: A systematic review. *Osteoporos. Int.* **20,** 507–518.

Patel, M. S., and Karsenty, G. (2002). Regulation of bone formation and vision by LRP5. *N. Engl. J. Med.* **346,** 1572–1574.

Rabe, K. F., Hurd, S., Anzueto, A., Barnes, P. J., Buist, S. A., Calverley, P., Fukuchi, Y., Jenkins, C., Rodriguez-Roisin, R., van Weel, C., and Zielinski, J. (2007). Global strategy for the diagnosis, management, and prevention of chronic obstructive pulmonary disease: GOLD executive summary. *Am. J. Respir. Crit. Care Med.* **176,** 532–555.

Raisz, L. G. (2005). Pathogenesis of osteoporosis: Concepts, conflicts, and prospects. *J. Clin. Invest.* **115,** 3318–3325.

Sadeghi, K., Wessner, B., Laggner, U., Ploder, M., Tamandl, D., Friedl, J., Zugel, U., Steinmeyer, A., Pollak, A., Roth, E., Boltz-Nitulescu, G., and Spittler, A. (2006). Vitamin D3 down-regulates monocyte TLR expression and triggers hyporesponsiveness to pathogen-associated molecular patterns. *Eur. J. Immunol.* **36,** 361–370.

Sambrook, P., and Cooper, C. (2006). Osteoporosis. *Lancet* **367,** 2010–2018.

Schurch, M. A., Rizzoli, R., Mermillod, B., Vasey, H., Michel, J. P., and Bonjour, J. P. (1996). A prospective study on socioeconomic aspects of fracture of the proximal femur. *J. Bone Miner. Res.* **11,** 1935–1942.

Scragg, R., Sowers, M., and Bell, C. (2004). Serum 25-hydroxyvitamin D, diabetes, and ethnicity in the Third National Health and Nutrition Examination Survey. *Diab. Care* **27,** 2813–2818.

Sethi, S., Mallia, P., and Johnston, S. L. (2009). New paradigms in the pathogenesis of chronic obstructive pulmonary disease II. *Proc. Am. Thorac. Soc.* **6,** 532–534.

Sin, D. D., Man, J. P., and Man, S. F. (2003). The risk of osteoporosis in Caucasian men and women with obstructive airways disease. *Am. J. Med.* **114,** 10–14.

Sinotte, M., Diorio, C., Berube, S., Pollak, M., and Brisson, J. (2009). Genetic polymorphisms of the vitamin D binding protein and plasma concentrations of 25-hydroxyvitamin D in premenopausal women. *Am. J. Clin. Nutr.* **89,** 634–640.

Speeckaert, M., Huang, G., Delanghe, J. R., and Taes, Y. E. (2006). Biological and clinical aspects of the vitamin D binding protein (Gc-globulin) and its polymorphism. *Clin. Chim. Acta* **372,** 33–42.

Suda, T., Takahashi, N., Udagawa, N., Jimi, E., Gillespie, M. T., and Martin, T. J. (1999). Modulation of osteoclast differentiation and function by the new members of the tumor necrosis factor receptor and ligand families. *Endocr. Rev.* **20,** 345–357.

Sutherland, E. R., Goleva, E., Jackson, L. P., Stevens, A. D., and Leung, D. Y. (2010). Vitamin D levels, lung function, and steroid response in adult asthma. *Am. J. Respir. Crit. Care Med.* **181,** 699–704.

Uitterlinden, A. G., Fang, Y., Van Meurs, J. B., Pols, H. A., and Van Leeuwen, J. P. (2004). Genetics and biology of vitamin D receptor polymorphisms. *Gene* **338,** 143–156.

van Etten, E., and Mathieu, C. (2005). Immunoregulation by 1, 25-dihydroxyvitamin D3: Basic concepts. *J. Steroid Biochem. Mol. Biol.* **97,** 93–101.

van Staa, T. P., Leufkens, H. G., and Cooper, C. (2002). The epidemiology of corticosteroid-induced osteoporosis: A meta-analysis. *Osteoporos. Int.* **13,** 777–787.

Vieth, R. (2007). Vitamin D toxicity, policy, and science. *J. Bone Miner. Res.* **22**(Suppl. 2), V64–V68.

Vrieze, A., de Greef, M. H., Wijkstra, P. J., and Wempe, J. B. (2007). Low bone mineral density in COPD patients related to worse lung function, low weight and decreased fat-free mass. *Osteoporos. Int.* **18,** 1197–1202.

Wang, T. T., Nestel, F. P., Bourdeau, V., Nagai, Y., Wang, Q., Liao, J., Tavera-Mendoza, L., Lin, R., Hanrahan, J. W., Mader, S., and White, J. H. (2004). Cutting edge: 1, 25-Dihydroxyvitamin D3 is a direct inducer of antimicrobial peptide gene expression. *J. Immunol.* **173,** 2909–2912.

Wang, T. J., Pencina, M. J., Booth, S. L., Jacques, P. F., Ingelsson, E., Lanier, K., Benjamin, E. J., D'Agostino, R. B., Wolf, M., and Vasan, R. S. (2008). Vitamin D deficiency and risk of cardiovascular disease. *Circulation* **117,** 503–511.

Wicherts, I. S., van Schoor, N. M., Boeke, A. J., Visser, M., Deeg, D. J., Smit, J., Knol, D. L., and Lips, P. (2007). Vitamin D status predicts physical performance and its decline in older persons. *J. Clin. Endocrinol. Metab.* **92,** 2058–2065.

Wright, R. J. (2005). Make no bones about it: Increasing epidemiologic evidence links vitamin D to pulmonary function and COPD. *Chest* **128,** 3781–3783.

Xystrakis, E., Kusumakar, S., Boswell, S., Peek, E., Urry, Z., Richards, D. F., Adikibi, T., Pridgeon, C., Dallman, M., Loke, T. K., Robinson, D. S., Barrat, F. J., *et al.* (2006). Reversing the defective induction of IL-10-secreting regulatory T cells in glucocorticoid-resistant asthma patients. *J. Clin. Invest.* **116,** 146–155.

Zhou, W., Heist, R. S., Liu, G., Neuberg, D. S., Asomaning, K., Su, L., Wain, J. C., Lynch, T. J., Giovannucci, E., and Christiani, D. C. (2006). Polymorphisms of vitamin D receptor and survival in early-stage non-small cell lung cancer patients. *Cancer Epidemiol. Biomarkers Prev.* **15,** 2239–2245.

Zhou, W., Heist, R. S., Liu, G., Asomaning, K., Neuberg, D. S., Hollis, B. W., Wain, J. C., Lynch, T. J., Giovannucci, E., Su, L., and Christiani, D. C. (2007). Circulating 25-hydroxyvitamin D levels predict survival in early-stage non-small-cell lung cancer patients. *J. Clin. Oncol.* **25,** 479–485.

CHAPTER EIGHTEEN

Vitamin D as a T-cell Modulator in Multiple Sclerosis

Joost Smolders*,† *and* Jan Damoiseaux‡

Contents

Abstract

Vitamin D is a potent immune modulator, keeping the T-cell compartment in a more tolerogenic state. Multiple sclerosis (MS), a disease in which an autoreactive T-cell response contributes to inflammation in the central nervous system, has been associated with vitamin D deficiency. The effects of vitamin D on the immune system are believed to be an important driver of this

* School for Mental Health and Neuroscience, Maastricht University Medical Center, Maastricht, The Netherlands
† Department of Internal Medicine, Division of Clinical and Experimental Immunology, Maastricht University Medical Center, Maastricht, The Netherlands
‡ Laboratory of Clinical Immunology, Maastricht University Medical Center, Maastricht, The Netherlands

Vitamins and Hormones, Volume 86
ISSN 0083-6729, DOI: 10.1016/B978-0-12-386960-9.00018-6

association. In this chapter, we elaborate on vitamin D as a modulator of the T-cell response. This discussion will be placed in the perspective of MS as a T-cell-mediated disease and in the perspective of the numerous association studies on vitamin D deficiency and multiple health outcomes. We conclude that there is a firm experimental and epidemiological basis supporting the model of vitamin D as a physiological immune modulator, on which intervention studies assessing clinical and immunological outcome measures should be designed.

I. Introduction

In the past years, vitamin D changed colors from merely a necessity for maintaining a healthy calcium metabolism to a potential preventive agent or cure for several adverse health outcomes and diseases. In multiple sclerosis (MS), vitamin D has become a major topic of interest for several research groups worldwide. Experimental evidence suggests that the interaction between vitamin D and the immune system, and in particular the T-cell compartment, may be the key to a new treatment modality for MS patients (Hayes *et al.*, 1997). The aim of this chapter is to discuss the interaction between the peripheral T-cell response and vitamin D reflected against the immune pathogenesis of MS. Finally, we combine immunological and epidemiological studies in a working model and discuss the present uncertainties and relevant targets for further research.

II. Multiple Sclerosis

A. Disease characteristics

MS is an invalidating disease of the central nervous system (CNS). The prevalence of MS is about 100 per 100,000 subjects. Similarly to most other autoimmune diseases, MS affects more females than males. The female/male ratio has increased during the past decades and is now estimated to be about 2.0 (Orton *et al.*, 2006). The age at disease onset is typically between 20 and 50 years of age, although MS can also sporadically have its onset during childhood or in the elderly. At onset, patients most frequently experience subacute attacks of neurological impairment, which resolve spontaneously after several days. At this stage, the disease is called relapsing remitting MS (RRMS). Although impairment resolves completely at disease onset, in later stage of disease recovery is not complete and impairment accumulates. Although some patients only experience a limited amount of disability throughout their disease courses, many will in time develop a gradually worsening of symptoms without attacks. In this stage, the disease is called secondary progressive MS (SPMS). A small proportion of patients experiences progressive disability from disease onset onward without exacerbations, and in these patients, the disease is called primary progressive MS (PPMS) (Compston and Coles, 2002). At disease onset, there have been only few tools identified to predict the severity of the clinical course of an individual patient. The impairment which patients experience is diverse in quantity and quality and can arise from dysfunction of each component of the CNS. Although loss of motor function and subsequent loss of mobility are most well recognized, symptoms can also include visual impairment, sensory impairment, balance disorders, bowel dysfunction, sexual dysfunction, etc.

B. The T-cell compartment in multiple sclerosis

Pathological and radiological studies of the CNS of MS patients revealed that pathogenesis is characterized by two phenomena: (i) focalized inflammation of CNS tissue and (ii) loss of neurons (Compston and Coles, 2002). Although the causality of these phenomena has often been disputed, there is increasing consensus that inflammation is the primary driver of the disease process of MS. Evidence of a disturbed T-cell homeostasis in MS patients is mounting, and at present, large genetic screens revealed almost exclusively immune-related risk alleles for developing MS. Further, even in patients with progressive disease, compartmentalized inflammation of the CNS remains a key characteristic in the pathological image of MS. Many clinical and experimental studies have addressed the immune pathogenesis of MS (reviewed in Bar-Or, 2008; Goverman, 2009).

The attack of the immune system on the CNS starts in the peripheral lymphoid organs, where antigen presenting cells (APC) present an epitope to naïve T cells. The nature of this epitope is uncertain, but a viral protein mimicking CNS proteins, soluble factors leaking from the CNS, and CNS proteins actively transferred by dendritic cells (DCs) from the CNS have been proposed. Autoreactive $CD4^+$ T cells lose their tolerant state for self-antigens, are primed, and enter the circulation. These cells adopt a proinflammatory cytokine profile, including production of interferon gamma (IFN-γ) by T helper type 1 (Th1) cells and interleukin 17 (IL-17) by Th17 cells. Patient-control studies revealed that peripheral regulatory mechanisms to maintain T-cell tolerance are impaired in MS patients. In a healthy T-cell compartment, regulatory $CD4^+$ T cells (Tregs) are capable of controlling the quality and quantity of the immune response. In patients with a number of autoimmune diseases, including MS, these Tregs have been found to be less effective suppressors of T-cell responses, while their number in the circulation is not affected (Haas *et al.*, 2005; Venken *et al.*, 2006; Viglietta *et al.*, 2004). This defective control mechanism enables the activation of autoreactive T cells. The autoreactive T cells attach to the very late antigen 4 (VLA-4) receptors on the blood–brain barrier and actively enter the CNS by secreting metalloproteinases. In the CNS, they are reactivated by resident APC, including macrophages and microglia cells. Subsequently, the T cells contribute to a focalized inflammatory reaction, in which the myelin sheet surrounding neurons is degraded.

C. Treatment of multiple sclerosis

The registered MS drugs so far are mostly either modulators or suppressors of the peripheral T-cell compartment. Beta Interferons and Glatiramer Acetate skew the balance between proinflammatory Th1 and anti-inflammatory Th2 cells toward a Th2 phenotype and promote the suppressive function of Tregs as well as the induction of naïve Tregs (de Andres *et al.*, 2007; Schrempf and Ziemssen, 2007). Therapies like mitoxantrone and cyclophosphamide are cytotoxic for T cells in the periphery (Neuhaus *et al.*, 2005). The newer therapy Natalizumab (anti-VLA-4 antibodies) prevents T cells from entering the CNS (Miller *et al.*, 2003). Regarding the severe side effects of the immune suppressive therapies, most patients start with immune-modulating drugs. These drugs reduce the number of MS exacerbations with 30%, but at the cost of several side effects. In the past years, attention has been drawn on vitamin D as a potential physiological promoter of T-cell homeostasis and, subsequently, as a potential therapy in MS.

III. Vitamin D

A. Sources of vitamin D

Vitamins are defined as substances of whom we are dependent upon our environment and which are vital for biological processes in the body, apart from their caloric value. While most vitamins are acquired via dietary intake, vitamin D is a unique vitamin in this perspective. The largest part is synthesized in the skin under the influence of ultraviolet B (UVB) radiation. Out of 7-dehydrocholesterol, UVB radiation forms pre-vitamin D, which transforms spontaneously as a result of body temperature to cholecalciferol or vitamin D_3. The vitamin D which is acquired via the diet contains both cholecalciferol, derived from animal products and ergocalciferol (vitamin D_2), which is derived from plant products. It is uncertain whether these forms of vitamin D differ in biological function. The contribution of dietary vitamin D intake to the total daily amount of vitamin D acquired is modest. However, depending on the geographical latitude, the amount of vitamin D effective UVB-radiation is limited through winter in large areas on the globe (Kimlin, 2008). In British children and elders, it was shown that vitamin D intake only predicts vitamin D status during winter and not in the other seasons (Bates *et al.*, 2003; Davies *et al.*, 1999).

B. Vitamin D metabolism

In the circulation, only small amounts of vitamin D are present. This molecule has a biological half-life of 12–16 h (Smith and Goodman, 1971), and fluctuates depending on the exposure to either sunlight or dietary intake (Hollis *et al.*, 2007). It is entirely bound to a specialized carrier protein, vitamin D-binding protein (DBP). The vitamin D is almost instantly hydroxylated in the liver by 25-hydroxylases (CYP2R1, CYP27A1, and CYP3A4) towards 25-hydroxyvitamin D (25(OH)D) (Fig. 18.1). This is the most abundant metabolite in the circulation and is most accepted to reflect the overall vitamin D status of an individual. It has a half-life of 20–90 days and is bound for about 90% to DBP

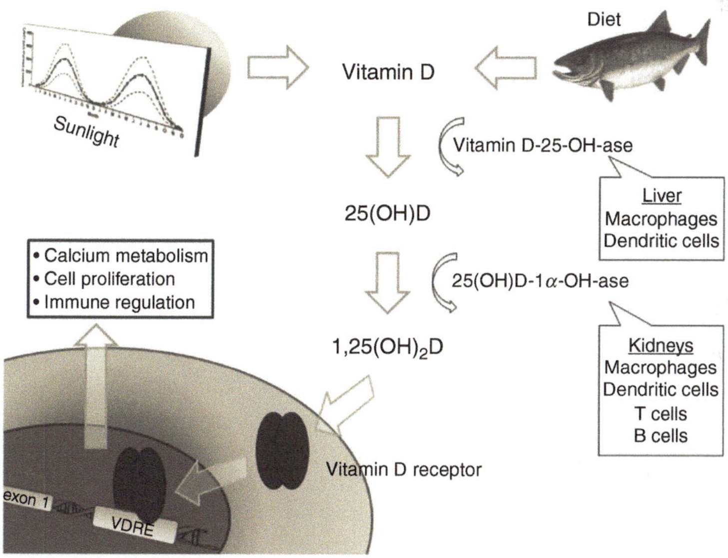

Figure 18.1 Vitamin D metabolism and action. Vitamin D is acquired via diet and via photosynthesis in the skin, dependent on the amount of intake and sun exposure, respectively. In the body, vitamin D is instantly hydroxylized in 25-hydroxyvitamin D (25(OH)D), the most abundant vitamin D metabolite. This metabolite can be further hydroxylized in the biologically active form, 1,25-dihydroxyvitamin D (1,25(OH)$_2$D). This metabolite interacts with the vitamin D receptor, which binds to vitamin response elements (VDRE) in the nucleus and induces transcription or transrepression of vitamin D responsive genes. This interaction affects calcium metabolism, cell proliferation, and immune regulation.

(Mawer *et al.*, 1969; Smith and Goodman, 1971). The other 10% is primarily bound to other serum proteins including albumin, and only a small fraction of about 0.40% is freely available. Although 25(OH)D is the most abundant vitamin D metabolite, it is not biologically active. Another hydroxylation step by 1-α-hydroxylase (CYP27B1) is required to form the biologically active metabolite of vitamin D, 1,25-dihydroxyvitamin D (1,25 $(OH)_2D$). The serum levels of 1,25$(OH)_2D$ are mostly dependent on expression of 1-α-hydroxylase in the kidneys upon signals from calcium metabolism (Jongen *et al.*, 1984). The biological effects of 1,25$(OH)_2D$ result from either direct actions at the cell membrane, or via modulation of gene transcription via intracellular binding to the vitamin D receptor (VDR). When bound to 1,25$(OH)_2D$, the VDR forms heterodimers with the retinoid X receptor (RXR) and moves to the nucleus of the cell. Here, it binds to a vitamin D response element and causes transcription or transrepression of vitamin responsive genes (reviewed in Smolders *et al.*, 2009a).

C. Vitamin D deficiency and calcium metabolism

The role of vitamin D in calcium metabolism is most well known. Vitamin D was discovered in the beginning of the twentieth century as the active substance in cod liver oil. Cod liver oil was identified as the cure of rickets in children. Vitamin D is an essential component for maintaining a stable calcium level in the circulation. If the serum calcium level drops, chief cells in the parathyroid gland start secreting parathyroid hormone (PTH). Besides some direct effects on bone metabolism, PTH predominantly catalyzes, via CYP27B1, the hydroxylation of 25(OH)D to 1,25$(OH)_2D$ in the kidneys. Elevated serum 1,25$(OH)_2D$ levels lead to an increased uptake of calcium from the intestines, increased resorption of calcium in the proximal tubules of the kidneys, and an increased osteoclast activity. The subsequent rise of serum calcium restores the balance between serum calcium and PTH. The availability of too little of the precursor 25(OH)D to be hydroxylized in 1,25$(OH)_2D$ results in a decompensation of this system. As a stable serum calcium level is vital for many processes in the body, calcium is retrieved from the skeleton to compensate for the loss of calcium via kidneys and intestine. Therefore, a poor vitamin D status has been associated with loss of bone mineral density (BMD; Bischoff-Ferrari *et al.*, 2004) and increased risk of fractures (Cauley *et al.*, 2009; Lopes *et al.*, 2009). Supplementation of vitamin D with or without calcium has been shown to improve BMD (Tang *et al.*, 2007) and to decrease fracture risk (Bischoff-Ferrari *et al.*, 2005) in the elderly. The latter effect may be due to an increased BMD, but additionally, supplementation of vitamin D also decreases the risk of falling (Bischoff-Ferrari *et al.*, 2009). The decreased risk of falling may be attributable to a favorable effect of vitamin D on muscle strength (Stewart *et al.*, 2009).

D. Extra-calcemic consequences of vitamin D deficiency

Apart from its association with osteoporosis and osteopenia, a poor vitamin D status has also been associated with an increased risk on numerous other diseases, which cluster around the main themes of cardiovascular diseases, cancer, and (auto)immune diseases. Two large prospective studies found a poor vitamin D status to be associated with an increased risk on myocardial infarction (Giovannucci *et al.*, 2008) and peripheral arterial disease (Melamed *et al.*, 2008a). A recent extensive systematic review on association studies on serum 25(OH)D levels and blood pressure concluded vitamin D status to be negatively correlated with systolic and diastolic blood pressure (Pilz *et al.*, 2009a). The incidence of breast cancer prospectively correlated negatively with serum 25(OH)D levels (Abbas *et al.*, 2008) as well as the incidence of colon cancer (Yin *et al.*, 2009a). Further, vitamin D status correlated negatively with the incidence of nonmelanoma skin cancer (Tang *et al.*, 2010) and positively with the survival of melanoma skin cancer patients (Newton-Bishop *et al.*, 2009). The effect of vitamin D status in prostate cancer is less certain (Yin *et al.*, 2009b). Taken into account the large part of cardiovascular diseases and cancers in overall mortality, it is intriguing that in two large population studies, vitamin D status was prospectively associated with all-cause mortality (Melamed *et al.*, 2008b; Pilz *et al.*, 2009b). A large number of autoimmune diseases has been associated with correlates of a poor vitamin D status with varying consistency, including diabetes mellitus type 1 (Hyppönen *et al.*, 2001), rheumatoid arthritis (Cutolo *et al.*, 2006), systemic lupus erythematodes (Müller *et al.*, 1995), and vasculitis (Gatenby *et al.*, 2009). In MS, a limited vitamin D exposure has also been associated with an increased disease incidence, as has been reviewed extensively (Ascherio *et al.*, 2010; Smolders *et al.*, 2008a). In short, decreased sun exposure during adolescence (Islam *et al.*, 2007; Kampman *et al.*, 2007), a decreased dietary intake of vitamin D (Munger *et al.*, 2004), and decreased serum levels of 25(OH)D during adolescence (Munger *et al.*, 2006) have been associated with an increased risk on developing MS in later life. Additionally, in MS patients, the amount of disability and the odds on remaining relapse-free correlated negatively with vitamin D status (Smolders *et al.*, 2008b; van der Mei *et al.*, 2007), and serum 25(OH)D levels were lower during relapses of MS when compared with periods of remission (Correale *et al.*, 2009; Soliu-Hänninen *et al.*, 2005, 2008). Two recent, prospective studies showed an inverse linear relationship between serum 25 (OH)D levels and the hazard of relapses in adults and children with relapsing remitting MS (Mowry *et al.*, 2010; Simpson *et al.*, 2010). Interestingly, a consistent seasonal fluctuation in the birth dates of MS patients is present, which deviates from healthy control data (Willer *et al.*, 2005). This data reveal a large proportion of patients born in spring (April/May) and a low proportion born in autumn (November).

Altogether, the presented evidence forms a consistent picture in which a higher vitamin D status is associated with a better prognosis on several health outcomes. However, the discussion about causation remains. In the past years, the scientific community gathered increasing amounts of evidence that vitamin D is of vital importance for more biological processes than the maintenance of calcium metabolism alone, including cell proliferation and immune regulation. These often basal scientific studies provide further building stones for the identification of biological mechanisms underlying the reported associations. In the case of MS and other autoimmune diseases, the interaction between vitamin D and immune regulation is of special interest. Several studies suggest that this interaction is a good candidate to underlie the reported associations (Hayes *et al.*, 1997).

IV. Vitamin D and T-cell Regulation in MS

A. Vitamin D receptor expression by immune cells

Numerous immune cells express the VDR. First, the expression of VDR mRNA by monocytes and activated B and T cells was recognized (Provvedini *et al.*, 1983). Measured by ELISA, both $CD4^+$ and $CD8^+$ T cells expressed VDR protein, which was upregulated upon activation and exposition to $1,25(OH)_2D$ (Veldman *et al.*, 2000). In resting naïve T cells, VDR protein levels were absent but upregulated on stimulation with anti-CD3 and anti-CD28 via the p38 TCR-signaling pathway (Von Essen *et al.*, 2010). In purified resting $CD4^+$ T cells, VDR mRNA expression was almost absent but was upregulated upon activation with phytohemagglutinin (PHA) or anti-CD3 (Correale *et al.*, 2009). Addition of $1,25(OH)_2D$ further upregulated VDR mRNA expression. Resting mature myeloid and plasmacytoid DCs, as well as immature myeloid DCs and monocytes expressed similarly high levels of VDR mRNA, which were not further enhanced by addition of $1,25(OH)_2D$ (Penna *et al.*, 2007). Others observed low, but detectable, levels of VDR expression in monocytes, which were instantly upregulated by a DC differentiation cocktail comprising granulocyte-macrophage colony-stimulating factor (GM-CSF) and IL-4 (Széles *et al.*, 2009). Resting B cells express undetectable amounts of VDR mRNA, but after activation or exposure to $1,25(OH)_2D$, expression of the VDR is upregulated (Chen *et al.*, 2007).

It can be concluded that APC express the receptor for $1,25(OH)_2D$, irrespective of activation or $1,25(OH)_2D$ exposition, while resting lymphocytes express very low amounts of VDR, which is upregulated on activation or exposition to $1,25(OH)_2D$. Therefore, immune cells appear to be a target for $1,25(OH)_2D$. Additionally, lymphocytes appear to become more susceptible for the actions of $1,25(OH)_2D$ when activated.

B. Metabolism of vitamin D by immune cells

The largest proportion of the vitamin D metabolites present in the circulation, lymphoid organs, and tissues comprises 25(OH)D. Only a small part (0.1%) consists of the biologically active metabolite 1,25$(OH)_2$D. Numerous immune cell types, however, have the ability to express 25(OH)D-1-α-hydroxylase (CYP27B1) and actively form 1,25$(OH)_2$D. Activated T cells upregulate the expression of CYP27B1, either on activation with anti-CD3 and anti-CD28 in a T cell/DC coculture (Sigmundsdottir *et al.*, 2007), or on activation with PHA in a $CD4^+$ T-cell monoculture (Correale *et al.*, 2009). *In vitro*, this upregulation also results in the formation of 1,25$(OH)_2$D out of 25(OH)D (Correale *et al.*, 2009; Sigmundsdottir *et al.*, 2007). Several APC, including macrophages and DC, also express high levels of CYP27B1. Resting blood DCs synthesize limited amounts of 1,25 $(OH)_2$D, which is dramatically upregulated by activation with LPS, accompanied by an upregulation of CYP27B1 expression (Fritsche *et al.*, 2003). The presence of 1,25$(OH)_2$D inhibits the expression of CYP27B1. In addition, human resting monocytes do not express CYP27B1, whereas *in vitro* differentiated macrophages and DC do express CYP27B1 and subsequently form 1,25$(OH)_2$D out of 25(OH)D (Gottfried *et al.*, 2006; Széles *et al.*, 2009). B cells are also able to form 1,25$(OH)_2$D out of 25(OH) D upon activation with several activation cocktails (Chen *et al.*, 2007; Heine *et al.*, 2008). Additionally, B cells express 1,25$(OH)_2$D-24-hydroxylase (CYP24A1) on exposure to 1,25$(OH)_2$D when in an activated state (anti-IgG/anti-CD40/IL-21) (Chen *et al.*, 2007; Heine *et al.*, 2008). Also, monocytes, macrophages, and DC (Gottfried *et al.*, 2006; Penna *et al.*, 2007), as well as T cells (Correale *et al.*, 2009) express CYP24A1 upon exposure to 1,25$(OH)_2$D. To evoke catabolism of 1,25$(OH)_2$D, activation of these cells is not mandatory.

In summary, activation of an immune response is accompanied by a local induction of 1,25$(OH)_2$D synthesis out of the locally available 25(OH)D (Fig. 18.2). When 1,25$(OH)_2$D is abundantly present, both activated and resting immune cells catabolize this metabolite. The observations that almost all immune cells carry the VDR and metabolize its ligand upon activation suggest that vitamin D might have an important autocrine function for immune regulation. Interestingly, CYP27A1, the enzyme which catalyzes the vitamin D-25-hydroxylation, is also expressed by macrophages and DCs upon activation, resulting in a local formation of 25(OH)D (Gottfried *et al.*, 2006; Sigmundsdottir *et al.*, 2007). The relevance of this mechanism in the periphery, where 25(OH)D is abundantly available, is probably limited. However, in the skin, where vitamin D_3 itself is mostly present, this mechanism is important to induce effective 1,25$(OH)_2$D synthesis.

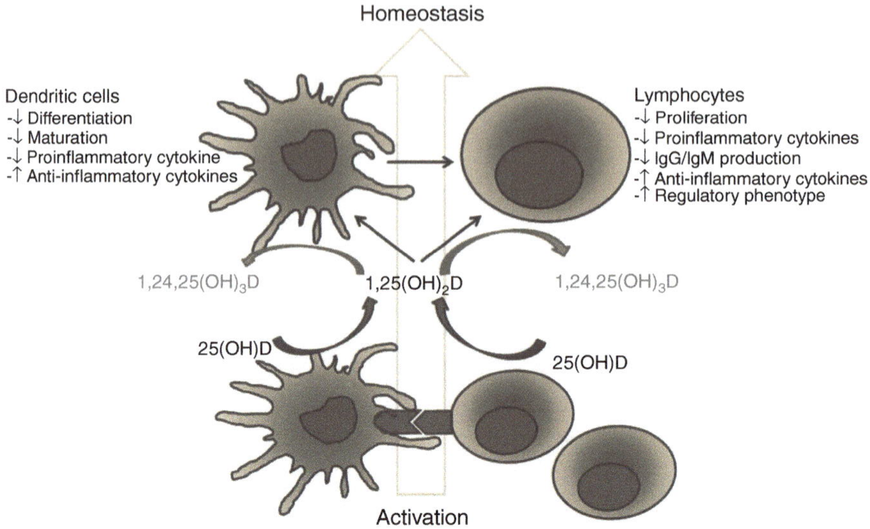

Figure 18.2 Interaction between vitamin D and the immune response. At sites of immune activation, expression of CYP27B1 and subsequent formation of 1,25$(OH)_2$D out of 25(OH)D are induced in activated immune cells. This results in a microenvironment of high local levels of 1,25$(OH)_2$D. Binding of 1,25$(OH)_2$D to the VDR, which is present in almost every immune cell, results in a functional modulation of APC/DC and activated B and T cells. Vitamin D exerts its effects on lymphocytes both directly and via modulation of APC/DC. When exposed to 1,25$(OH)_2$D, lymphocytes and DCs express CYP24A1, catalyzing the inactivation of 1,25$(OH)_2$D. Altogether, activation of an immune response is accompanied by local activation of 25(OH)D, subsequently establishing an increased level of homeostasis.

C. *In vitro* effects of 1,25$(OH)_2$D on the immune response

As activated immune cells synthesize 1,25$(OH)_2$D and express the VDR, 1,25$(OH)_2$D is likely to affect the immune response. Several studies investigated the effect of 1,25$(OH)_2$D exposition on the immune response *in vitro*. Studies on lymphocytes can be divided in studies which assessed the effect of 1,25$(OH)_2$D on proliferation, cytokine production, and the phenotype of cells. Unless stated otherwise, all data concern studies with human cells. Results are summarized in Table 18.1.

Addition of 1,25$(OH)_2$D to cell cultures directly inhibits proliferation of peripheral blood mononuclear cells (PBMC), T cells, and $CD4^+$ T cells on several mitogenic (Correale *et al.*, 2009; Fritsche *et al.*, 2003; Lemire *et al.*, 1984; Rigby *et al.*, 1984) and antigen-specific stimuli (Correale *et al.*, 2009). Purified $CD45RO^+$ T cells were more responsive to 1,25$(OH)_2$D suppression than $CD45RA^+$ T cells, suggesting a predominant suppression of memory T cells (Müller and Bendtzen, 1992). Interestingly, monocultures of T cells stimulated with anti-CD3 and anti-CD28 could not be suppressed

Table 18.1 Direct *in vitro* effects of $1,25(OH)_2D$ on proliferation and cytokine production of immune cells

Cell population	Stimulus	Proliferation	Proinflammatory cytokines/chemokines	Anti-inflammatory cytokines/ chemokines	Phenotypic markers	Reference
PBMC	PWM, PHA, DO, or SAC	Inhibited	↓IFN-γ, ↓GM-CSF, ↓IL-2, ↓IgM, ↓IgG, ↓IgA	–	–	Rigby *et al.* (1984), Lemire *et al.* (1984), Bhalla *et al.* (1986), Reichel *et al.* (1987), Tobler *et al.* (1987), Iho *et al.* (1986), Chen *et al.* (1987), Shiozawa *et al.* (1987), Müller *et al.* (1992b)
	Mixed-lymphocyte reaction	Inhibited	↓IFN-γ	–	–	Fritsche *et al.* (2003), Penna and Adorini (2000)
	Tetanus toxoid in vaccinated subjects	Inhibited	↓IL-2	–	–	Bhalla *et al.* (1986)
	Epstein–Bar Virus	Unaffected	=IgM, =IgG, =IgA	–	–	Müller *et al.* (1992b)
T cells (purified or enriched populations)	Anti-CD3 coated with(out) anti-CD28 monoculture	Unaffected	=IFN-γ	–	–	Penna and Adorini (2000)
	PHA	Inhibited	↓IFN-γ, ↓GM-CSF	–	–	Reichel *et al.* (1987), Tobler *et al.* (1987)
CD4+ T cells	PHA monoculture	Inhibited	[↓IL-6, ↓IL-17][a]	[↑IL-10][a]	–	Correale *et al.* (2009)
	Cognate antigen with irradiated PBMC	Inhibited	[↓IL-6, ↓IL-17][a]	[↑IL-10][a]	–	Correale *et al.* (2009)
	Anti-CD3, anti-CD28 monoculture	Unaffected	↓IFN-γ, ↓IL-2, ↓IL-17, ↓IL-21	↑IL-4, ↑IL-5, ↑IL-10	↑FoxP3, ↑CTLA-4, ↑$CD25^+FoxP3^+$	Barrat *et al.* (2002), Jeffery *et al.* (2009), Correale *et al.* (2009)
	Anti-CD3 coated monoculture	–	↓IL-6, ↓IL-17	↑IL-10	–	Correale *et al.* (2009)
	Anti-CD3 with autologous monocytes	Slightly inhibited	↓IFN-γ, ↓IL-2, ↓IL-17, ↓IL-21	↑IL-10	↑CTLA-4, =FoxP3	Jeffery *et al.* (2009)
	OVA + APC	–	↓IFN-γ	↑IL-4, ↑IL-5, ↑IL-10	–	Barrat *et al.* (2002), Boonstra *et al.* (2001)

(continued)

Table 18.1 *(continued)*

Cell population	Stimulus	Proliferation	Proinflammatory cytokines/chemokines	Anti-inflammatory cytokines/ chemokines	Phenotypic markers	Reference
CD8+ T cells	Con-A	Slightly promoted	–	–	–	Veldman *et al.* (2000)
	PHA	–	↓IL-2, ↓IFN-γ	↑/↓IL-4, ↑IL-13	–	Thien *et al.* (2005), Pichler *et al.* (2002)
Monocytes[b]	IL-4, GM-CSF (exposed to 1,25$(OH)_2$D during 6–7 days differentiation towards M-DC)	–	–	–	↓CD1a, ↑CD14, ↑CD32,=/↓CD40, =CD54, =/↓ CD86, ↑MR, ↑MHC-I, =/↓ MHC-II	Penna and Adorini (2000), van Halteren *et al.* (2002), Piemonti *et al.* (2000)
	LPS, CD40L (exposed to 1,25$(OH)_2$D during 7 days differentiation towards M-iDC on GM-CSF + IL-4)	–	↓IL-12 p70	=IL-10	↓CD1a, ↑CD14, ↑CD32, =/↓ CD40, =CD54, =/↓CD80, ↓CD83, ↓CD86, ↑MR, ↓MHC-I, ↓MHC-II	Piemonti *et al.* (2000)
Immature M-DC (derived from isolated monocytes)	IL-4, GM-CSF (exposed to 1,25$(OH)_2$D after 7 days differentiation towards M-DC on GM-CSF + IL-4)	–	–	–	↓CD1a, ↑CD14, ↓/= CD40, =CD80, ↓CD86, =MHC-I, ↓MHC-II	Piemonti *et al.* (2000)
	LPS, CD40L (exposed to 1,25$(OH)_2$D, GM-CSF and IL-4 after 7 days differentiation towards M-iDC on GM-CSF + IL-4).	–	–	–	↓CD40, ↓CD80, ↓CD83, ↓CD86, ↓MHC-I , ↓MHC-II	Piemonti *et al.* (2000)

	LPS, CD40L (exposed to $1,25(OH)_2D$ during maturation)	–	↓IL-12p70, ↓IL-12 p75	↑IL-10	=CD1a, ↑CD14, =/↓ CD40, =CD54, ↓CD58, =/↓ CD80, =/↓CD83, =/↓CD86, ↑MR, =/↓MHC-II	Penna and Adorini (2000), van Halteren (2002)
Blood derived M-DC	Unstimulated and CD40L	–	↓CCL17, ↓IL-12 p75	↑CCl22	↓CD40, ↓CD80, ↓CD86, ↓MHC-II, ↑ILT3	Penna *et al.* (2007)
B cells	Anti-IgM, anti-CD40, IL-21	Inhibited	↓IgG	–	↑CD38, ↓IgG, ↑IgM	Chen *et al.* (2007)
	B cell cross-linking, anti-CD40, IL-4	Unaffected	IgG unaffected	↑IL-10	↑CD38	Heine *et al.* (2008)

Direct effects of $1,25(OH)_2D$ on immune cells as observed in *in vitro* cultures. The effect of $1,25(OH)_2D$ on proliferation, cytokine/chemokine/antibody production, and phenotype of the given cell populations when added to cultures with the given stimuli are designated as ↑: increased; ↓: decreased; =: not significantly different. Abbreviations used: CCL: chemokine (C-C motive) ligand; Con-A: Concanavalin A; DO: dermatophyton O; ILT3: immunoglobulin-like transcript 3; IL: interleukin; M-DC: myeloid dendritic cell; PBMC: peripheral blood mononuclear cell; PHA: Phytohemagglutinin; PWM: Pokeweed Mitogen; SAC: *Staphylococcus aureus* Cowan I.

[a] These results were not shown, but described in the paper by Correale *et al.* (2009).

[b] Older studies on monocytes are not included in the present table, since phenotyping differs from the current studies. These studies comprise: Ohta *et al.* (1985), Bhalla *et al.* (1986), Rigby *et al.* (1990), d'Ambrosio *et al.* (1998), and Müller *et al.* (1992b).

directly by 1,25$(OH)_2$D (Jeffery *et al.*, 2009; Penna and Adorini, 2000). Additionally, proliferation of purified naïve T cells of chronic hemodialysis patients on anti-CD3 and anti-CD28 has even been reported to be promoted by 1,25$(OH)_2$D (Von Essen *et al.*, 2010). It can be concluded that 1,25$(OH)_2$D can directly suppress proliferation of PBMC and $CD4^+$ T cells unless the stimulus is too strong (anti-CD3 and anti-CD28), and rather suppresses proliferation of memory than naïve T cells. Addition of the precursor 25(OH)D also suppresses proliferation of PBMC in mixed lymphocyte reactions (Fritsche *et al.*, 2003) and PHA-driven proliferation of $CD4^+$ T cells in monoculture (Correale *et al.*, 2009). The metabolism of 25 (OH)D by CYP27B1 upon activation, therefore, seems to have autocrine effects, modulating the functional behavior of the lymphocytes. As 25(OH) D is also the most abundantly available vitamin D metabolite *in vivo*, the latter experimental model might also be the most relevant for studying vitamin D and lymphocyte interactions. Catabolites of vitamin D, 24,25 $(OH)_2$D, and 25,26$(OH)_2$D do not induce suppression of proliferation (Correale *et al.*, 2009).

Much attention has been paid to the effects of 1,25$(OH)_2$D exposition on the cytokine production by activated T cells *in vitro*. Addition of 1,25 $(OH)_2$D suppressed proinflammatory cytokine production in cultures of PBMC, T cells, or $CD4^+$ T cells stimulated with mitogens (Müller *et al.*, 1991a,b; Reichel *et al.*, 1987; Rigby *et al.*, 1984; Tobler *et al.*, 1987), with T-cell receptor agonists (Correale *et al.*, 2009), or specific antigens (Boonstra *et al.*, 2001; Jeffery *et al.*, 2009). Cytokines suppressed by 1,25 $(OH)_2$D included IFN-γ, IL-2, IL-6, IL-17, IL-21, and GM-CSF. In addition to the suppression of proinflammatory cytokines, the production of anti-inflammatory cytokines seemed to be promoted. Addition of 1,25 $(OH)_2$D to T-cell monocultures or DC cocultures, stimulated with T-cell receptor agonists (Barrat *et al.*, 2002; Boonstra *et al.*, 2001; Correale *et al.*, 2009) or specific antigens (Barrat *et al.*, 2002; Boonstra *et al.*, 2001), resulted in increased production of IL-4, IL-5, and IL-10. These studies show that exposition of activated T cells to 1,25$(OH)_2$D results in a skewing of proinflammatory toward anti-inflammatory cytokine production. The effects seen in monocultures reveal that there is a direct interaction between vitamin D and T cells.

The shift in proliferation and cytokine production of $CD4^+$ T cell has also been reflected in phenotypic changes. Culture of PBMC in the presence of 1,25$(OH)_2$D resulted in a dramatically increased proportion of functionally active Tregs ($CD25^+FoxP3^+$ $CD4^+$ T cells) (Correale *et al.*, 2009). In addition, in an anti-CD3 and anti-CD28-driven monoculture of $CD4^+$ T cells, 1,25$(OH)_2$D treatment induced FoxP3 and CTLA-4 expression (Jeffery *et al.*, 2009), again suggesting the induction of Tregs. Interestingly, the upregulation of FoxP3 was completely abrogated by the stimulation with autologous monocytes and anti-CD3, which was again restored by addition of IL-2 (Jeffery *et al.*, 2009). Altogether, 1,25$(OH)_2D$ appears to induce a regulatory T-cell phenotype in activated $CD4^+$ T cells. The combination of proliferation, cytokine production, and phenotypic analysis shows that vitamin D induces directly a more tolerogenic $CD4^+$ T-cell compartment (Fig. 18.2).

Direct effects of 1,25$(OH)_2D$ on $CD8^+$ T cells are uncertain. $CD8^+$ T cells do express the VDR protein and, in contrast to $CD4^+$ T cells, exposition to 1,25$(OH)_2D$ modestly improved proliferation rate (Veldman *et al.*, 2000). However, the cytotoxicity of $CD8^+$ T cells, as measured in a ^{51}Cr release assay, was inhibited by 1,25$(OH)_2D$ (Meehan *et al.*, 1992). The effects on cytokine production match these of the $CD4^+$ T cells, with an inhibition of IL-2 and IFN-γ and promotion of IL-4 and IL-13 (Thien *et al.*, 2005). In cord blood samples cultured under the same conditions, however, IL-4 production by $CD8^+$ T cells was suppressed by 1,25$(OH)_2D$ (Pichler *et al.*, 2002). It can be concluded that the effect of 1,25$(OH)_2D$ on $CD8^+$ T cells has not been very consistent so far, probably because $CD8^+$ T cells have received only little attention yet.

Besides the direct effects on the T-cell compartment, 1,25$(OH)_2D$ also affects the maturation and cytokine production of APC. In older studies, monocytes cultured with proinflammatory stimuli and 1,25$(OH)_2D$ display a VDR-dependent loss of maturation markers (Griffin *et al.*, 2000; Rigby *et al.*, 1990) and a loss of IL-6, IL-12, and tumor necrosis factor α (TNF-α) production (d'Ambrosio *et al.*, 1998; Müller *et al.*, 1992). Treatment with 25 (OH)D gives the same effects, albeit to a lesser extent. Alternatively, however, treatment of monocytes and macrophages with only 1,25 $(OH)_2D$ has been reported to increase the production of the proinflammatory cytokine IL-1 and cathelicidin antimicrobial peptide (Bhalla *et al.*, 1986; Gombart *et al.*, 2005). A promotion of monocyte proliferation has also been reported (Ohta *et al.*, 1985). Therefore, regarding monocytes and macrophages, the effects of vitamin D seem to depend on the way these cells are challenged. However, when monocytes are cultured supporting DC differentiation, the effect of 1,25$(OH)_2D$ becomes more consistent. Addition of 1,25$(OH)_2D$ to monocyte cultures hinders their differentiation to immature myeloid DC (Penna and Adorini, 2000; Piemonti *et al.*, 2000; van Halteren *et al.*, 2002). Additionally, fully differentiated immature myeloid DC can also lose their DC phenotype after exposition to 1,25$(OH)_2D$, reflected by a loss of CD1a and upregulation of CD14 (Piemonti *et al.*, 2000). Different maturation protocols of immature myeloid DC to mature DC are also inhibited by 1,25$(OH)_2D$, as reflected by surface markers of maturation (Griffin *et al.*, 2001; Penna and Adorini, 2000; Piemonti, 2000; van Halteren *et al.*, 2002). Interestingly, also functional consequences have been described. As suggested by the preservation of the mannose receptor and CD32, the antigen uptake capacity of the 1,25$(OH)_2D$-matured myeloid DC is improved (Piemonti *et al.*, 2000). DC, which reaches a mature stage under 1,25$(OH)_2$D, produces almost no IL-12 and more IL-10 (Penna and Adorini, 2000; van Halteren *et al.*, 2002). 1,25$(OH)_2$D treatment also induces apoptosis in mature myeloid DC (Penna and Adorini, 2000). It can be concluded that 1,25(OH)2D dramatically hampers maturation and affects function of myeloid DC. However, the phenotype and functionality of blood-isolated plasmacytoid DC are not affected by 1,25$(OH)_2$D (Penna *et al.*, 2007).

Therefore, besides direct effects of 1,25$(OH)_2$D on the T-cell compartment, vitamin D might also modulate the T-cell response via the APC compartment. Indeed, pretreatment of monocytes with 1,25$(OH)_2$D inhibited proliferation of T cells on tetanoid toxin in a coculture (Rigby *et al.*, 1990). Interestingly, 25(OH)D pretreatment also induced inhibition of proliferation, albeit to a lesser extent. Pretreatment of P-DC with 1,25 $(OH)_2$D did not affect T-cell function in a subsequent coculture (Penna *et al.*, 2007). Maturation of myeloid DC in the presence of 1,25$(OH)_2$D reduced the level of allogenic T-cell activation by mature DC in a mixed lymphocyte reaction (Griffin *et al.*, 2000; Penna and Adorini, 2000; Piemonti *et al.*, 2000). Pretreatment of antigen-loaded immature myeloid DC with 1,25$(OH)_2$D completely blocked the subsequent production of cytokines by autoreactive T-cell clones, although proliferation was not affected (Van Halteren *et al.*, 2002). Culture of mature 1,25$(OH)_2$D-treated myeloid DC with the T-cell clones and the antigen reduced both cytokine production and proliferation and stimulated apoptosis of T cells, when compared to culture with untreated DC (van Halteren *et al.*, 2002). When T cells were, after coculture with 1,25$(OH)_2$D-treated myeloid DC, reexposed to mature myeloid DC, a large proportion appeared to have become hyporesponsive (Penna and Adorini, 2000; Piemonti *et al.*, 2000). In conclusion, the effects of 1,25$(OH)_2$D on myeloid DC also affect their capacity to evoke an (autoreactive) immune response. Besides direct effects on the $CD4^+$ T-cell compartment, 1,25$(OH)_2$D also modulates the T-cell response via APC (Fig. 18.2).

As the focus of this chapter is on T cells, B cells have not been discussed yet. However, direct exposure of B cells to 1,25$(OH)_2$D has also been a topic of interest. Proliferation of PBMC and B cells on different combinations of B cell specific and aspecific stimuli is inhibited by 1,25$(OH)_2$D (Chen *et al.*, 2007; Iho *et al.*, 1986; Lemire *et al.*, 1984). However, 1,25 $(OH)_2$D exposition also induced apoptosis of proliferating B cells (Chen *et al.*, 2007). Further, phenotypic changes were noticed (Chen *et al.*, 1987, 2007; Heine *et al.*, 2008), and differentiation to plasma cells was inhibited (Chen *et al.*, 2007). The subsequent synthesis of IgM and IgG by PBMC and B cells on different stimuli was inhibited (Chen *et al.*, 1987, 2007; Iho *et al.*, 1986; Lemire *et al.*, 1984). When isolated $CD19^+$ B cells were stimulated by B cell receptor cross-linking, anti-CD40 and IL-4, 1,25$(OH)_2$D induced the secretion of IL-10 (Heine *et al.*, 2008). Interestingly, the cells cultured by this protocol excreted no IgG, and their proliferation was unaffected by 1,25(OH)$_2$D. Although 1,25(OH)$_2$D has direct effects on the B cells, several authors argued that indirect modulation of the B cell response might be more likely in physiological conditions. Much lower doses of 1,25(OH)$_2$D were needed to inhibit PHA-driven T-cell proliferation compared to pokeweed mitogen-driven B cell proliferation (Shiozawa *et al.*, 1987). In addition, PBMC depletion of either monocytes/macrophages (Chen *et al.*, 1987, Müller *et al.*, 1991a,b) or T cells (Müller *et al.*, 1991a,b) dramatically abrogated the reduction of IgG synthesis by 1,25 (OH)$_2$D. Direct stimulation of antibody production by Epstein–Bar virus was also not affected by 1,25(OH)$_2$D (Müller *et al.*, 1991a,b). Nevertheless, the B cell appears to be a potential direct target of 1,25(OH)$_2$D when exposed to a number of stimuli. The role of 1,25(OH)$_2$D in the induction of IL-10 producing regulatory B cells *in vivo* adds an exciting new area to the field of vitamin D and autoimmune diseases.

It can be concluded that, both directly and indirectly, 1,25(OH)$_2$D skews the CD4$^+$ T-cell compartment to a less inflammatory response (Smolders *et al.*, 2008a). *In vitro* assays showed that this skewing can be effectuated directly or via modulation of APC (Fig. 18.2). The interaction between CD8$^+$ T cells and vitamin D is at present not fully understood and requires further attention. In T-cell-mediated autoimmune diseases, the inhibition of IFN-γ producing Th1 and IL-17 producing Th17 cells in combination with promotion of Tregs can be of benefit for relieving disease activity.

D. Effects of 1,25(OH)$_2$D in EAE

The effects of 1,25(OH)$_2$D on the immune response have been assessed in rodents with experimental autoimmune encephalomyelitis (EAE). Although much criticized for being more an inflammatory than a neurodegenerative disease, EAE is the most widely used animal model for MS. In EAE, treatment with 1,25(OH)$_2$D prevents (Cantorna *et al.*, 1996; Lemire and Archer, 1991; Van Etten *et al.*, 2003) or induces a remission of EAE (Cantorna *et al.*, 1996; Muthian *et al.*, 2006). Knockout models revealed the VDR (Meehan and DeLuca, 2002a) and IL-10/IL-10-receptor signaling (Spach *et al.*, 2006) to be mandatory, and CD8$^+$ T cells to be of no critical importance to achieve these therapeutic effects (Meehan and DeLuca, 2002b). Additionally, no suppression of EAE activity was observed in RAG knockout mice, in which EAE was induced by encephalitic T-cell transfer (Nashold *et al.*, 2001). These observations suggest that via the VDR, an RAG-dependent IL-10 producing lymphocyte is an important mediator of the effects of vitamin D. The regulatory CD25$^+$FoxP3$^+$ T cell is the most likely candidate, although the induction of regulatory B cells also remains a theoretical option. Reports on effects of 1,25(OH)$_2$D therapy on cytokine production by lymphocytes in peripheral tissues and the spleen are conflicting (reviewed in Smolders *et al.*, 2008a).

Remarkably, supplementation of vitamin D_3 in EAE animals was only efficacious in female mice with intact ovaries (Spach and Hayes, 2005). Although in human MS a marked discrepancy between male and female patients is present (Eikelenboom *et al.*, 2009), a marked difference between the sexes has not been observed consistently in the interaction between 25 (OH)D or correlates of vitamin D status and MS. The exact differences in vitamin D metabolism and immune regulation between humans and rodents underlying this discrepancy are at present uncertain.

It can be concluded that animals with an immune-mediated inflammation of the CNS benefit clinically from treatment with $1,25(OH)_2D$, and that modulation of the autoreactive T-cell response is likely to be the most important driver of this effect.

E. Correlation between vitamin D status and the T-cell compartment in MS

In vitro, evidence shows compellingly that vitamin D is a potent immune modulator, and the animal model EAE suggests that subjects with inflammation in their CNS might benefit from vitamin D supplementation. In MS patients, however, the relationship between vitamin D status and markers of immune regulation has been marginally assessed. As vitamin D status has a seasonal fluctuating pattern, it is interesting that a comparable fluctuation of the regulatory cytokine IL-10 in the circulation has been observed (Stewart *et al.*, 2007). Additionally, the proinflammatory cytokines TNF-α and IFN-γ displayed an inverse seasonal fluctuation (Balashov *et al.*, 1998; Killestein *et al.*, 2002). However, a direct correlation with vitamin D status was not assessed.

At present, two studies assessed directly the association between vitamin D status and the composition of the T-cell compartment in MS patients (Royal *et al.*, 2009; Smolders *et al.*, 2009b). In our laboratory, we assessed a correlation between several characteristics of the T-cell compartment and serum 25(OH)D levels in a homogeneous cohort of 29 Caucasian patients with RRMS less than 5 years from disease onset (Smolders *et al.*, 2009b). The ability of $CD4^+CD25^+CD127^-$ Tregs to suppress $CD4^+$ T-cell proliferation was assessed in a proliferation suppression assay. The serum levels of 25(OH)D correlated positively with the amount of suppression (Fig. 18.3A). The numbers of either $CD4^+CD25^+FoxP3^+$ or $CD4^+CD25^+CD127^-$ Tregs did not correlate with vitamin D status. This is an interesting finding, as Treg function rather than number has been reported to be impaired in MS patients when compared to healthy controls (Viglietta *et al.*, 2004; Venken *et al.*, 2006). In addition to our study, Royal *et al.* (2009) assessed a correlation between $CD4^+CD25^+FoxP3^+$

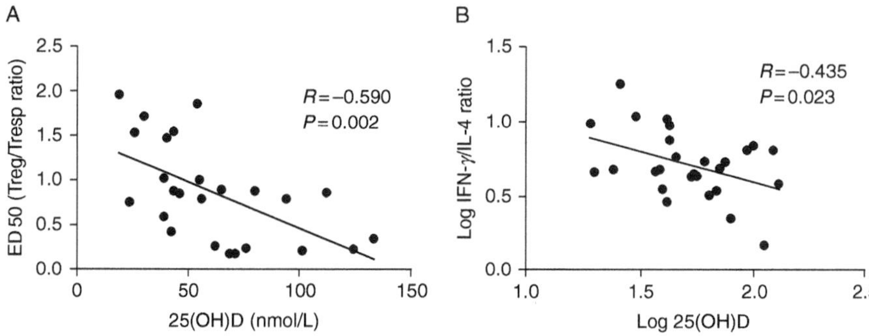

Figure 18.3 Correlation of vitamin D status with the T-cell compartment in patients with multiple sclerosis. (A) Correlation between regulatory T-cell function and vitamin D status. ED50: relative proportion of $CD4^+CD25^+CD127^-$ T cells needed to suppress 50% of anti-CD3 driven proliferation of $CD4^+CD25^-$ T responder cells in a 5-day CFSE-based proliferation suppression assay. The suppressive function of the Treg is better in patients with higher serum 25(OH)D values. (B) Correlation between vitamin D status and IFN-γ^+/IL-4^+ $CD4^+$ T-cell ratio (Th1/Th2 balance), as measured by intracellular flow cytometry. A higher vitamin D status correlates with a Th1/Th2 balance which is more directed toward Th2 (Adapted from Smolders *et al.*, 2009b).

Tregs with vitamin D status in a cohort of 30 Caucasian and African American RRMS patients. In a linear regression model, serum 25(OH)D levels predicted the number of Tregs negatively. The ratio between the serum levels of 1,25$(OH)_2$D and 25(OH)D was a positive predictor of the number of Tregs. We could not reproduce these associations in our dataset (Smolders *et al.*, 2010). Additionally, the relevance of this ratio for immune regulation locally in the CNS or the draining lymph nodes is uncertain. The extensive local production of 1,25$(OH)_2$D by activated immune cells as described in Section II.B is most likely to outweigh the low level of 1,25 $(OH)_2$D present in the circulation.

In our study, we related vitamin D status with the intracellular cytokine profiles of $CD4^+$ T cells (Smolders *et al.*, 2009b). The ratio between IFN-γ and IL-4 producing cells, that is, the Th1/Th2-balance, correlated negatively with vitamin D status in our cohort (Fig. 18.3B). The absolute number of IL-$17^+$$CD4^+$ T cells did not correlate with serum 25(OH)D levels. This shift of the T-cell compartment from Th1 to Th2 is in concordance with experimental studies. In experimental studies, however, an effect of 1,25$(OH)_2$D on Th17 cells was most eminent (Correale *et al.*, 2009). This discrepancy might be driven by the fact that all patients in our study were for at least 6 weeks in remission of disease (median 1.0 years), while in all experimental work an outspoken proinflammatory environment was created. Royal *et al.* (2009) found that the proportion of naïve $CXCR3^+$ $CD4^+$ T cells in the circulation correlated positively with vitamin D status. Although the proportion of memory $CXCR3^+$ $CD4^+$

T cells did not correlate with vitamin D status, the ratio between naïve and memory $CXCR3^+CD4^+$ T cells correlated positively with serum 25(OH) D levels. $CD4^+$ and especially $CD8^+$ $CXCR3^+$ T cells have been proposed as the T cells which home in the CNS of patients with MS (Sørensen *et al.*, 2002). In the circulation, lower proportions of $CXCR3^+$ $CD4^+$T cells were found in MS patients when compared to healthy controls. The significance of the naïve/memory $CXCR3^+CD4^+$ T cells for MS requires consolidation as well as its association with vitamin D status.

F. Supplementation of vitamin D in MS

At present, studies assessing the effects of vitamin D supplementation in MS are scarce. Some studies assessed retrospectively either an effect on the risk of developing MS (Munger *et al.*, 2004) or an effect on disease activity (Nordvik *et al.*, 2000) but failed to show conclusive results. One study assessed the effect of vitamin D supplementation on immunological outcome measures. Six-month daily supplementation of 1000 IU (25 μg) vitamin D_3 resulted in elevated expression of the regulatory cytokine transforming growth factor beta (TGF-β) and decreased expression of IL-2 in PBMC (Mahon *et al.*, 2003). It is, however, likely that the doses used for supplementation were too low to really have an impact on immune regulation. A safety study showed that supplementation of vitamin D_3 up to 7000 μg (280,000 IU) per week was safe in patients with MS and did not provoke hypercalcemia or hypercalciuria (Kimball *et al.*, 2007). It is uncertain if such high doses are mandatory to achieve clinical or immunological effectiveness, but it illustrates that there is a considerable safety zone when supplementing supraphysiological doses of vitamin D.

Some authors suggested that treatment with either $1,25(OH)_2D$ or calcium *per se* might be better alternatives. Serum PTH levels rather than 25(OH)D levels were correlated with MS activity in a Scandinavian cohort (Soilu-Hänninen *et al.*, 2008). Additionally, most studies on vitamin D efficacy in EAE were performed with $1,25(OH)_2D$, inducing a hypercalcemia in many animals. These effects of vitamin D on calcium homeostasis have been argued to be of vital importance for its effects on EAE (Becklund *et al.*, 2009; Cantorna *et al.*, 1999). In a pilot study in MS patients, 2 out of 15 patients developed a hypercalcemia on a 1-year 2.5 μg/day 1,25 $(OH)_2D$-regimen (Wingerchuk *et al.*, 2005). The other patients displayed no or only a mild hypercalcemia, which could be relieved with dose adjustments. Regrettably, the presence of a hypercalciuria was not assessed.

It has long been recognized that MS patients are at risk for developing a critically diminished BMD. Therefore, a sufficient intake of both calcium and vitamin D should be warranted. When regarding vitamin D as a potential disease modulator in MS, it remains to be seen whether serum

$1,25(OH)_2D$ and calcium levels are of critical interest. In the whole spectrum of health outcomes that have been associated with a poor vitamin D status, a more or less inverse linear relationship between vitamin D status and risk for adverse disease outcome has been described (Section III.D). At higher serum 25(OH)D levels, calcium metabolism is optimal and therefore not significantly affected by vitamin D. Additionally, it is not likely that the small amounts of $1,25(OH)_2D$ present in the circulation outweigh the $1,25(OH)_2D$ synthesized out of the 1000 times higher level of 25(OH)D at sites of immune activation. This idea is supported by the notion that we did not find a correlation between serum PTH, calcium, and $1,25(OH)_2D$ with Th1/Th2-balance and Treg function in patients with MS, in contrast to serum 25(OH)D levels (Smolders *et al.*, 2010).

V. Concluding Remarks

Vitamin D deficiency has been associated with an increased risk for developing MS and with an increased disease activity. Drugs that promote T-cell homeostasis have a beneficial effect on the disease activity of MS. Vitamin D has been shown to inhibit Th1 and Th17, promote Treg function and development *in vitro*, prevent and cure the MS animal model EAE, and be positively correlated with the level of T-cell homeostasis in patients with MS. These finding make supplementation of vitamin D a potential treatment modality in MS.

There are, however, several drawbacks. First of all, the most potent source of vitamin D is sunlight exposure. It is uncertain whether all associations observed in epidemiological studies really reflect the link between vitamin D and MS, or rather between MS and UV-exposure *per se*, exposition to bacteria, physical activity levels, etc. The same holds for association studies on vitamin D status and the T-cell compartment in MS patients. Second, exposition of animals with EAE to high doses of $1,25(OH)_2D$ has potent effects, but the translation to MS is difficult. Treatment of humans with high doses of $1,25(OH)_2D$ is not possible, due to severe side effects. Additionally, supplementation of EAE animals with vitamin D does not have the impressive efficacy as observed in animals treated with $1,25(OH)_2D$. Third, at present, no single large trial showed an actual effect of vitamin D supplementation in MS, although some pilots presented at scientific meetings show promising results.

There is a need for controlled studies, assessing the effects of vitamin D supplementation on both immunological and clinical outcome measures in MS patients. The massive body of immunological and epidemiological evidence indicates that vitamin D could play a vital role in the physiologic regulation of T-cell homeostasis. Correction of the abundantly present vitamin D deficiency among western populations could decrease the rising incidence of several vitamin D-associated diseases, including MS. Further, it might also reduce the need to treat MS patients with invasive and potentially dangerous immune suppressive and modulating therapies.

REFERENCES

Abbas, S., Linseisen, J., Slanger, T., Kropp, S., Mutschelknauss, E. J., Flesch-Janys, D., and Chang-Claude, J. (2008). Serum 25-hydroxyvitamin D and risk of post-menopausal breast cancer: Results of a large case-control study. *Carcinogenesis* **29,** 93–99.

Ascherio, A., Munger, K. L., and Simon, C. (2010). Vitamin D and multiple sclerosis. *Lancet Neurol.* **9,** 599–612.

Balashov, K. E., Olek, M. J., Smith, D. R., Khoury, S. J., and Weiner, H. L. (1998). Seasonal variation of interferon-gamma production in progressive multiple sclerosis. *Ann. Neurol.* **44,** 824–828.

Bar-Or, A. (2008). The immunology of multiple sclerosis. *Semin. Neurol.* **28,** 29–45.

Barrat, F. J., Cua, D. J., Boonstra, A., Richards, D. F., Crain, C., Savelkoul, H. F., de Waal-Malefyt, R., Coffman, R. L., Hawrylowicz, C. M., and O'Garra, A. (2002). In vitro generation of interleukin 10-producing regulatory CD4(+) T cells is induced by immunosuppressive drugs and inhibited by T helper type 1 (Th1)- and Th2-inducing cytokines. *J. Exp. Med.* **195,** 603–616.

Bates, C. J., Carter, G. D., Mishra, G. D., O'Shea, D., Jones, J., and Prentice, A. (2003). In a population study, can parathyroid hormone aid the definition of adequate vitamin D status? A study of people aged 65 years and over from the British National Diet and Nutrition Survey. *Osteoporos. Int.* **14,** 152–159.

Becklund, B. R., Hansen, D. W., and Deluca, H. F. (2009). Enhancement of 1, 25-dihydroxyvitamin D3-mediated suppression of experimental autoimmune encephalomyelitis by calcitonin. *Proc. Natl. Acad. Sci. USA* **106,** 5276–5281.

Bhalla, A. K., Amento, E. P., and Krane, S. M. (1986). Differential effects of 1, 25-dihydroxyvitamin D3 on human lymphocytes and monocyte/macrophages: Inhibition of interleukin-2 and augmentation of interleukin-1 production. *Cell. Immunol.* **98,** 311–322.

Bischoff-Ferrari, H. A., Dietrich, T., Orav, E. J., and Dawson-Hughes, B. (2004). Positive association between 25-hydroxy vitamin D levels and bone mineral density: A population-based study of younger and older adults. *Am. J. Med.* **116,** 634–639.

Bischoff-Ferrari, H. A., Willett, W. C., Wong, J. B., Giovannucci, E., Dietrich, T., and Dawson-Hughes, B. (2005). Fracture prevention with vitamin D supplementation, a meta-analysis of randomized controlled trials. *JAMA* **293,** 2257–2264.

Bischoff-Ferrari, H. A., Dawson-Hughes, B., Orav, J. E., Stuck, A. E., Theiler, R., Wong, J. B., Egli, A., Kiel, D. P., and Henschkowski, J. (2009). Fall prevention with supplemental and active forms of vitamin D: A meta-analysis of randomized controlled trials. *BMJ* **339,** b3692.

Boonstra, A., Barrat, F. J., Crain, C., Heath, V. L., Savelkoul, H. F., and O'Garra, A. (2001). 1alpha, 25-Dihydroxyvitamin d3 has a direct effect on naive CD4(+) T cells to enhance the development of Th2 cells. *J. Immunol.* **167,** 4974–4980.

Cantorna, M. T., Hayes, C. E., and DeLuca, H. F. (1996). 1, 25-Dihydroxyvitamin D3 reversibly blocks the progression of relapsing encephalomyelitis, a model of multiple sclerosis. *Proc. Natl. Acad. Sci. USA* **93,** 7861–7864.

Cantorna, M. T., Humpal-Winter, J., and DeLuca, H. F. (1999). Dietary calcium is a major factor in 1, 25-dihydroxycholecalciferol suppression of experimental autoimmune encephalomyelitis in mice. *J. Nutr.* **129,** 1966–1971.

Cauley, J. A., Parimi, N., Ensrud, K. E., Bauer, D. C., Cawthon, P. M., Cummings, S. R., Hoffman, E. R., Shikany, J. M., Barrett-Connor, E., and Orwoll, E. (2009). Serum 25 hydroxyvitamin D and the risk of hip and non-spine fractures in older men. *J. Bone Min. Res.* **25,** 545–553.

Chen, W. C., Vayuvegula, B., and Gupta, S. (1987). 1, 25-Dihydroxyvitamin D3-mediated inhibition of human B cell differentiation. *Clin. Exp. Immunol.* **69,** 639–646.

Chen, S., Sims, G. P., Chen, X. X., Gu, Y. Y., Chen, S., and Lipsky, P. E. (2007). Modulatory effects of 1, 25-dihydroxyvitamin D3 on human B cell differentiation. *J. Immunol.* **179,** 1634–1647.

Compston, A., and Coles, A. (2002). Multiple sclerosis. *Lancet* **359,** 1221–1231.

Correale, J., Ysrraelit, M. C., and Gaitán, M. I. (2009). Immunomodulatory effects of vitamin D in multiple sclerosis. *Brain* **132,** 1146–1160.

Cutolo, M., Otsa, K., Laas, K., Yprus, M., Lehtme, R., Secchi, M. E., Sulli, A., Paolino, S., and Seriolo, B. (2006). Circannual vitamin d serum levels and disease activity in rheumatoid arthritis: Northern versus Southern Europe. *Clin. Exp. Rheumatol.* **24,** 702–704.

D'Ambrosio, D., Cippitelli, M., Cocciolo, M. G., Mazzeo, D., Di Lucia, P., Lang, R., Sinigaglia, F., and Panina-Bordignon, P. (1998). Inhibition of IL-12 production by 1, 25-dihydroxyvitamin D3. Involvement of NF-kappaB downregulation in transcriptional repression of the p40 gene. *J. Clin. Invest.* **101,** 252–262.

Davies, P. S., Bates, C. J., Cole, T. J., Prentice, A., and Clarke, P. C. (1999). Vitamin D: Seasonal and regional differences in preschool children in Great Britain. *Eur. J. Clin. Nutr.* **53,** 195–198.

de Andres, C., Aristimuno, C., de Las Heras, V., Martinez-Gines, M. L., Bartolome, M., Arroyo, R., *et al.* (2007). Interferon beta-1a therapy enhances CD4+ regulatory T-cell function: An ex vivo and in vitro longitudinal study in relapsing-remitting multiple sclerosis. *J. Neuroimmunol.* **182,** 204–211.

Eikelenboom, M. J., Killestein, J., Kragt, J. J., Uitdehaag, B. M., and Polman, C. H. (2009). Gender differences in multiple sclerosis: Cytokines and vitamin D. *J. Neurol. Sci.* **286,** 40–42.

Fritsche, J., Mondal, K., Ehrnsperger, A., Andreesen, R., and Kreutz, M. (2003). Regulation of 25-hydroxyvitamin D3–1 alpha-hydroxylase and production of 1 alpha, 25-dihydroxyvitamin D3 by human dendritic cells. *Blood* **102,** 3314–3316.

Gatenby, P. A., Lucas, R. M., Engelsen, O., Ponsonby, A. L., and Clements, M. (2009). Antineutrophil cytoplasmic antibody-associated vasculitides: Could geographic patterns be explained by ambient ultraviolet radiation? *Arthritis Rheum.* **61,** 1417–1424.

Giovannucci, E., Liu, Y., Hollis, B. W., and Rimm, E. B. (2008). 25-Hydroxyvitamin D and risk of myocardial infarction in men A prospective study. *Arch. Intern. Med.* **168,** 1174–1180.

Gombart, A. F., Borregaard, N., and Koeffler, H. P. (2005). Human cathelicidin antimicrobial peptide (CAMP) gene is a direct target of the vitamin D receptor and is strongly up-regulated in myeloid cells by 1, 25-dihydroxyvitamin D3. *FASEB J.* **19,** 1067–1077.

Gottfried, E., Rehli, M., Hahn, J., Holler, E., Andreesen, R., and Kreutz, M. (2006). Monocyte-derived cells express CYP27A1 and convert vitamin D3 into its active metabolite. *Biochem. Biophys. Res. Commun.* **349,** 209–213.

Goverman, J. (2009). Autoimmune T cell responses in the central nervous system. *Nat. Rev. Immunol.* **9,** 393–407.

Griffin, M. D., Lutz, W. H., Phan, V. A., Bachman, L. A., McKean, D. J., and Kumar, R. (2000). Potent inhibition of dendritic cell differentiation and maturation by vitamin D analogs. *Biochem. Biophys. Res. Commun.* **270,** 701–708.

Griffin, M. D., Lutz, W., Phan, V. A., Bachman, L. A., McKean, D. J., and Kumar, R. (2001). Dendritic cell modulation by 1alpha, 25 dihydroxyvitamin D3 and its analogs: A vitamin D receptor-dependent pathway that promotes a persistent state of immaturity in vitro and in vivo. *Proc. Natl. Acad. Sci. USA* **98,** 6800–6805.

Haas, J., Hug, A., Viehöver, A., Fritzsching, B., Falk, C. S., Filser, A., Vetter, T., Milkova, L., Korporal, M., Fritz, B., Storch-Hagenlocher, B., Krammer, P. H., *et al.* (2005). Reduced suppressive effect of $CD4^{+}CD25^{high}$ regulatory T cells on the T cell immune response against myelin oligodendrocyte glycoprotein in patients with multiple sclerosis. *Eur. J. Immunol.* **35,** 3343–3352.

Hayes, C. E., Cantorna, M. T., and DeLuca, H. F. (1997). Vitamin D and multiple sclerosis. *Proc. Soc. Exp. Biol. Med.* **216,** 21–27.

Heine, G., Niesner, U., Chang, H. D., Steinmeyer, A., Zügel, U., Zuberbier, T., Radbruch, A., and Worm, M. (2008). 1, 25-dihydroxyvitamin D(3) promotes IL-10 production in human B cells. *Eur. J. Immunol.* **38,** 2210–2218.

Hollis, B. W., Wagner, C. L., Drezner, M. K., and Binkley, N. C. (2007). Circulating vitamin D_3 and 25-hydroxyvitamin D in humans: An important tool to define adequate nutritional vitamin D status. *J. Steroid Biochem. Mol. Biol.* **103,** 631–634.

Hyppönen, E., Läärä, E., Reunanen, A., Järvelin, M. R., and Virtanen, S. M. (2001). Intake of vitamin D and risk of type 1 diabetes: A birth-cohort study. *Lancet* **358,** 1500–1503.

Iho, S., Takahashi, T., Kura, F., Sugiyama, H., and Hoshino, T. (1986). The effect of 1, 25-dihydroxyvitamin D3 on in vitro immunoglobulin production in human B cells. *J. Immunol.* **136,** 4427–4431.

Islam, T., Gauderman, W., Cozen, W., and Mack, T. (2007). Childhood sun exposure influences risk of multiple sclerosis in monozygotic twins. *Neurology* **69,** 381–388.

Jeffery, L. E., Burke, F., Mura, M., Zheng, Y., Qureshi, O. S., Hewison, M., Walker, L. S., Lammas, D. A., Raza, K., and Sansom, D. M. (2009). 1, 25-Dihydroxyvitamin D3 and IL-2 combine to inhibit T cell production of inflammatory cytokines and promote development of regulatory T cells expressing CTLA-4 and FoxP3. *J. Immunol.* **183,** 5458–5467.

Jongen, M. J. M., van der Vijgh, W. J. F., Lips, P., and Netelenbos, J. C. (1984). Measurement of vitamin D metabolites in anephric subjects. *Nephron* **36,** 230–234.

Kampman, M., Wilsgaard, T., and Mellgren, S. (2007). Outdoor activities and diet in childhood and adolescence relate to MS risk above the Arctic circle. *J. Neurol.* **254,** 471–477.

Killestein, J., Rep, M. H., Meilof, J. F., Ader, H. J., Uitdehaag, B. M., Barkhof, F., van Lier, R. A., and Polman, C. H. (2002). Seasonal variation in immune measurements and MRI markers of disease activity in MS. *Neurology* **58,** 1077–1080.

Kimball, S. M., Ursell, M. R., O'Connor, P., and Vieth, R. (2007). Safety of vitamin D3 in adults with multiple sclerosis. *Am. J. Clin. Nutr.* **86,** 645–651.

Kimlin, M. G. (2008). Geographical location and vitamin D synthesis. *Mol. Aspects Med.* **29,** 453–461.

Lemire, J. M., and Archer, D. C. (1991). 1, 25-Dihydroxyvitamin D3 prevents the in vivo induction of murine experimental autoimmune encephalomyelitis. *J. Clin. Invest.* **87,** 1103–1107.

Lemire, J. M., Adams, J. S., Sakai, R., and Jordan, S. C. (1984). 1 alpha, 25-dihydroxyvitamin D3 suppresses proliferation and immunoglobulin production by normal human peripheral blood mononuclear cells. *J. Clin. Invest.* **74,** 657–661.

Lopes, J., Danilevicius, C., Takayama, L., Caparbo, V., Scazufca, M., Bonfá, E., and Pereira, R. (2009). Vitamin D insufficiency: A risk factor to vertebral fractures in community-dwelling elderly women. *Maturitas* **64,** 218–222.

Mahon, B. D., Gordon, S. A., Cruz, J., Cosman, F., and Cantorna, M. T. (2003). Cytokine profile in patients with multiple sclerosis following vitamin D supplementation. *J. Neuroimmunol.* **134,** 128–132.

Mawer, E. B., Lumb, G. A., and Stanbury, S. W. (1969). Long biological half-life of vitamin D_3 and its polar metabolites in human serum. *Nature* **222,** 482–483.

Meehan, T. F., and DeLuca, H. F. (2002a). CD8(+) T cells are not necessary for 1alpha, 25-dihydroxyvitamin D(3) to suppress experimental autoimmune encephalomyelitis in mice. *Proc. Natl. Acad. Sci. USA* **99,** 5557–5560.

Meehan, T. F., and DeLuca, H. F. (2002b). The vitamin D receptor is necessary for 1alpha, 25-dihydroxyvitamin D(3) to suppress experimental autoimmune encephalomyelitis in mice. *Arch. Biochem. Biophys.* **408,** 200–204.

Meehan, M. A., Kerman, R. H., and Lemire, J. M. (1992). 1, 25-Dihydroxyvitamin D3 enhances the generation of nonspecific suppressor cells while inhibiting the induction of cytotoxic cells in a human MLR. *Cell. Immunol.* **140,** 400–409.

Melamed, M. L., Michos, E. D., Post, W., and Astor, B. (2008a). 25-hydroxyvitamin D levels and the risk of mortality in the general population. *Arch. Intern. Med.* **168,** 1629–1637.

Melamed, M. L., Muntner, P., Michos, E. D., Uribarri, J., Weber, C., Sharma, J., and Raggi, P. (2008b). Serum 25-hydroxyvitamin D levels and the prevalence of peripheral arterial disease. *Arterioscler. Thromb. Vasc. Biol.* **28,** 1179–1185.

Miller, D. H., Khan, O. A., Sheremata, W. A., Blumhardt, L. D., Rice, G. P., Libonati, M. A., *et al.* (2003). A controlled trial of natalizumab for relapsing multiple sclerosis. *N. Engl. J. Med.* **348,** 15–23.

Mowry, E. M., Krupp, L. B., Milazzo, M., Chabas, D., Strober, J. B., Belman, A. L., *et al.* (2010). Vitamin D status is associated with relapse rate in pediatric-onset multiple sclerosis. *Ann. Neurol.* **67,** 618–624.

Müller, K., and Bendtzen, K. (1992). Inhibition of human T lymphocyte proliferation and cytokine production by human 1, 25-dihydroxyvitamin D3. Differential effects on CD45-RA^- and CD45-RO^- cells. *Autoimmunity* **14,** 37–43.

Müller, K., Heilmann, C., Poulsen, L. K., Barington, T., and Bendtzen, K. (1991a). The role of monocytes and T cells in 1, 25-dihydroxyvitamin D3 mediated inhibition of B cell function in vitro. *Immunopharmacology* **21,** 121–128.

Müller, K., Diamant, M., and Bendtzen, K. (1991b). Inhibition of production and function of interleukin-6 by 1, 25-dihydroxyvitamin D3. *Immunol. Lett.* **28,** 115–120.

Müller, K., Haahr, P. M., Diamant, M., Rieneck, K., Kharazmi, A., and Bendtzen, K. (1992). 1, 25-Dihydroxyvitamin D3 inhibits cytokine production by human blood monocytes at the post-transcriptional level. *Cytokine* **4,** 506–512.

Müller, K., Kriegbaum, N. J., Baslund, B., Sørensen, O. H., Thymann, M., and Bentzen, K. (1995). Vitamin D3 metabolism in patients with rheumatic diseases: Low serum levels of 25-hydroxyvitamin D3 in patients with systemic lupus erythematosus. *Clin. Rheumatol.* **14,** 397–400.

Munger, K. L., Zhang, S. M., O'Reilly, E., Hernán, M. A., Olek, M. J., Willett, W. C., and Ascherio, A. (2004). Vitamin D intake and incidence of multiple sclerosis. *Neurology* **62,** 60–65.

Munger, K., Levin, L., Hollis, B., Howard, N., and Ascherio, A. (2006). Serum 25-hydroxyvitamin D levels and risk of multiple sclerosis. *JAMA* **296,** 2832–2838.

Muthian, G., Raikwar, H. P., Rajasingh, J., and Bright, J. J. (2006). 1, 25 Dihydroxyvitamin-D3 modulates JAK-STAT pathway in IL-12/IFNgamma axis leading to Th1 response in experimental allergic encephalomyelitis. *J. Neurosci. Res.* **83,** 1299–1309.

Nashold, F. E., Hoag, K. A., Goverman, J., and Hayes, C. E. (2001). Rag-1-dependent cells are necessary for 1, 25-dihydroxyvitamin D(3) prevention of experimental autoimmune encephalomyelitis. *J. Neuroimmunol.* **119,** 16–29.

Neuhaus, O., Wiendl, H., Kieseier, B. C., Archelos, J. J., Hemmer, B., Stuve, O., *et al.* (2005). Multiple sclerosis: Mitoxantrone promotes differential effects on immunocompetent cells in vitro. *J. Neuroimmunol.* **168,** 128–137.

Newton-Bishop, J. A., Beswick, S., Randerson-Moor, J., Chang, Y. M., Affleck, P., Elliott, F., Chan, M., Leake, S., Karpavicius, B., Haynes, S., Kukalizch, K., Whitaker, L., *et al.* (2009). Serum 25-hydroxyvitamin D3 levels are associated with breslow thickness at presentation and survival from melanoma. *J. Clin. Oncol.* **27,** 5439–5444.

Nordvik, I., Myhr, K. M., Nyland, H., and Bjerve, K. S. (2000). Effect of dietary advice and n-3 supplementation in newly diagnosed MS patients. *Acta Neurol. Scand.* **102,** 143–149.

Ohta, M., Okabe, T., Ozawa, K., Urabe, A., and Takaku, F. (1985). 1 alpha, 25-Dihydroxyvitamin D3 (calcitriol) stimulates proliferation of human circulating monocytes in vitro. *FEBS Lett.* **185,** 9–13.

Orton, S. M., Herrera, B. M., Yee, I. M., Valdar, W., Ramagopalan, S. V., Sadovnick, A. D., and Eber, G. C., Canadian Collaborative Study Group (2006). Sex ratio of multiple sclerosis in Canada: A longitudinal study. *Lancet Neurol.* **5,** 932–936.

Penna, G., and Adorini, L. (2000). 1 Alpha, 25-dihydroxyvitamin D3 inhibits differentiation, maturation, activation, and survival of dendritic cells leading to impaired alloreactive T cell activation. *J. Immunol.* **164,** 2405–2411.

Penna, G., Amuchastegui, S., Giarratana, N., Daniel, K. C., Vulcano, M., Sozzani, S., and Adorini, L. (2007). 1, 25-Dihydroxyvitamin D3 selectively modulates tolerogenic properties in myeloid but not plasmacytoid dendritic cells. *J. Immunol.* **178,** 145–153.

Pichler, J., Gerstmayr, M., Szépfalusi, Z., Urbanek, R., Peterlik, M., and Willheim, M. (2002). 1 alpha, 25(OH)2D3 inhibits not only Th1 but also Th2 differentiation in human cord blood T cells. *Pediatr. Res.* **52,** 12–18.

Piemonti, L., Monti, P., Sironi, M., Fraticelli, P., Leone, B. E., Dal Cin, E., Allavena, P., and Di Carlo, V. (2000). Vitamin D3 affects differentiation, maturation, and function of human monocyte-derived dendritic cells. *J. Immunol.* **164,** 4443–4451.

Pilz, S., Dobnig, H., Nijpels, G., Heine, R. J., Stehouwer, C. D., Snijder, M. B., van Dam, R. M., and Dekker, J. M. (2009a). Vitamin D and mortality in older men and women. *Clin. Endocrinol. (Oxf)* **71,** 666–672.

Pilz, S., Tomaschitz, A., Ritz, E., and Pieber, T. R. (2009b). Vitamin D status arterial hypertension: A systematic review. *Nat. Rev. Cardiol.* **6,** 621–630.

Provvedini, D. M., Tsoukas, C. D., Deftos, L. J., and Manolagas, S. C. (1983). 1, 25-Dihydroxyvitamin D3 receptors in human leukocytes. *Science* **221,** 1181–1183.

Reichel, H., Koeffler, H. P., Tobler, A., and Norman, A. W. (1987). 1 alpha, 25-Dihydroxyvitamin D3 inhibits gamma-interferon synthesis by normal human peripheral blood lymphocytes. *Proc. Natl. Acad. Sci. USA* **84,** 3385–3389.

Rigby, W. F., Stacy, T., and Fanger, M. W. (1984). Inhibition of T lymphocyte mitogenesis by 1, 25-dihydroxyvitamin D3 (calcitriol). *J. Clin. Invest.* **74,** 1451–1455.

Rigby, W. F., Waugh, M., and Graziano, R. F. (1990). Regulation of human monocyte HLA-DR and CD4 antigen expression, and antigen presentation by 1, 25-dihydroxyvitamin D3. *Blood* **76,** 189–197.

Royal, 3rd, W., Mia, Y., Li, H., and Naunton, K. (2009). Peripheral blood regulatory T cell measurements correlate with serum vitamin D levels in patients with multiple sclerosis. *J. Neuroimmunol.* **213,** 135–141.

Schrempf, W., and Ziemssen, T. (2007). Glatiramer acetate: Mechanisms of action in multiple sclerosis. *Autoimmun. Rev.* **6,** 469–475.

Shiozawa, S., Shiozawa, K., Tanaka, Y., and Fujita, T. (1987). 1 alpha, 25-Dihydroxyvitamin D3 inhibits proliferative response of T- and B lymphocytes in a serum-free culture. *Int. J. Immunopharmacol.* **9,** 719–723.

Sigmundsdottir, H., Pan, J., Debes, G. F., Alt, C., Habtezion, A., Soler, D., and Butcher, E. C. (2007). DCs metabolize sunlight-induced vitamin D3 to 'program' T cell attraction to the epidermal chemokine CCL27. *Nat. Immunol.* **8,** 285–293.

Simpson, S., Jr., Taylor, B., Blizzard, L., Ponsonby, A. L., Pittas, F., Tremlett, H., *et al.* (2010). Higher 25-hydroxyvitamin D is associated with lower relapse risk in MS. *Ann. Neurol.* **68,** 193–203.

Smith, J. E., and Goodman, D. S. (1971). The turnover and transport of vitamin D and of a polar metabolite with the properties of 25-hydroxycholecalciferol in human plasma. *J. Clin. Invest.* **50,** 2159–2167.

Smolders, J., Damoiseaux, J., Menheere, P., and Hupperts, R. (2008a). Vitamin D as an immune modulator in multiple sclerosis, a review. *J. Neuroimmunol.* **194,** 7–17.

Smolders, J., Menheere, P., Kessels, A., Damoiseaux, J., and Hupperts, R. (2008b). Association of vitamin D metabolite levels with relapse rate and disability in multiple sclerosis. *Mult. Scler.* **14,** 1220–1224.

Smolders, J., Peelen, E., Thewissen, M., Menheere, P., Cohen Tervaert, J. W., Hupperts, R., and Damoiseaux, J. (2009a). The relevance of vitamin D receptor gene polymorphisms for vitamin D research in multiple sclerosis. *Autoimmun. Rev.* **8,** 621–626.

Smolders, J., Thewissen, M., Peelen, E., Menheere, P., Cohen Tervaert, J. W., Damoiseaux, J., and Hupperts, R. (2009b). Vitamin D status is positively correlated with regulatory T cell function in patients with multiple sclerosis. *PLoS ONE* **4,** e6635.

Smolders, J., Menheere, P., Thewissen, M., Peelen, E., Cohen Tervaert, J. W., Hupperts, R., and Damoiseaux, J. (2010). Regulatory T cell function correlates with serum 25-hydroxyvitamin D, but not with 1, 25-dihydroxyvitamin D, parathyroid hormone and calcium levels in patients with relapsing remitting multiple sclerosis. *J. Steroid Biochem. Mol. Biol.* **121,** 243–246.

Soilu-Hänninen, M., Laaksonen, M., Laitinen, I., Eralinna, J. P., Lilius, E. M., and Mononen, I. (2008). A longitudinal study of serum 25-hydroxyvitamin D and intact PTH levels indicate the importance of vitamin D and calcium homeostasis regulation in multiple sclerosis. *J. Neurol. Neurosurg. Psychiatry* **79,** 152–157.

Soilu-Hänninen, M., Airas, L., Mononen, I., Heikkilä, A., Viljanen, M., and Hänninen, A. (2005). 25-Hydroxyvitamin D levels in serum at the onset of multiple sclerosis. *Mult. Scler.* **11,** 266–271.

Sørensen, T. L., Trebst, C., Kivisäkk, P., Klaege, K. L., Majmudar, A., Ravid, R., Lassmann, H., Olsen, D. B., Strieter, R. M., Ransohoff, R. M., and Sellebjerg, F. (2002). Multiple sclerosis: a study of CXCL10 and CXCR3 co-localization in the inflamed central nervous system. *J. Neuroimmunol.* **127,** 59–68.

Spach, K. M., and Hayes, C. E. (2005). Vitamin D3 confers protection from autoimmune encephalomyelitis only in female mice. *J. Immunol.* **175,** 4119–4126.

Spach, K. M., Nashold, F. E., Dittel, B. N., and Hayes, C. E. (2006). IL-10 signaling is essential for 1, 25-dihydroxyvitamin D3-mediated inhibition of experimental autoimmune encephalomyelitis. *J. Immunol.* **177,** 6030–6037.

Stewart, N., Taylor, B., Ponsonby, A. L., Pittas, F., van der Mei, I., Woods, G., and Walters, H. (2007). The effect of season on cytokine expression in multiple sclerosis and healthy subjects. *J. Neuroimmunol.* **188,** 181–186.

Stewart, J. W., Alekel, D. L., Ritland, L. M., Van Loan, M., Gertz, E., and Genschel, U. (2009). Serum 25-hydroxyvitamin D is related to indicators of overall physical fitness in healthy postmenopausal women. *Menopause* **16,** 1093–1101.

Széles, L., Keresztes, G., Töröcsik, D., Balajthy, Z., Krenács, L., Póliska, S., Steinmeyer, A., Zuegel, U., Pruenster, M., Rot, A., and Nagy, L. (2009). 1, 25-Dihydroxyvitamin D3 is an autonomous regulator of the transcriptional changes leading to a tolerogenic dendritic cell phenotype. *J. Immunol.* **182,** 2074–2083.

Tang, B., Eslick, G., Nowson, C., Smith, C., and Bensoussan, A. (2007). Use of calcium or calcium in combination with vitamin D supplementation to prevent fractures and bone loss in people aged 50 years and older: a meta-analysis. *Lancet* **370,** 657–666.

Tang, J. Y., Parimi, N., Wu, A., John Boscardin, W., Shikany, J. M., Chren, M. M., Cummings, S. R., Epstein, E. H., and Bauer, D. C. (2010). Inverse association between serum 25(OH) vitamin D levels and non-melanoma skin cancer in elderly men. *Cancer Causes Control* **21,** 387–391.

Thien, R., Baier, K., Pietschmann, P., Peterlik, M., and Willheim, M. (2005). Interactions of 1 alpha, 25-dihydroxyvitamin D3 with IL-12 and IL-4 on cytokine expression of human T lymphocytes. *J. Allergy Clin. Immunol.* **116,** 683–689.

Tobler, A., Gasson, J., Reichel, H., Norman, A. W., and Koeffler, H. P. (1987). Granulocyte-macrophage colony-stimulating factor. Sensitive and receptor-mediated regulation by 1, 25-dihydroxyvitamin D3 in normal human peripheral blood lymphocytes. *J. Clin. Invest.* **79,** 1700–1705.

Van der Mei, I., Ponsonby, A., Dwyer, T., Blizzard, L., Taylor, B. V., Kilpatrick, T., Butzkueven, H., and McMichael, A. J. (2007). Vitamin D levels in people with multiple sclerosis and community controls in Tasmania, Australia. *J. Neurol.* **254,** 581–590.

Van Etten, E., Branisteanu, D. D., Overbergh, L., Bouillon, R., Verstuyf, A., and Mathieu, C. (2003). Combination of a 1, 25-dihydroxyvitamin D3 analog and a bisphosphonate prevents experimental autoimmune encephalomyelitis and preserves bone. *Bone* **32,** 397–404.

van Halteren, A. G., van Etten, E., de Jong, E. C., Bouillon, R., Roep, B. O., and Mathieu, C. (2002). Redirection of human autoreactive T-cells Upon interaction with dendritic cells modulated by TX527, an analog of 1, 25 dihydroxyvitamin D(3). *Diabetes* **51,** 2119–2125.

Veldman, C. M., Cantorna, M. T., and DeLuca, H. F. (2000). Expression of 1, 25-dihydroxyvitamin D(3) receptor in the immune system. *Arch. Biochem. Biophys.* **374,** 334–338.

Venken, K., Hellings, N., Hensen, K., Rummens, J. L., Medaer, R., D'hooghe, M. B., Dubois, B., Raus, J., and Stinissen, P. (2006). Secondary progressive in contrast to relapsing-remitting multiple sclerosis patients show a normal $CD4^+CD25^+$ regulatory T-cell function and FOXP3 expression. *J. Neurosci. Res.* **83,** 1432–1446.

Viglietta, V., Baecher-Allan, C., Weiner, H., and Hafler, D. (2004). Loss of functional suppression by $CD4^+CD25^+$ regulatory T cells in patients with multiple sclerosis. *J. Exp. Med.* **199,** 971–979.

Von Essen, M. R., Kongsbak, M., Schjerling, P., Olgaard, K., Ødum, N., and Geisler, C. (2010). Vitamin D controls T cell receptor signaling and activation of human T cells. *Nat. Immunol.* **11,** 344–349.

Willer, C. J., Dyment, D. A., Sadovnick, A. D., Rothwell, P. M., Murray, T. J., and Ebers, G. C., Canadian Collaborative Study Group (2005). Timing of birth and risk of multiple sclerosis: Population based study. *BMJ* **330,** 120.

Wingerchuk, D. M., Lesaux, J., Rice, G. P., Kremenchutzky, M., and Ebers, G. C. (2005). A pilot study of oral calcitriol (1, 25-dihydroxyvitamin D3) for relapsing–remitting multiple sclerosis. *J. Neurol. Neurosurg. Psychiatry* **76,** 1294–1296.

Yin, L., Grandi, N., Raum, E., Haug, U., Arndt, V., and Brenner, H. (2009a). Meta-analysis: Longitudinal studies of serum vitamin D and colorectal cancer risk. *Aliment. Pharmacol. Ther.* **13,** 113–125.

Yin, L., Raum, E., Haug, U., Arndt, V., and Brenner, H. (2009b). Meta-analysis of longitudinal studies: Serum vitamin D and prostate cancer risk. *Cancer Epidemiol.* **33,** 435–445.

CHAPTER NINETEEN

Vitamin D in Solid Organ Transplantation with Special Emphasis on Kidney Transplantation

Ursula Thiem *and* Kyra Borchhardt

Contents

Abstract

Within the past decades, vitamin D was identified as having additional physiological functions far beyond calcium homeostasis and bone metabolism. Stimulated by the discovery of the vitamin D receptor in a broad range of tissues as well as the expression of 1α-hydroxylase, the enzyme responsible for the activation of vitamin D, it became evident that the actions of vitamin D are not restricted to cells involved in mineral and bone metabolism. In fact, it affects proliferation, differentiation, and function of a large number of different cell types including cells of the immune system. Vitamin D receptor agonists were found to exert immunosuppressive effects on the adaptive immune system,

Division of Nephrology and Dialysis, Department of Internal Medicine III, Medical University of Vienna, Währinger Gürtel, Vienna, Austria

Vitamins and Hormones, Volume 86
ISSN 0083-6729, DOI: 10.1016/B978-0-12-386960-9.00019-8

thus being able to mediate immunologic tolerance. However, they promote the innate immune system and thereby improve the ability of the host to combat invading pathogens.

This review summarizes our current understanding of vitamin D as an immunomodulatory agent with special emphasis on its clinical implications in the transplant setting.

I. Vitamin D

A. Sources and metabolism

Vitamin D can be obtained either from the diet or by endogenous production in the skin. Ultraviolet B radiation induces the conversion of 7-dehydrocholesterol to previtamin D_3 in the skin which immediately isomerizes to vitamin D_3 in a thermal process (Holick *et al.*, 1980). The cutaneous synthesis is the main source of vitamin D_3, as there are only few foods containing substantial amounts of vitamin D. Vitamin D in the diet is available in two distinct forms, either ergocalciferol (vitamin D_2), which is produced from ergosterol in response to ultraviolet radiation in a variety of plants and yeast and can be obtained from sundried mushrooms, or cholecalciferol (vitamin D_3), which is mainly found in oily fish such as salmon, mackerel, and sardines (Holick, 2007).

From the skin or after intestinal absorption, vitamin D (hereafter "D" stands for D_2 and D_3) finds its way into the circulation, where it requires transport bound to plasma proteins due to its lipophilic properties. The major carrier protein for vitamin D metabolites is vitamin D binding protein. Both vitamin D_3 from the skin and vitamin D obtained from the diet are activated in a two-step hydroxylation process. First, the conversion to 25-hydroxyvitamin D [25(OH)D] is performed by the enzyme 25-hydroxylase predominantly in the liver. As the first hydroxylation step is poorly regulated and primarily substrate dependent, 25(OH)D reflects both the endogenous production and the dietary intake of vitamin D, and is therefore regarded the most reliable indicator of vitamin D status. 25(OH)D is further metabolized to 1,25-dihydroxyvitamin D [1,25$(OH)_2$D] mainly in the kidney, but also at extrarenal sites. The enzyme responsible for the second hydroxylation, 1α-hydroxylase (CYP27B1), mainly occurs in the proximal tubule cells of the kidney, and its activity is tightly regulated by calcium and phosphate levels, parathyroid hormone (PTH), and 1,25$(OH)_2$D itself. The most active, naturally occurring vitamin D derivative is calcitriol [1,25$(OH)_2D_3$] (Dusso *et al.*, 2005). In the following, it will therefore be used to refer to the active hormonal form of vitamin D. To ensure that the reader is clear on the difference between the vitamin D metabolites, a summary of the vitamin D nomenclature is provided in

Table 19.1 Vitamin D nomenclature

Vitamin D	Ergocalciferol (vitamin D_2) Cholecalciferol (vitamin D_3)
25-hydroxyvitamin D [25(OH)D]	Ercalcidiol [25(OH)D_2] Calcidiol [25(OH)D_3]
1,25-dihydroxyvitamin D [1,25$(OH)_2$D]	Ercalcitriol [1,25$(OH)_2D_2$] Calcitriol [1,25$(OH)_2D_3$]
Vitamin D receptor agonist (synthetic analogues)	Paricalcitol [19nor,1,25$(OH)_2D_2$] Maxacalcitol [22oxa,1,25$(OH)_2D_3$]
Vitamin D receptor agonist prodrugs[a]	Doxercalciferol [1(OH)D_2] Alfacalcidol [1(OH)D_3]

[a] Require 25-hydroxylation in the liver.

Table 19.1 (according to the vitamin D nomenclature suggested by Sprague and Coyne, 2010).

The primary function of 1,25$(OH)_2D_3$ is to keep the plasma calcium concentration within narrow limits. As serum calcium levels decrease, 1α-hydroxylase and thus 1,25$(OH)_2D_3$ production is directly stimulated. Additionally, low serum calcium levels trigger PTH release, which in turn increases 1α-hydroxylase activity. In order to raise calcium levels, 1,25 $(OH)_2D_3$ increases the absorption of renal calcium and intestinal calcium and phosphate by regulating different transport mechanisms in the kidney and the small intestine. Moreover, it induces osteoclast maturation and activity resulting in calcium and phosphate release from bone. As soon as normocalcemia is achieved, 1α-hydroxylase is no longer stimulated. Interestingly, 1,25$(OH)_2D_3$ itself inhibits the expression of 1α-hydroxylase and induces the enzyme responsible for the degradation of vitamin D derivatives, that is, 24-hydroxylase. Thus, important negative feedback mechanisms are provided that prevent excessive high levels of 1,25$(OH)_2D_3$ (Dusso *et al.*, 2005).

Most of the actions are mediated via the vitamin D receptor, a member of the nuclear receptors for steroid hormones, which acts as a ligand-activated transcription factor. After entering the target cell, 1,25$(OH)_2D_3$ binds to the vitamin D receptor which forms a heterodimer with the retinoid X receptor and subsequently binds to vitamin D responsive elements on the DNA and modulates gene transcription (Dusso *et al.*, 2005). The vitamin D receptor binds 1,25$(OH)_2D_3$ with high affinity. However, it has recently become evident that also 25(OH)D binds to the vitamin D receptor and regulates gene transcription synergistically with 1,25$(OH)_2D_3$ (Lou *et al.*, 2010). Besides these genomic mechanisms of action, it has been suggested that 1,25$(OH)_2D_3$ is also able to exert rapid nongenomic actions via a membrane vitamin D receptor (Marcinkowska, 2001). However, not only tissues involved in calcium homeostasis and bone metabolism respond to $1,25(OH)_2D_3$, nuclear vitamin D receptor expression was rather identified in virtually every human tissue (Bouillon *et al.*, 2008), suggesting a more widespread function of active vitamin D beyond its classical actions in mineral and bone metabolism. These nonclassical actions include modulation of immune function, regulation of cell proliferation and differentiation, and control of other hormonal systems (Bikle, 2010). Furthermore, the vitamin D activating enzyme 1α-hydroxylase is now known to be expressed in a much wider range of tissues than previously thought (Townsend *et al.*, 2005). Notably, the extrarenal 1α-hydroxylase is regulated differently. Unlike the renal form, it is not upregulated by calcium and PTH, but local production of $1,25(OH)_2D_3$ is dependent on adequate concentrations of the substrate 25(OH)D (Cross, 2007; van Etten *et al.*, 2008). Thus, maintaining adequate levels of 25(OH)D is important to optimize these nonclassical actions. An overview of the vitamin D metabolism and the actions of $1,25(OH)_2D_3$ is provided in Fig. 19.1.

B. Vitamin D metabolism in chronic kidney disease

In chronic kidney disease, $1,25(OH)_2D_3$ levels progressively decrease (Levin *et al.*, 2007). Different mechanisms are considered responsible for the impaired ability of the kidney to produce adequate amounts of $1,25(OH)_2D_3$ (summarized in Table 19.2). First, chronic renal failure entails loss in renal mass resulting in a decreased amount of 1α-hydroxylase being available for the conversion of 25(OH)D into its active metabolite. Further, 25(OH)D is known to undergo glomerular filtration and reuptake from the ultrafiltrate by the receptor megalin into the proximal tubule cell, where it is further metabolized to $1,25(OH)_2D_3$ (Nykjaer *et al.*, 1999). Thus, a decline in the glomerular filtration rate leads to a decreased delivery of 25(OH)D to the 1α-hydroxylase in the proximal tubule cell. Moreover, fibroblast growth factor 23 (FGF-23) was identified a contributing factor to reduced $1,25(OH)_2D_3$ production. FGF-23 is a phosphaturic hormone synthesized by bone which gradually increases with declining renal function (Gutierrez *et al.*, 2005). It enhances urinary phosphate excretion (Shimada *et al.*, 2004) and decreases intestinal phosphate absorption (Miyamoto *et al.*, 2005). Thus, oversecretion of FGF-23 in chronic kidney disease reflects a compensatory mechanism to maintain phosphate levels within a physiological range. FGF-23 was also found to directly inhibit the expression of 1α-hydroxylase and prevent further activation of 25(OH)D (Perwad *et al.*, 2007). Another contributing factor is low 25(OH)D status which is commonly observed in chronic kidney disease patients. The prevalence of inadequate 25(OH)D levels defined as 25(OH)D less than 75 nmol/L ranges from 70% to 93% in chronic kidney disease patients not yet on dialysis (Gonzalez *et al.*, 2004; LaClair *et al.*, 2005; Levin *et al.*, 2007; Rucker *et al.*, 2009) and only about

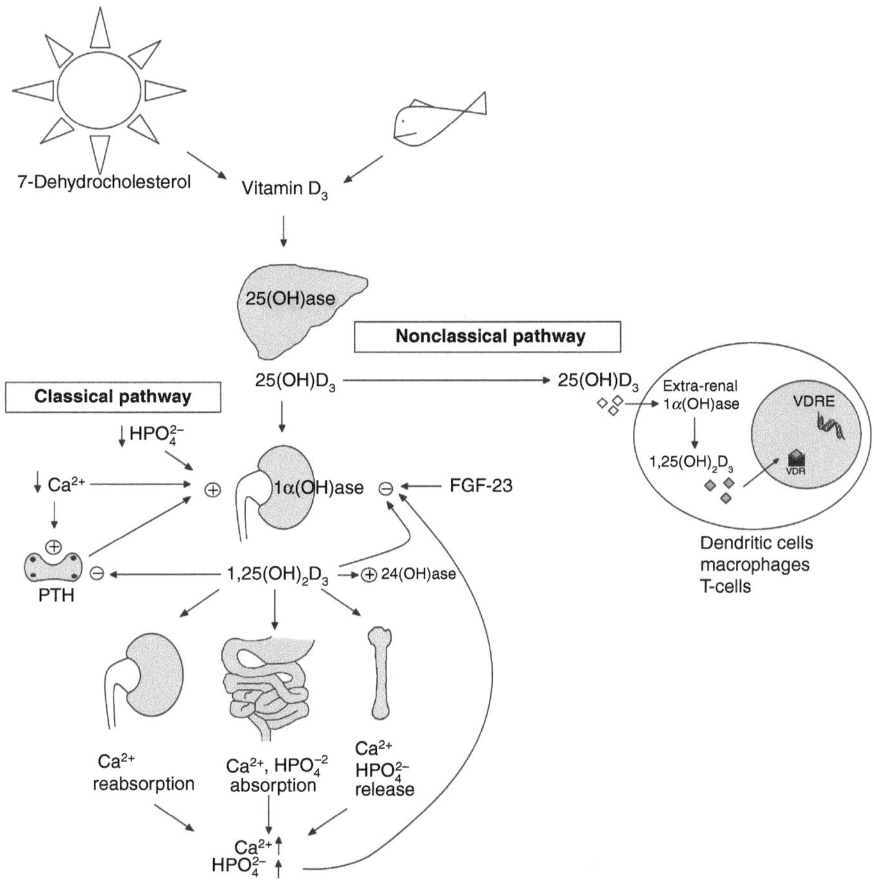

Figure 19.1 Vitamin D metabolism and actions. Abbreviations: 1α(OH)ase, 1α-hydroxylase; 1,25(OH)$_2$D$_3$, 1,25-dihydroxyvitamin D$_3$; 24(OH)ase, 24-hydroxylase; 25(OH)ase, 25-hydroxylase; 25(OH)D$_3$, 25-hydroxyvitamin D$_3$; Ca^{2+}, calcium; FGF-23, fibroblast growth factor 23; $HPO_4{}^{2-}$, phosphate; PTH, parathyroid hormone; VDR, vitamin D receptor; VDRE, vitamin D responsive element. The major source of vitamin D is endogenous synthesis from 7-dehydrocholesterol in the skin after UV radiation, only a small amount is obtained from the diet. Two hydroxylation steps are necessary to convert vitamin D$_3$ into its biologically active form. First, vitamin D$_3$ is converted by 25-hydroxylase to 25-hydroxyvitamin D$_3$ mainly in the liver. 25-hydroxyvitamin D$_3$ is further metabolized by 1α-hydroxylase mainly in the kidney to its biologically active form 1,25-dihydroxyvitamin D$_3$. The expression of 1α-hydroxylase and thus the production of 1,25-dihydroxyvitamin D$_3$ are tightly regulated. Serum calcium, phosphate, parathyroid hormone, and fibroblast growth factor 23 can either increase (+) or decrease (−) the renal production of 1,25-dihydroxyvitamin D$_3$. The classical actions of 1,25-dihydroxyvitamin D$_3$ include the regulation of calcium homeostasis. As serum calcium or phosphate levels decrease, 1,25-dihydroxyvitamin D$_3$ synthesis is stimulated and renal calcium and intestinal calcium and phosphate absorption as well as calcium and phosphate release from bone is increased. In order to prevent excessive high levels of 1,25-dihydroxyvitamin D$_3$, 1,25-dihydroxyvitamin D$_3$ itself as

Table 19.2 Contributing factors to low 1,25-dihydroxyvitamin D_3 levels in chronic kidney disease

- Loss of renal mass and 1α-hydroxylase
- Reduced glomerular filtration rate and inadequate delivery of 25-hydroxyvitamin D to the renal 1α-hydroxylase in the proximal tubule cell
- Increased levels of fibroblast growth factor 23 which directly inhibits 1α-hydroxylase
- 25-Hydroxyvitamin D deficiency due to
  - Reduced exposure to sunlight
  - Reduced cutaneous synthesis in the uremic state
  - Urinary loss of vitamin D binding protein

15% of chronic kidney disease patients were shown to have adequate 25 (OH)D levels at the time of transplantation (Ducloux *et al.*, 2008; Sadlier and Magee, 2007). Possible explanations for the high prevalence of inadequate 25(OH)D levels include reduced exposure to sunlight in the chronically ill (Thomas *et al.*, 1998) on the one hand, urinary loss of vitamin D binding protein in chronic kidney disease patients showing proteinuria on the other hand (Koenig *et al.*, 1992; Saha, 1994), as well as a reduction in the cutaneous synthesis of vitamin D_3 in the uremic state (Nessim *et al.*, 2007).

Together, these factors lead to a decreased amount of $1,25(OH)_2D_3$ available in chronic kidney disease. Additionally, hypocalcemia and hyperphosphatemia occur as a result of impaired kidney function, which together with low $1,25(OH)_2D_3$ levels constitute the major drivers in the development of PTH hypersecretion as a compensatory mechanism to maintain serum calcium levels within a physiological range. For this purpose, PTH acts on the bone to release calcium and phosphate, and acts on the kidney to reduce urinary calcium excretion and phosphate reabsorption, and induces 1α-hydroxylase and subsequent $1,25(OH)_2D_3$ production. As long as some renal function remains, the kidneys can respond to PTH to some extent but as kidney failure progresses, higher PTH concentrations are necessary to maintain calcium homeostasis. As secondary hyperparathyroidism progresses, parathyroid glands become hyperplastic and the expression of calcium-sensing receptor and vitamin D receptor in the parathyroid glands

well as high calcium and phosphate levels exert a negative feedback on the 1α-hydroxylase. Moreover, 1,25-dihydroxyvitamin D_3 induces 24-hydroxylase, the enzyme responsible for the degradation of vitamin D derivatives. 25-hydroxyvitamin D_3 is also activated at numerous extrarenal sites. Almost all cells of the immune system express 1α-hydroxylase and are therefore able to synthesize 1,25-dihydroxyvitamin D_3 locally from its precursor 25-hydroxyvitamin D_3. 1,25-dihydroxyvitamin D_3 subsequently binds to the vitamin D receptor in the nucleus where it interacts with vitamin D responsive elements and thus regulates gene transcription.

decreases making them resistant to calcium and 1,25$(OH)_2D_3$ regulation which finally results in an autonomous PTH excretion (Rodriguez *et al.*, 2005). However, secondary hyperparathyroidism is reversed in the majority of kidney transplant recipients.

C. Vitamin D metabolism after kidney transplantation

Despite successful kidney transplantation and restoration of renal function, abnormal mineral homeostasis might persist (Sprague *et al.*, 2008) and preexisting bone disease (Sherrard *et al.*, 1993) is often aggravated by immunosuppressive therapy (Weisinger *et al.*, 2006). A dramatic decrease of 25(OH)D levels within the first 3 months after kidney transplantation was reported, whereas 1,25$(OH)_2D_3$ levels almost doubled. Thereafter, 1,25 $(OH)_2D_3$ increased at a much slower pace (Evenepoel *et al.*, 2008). Moreover, during the first 3 months after transplantation, PTH levels initially markedly decrease but tend to stabilize at elevated levels after 1 year and remain elevated in the long-term posttransplant course in a subgroup of kidney transplant recipients. Calcium levels tend to increase after transplantation and stabilize at the upper limit of normal range within 6 months (Sprague *et al.*, 2008). Hypercalcemic episodes in patients with moderate to severe hyperparathyroidism at the time of transplantation were reported in 46% of cases after 1 year, 40% after 3 years, and 24% after 5 years posttransplant (Evenepoel *et al.*, 2004). Phosphate levels decrease rapidly after transplantation, and hypophosphatemia, if present, resolves within 2 months (Sprague *et al.*, 2008). Renal phosphate wasting after transplantation can be attributed to inappropriately high PTH and FGF-23 levels and was shown to regress by 1 year after kidney transplantation (Bhan *et al.*, 2006; Evenepoel *et al.*, 2008).

II. Vitamin D and the Immune System

Stimulated by the discovery of the vitamin D receptor as well as the enzymes responsible for the activation and degradation of vitamin D in different cells of the immune system, research during the recent 25 years has provided strong evidence of an immunomodulatory role of vitamin D receptor agonists besides its classical calcitropic actions.

The vitamin D receptor was identified in almost all cells of the immune system (Provvedini *et al.*, 1983), including neutrophils (Takahashi *et al.*, 2002), macrophages (Veldman *et al.*, 2000), and dendritic cells (Brennan *et al.*, 1987), as well as activated CD4+ and CD8+ T-lymphocytes (Veldman *et al.*, 2000), and B-cells (Chen *et al.*, 2007). Moreover, macrophages, dendritic cells (Fritsche *et al.*, 2003; Hewison *et al.*, 2007; Monkawa *et al.*, 2000), B-cells (Heine *et al.*, 2008), and also activated T-cells (Baeke *et al.*, 2010) express the enzyme 1α-hydroxylase which enables them to produce 1,25(OH)$_2$D$_3$ locally. The enzyme found in macrophages was shown to be identical to the renal form; however, it is not regulated by calcium and PTH but is under control of immune signals such as interferon (IFN)-γ and lipopolysaccharide. Moreover, no negative feedback by 1,25 (OH)$_2$D$_3$ itself could be observed (Overbergh *et al.*, 2000). Macrophages and dendritic cells were even found to express different cytochrome P-450 enzymes responsible for the 25-hydroxylation (Gottfried *et al.*, 2006; Sigmundsdottir *et al.*, 2007). Further, the major degrading enzyme, 24-hydroxylase, is expressed in monocytes, macrophages, and dendritic cells (Hewison *et al.*, 2003; Vidal *et al.*, 2002). The induction of 24-hydroxylase by 1,25(OH)$_2$D$_3$ is dependent on the activation and differentiation state of the cell. While 24-hydroxylase is highly induced by 1,25(OH)$_2$D$_3$ in undifferentiated monocytes, activated and differentiated macrophages were observed to be resistant to 1,25(OH)$_2$D$_3$ in the control of its own production and degradation (Vidal *et al.*, 2002).

Together, most of the cells of the immune system are able to produce 1,25(OH)$_2$D$_3$ locally from its circulating precursor 25(OH)D, some even from vitamin D$_3$, and they in turn can respond to locally synthesized 1,25 (OH)$_2$D$_3$.

Preclinical research revealed that vitamin D receptor agonists exert immunosuppressive activity on cells of the adaptive immune system, while stimulating the innate immune system. To understand the diverse immunomodulatory effects of vitamin D receptor agonists and the clinical implications in transplantation, basic immunologic concepts relevant to the development of graft rejection are detailed in the following section.

A. Basic immunologic concepts

Allograft rejection is mediated by different elements of the immune system, including antibody, complement, T-cells, and other cell types (Cornell *et al.*, 2008). T-lymphocytes and dendritic cells are of special interest in the connection with vitamin D and are therefore described in detail.

Central to the allograft response are CD4+ T-lymphocytes. They first need to be activated, which results from presentation of donor-derived antigens to the T-cell either by donor or recipient antigen presenting cells (Ingulli, 2010). Dendritic cells are considered the most important antigen presenting cells involved in this process. They occur in different stages of maturation in the circulation and are found in lymphoid and nonlymphoid organs. Immature dendritic cells are characterized by a high antigen-capture capacity. They continuously screen the surrounding environment for pathogens by means of pattern recognition receptors (Banchereau *et al.*, 2000). After uptake of donor-derived antigens, the antigens are processed by dendritic cells and subsequently presented to T-cells through major histocompatibility complex molecules ("signal 1"). Besides these alloantigen-specific signals, optimal activation of T-cells requires accessory antigen-nonspecific signals through costimulatory molecules provided by antigen presenting cells ("signal 2"). The expression of costimulatory molecules, such as B7.1 (CD80) or B7.2 (CD86), is increased during dendritic cell maturation leading to an improved capacity to stimulate T-cell response. In the absence of costimulation, T-cells become anergic, which means that the T-cell becomes unresponsive to activation by specific antigens (Ingulli, 2010).

Upon activation, T-lymphocytes proliferate and differentiate into diverse types of fully functional effector subsets, which differ in the cytokines they produce and thus in their function. These subpopulations were traditionally classified into T-helper 1 (Th1) and T-helper 2 (Th2) cells by Mosmann *et al.* (1986). More recent described subsets of T-lymphocytes include T-helper 17 (Th17) cells and regulatory T-cells (Tregs; Zhu *et al.*, 2010), both of which are considered to play an important role in allograft rejection. The major determinant in T-lineage decision is the cytokine environment. The activation and differentiation processes are depicted in Fig. 19.2.

In the presence of interleukin (IL)-12, which is mainly produced by activated cells of the innate immune system such as macrophages, CD4+ T-lymphocytes differentiate into Th1 cells. Also, IFN-γ plays an important role in the induction of Th1 cells. Th1 cells are characterized by secretion of the proinflammatory cytokine IFN-γ crucial for macrophage activation. They can also produce tumor necrosis factor (TNF)-α as well as IL-2, which is considered an autocrine growth factor for T-lymphocytes. Th1 cells are important for protection against intracellular pathogens and antitumor immunity, and are considered to play a major role in autoimmune disease (Zhu *et al.*, 2010). Moreover, Th1 cells are regarded to be involved in allograft rejection (Atalar *et al.*, 2009).

With respect to Th2 differentiation, IL-4 is the main factor involved. Th2 cells are associated with humoral immunity and are considered to have a more regulatory function through the production of IL-4, IL-5, IL-10, and IL-13. They are responsible for the eradication of extracellular pathogens and are the key mediators in allergic inflammatory response (Zhu *et al.*, 2010).

Differentiation of CD4+ T-cells into Th17 cells occurs under the influence of transforming growth factor (TGF)-β and IL-6. Th17 cells produce some of the members of the IL-17 family and are regarded crucial in pathogen clearance and controlling infections and are associated with the development of a variety of autoimmune diseases (Zhu *et al.*, 2010). Moreover, a role of Th17 cells in rejection is discussed (Atalar *et al.*, 2009).

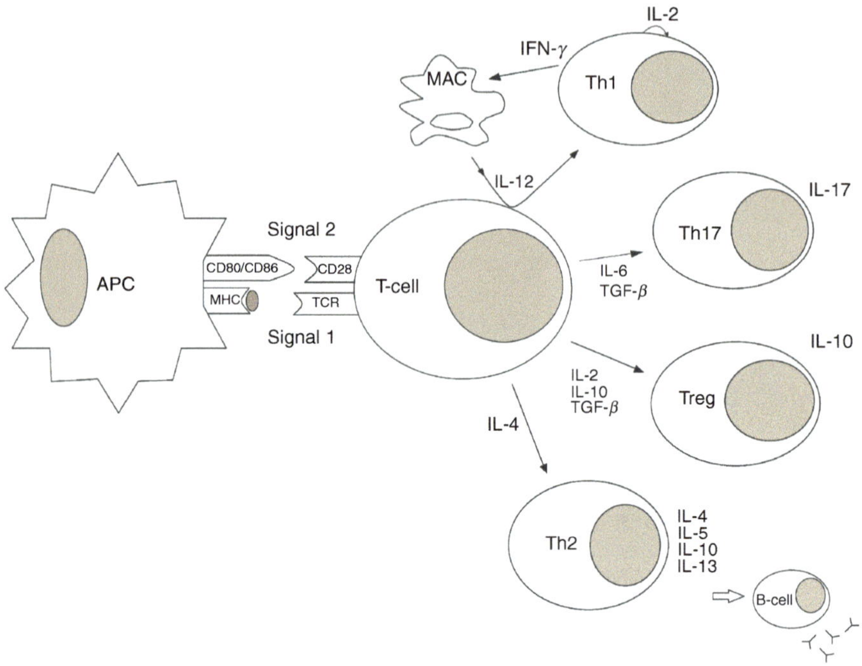

Figure 19.2 T-cell activation and differentiation. Abbreviations: APC, antigen presenting cell; IFN-γ, interferon-γ; IL, interleukin; MAC, macrophage; MHC, major histocompatibility complex; TCR, T-cell receptor; TGF-β, transforming growth factor-β. T-cell activation requires both an antigen-specific and an antigen-nonspecific signal provided by antigen presenting cells such as dendritic cells. Recognition of MHC–peptide complexes on dendritic cells by T-cell receptors constitutes "signal 1." The most important factor that constitutes "signal 2" is the interaction between costimulatory molecules expressed by dendritic cells such as CD80/CD86, CD40, and their ligands expressed by T-cells such as CD28 and CD154, respectively. After receptor activation and depending on the cytokine environment, naive T-cells can differentiate into diverse effector subsets which differ in the cytokine production and thus in their function.

For differentiation of Tregs, IL-2, TGF-β, and IL-10 were identified as the dominant inducing cytokines. Tregs are characterized by the combined expression of CD4 and CD25, as well as the transcription factor forkhead box P3 (FoxP3) necessary for the development and function of these cells. They are responsible for immune homeostasis and are able to mediate immunologic tolerance through production of inhibitory cytokines such as IL-10, as well as direct suppression of effector cells and modulation of dendritic cells (Sakaguchi *et al.*, 2008). In view of this, Tregs are considered an important target to achieve tolerance in solid organ transplantation (Sagoo *et al.*, 2008).

B. *In vitro* research

In vitro experiments revealed that vitamin D receptor agonists exert modulating effects on different cells of the immune system which may be exploited in the transplant setting. Vitamin D receptor agonists alter T-cell response through direct effects on T-cells and indirectly by modulation of the phenotype and function of dendritic cells.

In several studies, $1,25(OH)_2D_3$ and its analogues were shown to directly inhibit proliferation of human and murine T-cells after antigen stimulation (Bhalla *et al.*, 1984; Rigby *et al.*, 1984) and to directly target their transcription of different cytokines. Generally, the production of proinflammatory Th1-type cytokines such as IFN-γ and IL-2 is decreased after treatment with $1,25(OH)_2D_3$ (Cippitelli and Santoni, 1998; Takeuchi *et al.*, 1998), as are the cytokines produced by Th17 cells such as IL-17 and IL-21 (Borgogni *et al.*, 2008; Jeffery *et al.*, 2009). However, Th2-type cytokines, mainly IL-4, but also IL-5, and IL-10 are upregulated under the influence of $1,25(OH)_2D_3$ (Boonstra *et al.*, 2001). The production of the Th2 cytokine IL-4 is upregulated by $1,25(OH)_2D_3$ in most, but not all, studies (Staeva-Vieira and Freedman, 2002). The modulation of cytokine secretion patterns results in an overall shift away from a Th1 phenotype toward a more regulatory Th2 phenotype.

A more profound effect of $1,25(OH)_2D_3$ on the T-cell response is mediated indirectly via the modulation of dendritic cells. Several studies consistently showed that $1,25(OH)_2D_3$ induces dendritic cells with a potentially immunosuppressive phenotype (Berer *et al.*, 2000; Griffin *et al.*, 2000; Penna and Adorini, 2000; Piemonti *et al.*, 2000; Rosenblatt *et al.*, 2010; van Halteren *et al.*, 2002). *In vitro* treatment of dendritic cells with $1,25(OH)_2D_3$ or its analogues prevented differentiation and maturation of dendritic cells. These immature dendritic cells are characterized by a decreased expression of major histocompatibility complex class II molecules, and of costimulatory molecules, such as CD40, CD80, and CD86 (Gauzzi *et al.*, 2005; Pedersen *et al.*, 2009; Penna and Adorini, 2000), leading to an impaired capacity of antigen presentation and T-cell stimulation. Inhibition of dendritic cell maturation did not occur in cultures from mice genetically lacking the vitamin D receptor, suggesting vitamin D receptor-dependent pathways (Griffin *et al.*, 2000). Further, the cytokine secretion patterns are altered in dendritic cells treated with $1,25(OH)_2D_3$. While the secretion of IL-12 and IL-23 is diminished, thus leading to a decreased capacity to stimulate the development of Th1 and Th17 cells, respectively, the expression of IL-10 is enhanced, thereby favoring the emerge of a Th2 phenotype (Pedersen *et al.*, 2009; van Halteren *et al.*, 2002). Importantly, these $1,25(OH)_2D_3$ modulated dendritic cells are able to induce Tregs with suppressive activity (Penna *et al.*, 2005, 2007). Recently, Unger *et al.* showed that treatment of monocytes with either $1,25(OH)_2D_3$ or dexamethasone resulted in the induction of stable dendritic cells with a reduced level of costimulatory and MHC class II molecules which did not change after proinflammatory stimulation. Both $1{,}25(OH)_2D_3$- or dexamethasone-treated dendritic cells could convert CD4+ T-cells into IL-10-producing Tregs. $1{,}25(OH)_2D_3$-treated dendritic cells were found to express high levels of PD-L1 (programmed death-1 ligand) essential for the induction of Tregs. Blockade of PD-L1 during priming redirected T-cells to produce IFN-γ instead of IL-10 and abolished acquisition of regulatory capacity (Unger *et al.*, 2009).

Interestingly, $1{,}25(OH)_2D_3$ was found to directly regulate the transcription of different genes involved in the development of tolerogenity in dendritic cells, suggesting a mechanism of action which is independent from the inhibition of maturation and differentiation (Szeles *et al.*, 2009).

Together, vitamin D receptor agonists are able to shift the T-cell response away from an inflammatory Th1 phenotype toward a protective Th2 phenotype. By inducing dendritic cells with tolerogenic properties, vitamin D receptor agonists promote the development of Tregs with suppressive activity. An overview of the multiple immunomodulatory effects of vitamin D is depicted in Fig. 19.3.

These findings are not limited to *in vitro* experiments, but could be confirmed in different experimental models of transplantation.

C. Animal models of transplantation

The modulation of cytokine expression under the influence of vitamin D receptor agonists was observed in different animal models of transplantation (Gregori *et al.*, 2001; Redaelli *et al.*, 2001, 2002; Zhang *et al.*, 2003). $1{,}25(OH)_2D_3$ therapy was also found to be associated with improved graft function and survival (Hullett *et al.*, 1998; Lemire *et al.*, 1992; Redaelli *et al.*, 2001, 2002; Zhang *et al.*, 2003). Further, additive effects between $1{,}25(OH)_2D_3$ and other immunosuppressive drugs were observed in experimental models of heart, kidney, liver, and lung transplantation (Johnsson *et al.*, 1995; Redaelli *et al.*, 2001, 2002; Stammberger *et al.*, 2003; Zhang and Zheng, 2006). As such, vitamin D receptor agonists may be able to reduce the dose of other immunosuppressive drugs and thus their toxic side effects.

1. Kidney transplantation

In a rat model of kidney transplantation, both calcitriol and cyclosporine A (CsA) monotherapy were shown to prevent the secretion of the Th1 cytokines IL-2 and IL-12 in serum and allografts. A combination resulted in a stronger decline of IL-2 and IL-12 levels compared to CsA therapy alone. The expression levels of the Th2 cytokines IL-4 and IL-10 were only increased by calcitriol, but not by CsA monotherapy. However, a combination resulted in a significant increase of IL-10 expression levels, but not of IL-4. The explanations for these observations remain speculative but all

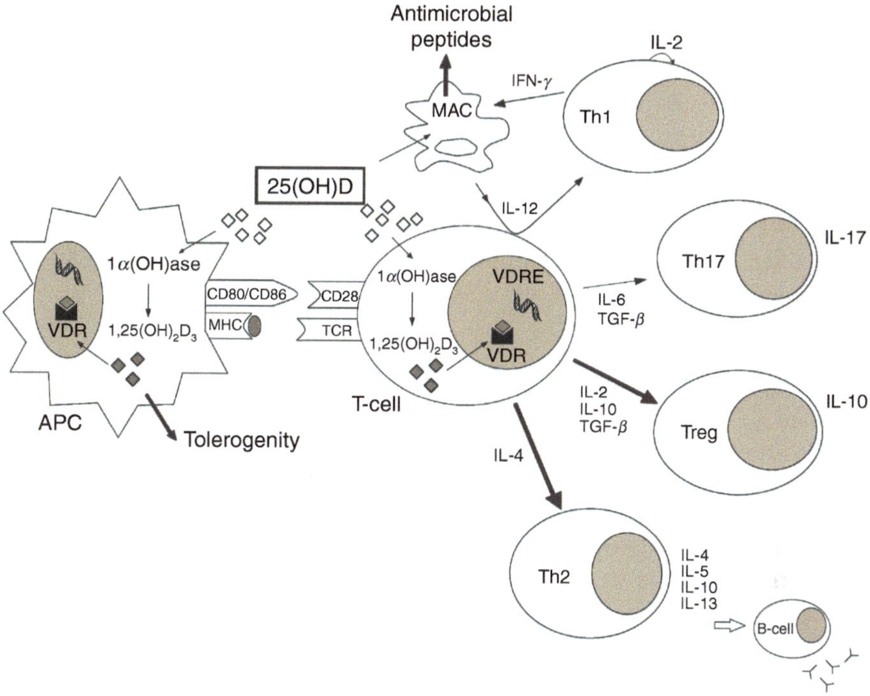

Figure 19.3 Immunomodulatory effects of 25-hydroxyvitamin D. Abbreviations: 1α(OH)ase, 1α-hydroxylase; 1,25(OH)$_2$D$_3$, 1,25-dihydroxyvitamin D$_3$; 25(OH)D, 25-hydroxyvitamin D; APC, antigen presenting cell; IFN-γ, interferon-γ; IL, interleukin; MAC, macrophage; MHC, major histocompatibility complex; TCR, T-cell receptor; TGF-β, transforming growth factor-β. Different immune cells express 1α-hydroxylase and are therefore able to produce 1,25-dihydroxyvitamin D$_3$ locally from its circulating precursor 25-hydroxyvitamin D. Almost all cells of the immune system express the vitamin D receptor and are thus able to respond to 1,25-dihydroxyvitamin D$_3$. Locally produced 1,25-dihydroxyvitamin D$_3$ modulates both the adaptive and the innate immune response. In T-lymphocytes, 1,25-dihydroxyvitamin D$_3$ directly modulates T-cell response by inhibition of inflammatory Th1 and Th17 cytokines and upregulation of Th2 cytokines, thus favoring the emerge of Th2 cells. Moreover, 1,25-dihydroxyvitamin D$_3$ induces antigen presenting cells with an immunosuppressive phenotype by inhibiting differentiation and maturation of these cells as well as the production of inflammatory cytokines, while stimulating the expression of anti-inflammatory cytokines. By this, 1,25-dihydroxyvitamin D$_3$ induces antigen presenting cells with tolerogenic properties which promote the development of regulatory T-cells with suppressive activity rather than effector T-cells. Together, 1,25-dihydroxyvitamin D$_3$ shifts the T-cell response away from an inflammatory Th1 response toward a protective Th2 and regulatory T-cell phenotype. While exerting suppressive activity on the adaptive immune system, 1,25-dihydroxyvitamin D$_3$ boosts the innate immune system by upregulation of the cathelicidin antimicrobial peptide in macrophages important for the immune defense of infections. (See Color Insert.)

together the results support the assumptions that calcitriol is a potent immunomodulatory agent in this experimental model of renal transplantation. Further, calcitriol monotherapy preserved graft function and significantly prolonged renal allograft survival (mean survival 9.6 ± 1.2 days) compared to the control group which did not receive immunosuppressive therapy (mean survival 5.7 ± 0.2 days). A combination of calcitriol and low-dose CsA increased allograft survival (mean survival 24 ± 0.9 days) compared to CsA administration alone (mean survival 13 ± 0.3 days). Moreover, a combination resulted in an additive effect on preventing deterioration of creatinine clearance and proteinuria compared to CsA alone (Redaelli *et al.*, 2002).

Another study investigated the effects of a vitamin D analogue (MC1288) with improved immunosuppressive capacity *in vitro* on allograft survival in a rhesus monkey model of kidney transplantation. *In vitro*, MC1288 was shown to suppress T-cell proliferation and IFN-γ production. However, the authors failed to demonstrate a difference in allograft survival (measured from the day of transplantation to the first rejection episode) between the rhesus monkeys treated with MC1288 and those without immunosuppressive treatment (Vierboom *et al.*, 2006).

2. Liver transplantation

In the field of liver transplantation, the effect of calcitriol on serum and intragraft cytokine expression was investigated in vascularized liver allografts in rats. The concentration of IL-2 and IL-12 in serum and in grafts significantly decreased under low-dose calcitriol therapy (0.1 μg/kg/day intraperitoneal) compared to no immunosuppressive therapy and remained at baseline levels under high-dose calcitriol (1 μg/kg/day intraperitoneal) or CsA therapy (2 mg/kg/day) 10 days posttransplant. IL-10 expression in the allografts significantly increased after low- or high-dose calcitriol therapy, whereas CsA did not show any influence on IL-10 expression. Serum IL-4 levels were undetectable, but calcitriol administration resulted in a strong expression of intragraft IL-4. CsA did not alter IL-4 levels either alone or in combination with calcitriol. Moreover, the rejection activity index 10 days after transplantation was significantly lower in calcitriol-treated rats compared to controls. Graft function was preserved and allograft survival was prolonged in recipients treated either with low- or high-dose calcitriol compared to no immunosuppressive therapy. A combination of calcitriol and CsA resulted in a strong additive effect and prolonged graft survival when compared to CsA alone (Redaelli *et al.*, 2001).

In another rat model of orthotopic liver transplantation, the effects of calcitriol on allograft survival and acute allograft rejection were studied. Survival time of recipients treated with calcitriol was similar to survival time of recipients treated with CsA and was significantly prolonged compared to those which did not receive immunosuppressive therapy. This benefit on survival was attributed to a marked inhibition of rejection that prevented deterioration of graft function. Moreover, a strong expression of IFN-γ in recipients without immunosuppressive therapy was observed, whereas the administration of CsA and calcitriol was found to be associated with a significant decrease of IFN-γ expression levels. A marked increase in IL-10 production in CsA and calcitriol-treated recipients was found (Zhang *et al.*, 2003).

When testing a combination of subtherapeutic doses of CsA and calcitriol in a rat model of liver transplantation in comparison to single or no immunosuppressive therapy, a combination of CsA and calcitriol led to an inhibition of cytokine production (IL-2 and IFN-γ) and alloantigen-mediated lymphocyte activation. Allograft rejection was minor and survival was prolonged in recipients treated with a combination of immunosuppressive drugs compared to single or no immunosuppression (Zhang and Zheng, 2006).

3. Cardiac transplantation

Using a cardiac allograft model in rats, the capacity of MC1288, a vitamin D analogue, and CsA in preventing allograft rejection was evaluated. A combination of MC1288 (0.1 μg/kg) and CsA (5 mg/kg) resulted in a significant prolongation of graft survival compared to MC1288 or CsA therapy alone. Adding LS-2616, an immunomodulatory agent which abolishes the immunosuppressive effects of CsA, did not result in an absolute counteraction of MC1288, indicating that MC1288 and CsA do not exert their immunosuppressive effects through the same mechanisms of action and thus suggesting an additive effect of MC1288 and CsA (Johnsson *et al.*, 1995).

Hullett *et al.* compared two vitamin D receptor agonists to CsA therapy in a mouse model of cardiac transplantation and showed that calcitriol and its analogue paricalcitol could inhibit rejection more effectively than a high-dose CsA regimen. The administration of calcitriol at a dose of 50 ng/day or its analogue paricalcitol at a dose of 200 ng/day markedly prolonged the survival of neonatal mouse heart allografts from 10 to 60 days and from 10 to 56 days, respectively. In comparison, CsA when given at 25 mg/kg/day increased heart muscle allograft survival from 10 to 36 days, showing calcitriol and its analogue to be superior to CsA in this setting (Hullett *et al.*, 1998).

However, one study, investigating a murine model of neonatal non-vascularized heart transplantation, did not show any significant prolongation in graft survival after treatment with calcitriol at a dose of 0.1 μg. Higher doses resulted in severe hypercalcemia and lead to the death of the experimental animals. Treatment with 1,25-dihydroxy-delta16-cholecalciferol, a calcitriol analogue, at a dose of 0.15 or 0.2 μg significantly prolonged allograft survival without deleterious side effects (Lemire *et al.*, 1992).

4. Lung transplantation

In a rat model of unilateral lung allotransplantation, the effect of calcitriol (0.5 μg/kg/day) combined with either CsA (2.5 mg/kg/day) or tacrolimus (40 μg/kg/day) compared to single immunosuppressive therapy was studied. Arterial PaO_2 on the fifth posttransplant day was used to evaluate graft function and was shown to be significantly lower in recipients treated with subtherapeutic dosages of single immunosuppressive drugs than in recipients treated with a combination of CsA and calcitriol, whereas tacrolimus in combination with calcitriol did not result in any benefit. These results indicated a significant improvement of graft function in recipients receiving a combination of calcitriol and CsA. However, the histopathological assessment did not show any differences between the treatment groups (Stammberger *et al.*, 2003).

5. Islet transplantation

Gregori *et al.* analyzed the ability of calcitriol alone or in combination with mycophenolate mofetil to induce transplantation tolerance in fully mismatched mouse islet allografts. The mean rejection time was prolonged in calcitriol-treated rats compared to vehicle-treated controls, and was comparable to mycophenolate mofetil-treated allograft recipients. A combination of calcitriol and mycophenolate mofetil resulted in a stronger prolongation of allograft acceptance. Calcitriol was shown to downregulate costimulatory molecules in dendritic cells and macrophages surrounding the graft, as well as their expression of IL-12 (Gregori *et al.*, 2001).

III. Vitamin D in Kidney Transplant Recipients

After kidney transplantation, vitamin D in its active form has different clinical applications, especially in the prevention of posttransplant bone loss (Palmer *et al.*, 2007) and in the treatment of normocalcemic persistent secondary hyperparathyroidism (De Sevaux *et al.*, 2002; El-Agroudy *et al.*, 2003; Lobo *et al.*, 1995; Torres *et al.*, 2004). However, one has to keep in mind that treatment with active vitamin D and its analogues will not compensate for inadequate 25(OH)D status which remains a common problem after kidney transplantation (Stavroulopoulos *et al.*, 2007). It is still important to correct 25(OH)D deficiency as 25(OH)D does not only serve as a substrate for 1α-hydroxylase in the kidney but also in several extrarenal tissues. Hence, these extrarenal tissues are dependent on adequate 25(OH)D substrate for adequate local $1,25(OH)_2D_3$ production.

A. Vitamin D deficiency and supplementation strategies

The definition of vitamin D deficiency is controversial and no general consensus on adequate 25(OH)D levels is available. However, vitamin D deficiency is defined by most experts as 25(OH)D levels less than 50 nmol/L (Holick, 2007).

As described above, low vitamin D status is frequently observed in chronic kidney disease patients and remains a common problem after renal transplantation. Vitamin D insufficiency [25(OH)D between 40 and 75 nmol/L] was reported to be present in 43%, deficiency [25(OH)D between 12 and 39 nmol/L] in 46%, and severe deficiency [25(OH)D less than 12 nmol/L] in 5% of long-term kidney transplant recipients with a median posttransplant time of 6 years (Stavroulopoulos *et al.*, 2007). The underlying causes of low vitamin D status in kidney transplant recipients are multifactorial. Considering the fact that endogenous production in the skin is the main source of vitamin D, the high prevalence of inadequate 25(OH) D levels can be mainly attributed to the avoidance of direct sun exposure because of the increased risk of skin cancer due to immunosuppressive therapy (Euvrard *et al.*, 2003). Querings *et al.* analyzed serum 25(OH)D levels in 31 kidney transplant recipients, who all protected themselves from sun exposure, compared to an age- and gender-matched control group without renal disease or other diseases requiring sun protection at the end of winter. Serum 25(OH)D levels were significantly lower in kidney transplant recipients compared to controls, with 10 out of 31 having undetectable serum 25(OH)D levels (Querings *et al.*, 2006). Moreover, other causes contributing to vitamin D deficiency include a decreased capacity of human skin to produce vitamin D_3 in elderly subjects compared to younger adults (Holick, 2004) and an enhanced catabolism of 25(OH)D by immunosuppressive drugs such as glucocorticoids (Pascussi *et al.*, 2005). Particularly, low 25(OH)D levels were observed in African American kidney transplant recipients (Tripathi *et al.*, 2008) which primarily result from the fact that increased pigmentation reduces vitamin D_3 production in the skin (Harris, 2006).

Despite the high prevalence of vitamin D deficiency among kidney transplant recipients, only few data on substitution strategies are available and there is no general consensus on treatment of vitamin D deficiency after kidney transplantation. The optimal treatment modality remains a subject of controversy, both in terms of the type of vitamin (vitamin D_2 or D_3) and dosage. While vitamin D_3 was reported to be more effective than vitamin D_2 in correcting low 25(OH)D levels by some authors (Armas *et al.*, 2004; Trang *et al.*, 1998), others claim equivalence in the treatment of vitamin D deficiency (Holick *et al.*, 2008; Rapuri *et al.*, 2004). In terms of dosage, it has recently become evident that the correction of low 25(OH)D concentrations and maintenance of adequate 25(OH)D levels require high doses of vitamin D (Holick, 2007). Courbebaisse *et al.* investigated the effects of a high-dose cholecalciferol therapy [50,000 International Units (IU) once a week for 8 weeks] in 47 kidney transplant recipients found to have 25(OH) D levels less than 75 nmol/L 3 months after transplantation compared to another group of 47 kidney transplant recipients who did not receive any vitamin D supplements. Cholecalciferol administration at this dosage was shown to be safe and effective in increasing serum 25(OH)D levels above 75 nmol/L in almost all study subjects, whereas only three study subjects in the control group were found to have 25(OH)D levels above 75 nmol/L 1 year after transplantation. For maintenance, treatment cholecalciferol was administered at a dose of 50,000 IU every 4 weeks for 4 more months. However, this emerged to be insufficient to keep serum 25(OH)D levels above 75 nmol/L in half of the study subjects (Courbebaisse *et al.*, 2009). These findings are in consistence with previous investigations by Wissing *et al.* who administered 25,000 IU once a month and failed to correct low 25 (OH)D levels in kidney transplant recipients, suggesting that a high dose of cholecalciferol is necessary to correct vitamin D deficiency and maintain adequate levels of 25(OH)D (Wissing *et al.*, 2005).

However, hypercalcemia is the hazard criterion for high-dose vitamin D therapy and all side effects of vitamin D are attributable to hypercalcemia. Still, one has to keep in mind that vitamin D is less likely to cause hypercalcemia compared to active vitamin D metabolites (Vieth, 2009). Currently, the tolerable upper intake level for vitamin D defined as the amount of vitamin D that can be consumed by adults on a long-term basis with no anticipation of harm is set at 2,000 IU/day. However, this is lower than justified by the scientific evidence that shows that prolonged intake of 10,000 IU/day is likely to pose no risk of adverse effects (Hathcock *et al.*, 2007). Therefore, the recommended tolerable upper intake level is suggested to be set at 10,000 IU/day.

B. Graft function and rejection

Early clinical trials reported beneficial effects of calcitriol therapy in kidney transplant recipients with respect to graft function and rejection. However, most of the currently published studies investigating the nonclassical effects of calcitriol in kidney transplant recipients are retrospective analyses that do not provide definitive evidence of the putative beneficial immunological effects.

An association between low vitamin D status and renal allograft function was observed in 64 kidney transplant recipients. Kidney transplant patients having 25(OH)D levels less than 50 nmol/L showed significantly higher creatinine and proteinuria levels after 1 year of follow-up compared to those with 25(OH)D levels above 50 nmol/L (Sezer *et al.*, 2009).

Tanaci *et al.* conducted a retrospective cohort study including a total of 70 kidney transplant recipients to evaluate the impact of calcitriol therapy on the incidence of acute rejection episodes and the amount of immunosuppressive drugs needed, as well as overall graft survival. Moreover, the safety of calcitriol therapy was assessed by analyzing serum calcium levels. Thirty-five of the studied kidney transplant recipients were treated with calcitriol (0.5 μg/day) due to osteoporosis. The mean follow-up time before and after calcitriol therapy was 12.2 ± 9.6 and 21.4 ± 7.3 months, respectively. The matched control group consisted of 35 kidney transplant patients without osteoporosis who did not receive calcitriol. Prior to the onset of calcitriol therapy, a significantly higher amount of acute rejection episodes in kidney transplant recipients with osteoporosis was observed compared to the control group. Accordingly, cumulative pulse steroid doses were significantly higher, which may have contributed to the observed osteoporosis in this study group. However, the difference in the number of acute rejection episodes and in cumulative pulse steroid doses between the two study groups disappeared after the initiation of calcitriol therapy. No differences were found in the maintenance steroid or CsA doses before and after calcitriol administration. After the initiation of calcitriol therapy, serum calcium levels increased continuously differing significantly from serum calcium levels in kidney transplant recipients without calcitriol exposure. The authors failed to demonstrate a difference in mean graft survival between the intervention and the control group, despite the difference in the number of acute rejection episodes (Tanaci *et al.*, 2003). This may be attributed to the fact that recovery of renal function after an acute rejection episode, either assessed by serum creatinine or proteinuria, is a better predictor of long-term graft survival than acute rejection *per se* (Djamali *et al.*, 2010; Meier-Kriesche *et al.*, 2004). If serum creatinine levels return to within 95% of baseline creatinine levels in kidney transplant with acute rejection by 1-year posttransplant, similar long-term graft survivals as those who never experienced acute rejection were demonstrated (Meier-Kriesche *et al.*, 2004).

In a small prospective study, Ardalan *et al.* investigated the effect of calcitriol therapy which was started in the donor and continued in recipient side compared to the conventional immunosuppressive therapy alone. The treatment group consisted of nine donors, who all received calcitriol at a dose of 0.5 μg/day orally for 5 days before donation. The recipients were treated with the same regimen for 1-month posttransplant and thereafter received 0.25 μg/day for 5 months. In the control group ($n = 10$), neither donors nor recipients received calcitriol. At baseline, there was no significant difference in the percentage of CD3+ CD4+ CD25+ T-lymphocytes between the calcitriol treated and the control group (14.2 ± 4.2% and 15.4 ± 4.5%, respectively). However, after 6 months, a significantly higher percentage of CD3+ CD4+ CD25+ T-lymphocytes was found in the treatment group (29.0 ± 6.3% and 12.1 ± 4.5% in the treatment and control group, respectively). Although only 19 kidney transplant recipients were included in this trial, a significant expansion of CD4+ CD25+ Tregs in the calcitriol-treated group could be demonstrated, providing strong evidence of the immunomodulatory properties of active vitamin D in kidney transplant recipients (Ardalan *et al.*, 2007).

Recently, a small prospective clinical trial investigated the expression of HLA-DR, a major histocompatibility complex class II cell surface receptor, and costimulatory molecules on peripheral blood leukocytes in kidney transplant recipients before and after 4 weeks of calcitriol therapy. A total of 24 patients who had undergone a transplantation 6–18 months before the study were treated with calcitriol at a dose of 0.5 μg/day over a time period of 4 weeks. A substantial decrease of HLA-DR, CD28, CD86, and CD40 expressed on white blood cells was found after calcitriol treatment. Neither did acute allograft dysfunction occur during the studied period, nor did mean serum creatinine levels change before and after intervention (Ahmadpoor *et al.*, 2009).

C. Chronic allograft injury

Within the past decade, modern immunosuppressive drug regimes have dramatically reduced the incidence of acute rejection. According to the US Renal Data System (2009) Annual Data Report, the incidence of acute rejection episodes within the first year after kidney transplantation is 12% in deceased donor recipients. Despite the advances in controlling acute allograft rejection, chronic allograft injury still poses a challenge in kidney transplantation and is regarded one of the major cause of kidney transplant failure (El-Zoghby *et al.*, 2009). The onset of chronic allograft injury occurs as early as 3 months after transplantation as a result of both immunologic and ischemic injuries. Moderate chronic allograft injury is present in about 25% of kidney transplant recipients at 1 year after transplantation, and in about 90% by 10 years (Nankivell *et al.*, 2003). Chronic allograft injury is clinically seen as progressive renal dysfunction and is characterized by fibrotic changes throughout the kidney including interstitial fibrosis, tubular atrophy, glomerulosclerosis, and intimal thickening of the graft blood vessels (Racusen *et al.*, 1999). The mechanisms responsible for the development of chronic allograft injury involve humoral and cellular immune response as well as a number of non-immunological factors such as chronic hypertension, calcineurin inhibitor toxicity, chronic obstruction to the ureter, and infection (Solez *et al.*, 2007).

1. Molecular mechanisms of chronic allograft injury

Particularly, TGF-β1 is regarded a key fibrogenetic cytokine involved in the development of chronic allograft injury. TGF-β1 stimulates the synthesis of several matrix molecules and is important in preventing matrix degradation, thus contributing to matrix accumulation and fibrosis (Jain *et al.*, 2000). After binding of TGF-β1 to its cell surface receptor, an intracellular signaling cascade is initiated involving a class of proteins called Smads. Receptor activation leads to the phosphorylation of the signaling proteins Smads 2/3 which subsequently form a heterodimer with Smad 4. This complex translocates to the nucleus where it regulates the transcription of genes involved in matrix accumulation and fibrosis. Smad 6 and Smad 7 are inhibitory signal proteins which function as negative feedback inhibitors for diverse molecules in the TGF-β superfamily (Zimmerman and Padgett, 2000).

In clinical studies, patients with chronic allograft injury were significantly linked with persistently higher plasma TGF-β1 levels (Harris *et al.*, 2007). Moreover, protocol renal allograft biopsies within the early post-transplant course showed upregulation of TGF-β after transplantation (Jain *et al.*, 2002) and revealed a clear increase of TGF-β expression in patients with histopathological features of chronic allograft injury (Sharma *et al.*, 1996). The expression of TGF-β in the allograft was associated with interstitial fibrosis (Baboolal *et al.*, 2002) as well as chronic vasculopathy (Viklicky *et al.*, 2003).

2. Interactions between vitamin D and transforming growth factor: Preclinical evidence

Several *in vitro* studies demonstrated cross-talk between the TGF-β and vitamin D signaling pathways (Subramaniam *et al.*, 2001; Yanagi *et al.*, 1999; Yanagisawa *et al.*, 1999), suggesting that vitamin D receptor agonists regulate TGF-β-mediated gene and protein expression and may therefore influence the effect of TGF-β in chronic allograft injury. Recently, 1,25 $(OH)_2D_3$ was found to inhibit TGF-β1-mediated proliferation in lung fibroblasts (Ramirez *et al.*, 2010), which is considered to play a central role in the development of posttransplant obliterative bronchiolitis.

An interaction between vitamin D receptor agonists and the Smad signaling cascade was also shown *in vivo* in rodent renal tissue (Aschenbrenner *et al.*, 2001). Moreover, in diverse rat models of kidney disease, $1,25(OH)_2D_3$ was reported to attenuate the development of glomerulosclerosis and progression of albuminuria accompanied by a lower expression of TGF-β1 in the kidney (Makibayashi *et al.*, 2001; Schwarz *et al.*, 1998). Studying a rat model of chronic allograft nephropathy, Hullett *et al.* observed that $1,25(OH)_2D_3$ therapy could preserve renal graft function and prolong allograft survival. Significant prolongation of graft survival was achieved with $1,25(OH)_2D_3$ at 1000 and 500 ng/rat/day compared to no immunosuppressive therapy, but not at 250 ng/rat/day, and was similar to graft survival in recipients treated with CsA. $1,25(OH)_2D_3$ also prevented histological changes typically found in chronic allograft injury by altering TGF-β1 and matrix regulating molecules. While a marked reduction in the

Smad 2 expression was observed, which is in accordance with previous findings (Li *et al.*, 2002), inhibitory Smad 7 expression was increased (Hullett *et al.*, 2005).

With respect to transplant vasculopathy, the mouse aortic allograft model is suitable to investigate immune-mediated vascular intimal thickening which is similar to the vascular lesions in human chronic allograft injury. The application of the nonhypercalcemic vitamin D receptor agonist BXL-628 in a mouse model of aortic transplantation resulted in a reduced leukocyte infiltration and an inhibition of intimal hyperplasia compared to dexamethasone or calcitriol therapy. Mice were treated with BXL-628 (30 μg/kg/five times a week), calcitriol (5 μg/kg/three times a week), dexamethasone, or a vehicle for 30 days. At day 60, posttransplant aortic allografts were harvested for histological analyses. Intimal hyperplasia was significantly reduced by dexamethasone, but to a higher extent by calcitriol and even more by BXL-628, which led to an ~80% reduction of intimal hyperplasia compared to vehicle-treated controls. This effect was attributed to a downregulation in the expression of different genes involved in muscle development such as desmin, transgelin, tropomyosin, alpha-actin, and myosin heavy chain 11 (Amuchastegui *et al.*, 2005).

Similarly, an inhibition of aortic intimal thickening was induced by the vitamin D receptor agonist MC1288 combined with CsA. However, the dosage used led to hypercalcemia and weight loss (Raisanen-Sokolowski *et al.*, 1997). MC1288 also reduced clinical and histological signs of chronic allograft injury in rat kidney allografts; however, chronic allograft damage index was only reduced in recipients treated with a combination of CsA and MC1288 (Kallio *et al.*, 1996).

3. Vitamin D in chronic allograft injury

In kidney transplant recipients with chronic allograft dysfunction, O'Herrin *et al.* undertook a case–control study to evaluate the impact of calcitriol therapy on renal function. Twenty-one kidney transplant recipients alone and five kidney–pancreas transplant recipients with chronic allograft dysfunction were included, all of them showing either increasing serum creatinine levels and/or biopsy-proven evidence of chronic allograft injury. All of them received calcitriol posttransplant, which was started at least 1 year after transplantation. The age- and gender-matched control group consisted of 45 kidney transplant recipients only and five kidney–pancreas transplant recipients. These patients did not receive calcitriol, but did have biopsy-proven chronic allograft injury and/or increasing serum creatinine levels after at least 1 year of graft function. All of the individuals received the same immunosuppressive regime. O'Herrin *et al.* found that calcitriol treatment was associated with a significant improvement in graft survival compared to no calcitriol treatment. Average serum creatinine levels increased in calcitriol-treated patients until the initiation of calcitriol therapy, then stabilized, indicating improved renal graft function. Moreover, a trend toward less acute rejection episodes could be observed in the calcitriol-treated group. There were no adverse events identified in association with calcitriol treatment (O'Herrin *et al.*, 2002).

Another retrospective study in 110 renal transplant recipients compared graft function of 57 osteoporotic patients treated with calcitriol to 53 nonosteoporotic patients who did not receive calcitriol. Mean time to start calcitriol therapy was 22.4 ± 6.8-months posttransplant. Prior to calcitriol therapy, creatinine levels were found to be similar in the two study groups. However, a significantly reduced increase in creatinine levels was observed in kidney transplant recipients treated with calcitriol after 2 years of therapy (1.7 ± 1.4 vs. 2.7 ± 2.5 mg/dL in the calcitriol- and nontreated group, respectively), suggesting a deceleration in the rate of loss of renal function. As regards acute rejection episodes, no significant difference was found between the two study groups. Still, the group treated with calcitriol was shown to require fewer pulse steroid doses. The authors postulate a synergistic effect of calcitriol with steroids, thus lower doses of steroids are needed to suppress an acute rejection attack (Sezer *et al.*, 2005). These findings could be corroborated after a follow-up period of 3 years (Uyar *et al.*, 2006). However, the authors may have failed to demonstrate a difference in the incidence of acute rejection episodes between the two study groups because of the delayed treatment after transplantation. The majority of acute rejection episodes occur within the first 90 days after transplantation (Heldal *et al.*, 2009; US Renal Data System, 2009).

D. Infections

Due to immunosuppressive therapy, transplant recipients are at higher risk of developing infections (Fishman, 2007). A connection between vitamin D status and the susceptibility to infectious diseases was observed by several epidemiological studies. Furthermore, clinical trials provide strong evidence of the beneficial effects of vitamin D therapy for tuberculosis, influenza, and viral upper respiratory tract infections (Yamshchikov *et al.*, 2009). These beneficial effects may also be exploited after organ transplantation.

1. Infection defense and the importance of antimicrobial peptides

The underlying molecular mechanisms of the immunomodulatory properties mediated by vitamin D in various infectious diseases include the interaction with cells of the innate immune system and the upregulation of specific endogenous antimicrobial peptides in these cells. The innate immune system is the first line of defense and combats pathogens in a nonspecific way. The cells of the innate immune system recognize invading pathogens via pattern recognition receptors. These receptors are able to detect conserved molecular patterns shared by different types of pathogens including bacterial or fungal products such as lipopolysaccharide or β-glucan, as well as viral nucleic acids. After activation, a cascade of immune responses is initiated including production of proinflammatory cytokines, induction of cell differentiation and apoptosis, and activation of the adaptive immune system that finally leads to the elimination or destruction of the foreign organisms. Besides, the response of the innate immune system involves the production of antimicrobial peptides, which exert direct antimicrobial activity (Medzhitov, 2007). In humans, there are three major families of antimicrobial peptides, which are α- and β-defensins, and cathelicidins. α-defensins are mainly found in neutrophil granules, while β-defensins are expressed by respiratory and intestinal epithelial cells as well as keratinocytes (Ganz, 2003). The human cathelicidin antimicrobial peptide encoded by the hCAP18 gene is mainly expressed in neutrophils and other leukocyte populations as well as at barrier sites such as respiratory and colonic epithelium, saliva, and skin (Durr *et al.*, 2006). Cathelicidin is a precursor protein that is cleaved by proteases during activation to release the active peptide LL-37 (Sorensen *et al.*, 2001). LL-37 has a broad activity against gram-positive and gram-negative bacteria as well as viruses and fungi. The antimicrobial mechanisms of LL-37 include lipopolysaccharide binding and thus prevention of immunostimulatory effects as well as cytotoxic and chemotactic activity (Durr *et al.*, 2006). In that, antimicrobial peptides act as potent, endogenous broad spectrum antibiotics and serve a critical role in the innate immune defense of infections.

2. Vitamin D and the innate immune system: Preclinical evidence

Vitamin D receptor agonists exert immunosuppressive activity on the adaptive immune system as described above; at the same time they boost the innate immune system and thus preserve important defense mechanisms against microbial infections.

Vitamin D responsive elements were identified in the promoters of the human cathelicidin antimicrobial peptide and defensin-β2 genes, which mediate $1,25(OH)_2D_3$-dependent gene expression (Wang *et al.*, 2004). Several *in vitro* experiments showed that vitamin D receptor agonists directly upregulate antimicrobial peptide gene expression in peripheral blood mononuclear cells and neutrophils, keratinocytes (Gombart *et al.*, 2005; Martineau *et al.*, 2007; Wang *et al.*, 2004), as well as bronchial epithelial cells (Yim *et al.*, 2007).

Liu *et al.* provided a key mechanism on how vitamin D may enhance innate immunity. They showed that toll-like-receptor activation of human macrophages by *Mycobacterium tuberculosis*-derived antigens leads to the upregulation of both the vitamin D receptor and 1α-hydroxylase. This enables the macrophages to produce $1,25(OH)_2D_3$ locally from its circulating precursor 25(OH)D. Intracellular generated $1,25(OH)_2D_3$ subsequently interacts with the vitamin D receptor which induces an enhanced expression of the antimicrobial peptide cathelicidin. Interestingly, macrophages cultured in vitamin D-deficient sera of African Americans are unable to upregulate LL-37 and kill *M. tuberculosis*. When adding 25(OH)D to the media, an enhanced production of LL-37 could be observed and effective killing of *M. tuberculosis* was restored (Liu *et al.*, 2006). These findings suggest that 25(OH)D levels affect an individual's ability to defense pathogens and that correction of vitamin D deficiency may improve one's resistance to certain infections.

In vivo, Cantorna *et al.* investigated the ability of $1,25(OH)_2D_3$-treated mice to resist to infection with *Candida albicans* and herpes simplex virus-1 (HSV-1) compared to nontreated or CsA-treated mice. Treatment with active vitamin D did not increase the susceptibility of mice to *C. albicans* infection. After intravenous injection of 5×10^6 *C. albicans*, recipients treated with CsA were significantly more susceptible to systemic *C. albicans* infections compared to the controls and the $1,25(OH)_2D_3$-treated animals. Three weeks after infection, 20% of the CsA-treated mice were alive, compared to 80% of the controls and 100% of the $1,25(OH)_2D_3$-treated mice. After the ocular infection with HSV-1, the viral infection disseminated and was lethal for 36% of the $1,25(OH)_2D_3$-treated mice and for 30% of the controls, whereas all the CsA-treated mice were dead by 10 days after infection. Thus, experimental data support the assumption that vitamin D is not a general immunosuppressant, but a selective modulator (Cantorna *et al.*, 1998).

Further, cathelicidin was found to play an important role in the protection against infections in the urinary tract. The examination of human renal biopsies showed that the cathelicidin antimicrobial peptide is constitutively expressed in the urinary tract. Exposure of the renal explants to *Escherichia coli* led to a rapid increase of the production of cathelicidin and its secretion into urine. To further investigate the role of the cathelicidin antimicrobial peptide in the protection of the urinary tract against infection *in vivo*, Chromek *et al.* studied a mouse model of ascendant pyelonephritis and compared the course of an ascending urinary tract infection in mice which lacked the cathelicidin gene to those with normal cathelicidin expression, and in neutrophil-depleted mice. After inoculation of the bladder with *E. coli*, cathelicidin-deficient animals had a greater number of bacteria adherent to bladder epithelium and developed both significantly more and more severe ascending infections compared to wild-type mice. Depletion of neutrophils did not change the susceptibility, suggesting a primary role of cathelicidin in mucosal immunity of the urinary tract (Chromek *et al.*, 2006).

3. Vitamin D in the prevention of infectious diseases

Epidemiologic studies demonstrated strong associations between low vitamin D status and the incidence of various infectious diseases. A case–control study in 1000 Ethiopians investigated the role of nutritional rickets in the development of pneumonia and revealed a 13-fold higher incidence of nutritional rickets in children with pneumonia than in controls (Muhe *et al.*, 1997). Moreover, several studies observed an inverse association between vitamin D status and the frequency of respiratory infections (Cannell *et al.*, 2006; Laaksi *et al.*, 2007). Ginde *et al.* examined the association between serum 25(OH)D levels and recent upper respiratory tract infections within a secondary analysis of the Third National Health and Nutrition Examination Survey including 18,883 participants. While upper respiratory tract infections were reported by 24% of participants with 25 (OH)D levels less than 25 nmol/L, 20% of those having 25(OH)D levels between 25 and 75 nmol/L did so. Seventeen percent of study subjects with 25(OH)D levels above 75 nmol/L reported upper respiratory tract infections (Ginde *et al.*, 2009).

In a *post hoc* analysis, Aloia and Li-Ng (2007) reported the incidence of common colds and influenza among 208 postmenopausal black women. The women were included in a 3-year randomized trial receiving either oral vitamin D_3 (800 IU the first 2 years, 2000 IU the third year) or placebo. Every 3 months, the study subjects were interviewed and asked whether they had experienced a cold or influenza in the previous 3 months. Twenty-six women taking the placebo reported respiratory tract symptoms, compared to seven taking 800 IU/day and only one taking 2000 IU of vitamin D_3/day (Aloia and Li-Ng, 2007).

A possible explanation for the mechanism of vitamin D in reducing the risk of infections included the production of the cathelicidin antimicrobial peptide. In fact, a significantly increased expression of hCAP18 in neutrophils of newborn rickets patients treated with 1α-hydroxyvitamin D_3 for 4 weeks compared to age-matched healthy controls without 1α-hydroxyvitamin D_3 intake was found (Misawa *et al.*, 2009). Moreover, to investigate the role of vitamin D in sepsis syndrome, a cross-sectional study of 25(OH)D status and its relationship to systemic LL-37 levels in a group of critically ill subjects including those with and without sepsis was performed (Jeng *et al.*, 2009). Almost all critically ill patients were found to have suboptimal levels of 25(OH)D associated with lower systemic levels of LL-37.

Gombart *et al.* investigated the association between baseline hCAP18 levels and death due to infections within 1 year after initiating hemodialysis in 279 individuals. It was shown that individuals in the lowest tertile of hCAP18 levels had a threefold increase in the odds of death due to infections. However, the authors could not find an association with 25(OH)D and hCAP18; a borderline positive association with 1,25$(OH)_2D_3$ and hCAP18 was observed. The authors state that this may be attributable to the high prevalence of vitamin D deficiency that was present in the majority of the study subjects. The strongest association was observed during active inflammation (Gombart *et al.*, 2009).

IV. Vitamin D in Other Transplant Recipients

Like in chronic kidney disease patients, vitamin D deficiency is commonly observed in patients with end-stage chronic liver disease (Crosbie *et al.*, 1999) as well as end-stage organ failure of the heart (Iqbal *et al.*, 2008; Shane *et al.*, 1997; Stein *et al.*, 2009) and lung (Forli *et al.*, 2004; Shane *et al.*, 1996). Especially, chronic liver disease patients are at high risk to develop severe vitamin D deficiency because of impaired 25-hydroxylation of vitamin D in the liver. Between 80% and 95% of chronic liver disease patients are reported to have 25(OH)D levels less than 50 nmol/L (Crosbie *et al.*, 1999; Stein *et al.*, 2009). Thirty percent of chronic liver disease patients were reported to have severe vitamin D deficiency (less than 25 nmol/L). Similar to kidney transplant recipients, inadequate 25(OH)D levels frequently persist after organ transplantation. At 1-year posttransplant, half of the lung transplant recipients and almost three-quarter of the heart transplant recipients were found to have inadequate 25(OH)D levels, defined as 25(OH)D less than 75 nmol/L (Forli *et al.*, 2010). In liver transplant recipients, 25(OH)D levels were found to steadily increase within the first postoperative year and only 14% of the patients showed severe vitamin D deficiency at 1 year (Monegal *et al.*, 2001). However, vitamin D supplementation in patients after solid organ transplantation has received little specific attention to date. Most of the studies on vitamin D in solid organ transplant recipients evaluate the effects on posttransplant bone loss (Cohen *et al.*, 2004; Ebeling, 2009). To our knowledge, only two studies are available which target the nonclassical effects of vitamin D.

Bitetto *et al.* retrospectively analyzed the association between acute liver allograft rejection and pretransplant serum 25(OH)D concentrations or posttransplant vitamin D_3 therapy in 133 liver transplant recipients. All study subjects underwent two per protocol allograft biopsies after 1-month and 6-months posttransplant, and if indicated. Seventy-nine patients (59.3%) with known pretransplant osteopenia or osteoporosis received oral vitamin D_3 therapy at a dose of 800 IU/day in order to avoid further bone loss, in 53 (39.8%) of which vitamin D_3 therapy was started within the first postoperative month. Only 7.5% among the patients analyzed in this study were found to have optimal 25(OH)D (above 75 nmol/L) at the time of transplantation. Low vitamin D status at the time of transplantation was identified, a predictor of acute allograft rejection. Moreover, a significant linear association was observed between the absence of rejection episodes and vitamin D_3 therapy (Bitetto *et al.*, 2010).

In heart transplant recipients, an additive effect of immunosuppressive therapy and calcitriol was observed. Fifty-two out of 99 heart transplant recipients were randomly assigned to receive 0.5–1 μg of calcitriol, started within the first 2 postoperative weeks and given for a time period between

6 months and 2 years. Heart transplant recipients treated with calcitriol were found to require less oral CsA throughout the 2-year follow-up (29% and 28% lower total cumulative dose at 1 and 2 years, respectively; Briffa *et al.*, 2003).

V. Conclusion and Future Directions

Vitamin D receptor agonists play multiple biological roles beyond calcium and bone metabolism including modulation of immune functions. It became evident that 25(OH)D is not only exclusively activated in the kidney but also serves as a substrate in many other tissues. Almost all cells of the immune system are capable of active vitamin D synthesis and subsequently can respond to locally produced $1,25(OH)_2D_3$. Unlike renal $1,25(OH)_2D_3$ production, local active vitamin D synthesis is not underlying the control of calcium, phosphate, and PTH, but is dependent on adequate 25(OH)D levels alone (Liu *et al.*, 2006). It is therefore important to correct vitamin D deficiency, to optimize these nonclassical actions. Particularly, vitamin D deficiency is a common problem after solid organ transplantation (Forli *et al.*, 2010; Stavroulopoulos *et al.*, 2007). Strict sun protection is recommended to transplant recipients in order to reduce the risk of skin cancer (Euvrard *et al.*, 2003). However, it is commonly overlooked that strict sun protection involves the risk of developing severe vitamin D deficiency, as the major source of vitamin D is endogenous production in the skin through the action of the sun (Querings *et al.*, 2006). Therefore, it is of high importance and relevance to transplant recipients to detect and treat vitamin D deficiency, taking into consideration that the actions of vitamin D extend far beyond calcium and bone metabolism. In several studies, a connection between low vitamin D status and various severe health problems including different types of malignancies (e.g., colon, prostate, and breast cancer; Grant, 2002), cardiovascular diseases (Giovannucci *et al.*, 2008; Wang *et al.*, 2008), and increased susceptibility to infections (Ginde *et al.*, 2009) has been reported. Particularly with regard to transplant recipients, correction of low vitamin D status may have beneficial effects on allograft outcome, infection defense, cardiovascular and cancer risk, and the development of posttransplant diabetes (Courbebaisse *et al.*, 2010).

Interestingly, an increased incidence of acute rejection episodes and graft loss was observed in black kidney transplant recipients compared to whites (Brown *et al.*, 2010; Young and Gaston, 2000). Possible explanations include immunologic hyperresponsiveness in blacks (Kerman *et al.*, 1991, 1992) as well as an overexpression of TGF-β (Suthanthiran *et al.*, 1998) and costimulatory molecules on peripheral blood cells (Hutchings *et al.*, 2001).

It is therefore hypothesized that low vitamin D status might contribute to the inferior graft outcome in blacks (Zasloff, 2006).

These nonclassical effects, however, are so far mostly documented by experimental and observational studies or small interventional trials. Until now, there is one ongoing randomized, placebo-controlled trial in Vienna investigating the effects of high-dose cholecalciferol therapy in vitamin D-deficient kidney transplant recipients on graft function, allograft rejection, and posttransplant infections as primary endpoints (Thiem *et al.*, 2009). Another current ongoing study focuses on the treatment of hyperparathyroidism with doxercalciferol and evaluates graft function and rejection rate as secondary endpoints (www.clinicaltrials.gov; NCT00646282). Therefore, we stress the urgent need for larger placebo-controlled trials in transplant recipients, targeting clinical endpoints such as graft function, rejection episodes, infections, cancers, and cardiovascular events. Especially, the additive immunomodulatory effects of vitamin D with conventional immunosuppressive drugs require further investigation. Vitamin D may reduce the dose of other immunosuppressive drugs, which subsequently results in a reduction of toxic side effects (e.g., nephrotoxicity of calcineurin inhibitors) as well as infectious complications. This is of special relevance, considering the fact that infections are one of the leading causes of death in kidney transplant recipients (Tapiawala *et al.*, 2010). Vitamin D may also be able to attenuate the development of chronic allograft injury which poses a major unresolved problem in kidney transplant recipients.

REFERENCES

Ahmadpoor, P., Ilkhanizadeh, B., Ghasemmahdi, L., Makhdoomi, K., and Ghafari, A. (2009). Effect of active vitamin D on expression of co-stimulatory molecules and HLA-DR in renal transplant recipients. *Exp. Clin. Transplant.* **7,** 99–103.

Aloia, J. F., and Li-Ng, M. (2007). Re: Epidemic influenza and vitamin D. *Epidemiol. Infect.* **135,** 1095–1096, author reply 1097–1098.

Amuchastegui, S., Daniel, K. C., and Adorini, L. (2005). Inhibition of acute and chronic allograft rejection in mouse models by BXL-628, a nonhypercalcemic vitamin D receptor agonist. *Transplantation* **80,** 81–87.

Ardalan, M. R., Maljaei, H., Shoja, M. M., Piri, A. R., Khosroshahi, H. T., Noshad, H., and Argani, H. (2007). Calcitriol started in the donor, expands the population of CD4+CD25+ T cells in renal transplant recipients. *Transplant. Proc.* **39,** 951–953.

Armas, L. A., Hollis, B. W., and Heaney, R. P. (2004). Vitamin D2 is much less effective than vitamin D3 in humans. *J. Clin. Endocrinol. Metab.* **89,** 5387–5391.

Aschenbrenner, J. K., Sollinger, H. W., Becker, B. N., and Hullett, D. A. (2001). 1,25-(OH (2))D(3) alters the transforming growth factor beta signaling pathway in renal tissue. *J. Surg. Res.* **100,** 171–175.

Atalar, K., Afzali, B., Lord, G., and Lombardi, G. (2009). Relative roles of Th1 and Th17 effector cells in allograft rejection. *Curr. Opin. Organ Transplant.* **14,** 23–29.

Baboolal, K., Jones, G. A., Janezic, A., Griffiths, D. R., and Jurewicz, W. A. (2002). Molecular and structural consequences of early renal allograft injury. *Kidney Int.* **61,** 686–696.

Baeke, F., Korf, H., Overbergh, L., van Etten, E., Verstuyf, A., Gysemans, C., and Mathieu, C. (2010). Human T lymphocytes are direct targets of 1, 25-dihydroxyvitamin D(3) in the immune system. *J. Steroid Biochem. Mol. Biol.* **121,** 221–227.

Banchereau, J., Briere, F., Caux, C., Davoust, J., Lebecque, S., Liu, Y. J., Pulendran, B., and Palucka, K. (2000). Immunobiology of dendritic cells. *Annu. Rev. Immunol.* **18,** 767–811.

Berer, A., Stockl, J., Majdic, O., Wagner, T., Kollars, M., Lechner, K., Geissler, K., and Oehler, L. (2000). 1, 25-Dihydroxyvitamin D(3) inhibits dendritic cell differentiation and maturation in vitro. *Exp. Hematol.* **28,** 575–583.

Bhalla, A. K., Amento, E. P., Serog, B., and Glimcher, L. H. (1984). 1, 25-Dihydroxyvitamin D3 inhibits antigen-induced T cell activation. *J. Immunol.* **133,** 1748–1754.

Bhan, I., Shah, A., Holmes, J., Isakova, T., Gutierrez, O., Burnett, S. M., Juppner, H., and Wolf, M. (2006). Post-transplant hypophosphatemia: Tertiary 'hyper-phosphatoninism'? *Kidney Int.* **70,** 1486–1494.

Bikle, D. D. (2010). Vitamin D: Newly discovered actions require reconsideration of physiologic requirements. *Trends Endocrinol. Metab.* **21,** 375–384.

Bitetto, D., Fabris, C., Falleti, E., Fornasiere, E., Fumolo, E., Fontanini, E., Cussigh, A., Occhino, G., Baccarani, U., Pirisi, M., and Toniutto, P. (2010). Vitamin D and the risk of acute allograft rejection following human liver transplantation. *Liver Int.* **30,** 417–444.

Boonstra, A., Barrat, F. J., Crain, C., Heath, V. L., Savelkoul, H. F., and O'Garra, A. (2001). 1alpha, 25-Dihydroxyvitamin d3 has a direct effect on naive CD4(+) T cells to enhance the development of Th2 cells. *J. Immunol.* **167,** 4974–4980.

Borgogni, E., Sarchielli, E., Sottili, M., Santarlasci, V., Cosmi, L., Gelmini, S., Lombardi, A., Cantini, G., Perigli, G., Luconi, M., Vannelli, G. B., Annunziato, F., *et al.* (2008). Elocalcitol inhibits inflammatory responses in human thyroid cells and T cells. *Endocrinology* **149,** 3626–3634.

Bouillon, R., Carmeliet, G., Verlinden, L., van Etten, E., Verstuyf, A., Luderer, H. F., Lieben, L., Mathieu, C., and Demay, M. (2008). Vitamin D and human health: Lessons from vitamin D receptor null mice. *Endocr. Rev.* **29,** 726–776.

Brennan, A., Katz, D. R., Nunn, J. D., Barker, S., Hewison, M., Fraher, L. J., and O'Riordan, J. L. (1987). Dendritic cells from human tissues express receptors for the immunoregulatory vitamin D3 metabolite, dihydroxycholecalciferol. *Immunology* **61,** 457–461.

Briffa, N. K., Keogh, A. M., Sambrook, P. N., and Eisman, J. A. (2003). Reduction of immunosuppressant therapy requirement in heart transplantation by calcitriol. *Transplantation* **75,** 2133–2134.

Brown, K. L., Doshi, M. D., Singh, A., Mehta, K., Morawski, K., Cincotta, E., West, M. S., and Gruber, S. A. (2010). Does donor race still make a difference in deceased-donor African-American renal allograft recipients? *Am. J. Surg.* **199,** 305–309, discussion 309.

Cannell, J. J., Vieth, R., Umhau, J. C., Holick, M. F., Grant, W. B., Madronich, S., Garland, C. F., and Giovannucci, E. (2006). Epidemic influenza and vitamin D. *Epidemiol. Infect.* **134,** 1129–1140.

Cantorna, M. T., Hullett, D. A., Redaelli, C., Brandt, C. R., Humpal-Winter, J., Sollinger, H. W., and Deluca, H. F. (1998). 1, 25-Dihydroxyvitamin D3 prolongs graft survival without compromising host resistance to infection or bone mineral density. *Transplantation* **66,** 828–831.

Chen, S., Sims, G. P., Chen, X. X., Gu, Y. Y., and Lipsky, P. E. (2007). Modulatory effects of 1, 25-dihydroxyvitamin D3 on human B cell differentiation. *J. Immunol.* **179,** 1634–1647.

Chromek, M., Slamova, Z., Bergman, P., Kovacs, L., Podracka, L., Ehren, I., Hokfelt, T., Gudmundsson, G. H., Gallo, R. L., Agerberth, B., and Brauner, A. (2006). The antimicrobial peptide cathelicidin protects the urinary tract against invasive bacterial infection. *Nat. Med.* **12,** 636–641.

Cippitelli, M., and Santoni, A. (1998). Vitamin D3: A transcriptional modulator of the interferon-gamma gene. *Eur. J. Immunol.* **28,** 3017–3030.

Cohen, A., Sambrook, P., and Shane, E. (2004). Management of bone loss after organ transplantation. *J. Bone Miner. Res.* **19,** 1919–1932.

Cornell, L. D., Smith, R. N., and Colvin, R. B. (2008). Kidney transplantation: Mechanisms of rejection and acceptance. *Annu. Rev. Pathol.* **3,** 189–220.

Courbebaisse, M., Thervet, E., Souberbielle, J. C., Zuber, J., Eladari, D., Martinez, F., Mamzer-Bruneel, M. F., Urena, P., Legendre, C., Friedlander, G., and Prie, D. (2009). Effects of vitamin D supplementation on the calcium-phosphate balance in renal transplant patients. *Kidney Int.* **75,** 646–651.

Courbebaisse, M., Souberbielle, J. C., and Thervet, E. (2010). Potential nonclassical effects of vitamin D in transplant recipients. *Transplantation* **89,** 131–137.

Crosbie, O. M., Freaney, R., McKenna, M. J., and Hegarty, J. E. (1999). Bone density, vitamin D status, and disordered bone remodeling in end-stage chronic liver disease. *Calcif. Tissue Int.* **64,** 295–300.

Cross, H. S. (2007). Extrarenal vitamin D hydroxylase expression and activity in normal and malignant cells: Modification of expression by epigenetic mechanisms and dietary substances. *Nutr. Rev.* **65,** S108–S112.

De Sevaux, R. G., Hoitsma, A. J., Corstens, F. H., and Wetzels, J. F. (2002). Treatment with vitamin D and calcium reduces bone loss after renal transplantation: A randomized study. *J. Am. Soc. Nephrol.* **13,** 1608–1614.

Djamali, A., Samaniego, M., Torrealba, J., Pirsch, J., and Muth, B. L. (2010). Increase in proteinuria >200 mg/g after late rejection is associated with poor graft survival. *Nephrol. Dial. Transplant.* **25,** 1300-1306.

Ducloux, D., Courivaud, C., Bamoulid, J., Kazory, A., Dumoulin, G., and Chalopin, J. M. (2008). Pretransplant serum vitamin D levels and risk of cancer after renal transplantation. *Transplantation* **85,** 1755–1759.

Durr, U. H., Sudheendra, U. S., and Ramamoorthy, A. (2006). LL-37, the only human member of the cathelicidin family of antimicrobial peptides. *Biochim. Biophys. Acta* **1758,** 1408–1425.

Dusso, A. S., Brown, A. J., and Slatopolsky, E. (2005). Vitamin D. *Am. J. Physiol. Ren. Physiol.* **289,** F8–F28.

Ebeling, P. R. (2009). Approach to the patient with transplantation-related bone loss. *J. Clin. Endocrinol. Metab.* **94,** 1483–1490.

El-Agroudy, A. E., El-Husseini, A. A., El-Sayed, M., and Ghoneim, M. A. (2003). Preventing bone loss in renal transplant recipients with vitamin D. *J. Am. Soc. Nephrol.* **14,** 2975–2979.

El-Zoghby, Z. M., Stegall, M. D., Lager, D. J., Kremers, W. K., Amer, H., Gloor, J. M., and Cosio, F. G. (2009). Identifying specific causes of kidney allograft loss. *Am. J. Transplant.* **9,** 527–535.

Euvrard, S., Kanitakis, J., and Claudy, A. (2003). Skin cancers after organ transplantation. *N. Engl. J. Med.* **348,** 1681–1691.

Evenepoel, P., Claes, K., Kuypers, D., Maes, B., Bammens, B., and Vanrenterghem, Y. (2004). Natural history of parathyroid function and calcium metabolism after kidney transplantation: A single-centre study. *Nephrol. Dial. Transplant.* **19,** 1281–1287.

Evenepoel, P., Meijers, B. K., de Jonge, H., Naesens, M., Bammens, B., Claes, K., Kuypers, D., and Vanrenterghem, Y. (2008). Recovery of hyperphosphatoninism and renal phosphorus wasting one year after successful renal transplantation. *Clin. J. Am. Soc. Nephrol.* **3,** 1829–1836.

Fishman, J. A. (2007). Infection in solid-organ transplant recipients. *N. Engl. J. Med.* **357,** 2601–2614.

Forli, L., Halse, J., Haug, E., Bjortuft, O., Vatn, M., Kofstad, J., and Boe, J. (2004). Vitamin D deficiency, bone mineral density and weight in patients with advanced pulmonary disease. *J. Intern. Med.* **256,** 56–62.

Forli, L., Bollerslev, J., Simonsen, S., Isaksen, G. A., Kvamsdal, K. E., Godang, K., Gadeholt, G., Pripp, A. H., and Bjortuft, O. (2010). Dietary vitamin K2 supplement improves bone status after lung and heart transplantation. *Transplantation* **89,** 458–464.

Fritsche, J., Mondal, K., Ehrnsperger, A., Andreesen, R., and Kreutz, M. (2003). Regulation of 25-hydroxyvitamin D3-1 alpha-hydroxylase and production of 1 alpha, 25-dihydroxyvitamin D3 by human dendritic cells. *Blood* **102,** 3314–3316.

Ganz, T. (2003). Defensins: Antimicrobial peptides of innate immunity. *Nat. Rev. Immunol.* **3,** 710–720.

Gauzzi, M. C., Purificato, C., Donato, K., Jin, Y., Wang, L., Daniel, K. C., Maghazachi, A. A., Belardelli, F., Adorini, L., and Gessani, S. (2005). Suppressive effect of 1alpha, 25-dihydroxyvitamin D3 on type I IFN-mediated monocyte differentiation into dendritic cells: Impairment of functional activities and chemotaxis. *J. Immunol.* **174,** 270–276.

Ginde, A. A., Mansbach, J. M., and Camargo, C. A., Jr. (2009). Association between serum 25-hydroxyvitamin D level and upper respiratory tract infection in the Third National Health and Nutrition Examination Survey. *Arch. Intern. Med.* **169,** 384–390.

Giovannucci, E., Liu, Y., Hollis, B. W., and Rimm, E. B. (2008). 25-hydroxyvitamin D and risk of myocardial infarction in men: A prospective study. *Arch. Intern. Med.* **168,** 1174–1180.

Gombart, A. F., Borregaard, N., and Koeffler, H. P. (2005). Human cathelicidin antimicrobial peptide (CAMP) gene is a direct target of the vitamin D receptor and is strongly up-regulated in myeloid cells by 1, 25-dihydroxyvitamin D3. *FASEB J.* **19,** 1067–1077.

Gombart, A. F., Bhan, I., Borregaard, N., Tamez, H., Camargo, C. A., Jr., Koeffler, H. P., and Thadhani, R. (2009). Low plasma level of cathelicidin antimicrobial peptide (hCAP18) predicts increased infectious disease mortality in patients undergoing hemodialysis. *Clin. Infect. Dis.* **48,** 418–424.

Gonzalez, E. A., Sachdeva, A., Oliver, D. A., and Martin, K. J. (2004). Vitamin D insufficiency and deficiency in chronic kidney disease. A single center observational study. *Am. J. Nephrol.* **24,** 503–510.

Gottfried, E., Rehli, M., Hahn, J., Holler, E., Andreesen, R., and Kreutz, M. (2006). Monocyte-derived cells express CYP27A1 and convert vitamin D3 into its active metabolite. *Biochem. Biophys. Res. Commun.* **349,** 209–213.

Grant, W. B. (2002). An estimate of premature cancer mortality in the U.S. due to inadequate doses of solar ultraviolet-B radiation. *Cancer* **94,** 1867–1875.

Gregori, S., Casorati, M., Amuchastegui, S., Smiroldo, S., Davalli, A. M., and Adorini, L. (2001). Regulatory T cells induced by 1 alpha, 25-dihydroxyvitamin D3 and mycophenolate mofetil treatment mediate transplantation tolerance. *J. Immunol.* **167,** 1945–1953.

Griffin, M. D., Lutz, W. H., Phan, V. A., Bachman, L. A., McKean, D. J., and Kumar, R. (2000). Potent inhibition of dendritic cell differentiation and maturation by vitamin D analogs. *Biochem. Biophys. Res. Commun.* **270,** 701–708.

Gutierrez, O., Isakova, T., Rhee, E., Shah, A., Holmes, J., Collerone, G., Juppner, H., and Wolf, M. (2005). Fibroblast growth factor-23 mitigates hyperphosphatemia but accentuates calcitriol deficiency in chronic kidney disease. *J. Am. Soc. Nephrol.* **16,** 2205–2215.

Harris, S. S. (2006). Vitamin D and African Americans. *J. Nutr.* **136,** 1126–1129.

Harris, S., Coupes, B. M., Roberts, S. A., Roberts, I. S., Short, C. D., and Brenchley, P. E. (2007). TGF-beta1 in chronic allograft nephropathy following renal transplantation. *J. Nephrol.* **20,** 177–185.

Hathcock, J. N., Shao, A., Vieth, R., and Heaney, R. (2007). Risk assessment for vitamin D. *Am. J. Clin. Nutr.* **85,** 6–18.

Heine, G., Niesner, U., Chang, H. D., Steinmeyer, A., Zugel, U., Zuberbier, T., Radbruch, A., and Worm, M. (2008). 1, 25-dihydroxyvitamin D(3) promotes IL-10 production in human B cells. *Eur. J. Immunol.* **38,** 2210–2218.

Heldal, K., Hartmann, A., Leivestad, T., Svendsen, M. V., Foss, A., Lien, B., and Midtvedt, K. (2009). Clinical outcomes in elderly kidney transplant recipients are related to acute rejection episodes rather than pretransplant comorbidity. *Transplantation* **87,** 1045–1051.

Hewison, M., Freeman, L., Hughes, S. V., Evans, K. N., Bland, R., Eliopoulos, A. G., Kilby, M. D., Moss, P. A., and Chakraverty, R. (2003). Differential regulation of vitamin D receptor and its ligand in human monocyte-derived dendritic cells. *J. Immunol.* **170,** 5382–5390.

Hewison, M., Burke, F., Evans, K. N., Lammas, D. A., Sansom, D. M., Liu, P., Modlin, R. L., and Adams, J. S. (2007). Extra-renal 25-hydroxyvitamin D3-1alpha-hydroxylase in human health and disease. *J. Steroid Biochem. Mol. Biol.* **103,** 316–321.

Holick, M. F. (2004). Sunlight and vitamin D for bone health and prevention of autoimmune diseases, cancers, and cardiovascular disease. *Am. J. Clin. Nutr.* **80,** 1678S–1688S.

Holick, M. F. (2007). Vitamin D deficiency. *N. Engl. J. Med.* **357,** 266–281.

Holick, M. F., MacLaughlin, J. A., Clark, M. B., Holick, S. A., Potts, J. T., Jr., Anderson, R. R., Blank, I. H., Parrish, J. A., and Elias, P. (1980). Photosynthesis of previtamin D3 in human skin and the physiologic consequences. *Science* **210,** 203–205.

Holick, M. F., Biancuzzo, R. M., Chen, T. C., Klein, E. K., Young, A., Bibuld, D., Reitz, R., Salameh, W., Ameri, A., and Tannenbaum, A. D. (2008). Vitamin D2 is as effective as vitamin D3 in maintaining circulating concentrations of 25-hydroxyvitamin D. *J. Clin. Endocrinol. Metab.* **93,** 677–681.

Hullett, D. A., Cantorna, M. T., Redaelli, C., Humpal-Winter, J., Hayes, C. E., Sollinger, H. W., and Deluca, H. F. (1998). Prolongation of allograft survival by 1, 25-dihydroxyvitamin D3. *Transplantation* **66,** 824–828.

Hullett, D. A., Laeseke, P. F., Malin, G., Nessel, R., Sollinger, H. W., and Becker, B. N. (2005). Prevention of chronic allograft nephropathy with vitamin D. *Transpl. Int.* **18,** 1175–1186.

Hutchings, A., Purcell, W. M., and Benfield, M. R. (2001). Increased costimulatory responses in African-American kidney allograft recipients. *Transplantation* **71,** 692–695.

Ingulli, E. (2010). Mechanism of cellular rejection in transplantation. *Pediatr. Nephrol.* **25,** 61–74.

Iqbal, N., Ducharme, J., Desai, S., Chambers, S., Terembula, K., Chan, G. W., Shults, J., Leonard, M. B., and Kumanyika, S. (2008). Status of bone mineral density in patients selected for cardiac transplantation. *Endocr. Pract.* **14,** 704–712.

Jain, S., Furness, P. N., and Nicholson, M. L. (2000). The role of transforming growth factor beta in chronic renal allograft nephropathy. *Transplantation* **69,** 1759–1766.

Jain, S., Mohamed, M. A., Sandford, R., Furness, P. N., Nicholson, M. L., and Talbot, D. (2002). Sequential protocol biopsies from renal transplant recipients show an increasing expression of active TGF beta. *Transpl. Int.* **15,** 630–634.

Jeffery, L. E., Burke, F., Mura, M., Zheng, Y., Qureshi, O. S., Hewison, M., Walker, L. S., Lammas, D. A., Raza, K., and Sansom, D. M. (2009). 1, 25-Dihydroxyvitamin D3 and IL-2 combine to inhibit T cell production of inflammatory cytokines and promote development of regulatory T cells expressing CTLA-4 and FoxP3. *J. Immunol.* **183,** 5458–5467.

Jeng, L., Yamshchikov, A. V., Judd, S. E., Blumberg, H. M., Martin, G. S., Ziegler, T. R., and Tangpricha, V. (2009). Alterations in vitamin D status and anti-microbial peptide levels in patients in the intensive care unit with sepsis. *J. Transl. Med.* **7,** 28.

Johnsson, C., Binderup, L., and Tufveson, G. (1995). The effects of combined treatment with the novel vitamin D analogue MC 1288 and cyclosporine A on cardiac allograft survival. *Transpl. Immunol.* **3,** 245–250.

Kallio, E., Hayry, P., and Pakkala, S. (1996). MC1288, a vitamin D analogue, reduces short- and long-term renal allograft rejection in the rat. *Transplant. Proc.* **28,** 3113.

Kerman, R. H., Kimball, P. M., Van Buren, C. T., Lewis, R. M., and Kahan, B. D. (1991). Possible contribution of pretransplant immune responder status to renal allograft survival differences of black versus white recipients. *Transplantation* **51,** 338–342.

Kerman, R. H., Kimball, P. M., Van Buren, C. T., Lewis, R. M., Cavazos, D., Heydari, A., and Kahan, B. D. (1992). Influence of race on crossmatch outcome and recipient eligibility for transplantation. *Transplantation* **53,** 64–67.

Koenig, K. G., Lindberg, J. S., Zerwekh, J. E., Padalino, P. K., Cushner, H. M., and Copley, J. B. (1992). Free and total 1, 25-dihydroxyvitamin D levels in subjects with renal disease. *Kidney Int.* **41,** 161–165.

Laaksi, I., Ruohola, J. P., Tuohimaa, P., Auvinen, A., Haataja, R., Pihlajamaki, H., and Ylikomi, T. (2007). An association of serum vitamin D concentrations < 40 nmol/L with acute respiratory tract infection in young Finnish men. *Am. J. Clin. Nutr.* **86,** 714–717.

LaClair, R. E., Hellman, R. N., Karp, S. L., Kraus, M., Ofner, S., Li, Q., Graves, K. L., and Moe, S. M. (2005). Prevalence of calcidiol deficiency in CKD: A cross-sectional study across latitudes in the United States. *Am. J. Kidney Dis.* **45,** 1026–1033.

Lemire, J. M., Archer, D. C., Khulkarni, A., Ince, A., Uskokovic, M. R., and Stepkowski, S. (1992). Prolongation of the survival of murine cardiac allografts by the vitamin D3 analogue 1, 25-dihydroxy-delta 16-cholecalciferol. *Transplantation* **54,** 762–763.

Levin, A., Bakris, G. L., Molitch, M., Smulders, M., Tian, J., Williams, L. A., and Andress, D. L. (2007). Prevalence of abnormal serum vitamin D, PTH, calcium, and phosphorus in patients with chronic kidney disease: Results of the study to evaluate early kidney disease. *Kidney Int.* **71,** 31–38.

Li, J. H., Zhu, H. J., Huang, X. R., Lai, K. N., Johnson, R. J., and Lan, H. Y. (2002). Smad7 inhibits fibrotic effect of TGF-Beta on renal tubular epithelial cells by blocking Smad2 activation. *J. Am. Soc. Nephrol.* **13,** 1464–1472.

Liu, P. T., Stenger, S., Li, H., Wenzel, L., Tan, B. H., Krutzik, S. R., Ochoa, M. T., Schauber, J., Wu, K., Meinken, C., Kamen, D. L., Wagner, M., *et al.* (2006). Toll-like receptor triggering of a vitamin D-mediated human antimicrobial response. *Science* **311,** 1770–1773.

Lobo, P. I., Cortez, M. S., Stevenson, W., and Pruett, T. L. (1995). Normocalcemic hyperparathyroidism associated with relatively low 1:25 vitamin D levels post-renal transplant can be successfully treated with oral calcitriol. *Clin. Transplant.* **9,** 277–281.

Lou, Y. R., Molnar, F., Perakyla, M., Qiao, S., Kalueff, A. V., St-Arnaud, R., Carlberg, C., and Tuohimaa, P. (2010). 25-Hydroxyvitamin D(3) is an agonistic vitamin D receptor ligand. *J. Steroid Biochem. Mol. Biol.* **118,** 162–170.

Makibayashi, K., Tatematsu, M., Hirata, M., Fukushima, N., Kusano, K., Ohashi, S., Abe, H., Kuze, K., Fukatsu, A., Kita, T., and Doi, T. (2001). A vitamin D analog ameliorates glomerular injury on rat glomerulonephritis. *Am. J. Pathol.* **158,** 1733–1741.

Marcinkowska, E. (2001). A run for a membrane vitamin D receptor. *Biol. Signals Recept.* **10,** 341–349.

Martineau, A. R., Wilkinson, K. A., Newton, S. M., Floto, R. A., Norman, A. W., Skolimowska, K., Davidson, R. N., Sorensen, O. E., Kampmann, B., Griffiths, C. J., and Wilkinson, R. J. (2007). IFN-gamma- and TNF-independent vitamin D-inducible human suppression of mycobacteria: The role of cathelicidin LL-37. *J. Immunol.* **178,** 7190–7198.

Medzhitov, R. (2007). Recognition of microorganisms and activation of the immune response. *Nature* **449,** 819–826.

Meier-Kriesche, H. U., Schold, J. D., Srinivas, T. R., and Kaplan, B. (2004). Lack of improvement in renal allograft survival despite a marked decrease in acute rejection rates over the most recent era. *Am. J. Transplant.* **4,** 378–383.

Misawa, Y., Baba, A., Ito, S., Tanaka, M., and Shiohara, M. (2009). Vitamin D(3) induces expression of human cathelicidin antimicrobial peptide 18 in newborns. *Int. J. Hematol.* **90,** 561–570.

Miyamoto, K., Ito, M., Kuwahata, M., Kato, S., and Segawa, H. (2005). Inhibition of intestinal sodium-dependent inorganic phosphate transport by fibroblast growth factor 23. *Ther. Apher. Dial.* **9,** 331–335.

Monegal, A., Navasa, M., Guanabens, N., Peris, P., Pons, F., Martinez de Osaba, M. J., Ordi, J., Rimola, A., Rodes, J., and Munoz-Gomez, J. (2001). Bone disease after liver transplantation: A long-term prospective study of bone mass changes, hormonal status and histomorphometric characteristics. *Osteoporos. Int.* **12,** 484–492.

Monkawa, T., Yoshida, T., Hayashi, M., and Saruta, T. (2000). Identification of 25-hydroxyvitamin D3 1alpha-hydroxylase gene expression in macrophages. *Kidney Int.* **58,** 559–568.

Mosmann, T. R., Cherwinski, H., Bond, M. W., Giedlin, M. A., and Coffman, R. L. (1986). Two types of murine helper T cell clone. I. Definition according to profiles of lymphokine activities and secreted proteins. *J. Immunol.* **136,** 2348–2357.

Muhe, L., Lulseged, S., Mason, K. E., and Simoes, E. A. (1997). Case-control study of the role of nutritional rickets in the risk of developing pneumonia in Ethiopian children. *Lancet* **349,** 1801–1804.

Nankivell, B. J., Borrows, R. J., Fung, C. L., O'Connell, P. J., Allen, R. D., and Chapman, J. R. (2003). The natural history of chronic allograft nephropathy. *N. Engl. J. Med.* **349,** 2326–2333.

Nessim, S. J., Jassal, S. V., Fung, S. V., and Chan, C. T. (2007). Conversion from conventional to nocturnal hemodialysis improves vitamin D levels. *Kidney Int.* **71,** 1172–1176.

Nykjaer, A., Dragun, D., Walther, D., Vorum, H., Jacobsen, C., Herz, J., Melsen, F., Christensen, E. I., and Willnow, T. E. (1999). An endocytic pathway essential for renal uptake and activation of the steroid 25-(OH) vitamin D3. *Cell* **96,** 507–515.

O'Herrin, J. K., Hullett, D. A., Heisey, D. M., Sollinger, H. W., and Becker, B. N. (2002). A retrospective evaluation of 1, 25-dihydroxyvitamin D(3) and its potential effects on renal allograft function. *Am. J. Nephrol.* **22,** 515–520.

Overbergh, L., Decallonne, B., Valckx, D., Verstuyf, A., Depovere, J., Laureys, J., Rutgeerts, O., Saint-Arnaud, R., Bouillon, R., and Mathieu, C. (2000). Identification and immune regulation of 25-hydroxyvitamin D-1-alpha-hydroxylase in murine macrophages. *Clin. Exp. Immunol.* **120,** 139–146.

Palmer, S. C., McGregor, D. O., and Strippoli, G. F. (2007). Interventions for preventing bone disease in kidney transplant recipients. *Cochrane Database Syst. Rev.* **18,** CD005015.

Pascussi, J. M., Robert, A., Nguyen, M., Walrant-Debray, O., Garabedian, M., Martin, P., Pineau, T., Saric, J., Navarro, F., Maurel, P., and Vilarem, M. J. (2005). Possible involvement of pregnane X receptor-enhanced CYP24 expression in drug-induced osteomalacia. *J. Clin. Invest.* **115,** 177–186.

Pedersen, A. W., Holmstrom, K., Jensen, S. S., Fuchs, D., Rasmussen, S., Kvistborg, P., Claesson, M. H., and Zocca, M. B. (2009). Phenotypic and functional markers for 1alpha, 25-dihydroxyvitamin D(3)-modified regulatory dendritic cells. *Clin. Exp. Immunol.* **157,** 48–59.

Penna, G., and Adorini, L. (2000). 1 Alpha, 25-dihydroxyvitamin D3 inhibits differentiation, maturation, activation, and survival of dendritic cells leading to impaired alloreactive T cell activation. *J. Immunol.* **164,** 2405–2411.

Penna, G., Roncari, A., Amuchastegui, S., Daniel, K. C., Berti, E., Colonna, M., and Adorini, L. (2005). Expression of the inhibitory receptor ILT3 on dendritic cells is dispensable for induction of CD4+Foxp3+ regulatory T cells by 1, 25-dihydroxyvitamin D3. *Blood* **106,** 3490–3497.

Penna, G., Amuchastegui, S., Giarratana, N., Daniel, K. C., Vulcano, M., Sozzani, S., and Adorini, L. (2007). 1, 25-Dihydroxyvitamin D3 selectively modulates tolerogenic properties in myeloid but not plasmacytoid dendritic cells. *J. Immunol.* **178,** 145–153.

Perwad, F., Zhang, M. Y., Tenenhouse, H. S., and Portale, A. A. (2007). Fibroblast growth factor 23 impairs phosphorus and vitamin D metabolism in vivo and suppresses 25-hydroxyvitamin D-1alpha-hydroxylase expression in vitro. *Am. J. Physiol. Ren. Physiol.* **293,** F1577–F1583.

Piemonti, L., Monti, P., Sironi, M., Fraticelli, P., Leone, B. E., Dal Cin, E., Allavena, P., and Di Carlo, V. (2000). Vitamin D3 affects differentiation, maturation, and function of human monocyte-derived dendritic cells. *J. Immunol.* **164,** 4443–4451.

Provvedini, D. M., Tsoukas, C. D., Deftos, L. J., and Manolagas, S. C. (1983). 1, 25-dihydroxyvitamin D3 receptors in human leukocytes. *Science* **221,** 1181–1183.

Querings, K., Girndt, M., Geisel, J., Georg, T., Tilgen, W., and Reichrath, J. (2006). 25-hydroxyvitamin D deficiency in renal transplant recipients. *J. Clin. Endocrinol. Metab.* **91,** 526–529.

Racusen, L. C., Solez, K., Colvin, R. B., Bonsib, S. M., Castro, M. C., Cavallo, T., Croker, B. P., Demetris, A. J., Drachenberg, C. B., Fogo, A. B., Furness, P., Gaber, L. W., *et al.* (1999). The Banff 97 working classification of renal allograft pathology. *Kidney Int.* **55,** 713–723.

Raisanen-Sokolowski, A. K., Pakkala, I. S., Samila, S. P., Binderup, L., Hayry, P. J., and Pakkala, S. T. (1997). A vitamin D analog, MC1288, inhibits adventitial inflammation and suppresses intimal lesions in rat aortic allografts. *Transplantation* **63,** 936–941.

Ramirez, A. M., Wongtrakool, C., Welch, T., Steinmeyer, A., Zugel, U., and Roman, J. (2010). Vitamin D inhibition of pro-fibrotic effects of transforming growth factor beta1 in lung fibroblasts and epithelial cells. *J. Steroid Biochem. Mol. Biol.* **118,** 142–150.

Rapuri, P. B., Gallagher, J. C., and Haynatzki, G. (2004). Effect of vitamins D2 and D3 supplement use on serum 25OHD concentration in elderly women in summer and winter. *Calcif. Tissue Int.* **74,** 150–156.

Redaelli, C. A., Wagner, M., Tien, Y. H., Mazzucchelli, L., Stahel, P. F., Schilling, M. K., and Dufour, J. F. (2001). 1 alpha, 25-Dihydroxycholecalciferol reduces rejection and improves survival in rat liver allografts. *Hepatology* **34,** 926–934.

Redaelli, C. A., Wagner, M., Gunter-Duwe, D., Tian, Y. H., Stahel, P. F., Mazzucchelli, L., Schmid, R. A., and Schilling, M. K. (2002). 1alpha, 25-dihydroxyvitamin D3 shows strong and additive immunomodulatory effects with cyclosporine A in rat renal allotransplants. *Kidney Int.* **61,** 288–296.

Rigby, W. F., Stacy, T., and Fanger, M. W. (1984). Inhibition of T lymphocyte mitogenesis by 1, 25-dihydroxyvitamin D3 (calcitriol). *J. Clin. Invest.* **74,** 1451–1455.

Rodriguez, M., Nemeth, E., and Martin, D. (2005). The calcium-sensing receptor: A key factor in the pathogenesis of secondary hyperparathyroidism. *Am. J. Physiol. Ren. Physiol.* **288,** F253–F264.

Rosenblatt, J., Bissonnette, A., Ahmad, R., Wu, Z., Vasir, B., Stevenson, K., Zarwan, C., Keefe, W., Glotzbecker, B., Mills, H., Joyce, R., Levine, J. D., *et al.* (2010). Immunomodulatory effects of vitamin D: Implications for GVHD. *Bone Marrow Transplant.* **45,** 1463–1468.

Rucker, D., Tonelli, M., Coles, M. G., Yoo, S., Young, K., and McMahon, A. W. (2009). Vitamin D insufficiency and treatment with oral vitamin D3 in northern-dwelling patients with chronic kidney disease. *J. Nephrol.* **22,** 75–82.

Sadlier, D. M., and Magee, C. C. (2007). Prevalence of 25(OH) vitamin D (calcidiol) deficiency at time of renal transplantation: A prospective study. *Clin. Transplant.* **21,** 683–688.

Sagoo, P., Lombardi, G., and Lechler, R. I. (2008). Regulatory T cells as therapeutic cells. *Curr. Opin. Organ Transplant.* **13,** 645–653.

Saha, H. (1994). Calcium and vitamin D homeostasis in patients with heavy proteinuria. *Clin. Nephrol.* **41,** 290–296.

Sakaguchi, S., Yamaguchi, T., Nomura, T., and Ono, M. (2008). Regulatory T cells and immune tolerance. *Cell* **133,** 775–787.

Schwarz, U., Amann, K., Orth, S. R., Simonaviciene, A., Wessels, S., and Ritz, E. (1998). Effect of 1, 25 (OH)2 vitamin D3 on glomerulosclerosis in subtotally nephrectomized rats. *Kidney Int.* **53,** 1696–1705.

Sezer, S., Uyar, M., Arat, Z., Ozdemir, F. N., and Haberal, M. (2005). Potential effects of 1, 25-dihydroxyvitamin D3 in renal transplant recipients. *Transplant. Proc.* **37,** 3109–3111.

Sezer, S., Yavuz, D., Canoz, M. B., Ozdemir, F. N., and Haberal, M. (2009). Vitamin D status, bone mineral density, and inflammation in kidney transplantation patients. *Transplant. Proc.* **41,** 2823–2825.

Shane, E., Silverberg, S. J., Donovan, D., Papadopoulos, A., Staron, R. B., Addesso, V., Jorgesen, B., McGregor, C., and Schulman, L. (1996). Osteoporosis in lung transplantation candidates with end-stage pulmonary disease. *Am. J. Med.* **101,** 262–269.

Shane, E., Mancini, D., Aaronson, K., Silverberg, S. J., Seibel, M. J., Addesso, V., and McMahon, D. J. (1997). Bone mass, vitamin D deficiency, and hyperparathyroidism in congestive heart failure. *Am. J. Med.* **103,** 197–207.

Sharma, V. K., Bologa, R. M., Xu, G. P., Li, B., Mouradian, J., Wang, J., Serur, D., Rao, V., and Suthanthiran, M. (1996). Intragraft TGF-beta 1 mRNA: A correlate of interstitial fibrosis and chronic allograft nephropathy. *Kidney Int.* **49,** 1297–1303.

Sherrard, D. J., Hercz, G., Pei, Y., Maloney, N. A., Greenwood, C., Manuel, A., Saiphoo, C., Fenton, S. S., and Segre, G. V. (1993). The spectrum of bone disease in end-stage renal failure—An evolving disorder. *Kidney Int.* **43,** 436–442.

Shimada, T., Hasegawa, H., Yamazaki, Y., Muto, T., Hino, R., Takeuchi, Y., Fujita, T., Nakahara, K., Fukumoto, S., and Yamashita, T. (2004). FGF-23 is a potent regulator of vitamin D metabolism and phosphate homeostasis. *J. Bone Miner. Res.* **19,** 429–435.

Sigmundsdottir, H., Pan, J., Debes, G. F., Alt, C., Habtezion, A., Soler, D., and Butcher, E. C. (2007). DCs metabolize sunlight-induced vitamin D3 to 'program' T cell attraction to the epidermal chemokine CCL27. *Nat. Immunol.* **8,** 285–293.

Solez, K., Colvin, R. B., Racusen, L. C., Sis, B., Halloran, P. F., Birk, P. E., Campbell, P. M., Cascalho, M., Collins, A. B., Demetris, A. J., Drachenberg, C. B., Gibson, I. W., *et al.* (2007). Banff '05 Meeting Report: Differential diagnosis of chronic allograft injury and elimination of chronic allograft nephropathy ('CAN'). *Am. J. Transplant.* **7,** 518–526.

Sorensen, O. E., Follin, P., Johnsen, A. H., Calafat, J., Tjabringa, G. S., Hiemstra, P. S., and Borregaard, N. (2001). Human cathelicidin, hCAP-18, is processed to the antimicrobial peptide LL-37 by extracellular cleavage with proteinase 3. *Blood* **97,** 3951–3959.

Sprague, S. M., and Coyne, D. (2010). Control of secondary hyperparathyroidism by vitamin d receptor agonists in chronic kidney disease. *Clin. J. Am. Soc. Nephrol.* **5,** 512–518.

Sprague, S. M., Belozeroff, V., Danese, M. D., Martin, L. P., and Olgaard, K. (2008). Abnormal bone and mineral metabolism in kidney transplant patients—A review. *Am. J. Nephrol.* **28,** 246–253.

Staeva-Vieira, T. P., and Freedman, L. P. (2002). 1, 25-dihydroxyvitamin D3 inhibits IFN-gamma and IL-4 levels during in vitro polarization of primary murine CD4+ T cells. *J. Immunol.* **168,** 1181–1189.
Stammberger, U., Kubisa, B., Gugger, M., Ayuni, E., Claudio, R., Grodzki, T., and Schmid, R. A. (2003). Strong additive effect of 1, 25-dihydroxycholecalciferol and cyclosporine A but not tacrolimus in rat lung allotransplantation. *Eur. J. Cardiothorac. Surg.* **24,** 196–200, discussion 200.
Stavroulopoulos, A., Cassidy, M. J., Porter, C. J., Hosking, D. J., and Roe, S. D. (2007). Vitamin D status in renal transplant recipients. *Am. J. Transplant.* **7,** 2546–2552.
Stein, E. M., Cohen, A., Freeby, M., Rogers, H., Kokolus, S., Scott, V., Mancini, D., Restaino, S., Brown, R., McMahon, D. J., and Shane, E. (2009). Severe vitamin D deficiency among heart and liver transplant recipients. *Clin. Transplant.* **23,** 861–865.
Subramaniam, N., Leong, G. M., Cock, T. A., Flanagan, J. L., Fong, C., Eisman, J. A., and Kouzmenko, A. P. (2001). Cross-talk between 1, 25-dihydroxyvitamin D3 and transforming growth factor-beta signaling requires binding of VDR and Smad3 proteins to their cognate DNA recognition elements. *J. Biol. Chem.* **276,** 15741–15746.
Suthanthiran, M., Khanna, A., Cukran, D., Adhikarla, R., Sharma, V. K., Singh, T., and August, P. (1998). Transforming growth factor-beta 1 hyperexpression in African American end-stage renal disease patients. *Kidney Int.* **53,** 639–644.
Szeles, L., Keresztes, G., Torocsik, D., Balajthy, Z., Krenacs, L., Poliska, S., Steinmeyer, A., Zuegel, U., Pruenster, M., Rot, A., and Nagy, L. (2009). 1, 25-dihydroxyvitamin D3 is an autonomous regulator of the transcriptional changes leading to a tolerogenic dendritic cell phenotype. *J. Immunol.* **182,** 2074–2083.
Takahashi, K., Nakayama, Y., Horiuchi, H., Ohta, T., Komoriya, K., Ohmori, H., and Kamimura, T. (2002). Human neutrophils express messenger RNA of vitamin D receptor and respond to 1alpha, 25-dihydroxyvitamin D3. *Immunopharmacol. Immunotoxicol.* **24,** 335–347.
Takeuchi, A., Reddy, G. S., Kobayashi, T., Okano, T., Park, J., and Sharma, S. (1998). Nuclear factor of activated T cells (NFAT) as a molecular target for 1alpha, 25-dihydroxyvitamin D3-mediated effects. *J. Immunol.* **160,** 209–218.
Tanaci, N., Karakose, H., Guvener, N., Tutuncu, N. B., Colak, T., and Haberal, M. (2003). Influence of 1, 25-dihydroxyvitamin D3 as an immunomodulator in renal transplant recipients: A retrospective cohort study. *Transplant. Proc.* **35,** 2885–2887.
Tapiawala, S. N., Tinckam, K. J., Cardella, C. J., Schiff, J., Cattran, D. C., Cole, E. H., and Kim, S. J. (2010). Delayed graft function and the risk for death with a functioning graft. *J. Am. Soc. Nephrol.* **21,** 153–161.
Thiem, U., Heinze, G., Segel, R., Perkmann, T., Kainberger, F., Muhlbacher, F., Horl, W., and Borchhardt, K. (2009). VITA-D: Cholecalciferol substitution in vitamin D deficient kidney transplant recipients: A randomized, placebo-controlled study to evaluate the post-transplant outcome. *Trials* **10,** 36.
Thomas, M. K., Lloyd-Jones, D. M., Thadhani, R. I., Shaw, A. C., Deraska, D. J., Kitch, B. T., Vamvakas, E. C., Dick, I. M., Prince, R. L., and Finkelstein, J. S. (1998). Hypovitaminosis D in medical inpatients. *N. Engl. J. Med.* **338,** 777–783.
Torres, A., Garcia, S., Gomez, A., Gonzalez, A., Barrios, Y., Concepcion, M. T., Hernandez, D., Garcia, J. J., Checa, M. D., Lorenzo, V., and Salido, E. (2004). Treatment with intermittent calcitriol and calcium reduces bone loss after renal transplantation. *Kidney Int.* **65,** 705–712.
Townsend, K., Evans, K. N., Campbell, M. J., Colston, K. W., Adams, J. S., and Hewison, M. (2005). Biological actions of extra-renal 25-hydroxyvitamin D-1alpha-hydroxylase and implications for chemoprevention and treatment. *J. Steroid Biochem. Mol. Biol.* **97,** 103–109.

Trang, H. M., Cole, D. E., Rubin, L. A., Pierratos, A., Siu, S., and Vieth, R. (1998). Evidence that vitamin D3 increases serum 25-hydroxyvitamin D more efficiently than does vitamin D2. *Am. J. Clin. Nutr.* **68,** 854–858.

Tripathi, S. S., Gibney, E. M., Gehr, T. W., King, A. L., and Beckman, M. J. (2008). High prevalence of vitamin D deficiency in African American kidney transplant recipients. *Transplantation* **85,** 767–770.

Unger, W. W., Laban, S., Kleijwegt, F. S., van der Slik, A. R., and Roep, B. O. (2009). Induction of Treg by monocyte-derived DC modulated by vitamin D3 or dexamethasone: Differential role for PD-L1. *Eur. J. Immunol.* **39,** 3147–3159.

US Renal Data System, USRDS (2009). Annual Data Report: Atlas of Chronic Kidney Disease and End-Stage Renal Disease in the United States National Institutes of Health, National Institute of Diabetes and Digestive and Kidney Diseases, Bethesda, MD.

Uyar, M., Sezer, S., Arat, Z., Elsurer, R., Ozdemir, F. N., and Haberal, M. (2006). 1, 25-dihydroxyvitamin D(3) therapy is protective for renal function and prevents hyperparathyroidism in renal allograft recipients. *Transplant. Proc.* **38,** 2069–2073.

van Etten, E., Stoffels, K., Gysemans, C., Mathieu, C., and Overbergh, L. (2008). Regulation of vitamin D homeostasis: Implications for the immune system. *Nutr. Rev.* **66,** S125–S134.

van Halteren, A. G., van Etten, E., de Jong, E. C., Bouillon, R., Roep, B. O., and Mathieu, C. (2002). Redirection of human autoreactive T-cells Upon interaction with dendritic cells modulated by TX527, an analog of 1, 25 dihydroxyvitamin D(3). *Diabetes* **51,** 2119–2125.

Veldman, C. M., Cantorna, M. T., and DeLuca, H. F. (2000). Expression of 1, 25-dihydroxyvitamin D(3) receptor in the immune system. *Arch. Biochem. Biophys.* **374,** 334–338.

Vidal, M., Ramana, C. V., and Dusso, A. S. (2002). Stat1-vitamin D receptor interactions antagonize 1, 25-dihydroxyvitamin D transcriptional activity and enhance stat1-mediated transcription. *Mol. Cell. Biol.* **22,** 2777–2787.

Vierboom, M., Johnsson, C., t Hart, B., and Jonker, M. (2006). Monotherapy with the vitamin D analogue MC1288 does not result in prolonged kidney allograft survival in rhesus monkeys. *Transpl. Int.* **19,** 396–403.

Vieth, R. (2009). Vitamin D and cancer mini-symposium: The risk of additional vitamin D. *Ann. Epidemiol.* **19,** 441–445.

Viklicky, O., Matl, I., Voska, L., Bohmova, R., Jaresova, M., Lacha, J., Lodererova, A., Striz, I., Teplan, V., and Vitko, S. (2003). TGF-beta1 expression and chronic allograft nephropathy in protocol kidney graft biopsy. *Physiol. Res.* **52,** 353–360.

Wang, T. T., Nestel, F. P., Bourdeau, V., Nagai, Y., Wang, Q., Liao, J., Tavera-Mendoza, L., Lin, R., Hanrahan, J. W., Mader, S., and White, J. H. (2004). Cutting edge: 1, 25-dihydroxyvitamin D3 is a direct inducer of antimicrobial peptide gene expression. *J. Immunol.* **173,** 2909–2912.

Wang, T. J., Pencina, M. J., Booth, S. L., Jacques, P. F., Ingelsson, E., Lanier, K., Benjamin, E. J., D'Agostino, R. B., Wolf, M., and Vasan, R. S. (2008). Vitamin D deficiency and risk of cardiovascular disease. *Circulation* **117,** 503–511.

Weisinger, J. R., Carlini, R. G., Rojas, E., and Bellorin-Font, E. (2006). Bone disease after renal transplantation. *Clin. J. Am. Soc. Nephrol.* **1,** 1300–1313.

Wissing, K. M., Broeders, N., Moreno-Reyes, R., Gervy, C., Stallenberg, B., and Abramowicz, D. (2005). A controlled study of vitamin D3 to prevent bone loss in renal-transplant patients receiving low doses of steroids. *Transplantation* **79,** 108–115.

Yamshchikov, A. V., Desai, N. S., Blumberg, H. M., Ziegler, T. R., and Tangpricha, V. (2009). Vitamin D for treatment and prevention of infectious diseases: A systematic review of randomized controlled trials. *Endocr. Pract.* **15,** 438–449.

Yanagi, Y., Suzawa, M., Kawabata, M., Miyazono, K., Yanagisawa, J., and Kato, S. (1999). Positive and negative modulation of vitamin D receptor function by transforming growth factor-beta signaling through smad proteins. *J. Biol. Chem.* **274,** 12971–12974.

Yanagisawa, J., Yanagi, Y., Masuhiro, Y., Suzawa, M., Watanabe, M., Kashiwagi, K., Toriyabe, T., Kawabata, M., Miyazono, K., and Kato, S. (1999). Convergence of transforming growth factor-beta and vitamin D signaling pathways on SMAD transcriptional coactivators. *Science* **283,** 1317–1321.

Yim, S., Dhawan, P., Ragunath, C., Christakos, S., and Diamond, G. (2007). Induction of cathelicidin in normal and CF bronchial epithelial cells by 1, 25-dihydroxyvitamin D(3). *J. Cyst. Fibros.* **6,** 403–410.

Young, C. J., and Gaston, R. S. (2000). Renal transplantation in black Americans. *N. Engl. J. Med.* **343,** 1545–1552.

Zasloff, M. (2006). Fighting infections with vitamin D. *Nat. Med.* **12,** 388–390.

Zhang, A. B., and Zheng, S. S. (2006). Strong additive effect of calcitriol and cyclosporine A on lymphocyte proliferation in vitro and rat liver allotransplantations in vivo. *Chin. Med. J. (Engl.)* **119,** 2090–2095.

Zhang, A. B., Zheng, S. S., Jia, C. K., and Wang, Y. (2003). Effect of 1, 25-dihydroxyvitamin D3 on preventing allograft from acute rejection following rat orthotopic liver transplantation. *World J. Gastroenterol.* **9,** 1067–1071.

Zhu, J., Yamane, H., and Paul, W. E. (2010). Differentiation of effector CD4 T cell populations (*). *Annu. Rev. Immunol.* **28,** 445–489.

Zimmerman, C. M., and Padgett, R. W. (2000). Transforming growth factor beta signaling mediators and modulators. *Gene* **249,** 17–30.

Index

R

S

T

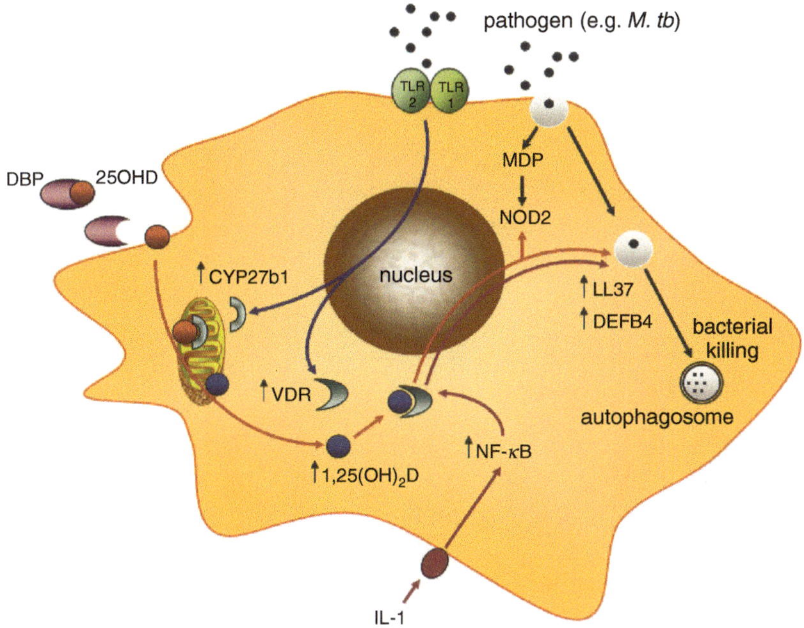

Martin Hewison, Figure 2.1 *Vitamin D and monocyte antibacterial responses.* Schematic representation showing mechanisms associated with the intracrine regulation of bacterial killing mechanisms by vitamin D in response to a pathogen such as *Mycobacterium tuberculosis*. Monocyte sensing of *M. tuberculosis* via toll-like receptor (TLR) 2 and 1 enhances expression of the vitamin D-activating enzyme 1α-hydroxylase (CYP27B1) and the vitamin D receptor (VDR). CYP27B1 catalyzes synthesis of active 1,25-dihydroxyvitamin D (1,25$(OH)_2$D) from substrate 25-hydroxyvitamin D (25OHD), the main circulating form of vitamin D. Bioavailability of 25OHD is dependent on vitamin D status and the action of serum vitamin D-binding protein (DBP). 1,25 $(OH)_2$D synthesized by monocyte CYP27B1 binds to VDR and regulates transcription of target genes such as the antimicrobial protein cathelicidin (LL37). Other antibacterial proteins such as β-defensin 2 (DEFB4) are also induced by 1,25$(OH)_2$D but require adjunct signaling via nuclear factor-kappa B (NF-κB), involving signaling via interleukin-1 (IL-1) or nucleotide-binding oligomerization domain containing 2 (NOD2) and muramyl dipeptide (MDP). Intracrine synthesis of 1,25$(OH)_2$D is also associated with the induction of autophagy, a cytoplasmic process known to enhance bacterial killing.

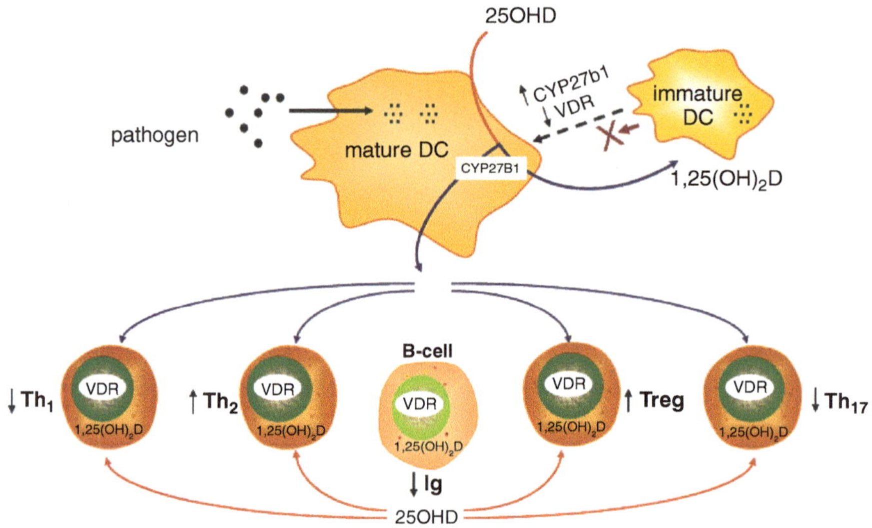

Martin Hewison, Figure 2.2 *Vitamin D, dendritic cell function and adaptive immunity.* Schematic representation showing the paracrine synthesis of 1,25-dihydroxyvitamin D (1,25(OH)$_2$D) by antigen-presenting dendritic cells (DCs) and the impact of this on the function of DCs as well and T- and B-cells. Mature DCs present antigen from pathogens to T- and B-cells. Mature DCs also express high levels of the vitamin D-activating enzyme 1α-hydroxylase (CYP27B1). 1,25(OH)$_2$D synthesized from 25-hydroxyvitamin D (25OHD) by mature DCs acts on immature DCs which express higher levels of the vitamin D receptor (VDR). Using this mechanism, paracrine synthesis of 1,25(OH)$_2$D acts to suppress maturation of DCs, thereby attenuating antigen presentation and enhancing a tolerogenic immune response. Paracrine synthesis of 1,25(OH)2D by DCs can also act on VDR-expressing T- and B-cells to promote a variety of adaptive immune responses. T- and B-cells have also been reported to express CYP27B1 and may therefore be regulated by vitamin D via intracrine conversion of 25OHD to 1,25(OH)$_2$D.

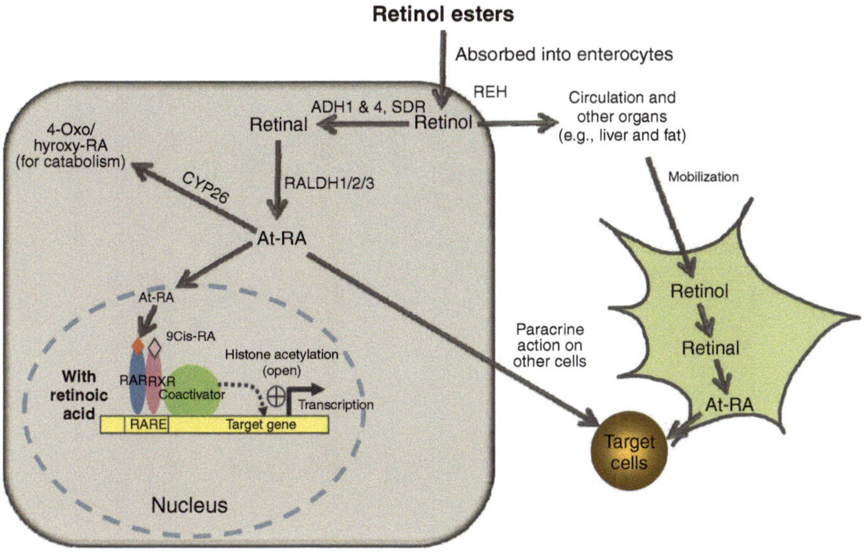

Chang H. Kim, Figure 4.1 *Metabolism and basic action mechanisms of retinoic acid.* Retinol is absorbed into enterocytes and transported into the liver in chylomicrons. Retinols and retinoids in the body are found as complexes with carrier proteins such as retinol binding protein (RBP) in blood and cellular RBP within cells. Retinol is metabolized into retinaldehyde by alcohol dehydrogenase (ADH) or short-chain dehydrogenase/reductase (SDR). Retinaldehyde is metabolized into retinoic acid (At-RA) by retinaldehyde dehydrogenases (RALDH). There are three types of RALDH proteins encoded by different genes (i.e. RALDH1, 2, and 3) and with different patterns of expression. Intestinal epithelial cells and dendritic cells constitutively express RALDH to produce RA. At-RA and its isoform 9-*cis*-RA activate RAR–RXR heterodimers which specifically bind retinoic acid response elements (RAREs) on chromosomes for regulation of gene expression. Receptor activation is necessary to recruit the coactivator and histone acetyltransferase complex to open the chromatin for initiation of gene transcription. RA, produced in certain cell types, can be secreted out of the cells for paracrine action as well as for autocrine action within the same cells. RA can be catabolized into 4-oxo or hydroxy-RA for degradation.

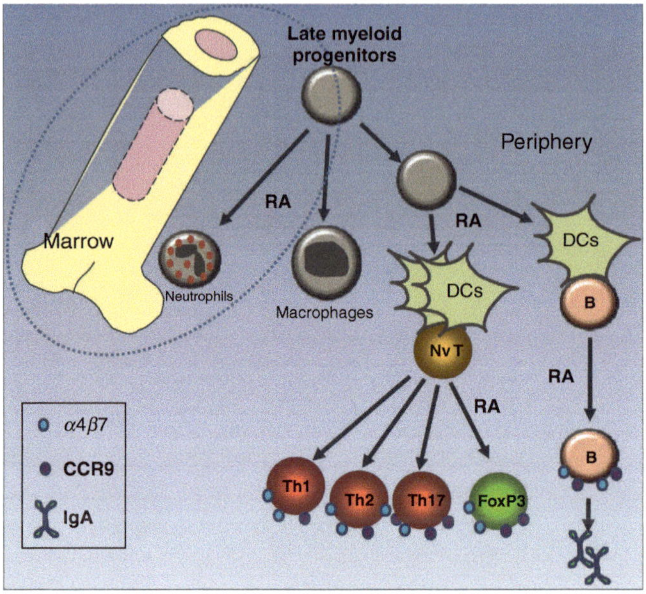

Chang H. Kim, Figure 4.2 *Key functions of retinoic acid in the immune system*. In the bone marrow, RA is required for terminal differentiation of myeloid cells such as neutrophils. Therefore, RA is required to maintain optimal phagocytic activities. Myeloid progenitor cells, migrated out to the periphery, become dendritic cells. RA acts on these differentiating dendritic cells and turn them into FoxP3$^+$ T cell-inducing tolerogenic DCs. When T cells are antigen-primed in the presence of RA at high enough concentrations ($\sim$10 nM), T cells become effector T cell such as Th1, Th2, and Th17 cells that express CCR9 and $\alpha4\beta7$, the two gut-homing receptors. It requires higher concentrations of RA to upregulate CCR9 than that required for $\alpha4\beta7$. These T cells play important roles in formation of immunity in the intestine and potentially other tissues as well. Certain mucosal DCs can produce RA and activate B cells for generation of IgA-producing B cells. RA helps induce both effector and regulatory (suppressive) lymphocytes. This is to assure immune tolerance on one hand and prevention of inflammatory diseases on the other hand. The intestine is a good example of tissues where the RA action is required because commensal bacteria constantly provide stimulatory signals for the immune system and can be inflammatory without appropriate tolerance mechanisms.

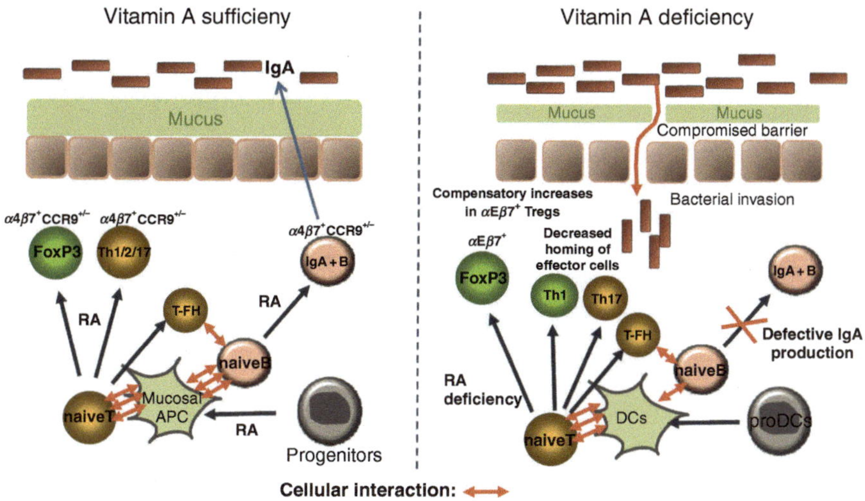

Chang H. Kim, Figure 4.3 *Vitamin A status and mucosal immune system.* When vitamin A intake is sufficient, RA is produced at high levels and promotes formation of epithelial tight junction, secretion of mucus, and expression of pIgR (*trans*-epithelial IgA transporter). Within the lamina propria, RA promotes the production of IgA by B cells, generation of tolerogenic antigen presenting cells, and differentiation of naïve T cells into gut-homing regulatory T cells and effector T cells. Consequently, the gut bacteria are under control by the host immunity and appropriate levels of immune tolerance are achieved at the same time. In vitamin A deficiency, secretion of mucus and integrity of epithelial cells are compromised, allowing the invasion of bacteria into the tissue. Moreover, IgA production and transportation across the epithelial barrier are decreased, resulting in dysregulation of mucosal immunity and potential changes in commensal flora. There is an increased risk for mucosal tissue inflammation in this condition. Interestingly, $FoxP3^{+}$ Tregs that express $\alpha E\beta7$ are highly enriched in the body, counteracting the increased risk of tissue inflammation. Another factor that can decrease the tissue inflammation is poor homing of immune cells into the gut due to defective expression of $\alpha4\beta7$ and CCR9. Despite the compensatory increase in $\alpha E\beta7^{+}$ Tregs, prolonged RA deficiency and decreased immunity lead to the inability to clear bacteria and, then, to chronic tissue inflammation.

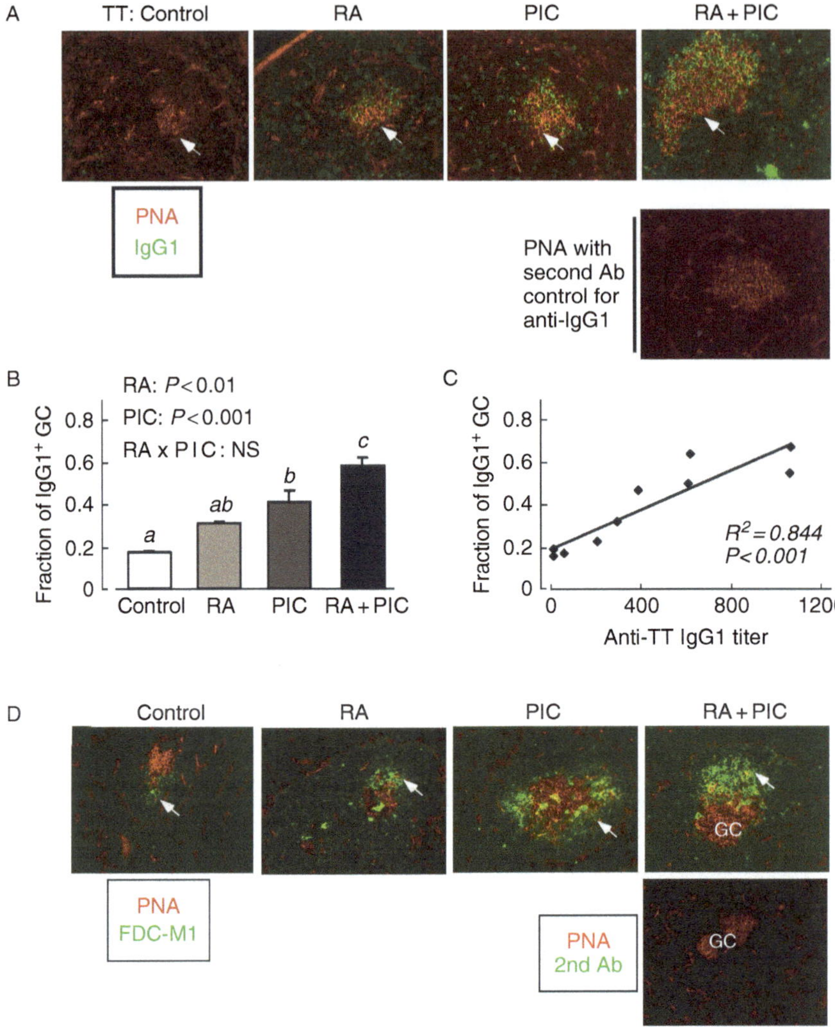

A. Catharine Ross *et al.*, Figure 5.3 RA and PIC promote TT-induced GC formation. Mice were immunized with tetanus toxoid (TT) and treated with RA orally for 5 days and with PIC at the time of antigen priming. (A) On day 10, fixed spleen sections were prepared and 7-μm sections were stained with biotinylated peanut agglutinin (PNA) followed by incubation with Alexa-568-Streptavidin (red) to detect GC, and with FITC-anti-mouse IgD to identify B-cell follicles (green). Results for nonimmunized mice showed no substantial GC formation. (B) The proportion of B-cell follicles containing a GC, determined by microscopic imaging and counting (Ma and Ross, 2009). The number and relative size of GC were determined by imaging a minimum of 20 GC in each spleen. Bars show mean ± SE, $n = 4$ mice/group. Different letters above bars within panels indicate significant differences ($P < 0.05$, $a < b$). Results of two-way ANOVA are also shown in each panel. (C) Linear regression analysis of the plasma anti-TT IgG response versus the proportion of follicles with a GC, determined for the same animals. (D) GC staining of the same spleen samples with biotinylated PNA (red stain), and monoclonal antibody against FDC (FDC-M1, green stain). (Figure modified from (Ma and Ross, 2009), with permission of Clinical and Vaccine Immunology.)

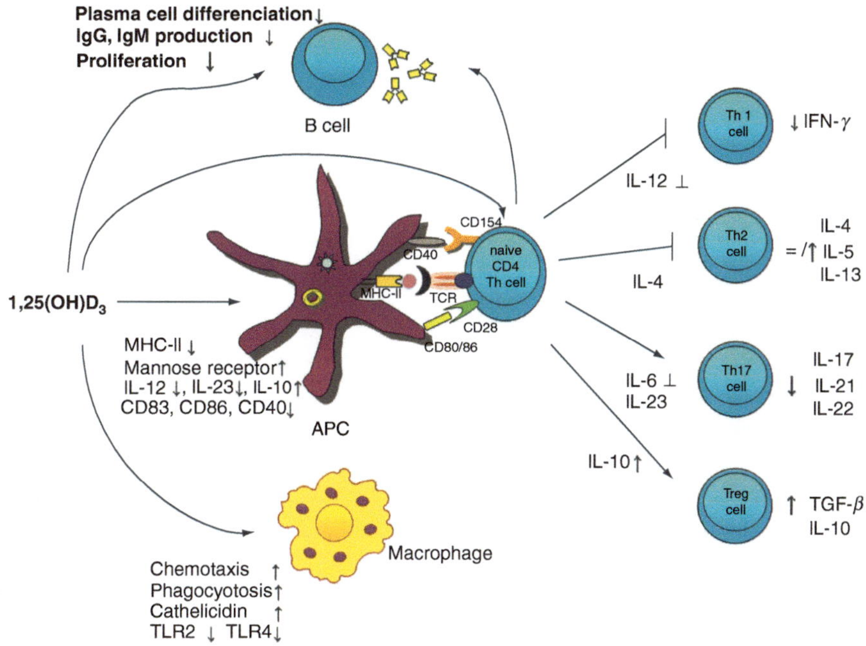

Eva Zold *et al.*, Figure 11.1 Vitamin D and adaptive immune cells: molecular actions—modulation of immunity.

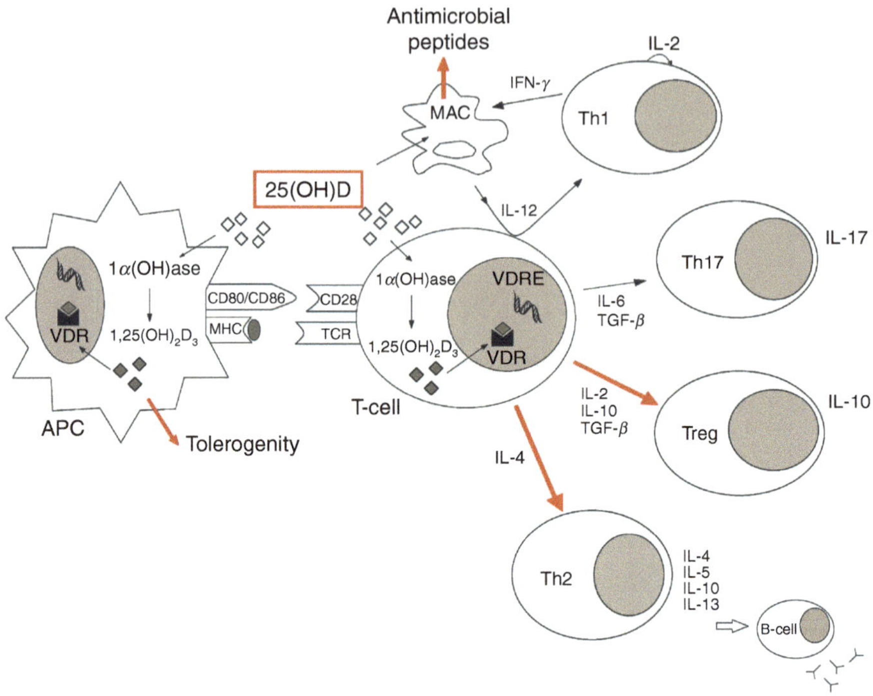

Ursula Thiem and Kyra Borchhardt, Figure 19.3 Immunomodulatory effects of 25-hydroxyvitamin D. Abbreviations: 1α(OH)ase, 1α-hydroxylase; $1,25(OH)_2D_3$, 1,25-dihydroxyvitamin D_3; 25(OH)D, 25-hydroxyvitamin D; APC, antigen presenting cell; IFN-γ, interferon-γ; IL, interleukin; MAC, macrophage; MHC, major histocompatibility complex; TCR, T-cell receptor; TGF-β, transforming growth factor-β. Different immune cells express 1α-hydroxylase and are therefore able to produce 1,25-dihydroxyvitamin D_3 locally from its circulating precursor 25-hydroxyvitamin D. Almost all cells of the immune system express the vitamin D receptor and are thus able to respond to 1,25-dihydroxyvitamin D_3. Locally produced 1,25-dihydroxyvitamin D_3 modulates both the adaptive and the innate immune response. In T-lymphocytes, 1,25-dihydroxyvitamin D_3 directly modulates T-cell response by inhibition of inflammatory Th1 and Th17 cytokines and upregulation of Th2 cytokines, thus favoring the emerge of Th2 cells. Moreover, 1,25-dihydroxyvitamin D_3 induces antigen presenting cells with an immunosuppressive phenotype by inhibiting differentiation and maturation of these cells as well as the production of inflammatory cytokines, while stimulating the expression of anti-inflammatory cytokines. By this, 1,25-dihydroxyvitamin D_3 induces antigen presenting cells with tolerogenic properties which promote the development of regulatory T-cells with suppressive activity rather than effector T-cells. Together, 1,25-dihydroxyvitamin D_3 shifts the T-cell response away from an inflammatory Th1 response toward a protective Th2 and regulatory T-cell phenotype. While exerting suppressive activity on the adaptive immune system, 1,25-dihydroxyvitamin D_3 boosts the innate immune system by upregulation of the cathelicidin antimicrobial peptide in macrophages important for the immune defense of infections.

Kolibri 360 GmbH
Ferdinand-Jühlke-Straße 7
99095 Erfurt, Deutschland
produktsicherheit@kolibri360.de